MECHANISMS OF DISEASE

An Introduction to Pathology

By

RUY PEREZ-TAMAYO, M.D.

Professor and Director of the
Department of Pathology of the School of Medicine,
National University of Mexico

ILLUSTRATED

W. B. SAUNDERS COMPANY / PHILADELPHIA AND LONDON / 1961

THIS BOOK IS MOST AFFECTIONATELY DEDICATED

TO

MY TEACHERS

ISAAC COSTERO

AND

LAUREN V. ACKERMAN

GUSTAVE J. DAMMIN

AVERILL A. LIEBOW

ROBERT A. MOORE

PREFACE

The general theme of this book is disease. The central idea, which appears once and again in every chapter, can be expressed as follows: *disease is life under abnormal conditions.* It follows from this concept that an adequate understanding of disease is not possible when studied only from an isolated point of view, as it is also impossible to learn what life is from a unilateral approach. However, didactic requirements impose a dissection of knowledge, in medicine and in any other scientific endeavor. In other words, to reach synthesis, which is the best of all knowledges, it is necessary to analyze. But analysis of facts is only one aspect of the complex process of learning, which can be separated into three different stages; Whitehead has called them the stages of romance, precision and generalization: "The stage of romance is the stage of first apprehension. The subject matter has the vividness of novelty. It holds within itself unexplored connections with possibilities half-disclosed by glimpses and half-concealed by the wealth of material. In this stage, knowledge is not dominated by a systematic procedure. Such system as there must be is created piecemeal *ad hoc.* We are in the presence of immediate cognizance of fact, only intermittently subjecting fact to systematic dissection. Romantic emotion is essentially the excitement consequent on the transition from the bare facts to the first realization of the import of their unexplored relationships. . . . The stage of precision also represents an addition to knowledge. In this stage width of relation is subordinated to exactness of formulation. It proceeds by forcing on the students acceptance of a given way of analyzing the facts bit by bit. . . . New facts are added but they are the facts that fit into the analysis. . . . The final stage of generalization is Hegel's synthesis. It is the return to romanticism with the added advantage of classified ideas and relevant technique. It is the fruition which has been the goal of the precise training. It is the final success." This extensive quotation from Whitehead's *The Aims of Education* finds a direct application in the study of pathology. It may be accepted that this field also goes through three similar stages, which would be (1) the general principles, where the student is presented with a broad view of the mechanisms of disease; (2) the analysis of specific disease entities, and (3) the study of patients, as isolated instances of different ailments. In other words, general pathology, special pathology and clinical medicine. Therefore, the most appropriate introduction to the understanding of disease is the study of the general principles of pathology.

This book was written with the purpose of presenting in a single volume a general survey of the mechanisms of disease. Since it was aimed to serve as a guide during the first stage of the study of pathology it was not considered necessary nor desirable to expand its size by including more data or adding other chapters. For the same reason, it was not limited to the facts obtained by a single method, be it cytologic, histologic, physiologic or biochemical. On the contrary, an effort was made to point out how all these data are integrated within the indivisible whole represented by the human being. In this sense, the book pretends to be more synthesis than analysis, more general than particular, more romantic than precise.

The material consists of two sections

which follow one another in a continuous sequence. The first section refers to the most general aspects of cellular pathology; therefore, it contains information usually treated in texts of general pathology. The second section has been arbitrarily selected from a much larger group of subjects and its purpose is to present a coherent view of disease as a disturbance in homeostasis. A growing body of information suggests that "The coordinated physiological processes which maintain most of the steady states in the organism . . ." belong to the general group of self-regulatory or "feedback" mechanisms. From the formation of adaptive enzymes to the regulation of posture, the principle seems to be an incipient failure in performance that tends to cancel itself. Disease, and many of the clinical manifestations of abnormal processes, are considered to be uncompensated disturbances of self-regulating mechanisms which bring about a loss of homeostasis. These concepts are enlarged in the Epilogue, where the nature of disease is explored with more detail and in a more philosophical vein.

Each chapter is followed by a list of references to the literature which will surely reveal the personal interests and biases of the author. An effort was made to document most of the important statements and to include those recent references examined personally which contain long bibliographical lists. It is customary to offer an apology to those authors whose work has not been included in the bibliography, and the present writer has no wish to break the custom. For that reason, the apology is here most humbly offered. But at the same time it is true that most of the publications left out were considered inadequate or were simply not consulted; the human brain, as the physical facilities of libraries, has limits that cannot be trespassed, and if these limits are added to the tyranny of time and the immensity of present-day literature, this fault of the book may be understood. Indeed, art is long and life is short.

ACKNOWLEDGMENTS

This book is an abridged adaptation of my "Principios de Patologia," published in Spanish in 1959. I have availed myself of the opportunity presented by this English edition to review the text, introduce new figures and bring the references up to date. It is a pleasure to acknowledge that, both for the Spanish and for this edition, I have been privileged with the generous and valuable advice of my friend and associate Dr. Herman Brandt, who cheerfully released me from most of my administrative and academic chores during the long months occupied in completing the text. It is no reiteration of a worn-out habit to state that without his help the book would be still in preparation; furthermore, several chapters were carefully reviewed and courteously but rigidly criticized by Dr. Brandt, thus eliminating many flagrant mistakes. That I did not always follow his worthy suggestions is something that both the reader and I may rightly regret, and that makes all inaccuracies and obscurities my sole responsibility. Dr. Luis F. Bojalil revised his section on Chemotherapy for this edition, and both to him and to Dr. Francisco Biagi I am grateful for contributing with their specialized knowledge on the host-parasite relation. Dr. Irmgard Montfort and Dr. Marcos Rojkind made many suggestions for the chapter on Connective Tissues and kindly obtained some bibliographical notes. I am grateful to Drs. Amado González and Juan M. Gutiérrez Vázquez for thoughtful and informative conversations and discussions on my brief and amateurish excursions into medical history and philosophy contained in the Introduction and, above all, in the Epilogue. For the selection of illustrations my thanks and deep appreciation belong to Drs. Fernando Flores Barroeta and Luis Salinas. Many authors and editors gave permission to use published material, and although this is recognized at the appropriate places I would like to leave record here of my gratitude for their kind courtesy. Drs. Edmundo Rojas and Edward S. Murphy lent me some valuable specimens for illustration of uncommon conditions. The credit for photographic work belongs to Mr. José Bautista, photographer to the Department of Pathology in our school, who has always responded to the most exacting demands.

The Spanish edition of this book was dedicated to my wife. It is at her prompting and with her authorization that the present edition is dedicated to my teachers. It is obvious that the list contains the names of some of the most distinguished pathologists and scholars of our times, but it has not been included for the purpose of presenting their authority as an excuse for my limitations. On the contrary, I am eager to state the specific reasons for mentioning their names. Dr. Isaac Costero introduced me to pathology and inspired an intense devotion to science and a great love for teaching, which at best can only be a pale reflection of the same qualities admired in him by the many generations of fortunate students that have come under his influence; in addition, his friendship and guidance in scientific and many other fields are here most gratefully recognized. Dr. Lauren V. Ackerman unveiled the privileged role of the pathologist in clinical medicine and generously gave me of his immense experience in tumors. Dr. Gustave J. Dammin personifies the synthesis of physician and investigator which should be the goal of all those interested in the healing arts; his friendship is one of my most treasured affections. Dr. Averill A. Liebow may be a little surprised to see his name in the list of my teachers, since my association with him was only too brief; nevertheless, in that short period I was deeply impressed with his scholarship and Olympian passion for truth, so I must beg his indulgence for my undeserved wish to be his student, and his forgiveness for listing his name with those of my other teachers. Dr. Robert A. Moore was one of the best teachers it was my fortune to work with, and I will always be grateful for the many "pearls" that were casually dropped on my lap. May these scholars receive this humble tribute as a small token of gratitude for what they attempted when I came under their influence.

Ruy Perez Tamayo

CONTENTS

PART II

Chapter *VI.* **General Pathology of Connective Tissues** 251

Chapter *VII.* **General Pathology of the Host-Parasite Relation** 313

INTRODUCTION

The word pathology means "branch of Medicine which studies diseases and the disturbances produced in the organism." It is, next to Therapeutics, the oldest division of the healing arts. According to Krumbhaar,[1] the term pathology "might be thought a more suitable name for our profession than 'medicine,' which presumably conquered through its euphemistic emphasis on the idea of healing contained in its derivation." In Spanish-speaking countries, the word pathology requires an adjective to be explicit, such as general pathology, internal pathology, etc., and the same holds for France or Germany. On the other hand, in English-speaking countries, and especially in the United States, the word pathology is usually taken to mean one specific and limited aspect of the entire field, i.e., pathologic anatomy.

The main concern here, however, is not with the word but with the concept; whatever designation is given to this field, the study of the causes, mechanisms and consequences of disease constitutes one of the most important aspects of medicine.

Only a few centuries ago, a sufficiently interested individual could learn most or all the facts of pathology. With time, however, the field became larger and more diverse, so that at present it is well nigh impossible to command it as a whole. Recent advances have been due not only to original contributions of many research workers in pathology, but also to other investigators with interests in associated or widely separate areas such as physics, chemistry, engineering, mathematics, etc. Concepts and techniques elaborated in each one of those fields have found application in the study of disease and have helped to state and/or solve problems that otherwise might still remain either unsuspected or ignored. With this continuous expansion of knowledge, specialization has become necessary. Both the amount of accumulated information and the different research techniques demand long years of study and training, as well as the continuous exercise of special abilities. This is true not only in pure research in biologic sciences but also in the practice of medicine. At the end of many years of training physicians are in danger of finding themselves on the road of those who know more and more of less and less. In order to avoid the negative aspects of super-specialization it is imperative to have a thorough grasping of the general principles of pathology.

The organism is formed by cells which are organized into tissues; the latter form organs, and these become associated in different systems. Both ends of this scale are open, since subcellular particles may be further subdivided into molecules and atoms, and man is only part of social groups of different sizes. Each level of organization has its own reactive features in disease, so that the study of pathology at a given level provides data which cannot be obtained nor replaced by information derived from higher or lower levels. Historically, the development of knowledge in pathology has gone from gross to microscopic changes, and is now moving into the submicroscopic and molecular levels. The study of such evolution is of interest not only in itself, but also because "nothing gives a better perspective of the subject than an appreciation of the steps by which it has reached its present state."

The historical growth of pathology can be considered in four broad stages, each one

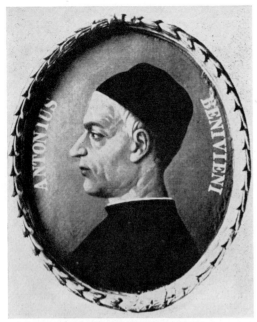

FIG. 1.   Antonio Benivieni.

HIERONYMVS BENIVENI,
VS IOHANNI ROSATO ME
DICO ET PHILOSOPHO.S.

c   VM POST Infperatā aman
tiſſimi fratris morteʒ, qua, prop
terea q, quicquid in me fugiētis
uitæ ex tam multis miſeriis ac langoribus
ſupererat, uno illo niteretur, nihil mihi in
terris potuit accidere grauius, cius per q̄
ſane honeſtam &omni doctrinaʒ genere lo
cupletem bibliothecam euoluerem, incidi
in pleraqʒ eius ingenii monumēta:quæ ille,
ut erat uir doctrina & ætate prouectior, ac
propterea multaʒ rerum uſu & experientia
pollens, cudebat quotidie. Lectitanti igiē
ea mihi, ac ſæpius ob memoriā illius reuol
uenti obtulit ſe ſe interea libellus quidam,
in quo uir ſūmo & ſtudio & diligentia præ
ditus, q̄cunqʒ trigeſimum, ſupra ſecundum
iam annum medenti illi admiratione digna
occurrerāt, & ex quoʒ cognitu uſus aliqs
poſſet exiſtere, ſtudioſiſſime prout quæqʒ ac
ciderant ſcriptitabat. Delectatus ſuʒ fateor
nouitate ipſa rerum & uarietate lectionis:
Measqʒ partis eſſe duxi, ea q̄libet impolita,
et quæ tumultuaria quadam, ut uidebanē,
feſtinatione ex tempore potius effuſa, q̄ a cu
a ii

FIG. 2.   First page of Benivieni's Book.

highlighted by a fundamental change in the idea of the seat of disease. Such stages may be labeled humoral, organic, tissue and cellular; the present times will probably be known to posterity as the beginning of the subcellular epoch.

A. Humoral Epoch. The beginning of the development of pathology extends from the earliest records of history to the fifteenth and sixteenth centuries, when the spirit of the Renaissance shook the Western World, creating among other things the freedom necessary to doubt the dogmatic authority of Galen without imminent danger of dying at the stake. Theories dominating this stage of knowledge were adopted from India and Egypt by the Greeks and were based on "spirits" and "humors." It is very difficult to give even an approximate idea of the complexity and fantasy of these theories, not only because at present it seems incredible that they were ever considered true, but also because they changed from one place to another according to popular folklore (*see* Epilogue). The study of anatomy was begun in the sixteenth century and this can be considered as the declination of "humoral" pathology, notwithstanding the heroic defenders of the same type of hypotheses which, more or less disguised, have been advanced during the twentieth century.

B. Organic Epoch. Most medical historians agree in considering Antonio Benivieni[2] (ca. 1440–1502) as the father of pathologic anatomy (Fig. 1), with that curious tendency to view the different branches of science as the sudden result of the work and vision of one man. Nevertheless, his book does appear to be the first dealing with anatomic changes in the different organs in relation to clinical symptoms. Benivieni lived in Florence, in the same picturesque epoch of Lorenzo de Medici and Machiavelli, dedicated to the practice of surgery. His observations would have remained unpublished had it not been for his brother Hyeronimus, who five years after Antonio's death collected all his writings and published them under the title *De Abditis Nonnullis ac Mirandis Morborum et Sanationum Causis* (Fig. 2). This is a most fascinating and charming document of the status of medicine in Italy in the early Renaissance,[3] full of interesting observations dealing not only with pathology but also with the practice of surgery and life in general. It contains the protocols of a little more than fifteen autopsies, performed with the purpose of ascertaining the seat of disease or the cause of death. There is in addition a short description of the clinical illness, in each case, but in most of them both the history and the autopsy findings are too brief to allow interpretation at a distance of four centuries. A good example of Benivieni's work is Case III, "Stones found in the coat of the liver."

"A woman of noble birth had been for long greatly tormented by pain in the region of the liver. She had consulted many physicians, but could not drive out the evil by any remedy. She therefore decided to try my help in conjunction with some others.

"Thus several of us met and discussed at great length from different aspects the hidden causes of this disease. As often happens in doubtful cases, we were divided. Some thought there was an abscess on the liver, others that it was itself diseased, but I personally believed that the fault lay in the covering membrane. A few days afterward the disease took stronger hold and she departed this life, even as we had foretold by common consent from unmistakable symptoms.

"I then had her dead body cut open. There were found in the lower part of the membrane round the liver, a collection of small stones varying in shape and colour. Some were round, some pointed, some square, according as position and chance had determined, and they were also marked with reddish, blue and white spots. These stones by their weight had caused the membrane to hang down in a bag a palm's length and two fingers wide. This we judged the cause of her death and decided that discussions upon what was hidden were vain and futile."

That autopsies were frequently resorted to in order to clarify diagnosis or uncover the cause of death can be surmised by Case XXXII, where Benivieni ". . . was eager to prove this theory by examination and sought to cut open the body, but his relations refused through some superstition or other, and I was unable to gratify my wish," and from Case XXXVII, a boy who died of "callus in the mesaraic veins" and whose autopsy was performed "with his father's consent." Nevertheless, Benivieni was part of his epoch and in his pages exorcisms and demons can be found next to anatomic findings; furthermore, Galen and Avicenna are quoted as maximal authorities.

Benivieni is extremely important in the evolution of pathology not only for his contributions in detail, but mainly because he began the use of a method that has continued to render useful information in the study of disease, namely clinicopathologic correlation.

Of great significance in the development of pathology as well as many other sciences was Jean Fernel[4] (ca. 1497–1558), philosopher, mathematician, philologist and physician (Fig. 3). Fernel was professor of medicine in Paris and in 1554 published his work *Universa Medicina* (Fig. 4) divided into three parts: physiology, pathology and therapeutics. This book was one of the most widely read texts of general medicine in the sixteenth and seventeenth centuries and it passed through more than thirty editions, reprintings and partial translations. The section on pathology consists of seven books divided into 120 chapters; diseases were separated into general and special groups, and the latter were considered under three headings: diseases involving organs placed above the diaphragm, diseases affecting subdiaphragmatic structures and external pathology. From a different standpoint, ailments were also classified as simple, if they involved only part of the organ; composed, if all the organ was affected; and complicated, if the relations between different organs were compromised. Autopsy records were occasionally presented, unfortunately in too brief a form to allow interpretation. This attempt to systematize disease followed a clinical criterion and the anatomic changes of organs were only referred to when related to some sign or symptom.

Early in the seventeenth century there appeared a group of physicians who, instead of limiting themselves to the publication of their own observations, collected all other available experience and printed it in enormous volumes. Most of the time these compilators exercised little or no critical judgment, so in their work it is difficult to distinguish fact from fancy. One of the most important members of this group of early reviewers was Teophilus Bonettus (1620–1671), who graduated from the

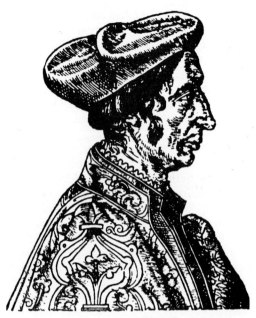

FIG. 3. Jean Fernel.

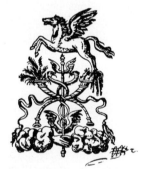

IO. FERNELII
AMBIANI,
Medicina.

AD HENRICVM .II. GALLIARVM
REGEM CHRISTIANISSIMVM.

LVTETIÆ PARISIORVM,
APVD ANDREAM WECHELVM, SVB
PEGASO, IN VICO BELLOVACO.

1 5 5 4

Cum Priuilegio Regis.

FIG. 2. TITLE-PAGE OF THE FIRST EDITION OF FERNEL'S 'MEDICINA'.

FIG. 4. Title page of Fernel's *Universa Medicina*.

University of Bologna and early in his career was appointed physician to the Duke of Longueville, a position which allowed much leisure for study. Unfortunately for him, a few months later Bonettus suffered an accident which left him almost deaf and caused him to retire from the practice of medicine. He could then dedicate all of his time to the fulfillment of his cherished ambition: to edit everything that was written up to that time on pathologic anatomy. His efforts appeared in book form in 1679, under the title of *Sepulchretum Anatomicum Sive Anatomia Practica*. This work is made up of 1700 pages and contains protocols of over 3000 autopsies, including those of Benivieni, Glisson, Willis, Vesalius, Riolan, Wepfer and scores of others. The book is important not only because it represents the greatest collection of facts in the entire history of pathology (with the exception of some modern German texts), but also because it served as a basis and stimulus for the work of Morgagni.[6]

The inauguration of pathologic anatomy as a science is marked by Giovanni Batista Morgagni (1682–1771) who started his brilliant career as associate professor of medicine at the University of Padua (Fig. 5). Four years later, however, he moved to the chair of anatomy in the same university and remained there for more than fifty years, loved and respected by all. Morgagni was a retiring, dignified scholar with an almost maniacal love for descriptive detail; a delicate gentleman, he refused to perform the autopsy of his colleague Vallisnieri and of a bishop with whom he had been linked in close friendship. His rare free hours he dedicated to classical culture and archeological studies; most of the time he spent working in anatomy and in clinical medicine. In his later years Morgagni came to be known as "his anatomical majesty," a title more expressive of his prestige than any chronologic list of his achievements.[7] In those times there were no journals in which scientific papers could be published (the present-day deluge of periodicals may make one a little envious of such an epoch) and authors would communicate their findings by means of letters which were read to small groups or scientific societies. When knowledge had matured enough it was ready to be printed in book form. Morgagni began his work by "sending some letters to my friend. And that he was pleased with them appears from two circumstances; the first, that he was continually soliciting me to send him more and more after that, till he drew me on so far as to the seventieth; the second, that when I begged them of him in order to revise their contents, he did not return them, till he had made me solemnly promise, that I would not abridge any part thereof."[8] Morgagni accepted and in 1761 his monumental work *De Sedibus et Causis Morborum per Anatomen Indagatis* appeared (Fig. 6), containing the clinical histories and autopsy protocols of more than 700 cases. All data, even the most insignificant features of the clinical history and especially of the autopsy findings, are to be found described with great prolixity and unparalleled detail, "without fear of abusing the patience of the reader." At every moment Morgagni tries to establish correlations between morphologic findings and clinical disturbances (there are two indices which list the clinical data with the correlated anatomic findings, and vice versa), thus inaugurating the practice of modern physicians who frequently attempt to express the symptoms in terms of anatomic changes. Morgagni went beyond the explanation of clinical manifestations and "unequivocally committed pathologic anatomic investigations to the revelation of the cause of disease. One can hardly understand why this precise, almost perfectionist scholar should not have recognized the fallacy of this claim. One may find an explanation for Morgagni's apparent conceptual simplicity if one gives thought to the philosophic climate of his period."[9] Klemperer is referring here to David Hume, the Scottish philosopher, whose idea of causality was the continuous association of perceptive data, thus justifying Morgagni's search for the cause of disease in anatomic correlations.

Many interesting observations fill the pages of *De Sedibus;* descriptions of aneurysms, cerebral hemorrhage, ovarian cysts, cirrhosis of the liver, etc., are masterful. The following quotation refers to a patient

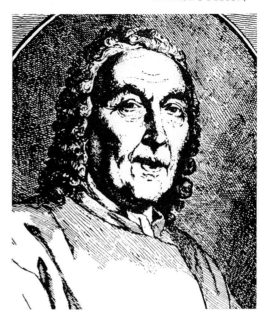

FIG. 5.   Giovanni Batista Morgagni.

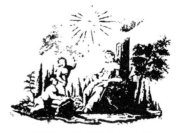

J O. B A P T I S T Æ
MORGAGNI
P. P. P. P.

DE SEDIBUS, ET CAUSIS
M O R B O R U M
PER ANATOMEN INDAGATIS
L I B R I   Q U I N Q U E.

DISSECTIONES, ET ANIMADVERSIONES, NUNC PRIMUM EDITAS COMPLECTUNTUR PROPEMODUM INNUMERAS, MEDICIS, CHIRURGIS, ANATOMICIS PROFUTURAS.

Multiplex præfixus eft Index rerum, & nominum accuratiſſimus.

T O M U S   P R I M U S
DUOS PRIORES CONTINENS LIBROS.

V E N E T I I S,
MDCCLXII.

Ex TYPOGRAPHIA REMONDINIANA.
SUPERIORUM PERMISSU, AC PRIVILEGIO.

FIG. 6.   Title page of Morgagni's *De Sedibus.*

with cirrhosis of the liver, splenomegaly, renal calculi, choroid plexus cysts and an old cerebral infarct:

"An old man of seventy, who had been very voracious in his diet, being seized with an apoplexy long before, and after that with a palsy of the whole right side of the body, was frequently agitated on the other side with convulsions. His senses were affected; and he sometimes discharged calculi with his urine. The abdomen being open'd after death, the omentum was seen to be far drawn upward, as to cover the whole anterior part of the stomach. But the left lobe of the liver, which is us'd to lie over a part of the stomach, scarcely touched it at all, in consequence of being drawn up by the diaphragm, to which it was firmly attached. Moreover, the stomach, although it was corrugated, was, however, when extended, much bigger than it generally is. And the spleen was evidently twice as big as it ought to have been, and of a very dark colour. In the left kidney were found four stones; one of the bigness of a chestnut, the others less. The thorax was not at all open'd. While the brain was taken out of the cranium, some serum, which was contained betwixt the dura and pia mater, flow'd out. In the left ventricle the plexus choroides had in it a body of the bigness of a horse-bean, made up of several hydatids: and under the same ventricle was a sinus, the sides of which consisted of the substance of the cerebrum, that was yellow and flaccid, and seemed also to be corrupted. . ."

Morgagni raised the level of pathologic anatomic description to a degree in which everything described is of value. But Morgagni's eternal contribution is based not only on the scientific facts that appeared in his book, which in themselves would have been sufficient to immortalize him, but on the general principle that organs are seats of diseases and that localization in different organs explains different symptoms. Despite the fact that Morgagni was professor of anatomy, his criterion was essentially clinical and his explanations were humoral. Sigerist[10] pays a fine tribute to Morgagni's genius with the following words:

"From every physician we expect tact and moral earnestness, but we expect them from the pathologist in a supreme degree. It is the dead who are brought to the latter, persons whom medical practitioners have failed to save. All too often an autopsy demonstrates an insufficiency of human knowledge. In such cases the pathologist must not play the part of judge, but must be a helper and an exhorter. It is well that a man of such high character, a man so profoundly impressed with his mission, should have stood on the threshold of the developing science of pathological anatomy."

This stage of knowledge of the science of disease closed with the firm establishment of the principle that symptoms are explained by anatomic alterations, which served as the basis for the fundamental work of Laennec, Bright, Skoda and many other clinician-anatomists of the nineteenth century. In addition, the usefulness of postmortem studies for the advance of medicine, as a corollary of clinicopathologic correlations, became a more widespread concept throughout the Western World, culminating in the great German school of pathology of the late nineteenth and early twentieth centuries.

C. Tissue Epoch. The next great step in pathology was taken by a young French physician, in the most stormy and productive epoch of France. Xavier Bichat (1771–1802) (Fig. 7) studied in Montpellier and Lyon, and was 18 years old at the fall of the Bastille. Bichat joined the army but his poor health did not allow his remaining there for long, and in 1793 he found himself in Paris. Medical schools had been reorganized; Latin had been abandoned as the official language; the traditional division between medicine and surgery was ended; and each "Ecole de Santé" had three hospitals at its disposal and a complete staff of full-time professors with teaching and research laboratories.[10] A protégé of Desault, who was professor of surgery at the School of Paris, Bichat applied himself with tremendous energy to the study of medicine and in 1800, when not yet 30 years old, he was appointed physician to the Hôtel Dieu. Bichat worked day and night in the wards, in the laboratory and in the autopsy room; it is said that in one year he performed more than 600 autopsies, and that his only rest was to change from one type of work to another. Soon the products of such formidable labor began to appear. The one of special interest here was called *Traité des Membranes,* and was published in 1800. In this book Bichat established that organs are formed of elements called "tissu," that similar tissues may form part of different organs, and that this is the reason for the appearance of identical symptoms when different organs are involved. Bichat mentions that there are twenty-one different types of

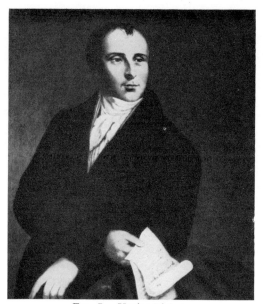

FIG. 7. Xavier Bichat.

science, while pathologic anatomy achieved a supremacy that had not been known before. Virchow was a student under Müller and Schönlein, and when his studies in Berlin were finished he became an assistant of Froriep, who was prosector at the Charité; in 1846, Froriep was called to Weimar and Virchow took his place. Nevertheless, this appointment was short-lived since Virchow's political activities were not in keeping with the Prussian government; the young pathologist was offered the first full-time chair of pathologic anatomy in Germany, that of Würzburg, and he accepted. There followed seven years of fruitful work on what later would become cellular pathology, and at the end of this period Virchow was back in Berlin. The influence of his former teacher, Johannes Müller, had helped to create a position of professor of pathologic anatomy which included an institute at the Charité.[11] Two years after Virchow had returned to Berlin, when he was 37 years old, he delivered a series of lectures which appeared in book form on August 8, under the title *Die Cellularpathologie in ihrer Begründung auf physiologische Geweblehre*. This is one of the most important books ever written in medicine, certainly the most prominent contribution to the advance of the healing arts in the nineteenth century. It is not only

tissues, characterized by several properties, which were studied by methods such as "the action of several chemical substances, heat, air, water, acids, alkalies, salt, desiccation, maceration, putrefaction, boiling water, etc." At no time did Bichat use the microscope, nor was it believed in that epoch that the cell was to play as important a role in pathology as was to be recognized later. Bichat died before he was 31 years old, leaving his fundamental contribution to the science of disease. His work is in striking contrast with that of Morgagni, who passed away when he was more than 90 years old and after a long working life of more than fifty years, leaving pathology solidly established on clinicopathologic correlations. Bichat labored only for eight years under the strain of tuberculosis and the weight of a self-imposed intense activity, but at his death he had succeeded in establishing the concept of tissues, through which organ pathology would pass to become cellular pathology, culminating its evolution of nineteen centuries.

D. Cellular Epoch. The next and last step in the search for the seat of disease was taken by the famous Rudolf Virchow (1821–1902) (Fig. 8). Through his work, pathology was definitely established as a

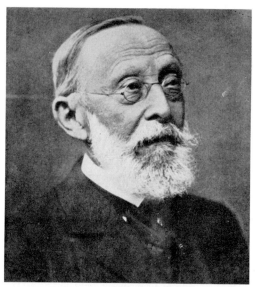

FIG. 8. Rudolf Virchow.

the culmination of the evolution of pathology; it is a new outlook on disease. Cameron[12] has written that Virchow's theory of disease rests on six propositions, which may be summarized as follows:

1. Cells are the units of life.
2. The tissues of the living organisms are built up from cells; organs in turn are composed of tissues. But the organism is essentially a cell state.
3. Cells receive their nutriment from blood vessels, abstracting nourishment from the blood of their specific vascular territories.
4. Cells, too, are units of disease. Unhealthy cells show impairments of their power of nutritive attraction and contribute noxious ingredients to the blood thus producing dyscrasias and metastatic disease.
5. Cells possess irritability as long as they are living. Response to irritation may be functional, nutritive, or formative.
6. Disturbance of function may result in exhaustion and fatigue; nutritional upset is shown by hypertrophy, cloudy swelling and inflammation or passive changes such as degenerations and necrobiosis. Formative disturbances give hyperplasia, pus formation, tuberculosis and neoplasms.

Not all of these six propositions have withstood the passing of one hundred years of research. The two that remain undisturbed are 2 and 5; the others are either modified or their apparent simplicity has been lost by a thousand discoveries and additions. However, "nothing has emerged to disturb the position of the cell as the centre of the theory of disease."

The gigantic step forward taken by Virchow has been admirably summarized by Klemperer:[9]

"Under the guidance of Morgagni's principles the art of healing had made an impressive advance in the preceding seventy years. For a long time, pathologic anatomy had been generally accepted as the foundation of scientific medicine also. 'The anatomical concept' of Morgagni, as Virchow called it many years later, had served the practice of diagnostic medicine, it had broken the shackles of humoral speculation regarding the essential nature of disease by disclosing its perceptible seat and, above all, conceptually it aimed at a union with rational contemplation of functional disorders. Anatomic pathology could provide the leadership which Mueller called for, but only if it became fully aware of its driving idea and strong enough to carry it through against decentralizing influences. It had to be free itself from the role of a handmaiden of clinical medicine without losing its full partnership in the task of interpretation of human disease; it had to develop as a universal concept of medicine and not as a narrow morphologic specialty. This was the historic mission which Virchow came to fulfill."

Virchow's concept goes beyond the narrow limits imposed by different techniques. It is not pathologic anatomy, or pathologic physiology, or pathologic biochemistry, or any other isolated avenue of research which can penetrate the intimate nature of disease, but rather the harmonic and complementary union of all these and still other specialties. The same Virchow said, "Let no physiologist, and no practitioner, forget that medicine unites within itself all knowledge of the laws which govern the body and the soul."[13] If disease is life under abnormal conditions, it can be comprehended only by the same integration of methods demanded for a full concept of life.

E. The Pathology of the Future. Recent years have witnessed a healthy and fascinating turn in pathologic research.[14] Armed with biochemical and biophysical techniques, investigators are now probing molecular structures in disease, so some changes that ten years ago were still described exclusively on morphologic terms are now understood in their biochemical and metabolic dimensions; cytochemistry is permitting correlations of structure with chemical composition of intranuclear and/or intracellular elements, both spatially and in time. The toxic actions of various substances are being explored with microchemical methods, and much has been learned of their effects on mitochondria and other subcellular particles, involving both chemical structure and metabolic functions.[15] This is obviously only the beginning, but at the same time it represents a foreshadowing of things to come. On the other hand, it does not represent, as some uninformed people would believe, the death of pathologic anatomy as a scientific pursuit of interest. The autopsy has still much to contribute in education and research, "a well conducted autopsy service not only provides a vital source of material for chemical as well as anatomic studies and an investigative tool (one of many in a modern department) but also constitutes a priceless, continuing and intimate contact with the natural history of disease."[16] And physicians who become detached from pathologic anatomy cease to understand disease; their efforts to deal with it are vain and ill-aimed, being directed against abnormal conditions they know little about or ignore entirely. The future will see not a decrease in the different methods used for the study of disease, but an integrated accretion of those derived from other disciplines into research and practice in medicine. Perhaps these last words may be considered optimistic; the present development of pathology, however, fully justifies the confident expectation of a greater understanding of disease in the future.

REFERENCES

1. Krumbhaar, E. B.: Pathology, Clio Medica, New York, Paul B. Hoeber, 1937.
2. Major, R. H.: Antonio di Pagolo Benivieni, Bull. Hist. Med. *3:*739, 1935.
3. Benivieni, A.: The Hidden Causes of Disease, transl., Charles Singer: Biogr. Esmond R. Long, Springfield, Charles C Thomas, 1954.
4. Sherrington, C.: The Endeavour of Jean Fernel, Cambridge University Press, 1946.
5. Long, E. R.: The penetration of pathological anatomy in the first half of the sixteenth century as illustrated by the *Medicina* of Jean Fernel, Tr. & Stud. Coll. Physicians Philadelphia *8:*228, 1941.
6. Long, E. R.: A History of Pathology, Baltimore, Williams and Wilkins, 1928.
7. Speert, H.: Giovanni Battista Morgagni and the hydatids of the broad ligament, Am. J. Clin. Path. *25:*1341, 1955.
8. Morgagni, G. B.: Seats and Causes of Diseases Investigated by Anatomy, New York, Hafner Publishing, 1960.
9. Klemperer, P.: The pathology of Morgagni and Virchow, Bull. Hist. Med. *32:*24, 1958.
10. Sigerist, H. E.: The Great Doctors, New York, Doubleday and Co., 1958.
11. Ackerknecht, E. H.: Rudolf Virchow. Doctor, Statesman, Anthropologist, Madison, University of Wisconsin Press, 1953.
12. Cameron, G. R.: Pathology of the Cell, London, Oliver and Boyd, 1952.
13. Virchow, R.: Die naturwissenschaftliche Methode und die Standpunkte in der Therapie, Virchows Arch. path. Anat. *2:*1, 1849.
14. Cameron, G. R.: New Pathways in Cellular Pathology, London, Edward Arnold, 1956.
15. Dawkins, M. J. R., and Rees, K. R.: A Biochemical Approach to Pathology, London, Edward Arnold, 1959.
16. Liebow, A. A.: The autopsy room as a hall of learning, Am. J. Med. *21:*485, 1956.

PART I

Chapter I

DEGENERATIVE AND

REGRESSIVE DISTURBANCES

OF CELLS AND TISSUES

I. INTRODUCTION

Disturbances known as degenerative, infiltrative and regressive are the classic field of pathologic anatomy. Since the publication of Rudolf Virchow's famous book *Die Cellularpathologie* on August 20, 1858, the cell has been conceived of as the seat of disease, although in some instances knowledge is incomplete and fragmentary. It is convenient, however, to describe several lesions at a higher level of organization, i.e., as they can be seen in tissues, the reason for this being that, although in principle all disturbances have their origin in the cell, sometimes the evidence of physiologic aberration is apparent only in extracellular structures. In general, degenerations refer to changes in cellular or tissue components, while infiltrations describe abnormalities secondary to the deposition of elements foreign to the cell or tissue where they occur; infiltrations are often intercellular. Regressive changes are the advanced, often irreversible stages of the two previously mentioned processes. Regressions frequently lead to death and disintegration of cells and tissues.

The list of degenerations is relatively short, especially when compared with the almost endless number of possible causal agents. That only few degenerations are distinguished may be understood because the chemical composition and metabolism of different cells are relatively similar, and also because the methods used for the study of degenerative processes have been mainly morphologic. The cell is a biochemical complex where a series of more or less constant functions are carried out which participate of the same enzymatic mechanisms, such as respiration, degradation of food principles, synthesis of fat and proteins, etc. In addition, in specialized organs such as the kidney, the liver and the brain, parenchymatous cells have other more specific functions which are also performed through enzymatic mechanisms. When the biochemical lesion causing a degenerative process affects the enzymes related to functions common to all cells, the resulting disturbances will have a similar morphology, will be nonspecific and will appear in different parts of the organism. For instance, cloudy swelling, which probably results from interference with the respiratory mechanisms, can occur in several organs such as liver, kidney, pancreas, myocardium, etc. On the other hand, when enzymes involved in more specialized functions are disturbed, the resulting degenerations will be more specific; for instance, the "alcoholic hyalin" or Mallory's body in Laennec's cirrhosis of the liver.

The fact that degenerations and regressions have been studied mainly from a morphologic standpoint can also account for their relatively short number. Cytochemical, biochemical and biophysical techniques are only beginning to be applied, and the results are not only fascinating, but also suggest that some changes with the same morphologic features may have an entirely different meaning in the physiology of the cell.[1]

Degenerations are frequently studied in connection with disturbances in metabolism. In fact, many of them are indicating an important metabolic change which may be recognized as either cause or consequence. However, degenerations also appear in cases where there is no generalized metabolic disturbance, and there are many abnormalities of metabolism which evolve without known morphologic changes. Another large group of causes of degenerative or regressive processes are toxic substances, using the term in its widest sense. Those most frequently found are bacterial toxins and chemical derivatives of some industrial processes. In these cases, morphologic changes are the result of toxic effects on the cell and not manifestations of general metabolic disturbances. Therefore, it seems better to accept degenerations and regressions only as signs of cellular injury, without linking them to specific etiologic agents, or metabolic alterations, but keeping in mind that they may be some of their manifestations.

Some recent studies suggest that certain histologic aspects classically considered as degenerative are only the morphologic expressions of cellular function. This opinion is held regarding cloudy swelling, hyaline droplet degeneration and some types of vacuolar degeneration. In these instances it is not possible to consider the anatomic change as a degenerative lesion, although the microscopic picture may be identical with cases undoubtedly accompanied by aberrations in cellular function. What happens is that, as a response to an exaggerated stimulus, the cell is working more than usual; it is difficult to believe that a "degenerated" cell may be capable of increasing its metabolic activity.

According to the nature of the causative agent, the cell involved, the intensity and duration of the noxious stimulus, etc., the resulting degenerations may be of slight significance or, on the other hand, they may represent a transitional stage between a nor-

Table 1. Degenerative and Regressive Disturbances of Cells and Tissues

	DEGENERATIVE PROCESSES	REGRESSIVE PROCESSES

Reversible	*Degenerations*
	Cloudy swelling
	Vacuolar degeneration
	  Watery vacuolation
	Hyaline degeneration
	  Hyaline droplet in
	    kidney
	  Crooke's change
	Fatty deposition
	
	Infiltrations
	Interstitial infiltration of
	  fatty tissue
	Fatty deposition
	Amyloidosis
	Mucoid degeneration
	Colloid degeneration (?)
		None

Irreversible	Hydropic degeneration
	Hyaline degeneration
	  Extracellular (collagen,
	    smooth muscle, etc.)
	  Intracellular (Russell
	    bodies, Mallory bodies,
	    etc.)
	Amyloidosis
		Necrosis
		Necrobiosis
		Autolysis
		Putrefaction

mal and a dying or dead cell. When degenerations belong to the first group, they are known as reversible and appear most of the time in the cytoplasm or in the intercellular substances. When degenerative processes are severe they fall in the category of irreversible changes and indicate that the cell is doomed or dead and that it will continue to complete disintegration. Table 1 is an attempt to group different degenerative, infiltrative, and regressive changes according to their severity and reversibility.

II. DEGENERATIVE AND INFILTRATIVE CHANGES

A. Cloudy Swelling and Vacuolar Degeneration. Cloudy swelling is one of the tissue changes most frequently met in histologic studies. It was originally described by Virchow in 1871, and ever since its nature and significance have been subjects of controversy. In fact, some pathologists were inclined to consider this disturbance not as a degenerative phenomenon but as the morphologic expression of normal cellular activity.[2] Still other investigators denied its existence and considered it a postmortem change. It is also known by the names of albuminous degeneration, parenchymatous degeneration or toxic decomposition.

The organs most frequently involved are myocardium, liver, kidney and striated muscle. Grossly there is an increase in size, opaque color, soft and friable consistency and on section the architecture of the organ is poorly visualized. Bell[3] states that this picture may occur in other degenerative conditions, such as fatty deposition, vacuolar degeneration and even edema; furthermore, sometimes cloudy swelling is found microscopically in organs grossly normal. Under the microscope, the cells appear increased in size, with indefinite boundaries and with the cytoplasm occupied by fine and uniform opaque droplets or granulations which may adopt a reticular arrangement. Such granulations can occupy the entire cytoplasm or arrange around the nucleus. The latter is often partially hidden by the opaque cytoplasm and almost never shows regressive changes (Fig. 1–1). The granulations are acidophilic, dissolve with acetic acid and give a positive xanthoproteic reaction; for all these reasons they have been considered as protein. The chemical analysis of organs affected with cloudy swelling gives contradictory results. While some authors consider that there is an increase in the amount of protein and water, others deny it. Some have even obtained opposite results in different experiments in the same organ and with the same etiologic agent. Fonnessu and Severi[4] studied the nucleic acid content of cells with experimental cloudy swelling induced by three different methods, and found that when the noxious agent was *Sal. typhimurium* there was no loss of ribonucleic acid, but with injury produced by mercuric chloride poisoning or ligation of the renal pedicle the content of nucleic acids was less than normal.

Perhaps the conflicting findings can be reconciled when the large variety of clinical and experimental situations producing cloudy swelling are considered:[5] the disturbance has been found in patients dead from extensive burns, intoxications, anoxia, anemia, hypoproteinemia, etc., or with hypertrophic organs, such as the heart and the kidney. Experimentally it has been produced in isolated cells by means of osmotic changes in the medium,[6] and it has been found in animal tissues subjected to inflammation, congestion, hypo- or hyperthermia, anoxia, compensatory hypertrophy, etc.

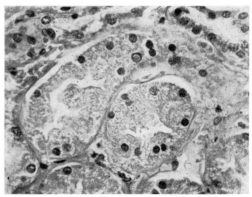

FIG. 1–1. Cloudy swelling of renal tubular cells. The cytoplasm is swollen and finely granular; cellular boundaries are lost; nuclei appear small and somewhat hyperchromatic.

The nature of the cytoplasmic granulations has been discussed, and the different opinions on the significance of cloudy swelling depend in part on the interpretation given to their origin. Initially, Virchow considered that cloudy swelling was the result of absorption of vascular exudate by parenchymatous cells ("parenchymatous inflammation"), and that the granules were coagulated or precipitated protein. Later, the same author accepted that there was a more active participation of the cell since it was abnormally metabolizing the material absorbed, thus inducing precipitation. Virchow considered as one and the same the changes in "parenchymatous inflammation" and compensatory hypertrophy. Other authors have thought that the granules are mitochondria and/or Golgi's apparatus, changed as a result of nuclear irritation. Still others believe that cloudy swelling is produced by water imbibition, secondary to changes in cellular permeability or in pH. This last hypothesis was quite popular for some time; proposed by the famous chemist Fischer, it suggested that an increase in intracytoplasmic H^+ ions would change the proteins and cause their precipitation, thus increasing intracellular hydrophilia and attracting water to the inside of the cell. However, it has never been demonstrated that intracellular pH can change as much as would be necessary for this precipitation. Furthermore, when these changes have been produced in the environment of living cells, cloudy swelling has always been irreversible.[7]

Harman[8] believes that mitochondria are the major components of the intracellular granulations in cloudy swelling. When a cell is exposed to hyposmolarity, toxemia, ischemia and starvation, the result is mitochondrial enspherulation and rarefaction with cloudy swelling. There is also a decrease in the amount of basophilic material from the cytoplasm, presumably out of the ribonucleic particles. Morphologically intact mitochondria have been isolated from the cell by means of different procedures (moderate hyperosmolarity with selected nonelectrolytes, careful pH adjustments, refrigeration, chelation, etc.). With native mitochondria so obtained it has been possible to reproduce the phenomena of cloudy swelling in the free, uncontaminated units. The result is swelling and the formation of distinctive spheres with crescent shaped marginal condensations. The morphologic transformations are attended by profound disturbances in the mitochondrial metabolic activities. There is a disruption of the organized sequence of the Krebs' cycle and an increase in oxidation of metabolites without simultaneous phosphorylation, so that the process of transfer of energy is impaired and the energy level of the units is depleted. This will be reflected in a decrease in the anabolic functions of the cell, with predominance of catabolism and eventual destruction of all structures. *In vitro* cloudy swelling of isolated mitochondria is not reversible because of gross fracture of structural units and depletion of ribonucleic acid constituents. The relation between the *in vitro* phenomenon, which seems like a very severe change, and cloudy swelling as commonly observed *in vivo*, which is considered as a benign, transient disturbance, remains to be established, although Harman makes the pertinent remark that no one has determined the survival of cells submitted to this change and that most observations have been made on postmortem material. It is true that occasionally the change is very extensive and that it is difficult to envision recovery should the disease causing cloudy swelling be cured. For this reason it is possible that *in vitro* and *in vivo* cloudy swelling may represent different metabolic disturbances of the cell with the same morphology.

It is usually admitted that cloudy swelling can advance to become "watery," "hydropic" or "vacuolar" degeneration, and that the last is probably a more advanced stage of the same degenerative, but still reversible, process. Organs involved show the same gross characteristics described for cloudy swelling or may be entirely normal. Under the microscope the cellular cytoplasm appears occupied by one or more empty vacuoles, which fail to take fat or glycogen stains but give a faintly positive reaction with protein dyes (Fig. 1–2). Some types of vacuoles produce a characteristic indentation in the nucleus, while others seem to include it or surround it completely.

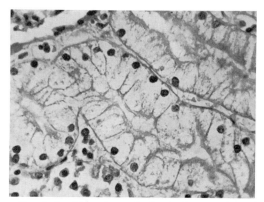

FIG. 1–2. Vacuolar or hydropic degeneration of renal tubular cells. The cell limits are preserved; the cytoplasm appears mostly empty; nuclei are unaffected.

The origin of the different types of vacuoles is unknown but probably varies according to the mechanism of production. By means of differential centrifugation and microchemical analysis, Judah and Christie[9] have shown that the composition of vacuoles produced in rat liver cells with CCl_4 is identical to that of mitochondria. Aterman[10] injected carboxymethyldextran, a synthetic polymer with iron in the molecule, and at the same time produced vacuolar degeneration in the liver cells of the rat; the presence of iron was determined within the liver vacuoles by a histologic technique, and was taken as evidence suggestive of the absorption of circulating elements. Additional experiments[11] with the intravenous injection of hypertonic saline, Evans blue and heparin confirmed the hematogenous origin of such vacuoles; anoxia was considered responsible for the formation of the vacuoles. The relation of these changes to mitochondria or to the physiology of the cell was not studied. Robinson[12] has also suggested that vacuolar degeneration may be the result of anoxia; according to this author, the cell utilizes part of the oxygen in limiting the entry of sodium and water into the cytoplasm, but when there is a decrease in oxygen the resistance to imbibition is lowered, sodium and water pass through the cell membrane in excess of the potassium lost and vacuoles are formed.[13] The observations of Aterman and Robinson underline the apparent non-specific nature of the phenomenon, which

can be produced perhaps by all agents interfering with the utilization of oxygen by the cell.

The functional significance of vacuolar or hydropic degeneration varies according to the situation in which it is found. Thus, when it follows cloudy swelling it is probably reversible, but after experimental intoxication with carbon tetrachloride the liver cells of the rat show vacuolar degeneration ("hydropic cells") with marked nuclear disturbances, which surely announce the death of the cell (Fig. 1–3). Dixon and McCullagh[14] induced this type of hydropic degeneration with CCl_4 and studied its nature by means of several histochemical techniques. The result was that cells affected in this way lose nearly all their cytoplasmic protein; the explanation suggested was that autolysis of protein may require the prior absorption of water by intact osmotic systems in the partially damaged cells, which would account for the substantial loss of protein from the swollen hydropic cells. In rats given alloxan, Dixon, et al.[15] studied the β-cells of pancreatic islets and found that loss of protein from these elements was a late event in necrosis, but that swelling with absorption of water appeared as a necessary prelude to autolysis of intracellular protein. In this case swelling is a manifestation of advanced and irreversible damage to the cell. When vacuolar degeneration appears in the proximal convoluted tubules of the kidney as a result of the injection of hypertonic solutions of sucrose (osmotic nephrosis) it is reversible and does not change renal func-

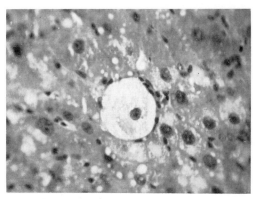

FIG. 1–3. Hydropic degeneration of rat liver cell produced by CCl_4.

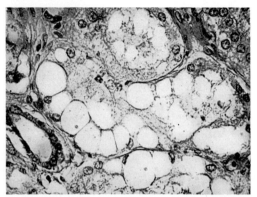

FIG. 1–4. Hypokalemic vacuolar nephropathy. Cell boundaries are preserved; nuclei are displaced towards the base of the cell; the cytoplasm is occupied by a single, empty vacuole. (Courtesy of the Editor, Revista Latino Americana de Anatomía Patológica.)

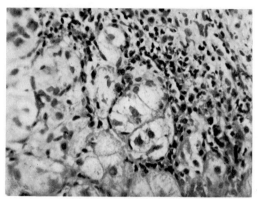

FIG. 1–5. Hydropic degeneration ("ballooning") of liver cells in viral hepatitis.

tion.[16] Another example is the "vacuolar nephropathy"[17] usually associated with hypokalemia and other disturbances in water and electrolyte metabolism[18] (Fig. 1–4), which is reversible but has definite physiologic consequences;[19] in experimental animals and in man there is Pitressin resistant isosthenuria and perhaps a decrease in PAH clearance. The experimental lesion produced by potassium deficiency in animals gives rise to a great variety of tubular lesions, mainly in the collecting tubules. Swelling of cells has been reported but it is not very prominent;[20] renal lesions appear to develop more rapidly and with greater severity in old than in young rats.[21] Histochemical studies have shown an increase in activity of several enzymes in the medullary tubules, interpreted by Wachstein and Neisel as a nonspecific compensatory phenomenon of the biochemical defect in cells deprived of potassium.[22] On the other hand, in viral hepatitis some of the liver cells show a peculiar type of vacuolation ("ballooning") (Fig. 1–5) which is very severe and is accompanied by profound nuclear changes.[23] Vacuolar degeneration appears in the liver during regeneration induced by partial hepatectomy, and in this case it seems to be transitory.[24] Examples could be multiplied but those quoted should suffice to illustrate the concept that the presence of empty, watery vacuoles in the cytoplasm may indicate very different physiologic effects, although morphologically they may be

identical. An excellent review of pathologic swelling and vacuolization of cells has been published by Manuelidis, with an analysis of these changes in both tissues and tissue cultures.[25]

B. Fatty Deposition.* From a general topographic standpoint and without considering specific disease entities, two different types of abnormal deposition of fat can be observed in the organism: interstitial infiltration of adipose tissue and intracellular fatty deposition. Interstitial infiltration exists when there is abnormal presence (or abnormal increase) of organized adipose tissue in the stroma of parenchymatous organs. On the other hand, fatty deposition is the presence of fat in abnormal amounts inside the cell, visible with the microscope and identifiable by means of special stains.

Interstitial infiltration of fat is seen mainly in the myocardium, pancreas, lymph nodes and striated muscle; it is usually accompanied by atrophy of the parenchyma. In the myocardium it is frequently observed in the right ventricle, near the atrioventricular groove or at the apex. In these areas, the

---

* Many terms are used in connection with this particular abnormality. In the following paragraphs adherence has been observed to the following definitions. *Interstitial infiltration of fatty tissue:* Abnormal presence (or abnormal increase) or organized adipose tissue in the interstitial spaces of parenchymatous organs. *Fatty deposition:* Appearance of visible droplets of liquid fats and cholesterol esters in the cytoplasm of normal or damaged cells. Other names, such as fatty degeneration, fatty accumulation, fatty metamorphosis, etc., carry causal connotations not always acceptable in the light of present knowledge.

adipose tissue of the epicardium penetrates among the bundles of myocardial fibers and appears as yellowish striations or bands separating the muscular fibers. In the pancreas, it is mainly observed in obese, atherosclerotic or diabetic patients, and it may reach great extensions, to the point that only a few islands of Langerhans and of acinar tissue are seen, separated by large areas of adipose tissue (pancreatic lipomatosis). This condition may also be seen in the kidney. Sometimes the atrophy of skeletal muscles is accompanied by interstitial adipose infiltration, as in pseudohypertrophic muscular dystrophy and other degenerative diseases; however, in some of these muscles atrophy may appear after interstitial accumulation of fat.[26] In general, the increase in interstitial adipose tissue is probably secondary to atrophy of the parenchyma and has little functional significance.

Normally, many cells in the body contain fat in the cytoplasm: adipocytes, adrenal cortical cells, adult nerve cells, corpus luteum cells of the ovary, interstitial cells of the testis, etc. In these elements, the decrease or absence of fat is abnormal. In all the other cells of the organism, the appearance of visible fat in the cytoplasm is always considered as abnormal, although the etiology, pathogenesis and functional significance may differ greatly from case to case. Fatty deposition is the degenerative process more closely associated with general disturbances of metabolism; still, the cell may be loaded with fat for purely local reasons, often toxic in nature, in the presence of normal general metabolism. In order to maintain this chapter at the cellular and tissue levels, general disturbances of metabolism will be presented in Chapter X; in this section only the following five aspects of fatty deposition will be discussed: (1) Gross and microscopic aspects of organs with fatty deposition; (2) Origin of intracellular lipid; (3) Causes of fatty deposition; (4) Functional meaning; and (5) The evolution of fatty deposition.

1. Gross and Microscopic Aspects of Organs with Fatty Deposition. This process is seen more often in parenchymatous organs such as liver, myocardium and kidneys. The gross picture will vary according to the amount of fat present but in general

there is slight increase in size of the organ and the surface is pale and yellowish in color. On section the consistency is decreased and friable and the architecture may be partially or completely lost; the tissues show an opaque, dull appearance and the knife retains a large amount of fat. The specific weight of the liver can change so much that when fatty deposition is intense a thin section may float on water.

Microscopically the cells show many vacuoles of variable size or one large vacuole distending the cytoplasm and displacing the nucleus towards the periphery; frequently, both types of vacuoles appear in the same organ and transitions can be observed between them (Figs. 1–6 and 1–7). The microscopic aspect of cells with fatty deposition is independent of the cause that brought about the change; there seems to be more relation between the causal agent and the topographic distribution of intra-

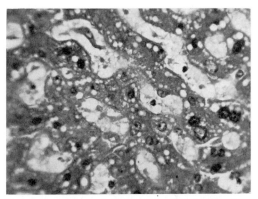

FIG. 1–6. Fatty deposition in liver cells, fine-droplet type.

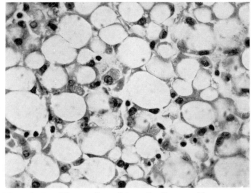

FIG. 1–7. Fatty deposition in liver cells, coarse-droplet type.

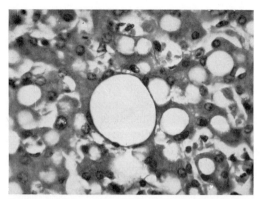

FIG. 1–8. Fatty deposition in liver cells showing one lipodiastema surrounded by several nuclei.

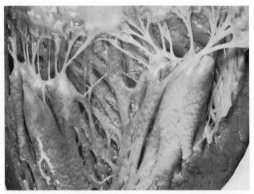

FIG. 1–9. Gross aspect of endocardium with "tigroid" fatty degeneration. This patient had an old occlusion of the left descending coronary artery.

cellular fat, especially in the liver. Therefore, it is not possible to accept, as Virchow suggested in 1849,[5] that the two types of vacuoles (small and large) have a different meaning; rather, they represent different stages of the same process. In the myocardium, fats appear usually around the nucleus, where normally a small amount of yellowish-brown pigment can be seen, especially in older people (Fig. 1–9). In the kidney, fat vacuoles occupy the basal part of the cytoplasm, displacing the nucleus toward the tubular lumen. Other aspects of cells showing fatty deposition are noted below.

Fats are histologically recognized by many staining reactions which once were thought to be more or less specific of the different types of lipids. However, recent histochemical studies have shown that the same technique may reveal fats of different structure, that fats with the same biochemical configuration are stained by different methods, and that no technique could reveal combined or "masked" fat.[27] Frequently, the results of histologic study and chemical extraction do not coincide. In spite of these qualitative and quantitative limitations, the identification of fats by means of histologic stains is adequate for routine studies.[28]

2. Origin of Intracellular Lipids. In 1849, Virchow[29] distinguished two kinds of fatty deposition in the liver and named them infiltration and degeneration. The first would have a microscopic aspect characterized by a single large drop of fat occupying the entire cytoplasm, displacing the nucleus and increasing the size of the cell. The second type would show multiple, small droplets in the cytoplasm without dislocation of the nucleus or enlargement of the cells; furthermore, in this second form there would be frequent regressive changes in the nucleus. This distinction was important because Virchow thought that each type had a different mechanism. In infiltration, the deposition of fat would be the result of a diet rich in lipids, the excess of which would be stored in the liver when the capacity of the other lipid depots of the organism was filled; therefore, it was not considered as a definite degenerative change, since cells were not damaged. On the other hand, fatty degeneration was the result of cellular injury and the multiple cytoplasmic vacuoles would contain lipids normally present in the cell but invisible because of their combined status; when the lesion was produced, these lipids would be released from their associations and become visible in the cytoplasm. The process was known as "unmasking." These classic concepts have been modified as the result of many investigations of lipid metabolism and although there are still large gaps in knowledge and many of the recently uncovered facts have yet to be organized into an explanation as simple and elegant as that of Virchow, it is better to adhere to them instead of repeating historically important but outdated theories.

Theoretically, fat in the cellular cytoplasm may have three different origins: (1) "unmasking," (2) deposition of exogenous fat from outside of the organ and (3) cellular synthesis. The majority of investigators agree that in fatty deposition the greater part of the cytoplasmic fat is almost always of exogenous origin, probably from the body depots, and the "unmasking" plays, if any, a secondary role; finally, synthesis has been found to be capable of contributing some of that fat. These conclusions are derived from the ingenious experiments of Lebedev and Rosenfeld, the observations of Lambert, and Lewis and Lewis, the studies of Dible and associates, and the recent tissue culture work of King, *et al*.

Lebedev[30] noted in 1883 that phosphorus poisoning does not result in fatty deposition in the liver if animals are fasted beforehand and have very little fat left in the depots for transport. This experiment was suggested by a case observed in autopsy of an emaciated man who died of phosphorus poisoning and failed to show fatty liver. Similar observations were made later by Dible and Gerrard.[31] In 1902 Rosenfeld[32] fasted dogs until practically all the body fat had been exhausted and then fed the animals on easily detected foreign fats, such as mutton tallow and linseed oil. When the subcutaneous tissues and other fat depots had accumulated large amounts of these foreign fats, the dogs were again fasted until depletion of liver fats was completed. Administration of phosphorus and other poisons produced fatty liver, in which most of the fat was foreign and of the type fed, passing by the circulation to the damaged liver cells. No data were found favoring "unmasking" as contributing to fatty deposition. Lewis and Lewis[33] and Lambert[34] studied the phenomenon of "lipophanerosis" in tissue cultures; the name is applied to the appearance of fat in the cytoplasm of cells, especially in anoxia. These authors observed that lipophanerosis was present only when the culture medium contained fat, but when the cells were explanted to a medium without lipids anoxia became apparent through other degenerative changes and there was no fatty deposition. In Lewis and Lewis' own words, ". . . growing cells in salt solutions differ from those in plasma in one very noticeable feature, namely, the absence of the accumulation of fat or oil globules within the cell body which is so characteristic of plasma cultures." Therefore, lipophanerosis would also have to be explained by transportation of fat to the cell and not through the appearance of normally present but invisible fat in the cytoplasm.

In a long series of careful experiments, Dible and associates[35, 36, 37] demonstrated that when fatty deposition is produced in the myocardium of the guinea pig by phosphorus poisoning, the amount of fat that can be chemically extracted is greater than normal. Furthermore, the type of fat obtained differs from that normally present and is identical with the fat of body depots. Other experiments were carried out on renal fatty deposition in fasting rabbits with similar results.[38]

All these observations suggest that fatty deposition is the result of accumulation of fat brought to cells by the blood from storage depots. However, "unmasking" may also play a role on some occasions, such as the experiments of Best, *et al.*,[39] who fed protein deficient diets to rats and observed the development of fatty livers without increase in the normal amount of fat of this organ. Furthermore, something similar occurs in wallerian degeneration of myelinized nerve fibers, in which myelin becomes stainable with fat stains which normally fail to reveal it.

Finally, King, *et al.*[40] have obtained interesting results with tissue cultures and radioactive isotopes; when strain L cells are placed in deficient media or poisoned with colchicine or other toxics, the amount of cholesterol and phospholipids is considerably increased. This result can only explained if there is synthesis of fat stimulated by adverse conditions; it will be interesting to observe the application of these studies *in vitro* to phenomena developing *in vivo*.

In a review of fatty deposition, Dixon[41] analyzed the intracellular events leading to the appearance of fat in the cytoplasm. According to this author, fat exists normally in two different forms within the cell: (a) in laminar or cylindric micelles such as mitochondria, where it is neither visible nor stainable with Sudan III or IV; it has no optic properties nor solubility characteristics of fat. Therefore, it may be considered as "masked" fat. The stability of micellar fat depends on the total concentration of fat in the cytoplasm, on the amount of phospholipids (which are responsible for its

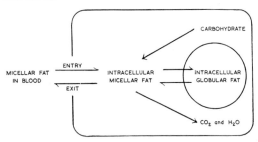

FIG. 1–10. Intracellular relation between micellar and globular fat. (Courtesy of Dr. K. C. Dixon and the Editor, Quarterly Journal of Experimental Physiology.)

laminated structure), on the concentration of cholesterol (which counteracts the emulsifying action of phospholipids) and of protein, which form lipoproteins and contribute to maintain micellar fat in a stable form. (b) Lipids can also exist in the form of spherical aggregates of liquid fat visible as cytoplasmic droplets with the optic properties and the solubility of fat. These droplets can be stained with Sudan III or IV and are surrounded by a unimolecular layer of phospholipids.

In many normal cells fat is found in micellar form; however, when the ratio of total fat to phospholipids is changed, either by an increase in total fat or a decrease in phospholipids, the micellar form can go into the globular form and appear as visible fat in the cytoplasm. The synthesis of phospholipids is directly related to the presence of lipotropic factors and requires adequate oxygenation and the provision of energy in the form of adenosine triphosphate (ATP). Other causes of fatty deposition would be an increase in cholesterol concentration or a decrease in proteins, which would diminish the stability of micellar fat and would favor the formation of spherical aggregates with scarce phospholipid (Fig. 1–10). This means that whatever the mechanism of fatty deposition (unmasking, accumulation of exogenous fat, synthesis) in the end it is always due to the transformation of micellar into globular fat. The different pathogenic forms of fatty deposition may be summarized as in Table 2.

3. Causes of Fatty Deposition. With the previous data it is possible to attempt a classification of the causes of fatty deposition in three groups, which would be: (a) dietary, (b) anoxic and (c) toxic.

Table 2. Pathogenesis of Fatty Deposition

A. Interference with micellar dispersion ("unmasking")

    a. Lack of phospholipids
    b. Lack of lipotropic agents
    c. Lack of oxygen and ATP
    d. Lack of protein
    e. Excess of cholesterol

B. Increase in the total amount of intracellular fat

    a. Increased entry of fat into the cell
    b. Diminished removal of fat from the cell
       1. Diminished oxidation
       2. Diminished removal as phospholipid
       3. Diminished mobilization as fat itself
    c. Increase in synthesis of fat by the cell

(Data from Dixon,[41] slightly modified)

A. DIETARY. Malnutrition causes mobilization of fat and so indirectly may be responsible for an increased entry of fat into the liver; at the same time, lack of choline and other lipotropic agents produces defective synthesis of phospholipids, thus inhibiting the transport of lipid to the body stores.[42] Lack of protein may interfere with the micellar dispersion of fat and enhance the transformation of micellar into globular fat. Meyer and Hartroft induced polyphagia in albino rats by means of hypothalamic damage and observed periportal fatty deposition in the liver which was not influenced by the administration of choline chloride; they suggested that this fatty change represents a physiologic response to increased metabolic demand since there were no signs of liver cell injury.[43] A similar but less well marked change was seen in rats with insulin-induced polyphagia. On the other hand, Deo and Ramalingaswami[44] produced periportal fatty deposition in the liver of rhesus monkeys by a protein-deficient diet which contained adequate amounts of choline chloride. Although not dietetic in origin, diabetes mellitus may also be considered under this heading since lack of insulin becomes manifest as fatty deposition, especially in the liver; the mechanism is probably mediated through an increase in cholesterol, which may promote deposition of fat by directly antagonizing the emulsifying action of phospholipid.

B. ANOXIC. Heart failure and anemia produce deposition of fat in the liver. This change is usually most pronounced in the central part of the liver lobules, although the topographic arrangement is better understood under the light of the "acinar" concept of liver structure of Rappoport, et al.[45] According to these authors, each one of the acini ensheathes the terminal branches of the entering vessels; therefore, the central region of the acini is represented by the peripheral areas of the classic lobules, and the outer region corresponds to the central and also the peripheral and midzonal portions of the lobules which are remote from the entering vessels. In anemia and heart failure fatty deposition occurs first in the cells situated at the periphery of the acini, which are most poorly supplied with oxygen. Lack of oxygen interferes with the energy-transfer mechanism and so interrupts the synthesis of phospholipids.

Anemia is also accompanied by fatty deposition in the myocardium, where it tends to be more pronounced in the inner parts of the ventricular walls, where the blood vessels are emptied of blood by compression during systole. The zonal distribution, however, is not explained by this phenomenon but probably represents more extensive accumulation of fat around the nuclei.[41]

C. TOXIC. Many poisons can induce deposition of fat in the cell. Dianzani and Scuro[46] showed that methylene blue, thionine and Janus green, which interfere with oxidative phosphorylation, even without inhibiting respiration, cause fatty deposition in liver cells. In these cases the mechanism may be a block in the synthesis of phospholipid. Carbon tetrachloride causes intense fatty deposition in the liver and also kills many cells. There is a peculiar topographic distribution within the lobule, where the peripheral cells are relatively uninjured; the midzonal cells show fatty deposition; and the central elements undergo hydropic degeneration.[14] This distribution again follows the "acinar" arrangement of Rappoport, et al., [45] thus suggesting anoxia as the fundamental mechanism of injury. Christie and Judah[47] advanced the view that the primary locus of action of carbon tetrachloride was the membranes of the liver mitochondria, and that the effect was inhibition of respiration. However, the cellular respiration of

slices of fatty liver of guinea pigs poisoned with carbon tetrachloride is not lower than in similar tissue from normal animals.[48] Dianzani[49] showed that the effect of carbon tetrachloride, phosphorus or a choline deficient diet was uncoupling of oxidative phosphorylation, loss of mitochondrial pyridine nucleotides and lowering of the liver content of adenosine triphosphate; therefore, the key lesion in toxic and nutritional fatty liver was envisioned as a loss of mitochondrial function. An inverse relationship was established by Frieden between the histochemical distribution of oxidative enzymes associated with mitochondria, and fatty deposition due to experimental intoxication with CCl_4 in rats and dogs.[50] On the other hand, Recknagel and Anthony[51] have presented evidence suggesting that the profound changes in mitochondrial activity induced by carbon tetrachloride occur *after* the appearance of fat in the cytoplasm; these authors submit that the toxic agent produces an unknown degenerative change which sets in motion a series of pathologic processes. One line of pathologic development leads to marked increase in fat; another leads to mitochondrial degeneration. In support of this view are the experiments of Calvert and Brody,[52] who observed that intraperitoneal administration of EDTA (ethylenediamine-tetra-acetate) to carbon tetrachloride-fed rats protected against mitochondrial degeneration but did not prevent the increase in liver fat.

Other poisons such as diphtheria toxin will also cause fatty deposition,[53] and the same may be observed with lecithinase (from *Cl. welchii* toxin). In these cases the mechanism may be inhibition of respiration caused by a direct attack on mitochondria.

4. Functional Significance of Fatty Deposition. What changes may appear in the physiology of the cells as a result of the deposition of fat is almost completely unknown, except that in some cases it has been established that an organ is capable of carrying out its functions normally in spite of fatty deposition. Experimentally produced fatty liver is difficult to analyze because most agents will injure the liver cell at the same time that they provoke an increase in intracellular fat. Bromsulphalein retention and increased serum bilirubin are observed in

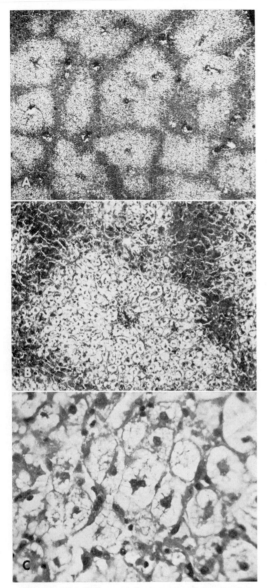

Fig. 1–11. Microscopic aspect of acute fatty metamorphosis of pregnancy. *A,* Low power view to illustrate preservation of periportal liver cells. *B,* A central vein surrounded by enlarged liver cells with foamy cytoplasm. *C,* Detail showing centrally placed nuclei and absence of necrosis.

fatty livers produced by ethionine, a choline-deficient diet, high fat-low protein diet, or CCl_4. These changes are possibly due to impaired sinusoidal circulation by fat-laden cells. Other changes, especially in blood enzymes, are interpreted as secondary to liver cell injury. Regeneration is not impaired by fatty deposition in the liver[53a]

(*see* Chapter III). On the other hand, in the literature there are several discussions of the role of fatty deposition in the liver or myocardium in the sudden death of people with no other anatomic changes.[54] These cases are difficult to evaluate; surely, there are other instances of sudden death without increased amounts of visible fat in cardiac or liver cells. In addition, many patients show these changes without any functional results. This only means that until more is known of the functional status of organs with fatty deposition it is better not to draw any conclusions. However, that the physiologic effects of deposition of fat may be quite different may be illustrated with the following examples. In the so-called lipoid nephrosis the renal tubular cells appear loaded with fat, and for a long time it was thought that the change was primary. Fatty deposition in the kidney was considered responsible for the symptoms and signs of the nephrotic syndrome. However, at present it is accepted that the primary lesion lies in the glomerular capillaries, which increase their permeability and permit the passage of large amounts of protein and lipids.[55, 56] The latter are reabsorbed and stored in the tubular cells. Fatty deposition in the liver, when unaccompanied by other degenerative changes, is compatible with normal liver function; nevertheless, there is a peculiar type of deposition of fat in the liver occurring in pregnant women during the last weeks of gestation, which gives rise to a clinical picture indistinguishable from acute hepatitis, with rapid and severe liver failure invariably causing death. This type of fatty liver differs from the ordinary variety in that the cells involved show no displacement of the nucleus; another interesting feature is the almost exclusive deposition of fat in the central part of the liver lobules (Fig. 1–11). All cases examined so far have had an acute course; Ober and LeCompte[57] suggested the term "acute fatty metamorphosis of pregnancy" for this picture.

In brief, it can be stated that although most cases of fatty deposition in organs are without functional consequence, there are some special situations in which the physiology of the cell is profoundly affected; possibly in these cases the presence of fat is incidental to a more important disturbance, but at present this is a matter of conjecture.

5. *Course of Fatty Deposition.* Perhaps the only organ in which the late effects of fatty deposition have been studied is the liver. In experimental dietary cirrhosis, a very interesting sequela is the formation of fatty cysts produced by rupture of the intercellular membranes of two neighboring fat-laden liver cells.[58] The repetition of this phenomenon leads to the formation of large cysts, which sometimes show more than sixty nuclei adherent to the wall; the cells so involved do not show atrophy. They are compressed in one direction and in tangential sections of the wall of the fatty cysts their cytoplasm appears normal and without additional droplets of fat.

The internal pressure of the fatty cyst is the same in small or large cysts. The maximal size may be 80 to 100μ; beyond this limit fatty cysts break into either a bile duct or a sinusoid capillary.[59] In the latter circumstance there may be fat embolism to the lung, kidney, heart or brain, though fatal cases of this sort of embolism are very rare.[60] After breaking, the cysts are filled with red blood cells and probably form most of the "ceroid" pigment, which has not been demonstrated in human material.[61] If the cysts do not break and there is a decrease in fatty deposition, there may be disappearance of lipids with complete restitution of normal liver plates. Some of the fatty cysts may remain in the liver parenchyma for a long time, as the only sign that there was fatty deposition in the past. Hartroft[59] has suggested that fat embolism secondary to rupture of fatty cysts may account for some of the complications of diabetes, such as intercapillary glomerulosclerosis.

Fatty deposition precedes and frequently accompanies that form of cirrhosis of the liver associated with chronic alcoholism and malnutrition (Laennec's cirrhosis);[62] compensated cirrhosis shows little or no fat in the liver cells. Based on observations of experiments and patients, Chaikoff and Connor[63, 64] suggested that fibrosis of the liver was a sequel to the deposition of fat, and many authors have followed them in this idea. Experimental dietetic cirrhosis, usually produced with choline deficient and lipid rich diets, begins as a heavy fatty deposition in the centrolobular areas which are later replaced by fibrous tissue. It has been said that compression of the sinusoids produced by enlarged liver cells and the consequent anoxia are the causes of parenchymatous damage and fibrosis;[65] if this is so, fatty deposition would be incidental to the development of cirrhosis and the stimulus for proliferation of fibrous tissue would be liver cell necrosis. Furthermore, the important factor would be the speed of deposition of fat and not the intensity of the change, and this seems to be the case in experimental animals. In human cirrhosis the evidence causally linking fatty deposition to fibrosis is even more tenuous and has been contested by several authors.[66] It is of interest that in infantile malnutrition (kwashiorkor) extreme degrees of fatty deposition in the liver are very common, and yet infantile cirrhosis is seldom, if ever, seen. The problem resolves itself in one question: Is the relation between fatty deposition and fibrosis of the liver one of cause and effect, or are both changes independent of each other but produced by the same cause? Until this question is definitely answered no final conclusion can be reached.

C. Hyaline Degenerations. Hyaline degeneration means a transformation of cellular and tissue components into amorphous structures similar to glass; the similarity is due both to the translucence and to the uniform and smooth aspect. The term "hyaline" was introduced by von Recklinghausen in reference to a heterogeneous group of changes which have their microscopic aspect in common. However, it is certain that this group includes disturbances of very diverse etiology, pathogenesis and functional significance. In some cases, hyalinization is caused by the deposition of material foreign to the tissues, and then it would be better to speak of hyaline infiltration; in other cases, hyalinization is produced by a drastic modification in the physico-chemical properties of inter- or intracellular components, and then degeneration is an adequate term. In general, it is better not to use "hyalin" as a name, since this habit might create the impression that there is such an entity; "hyalinosis" adds nothing to the concept mentioned above of hyaline degeneration.

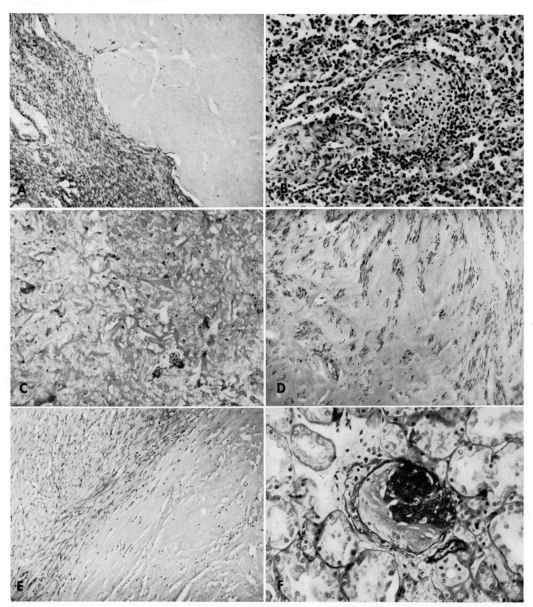

FIG. 1–12. Some instances of extracellular hyalinization. *A,* Normal corpus albicans in the ovary. *B,* Hyaline material in a lymphoid follicle of the spleen. *C,* Hyaline collagen fibers in scleroderma. *D,* Hyalinization in a uterine fibroleiomyoma. *E,* Old scar. *F,* Hyaline glomerulus in arteriolar nephrosclerosis.

For descriptive purposes only, it is convenient to separate hyaline degenerations into extra- and intracellular forms. Table 3 is a short and obviously incomplete list of the most frequent types.

Extracellular hyaline degenerations usually affect collagen fibers, although they may also appear in smooth and skeletal muscle.

The classic form appears in old scars and in organized inflammatory exudates, such as perihepatitis and perisplenitis. Collagen fibers are normally characterized as undulating, birefringent and longitudinally striated bundles of regular thickness; in hyalinization they become much thicker and irregular, fuse with each other losing a great part of

Table 3. Some Hyaline Degenerations

EXTRACELLULAR	INTRACELLULAR
Keloid	Hyaline droplets in kidney and adrenals
Corpus albicans	
Islands of Langerhans in diabetes	Russell's bodies in plasma cells
	Councilman bodies in liver cells
Diabetic nephropathy	
Arteriolosclerosis	Mallory's bodies in liver cells
Chronic glomerulonephritis	Crooke's change in the pituitary
Scleroderma	Hyaline globules in liver cells
	"Waxy" degeneration in muscle

their individuality, striation and birefringence. This change is seen normally in the corpus albicans of the ovary and in the center of lymph follicles of adult people; it is quite prominent in the late stages of scleroderma, in some uterine fibroleiomyomas and in the glomeruli of chronic glomerulonephritis (Fig. 1–12). It is also well exemplified

by keloids, which are nothing but exuberant scars,[67] where, in addition to the changes mentioned, the collagen bundles show variations in their tinctorial affinities (Fig. 1–13). In all the cases mentioned and in many others hyalinization probably represents a

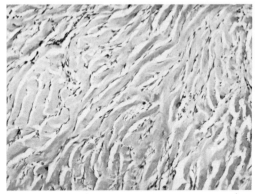

FIG. 1–13. Thick hyaline collagen bundles in keloid.

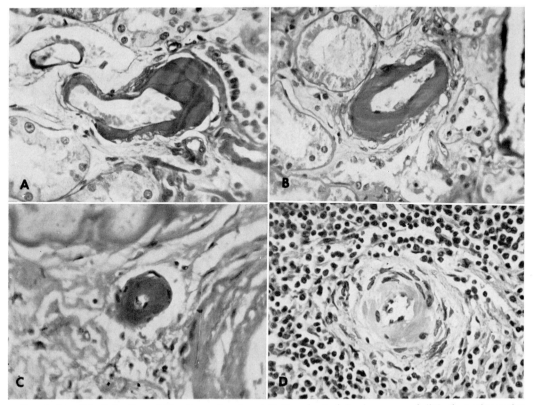

FIG. 1–14. Hyalinization of blood vessels. *A* and *B,* Renal arterioles in a case of diabetic nephropathy. *C,* Small arteriole in periadrenal tissue in a case of hypertension, *D,* Hyaline arteriole in the spleen of an elderly subject.

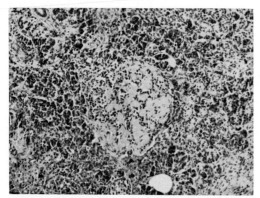

FIG. 1–15. Hyalinization of an island of Langerhans in diabetes. (Tissue courtesy of Dr. Edmundo Rojas.)

change in the physicochemical properties of collagen.

Hyaline degeneration of smooth muscle is usually limited to arterioles. It is normal in the media of intratrabecular arterioles in the spleen after the age of 20 years,[68, 69] and as a pathologic process it appears in the media of arterioles of many organs affected by sustained hypertension.[70] The change is usually well developed in the arterioles of the pancreas, kidney and peri-adrenal fat (Fig. 1–14). It has been suggested by Duguid and Anderson that hyaline arteriolosclerosis is nothing more than fibrin incorporated in the vessel wall.[71] By means of an immunohistochemical technique, Crawford and Woolf showed that splenic hyaline arteriolosclerosis contains fibrin, which was not clearly detected with the usual staining methods.[72] On the other hand, Smith[73] believes that this peculiar degeneration is caused by a change in the basal membrane of the arteriole, and his illustrations are very convincing. By means of histochemical studies, Muirhead, et al.[74] have found that hyaline arteriolosclerosis in the kidney of diabetic patients has the same composition of smooth muscle fibers. As mentioned before, it is possible that the same morphologic picture may have different origins and biochemical composition.

Other instances of extracellular hyaline degeneration may be mentioned. In patients with diabetes mellitus (and also in old people without diabetes[75]), hyaline changes may be prominent in the islands of Langerhans (Fig. 1–15). This change was first described by

Opie[76] and considered for some time as the cause of diabetes; however, more recently it has been accepted as a consequence of the generalized vascular disease of diabetics and, according to Moschowitz,[77] it is only the extension of hyaline arteriolosclerosis of intrapancreatic vessels into the sinusoid capillaries of the islands of Langerhans. Also in diabetic patients of long standing a hyaline substance is deposited in the renal glomeruli which may take three different forms: nodular, diffuse or exudative. The histologic picture is highly characteristic and was surprisingly not described until 1936, by Kimmelstiel and Wilson,[78] who recognized the nodular form and its frequent association with a mixed nephrotic syndrome of poor prognosis. In the nodular form, the hyaline material is deposited first in the subendothelial space of the glomerular capillaries, on the inner aspect of the basement membrane. The first result of this must be some degree of obstruction to the blood flow, since there is usually an "aneurysmatic" dilation of the uninvolved capillary segments. The deposition continues in layers (which may be seen with silver impregnations) until a nodular mass is formed where the remnants of nuclei can be seen; this mass is acidophilic and poorly birefringent. The fully developed lesions transform the glomerulus into a group of hyaline, acidophilic, round bodies with few, bloodless capillaries (Fig. 1–16); Bowman's capsule is also involved, sometimes with the formation of nodules but more frequently as a uniform, acidophilic thickening. The diffuse

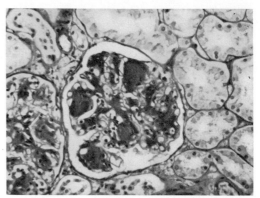

FIG. 1–16. Diabetic nephropathy (Kimmelstiel-Wilson), nodular type.

form was recognized by Bell[79] and is characterized by a more uniform deposition of hyaline material which gives the appearance of thickening of the basement membrane. According to Gellman, *et al.,* this would be the form most frequently associated with the clinical nephrotic syndrome[80] (Fig. 1–17). The exudative or lipohyaline form is vacuolated and more irregularly acidophilic; it contains polysaccharide, lipid and protein, and has been associated with extensive arteriolosclerosis and shock[81] (Fig. 1–18). The nature of the hyaline substance is unknown. Muirhead, *et al.*[82] found it to be histochemically similar to hyaline degeneration of the arteriolar media and suggested that it was derived from degenerated smooth muscle extending from the afferent arteriole into the glomerulus. Wilens, *et al.*[83] observed that the hyaline substance has a high content of fat, and Hartroft's idea that it may be the result of fat embolism secondary to the rupture of fatty cysts in the liver has been mentioned. Electron microscope studies of kidney biopsies of 7 patients with diabetes mellitus convinced Farquhar, *et al.*[84] that the hyaline material may be produced by the endothelial cell and that it is not derived from the circulation. It would be extremely important to establish the chemical nature of this type of hyaline degeneration, perhaps by means of mechanical isolation and chemical analysis of involved glomeruli, as it has been done for other purposes (Fernández de Cicero, *et al.*[85]).

Some types of extracellular hyalinization, especially the one mentioned in the islands of Langerhans, may take the stains used to identify amyloid (*vide infra*). Furthermore, on many occasions the histologic similarity to the latter form of infiltration may be striking, and as both may occur in similar areas of the organism great care must be exercised to avoid confusion.

Intracellular hyaline degenerations present very different problems. They are frequently found in parenchymatous organs with predominant secretory functions, but the exceptions to this are many and very important. In some cases intracellular hyalinizations indicate an irreversible change in the organization of cytoplasmic colloids and represent a sign that the cell is dead or

definitely doomed. On the other hand, there are other instances where the presence of intracellular hyaline formations is brought about by the transitory accumulation of foreign elements in the cytoplasm, which are eventually eliminated. In these cases, the cell returns to normal morphology and metabolism.

Intracellular hyalinizations indicating severe disruption in cytoplasmic organization are many; however, only a few of those more frequently observed will be mentioned here. Perhaps the best example is Russell's bodies, described in 1890 by William Russell of Edinburgh under the name of "the characteristic organism of cancer." Russell's bodies are spherical, acidophilic and birefringent, well limited masses appearing first in the cytoplasm of plasma cells as isolated or small groups (Fig. 1–19). They grow in

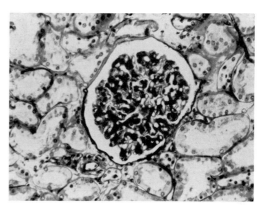

FIG. 1–17. Diabetic nephropathy (Kimmelstiel-Wilson), diffuse type.

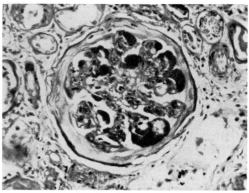

FIG. 1–18. Diabetic nephropathy (Kimmelstiel-Wilson), exudative or lipohyaline type.

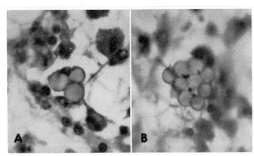

FIG. 1–19.   Russell bodies from a case of multiple myeloma.

size and, when multiple, decrease in number until the entire cytoplasm of the cell is replaced by the body; what happens then is conjecture but it seems that cell membrane is ruptured and Russell's bodies are released to the interstitial tissues, which is where they are found more frequently. It is unlikely that the plasma cell survives this process. Russell's bodies are found mainly in chronic inflammations with many plasma cells in the exudate, such as some mycoses and scleroma; they are also present in plasma cell myeloma. Pearse[86] and White[87] have used histochemical techniques to study experimentally produced Russell's bodies and agree in their conclusion that they are some type of glycoprotein, probably formed by plasma cells as a response to antigenic stimulation. Another form of intracellular hyaline degeneration is "waxy" or Zenker's degeneration, described by this author in the cytoplasm of striated muscles in cases of typhoid fever. It has also been observed in patients with pneumonia, tetanus, influenza, trichinosis and other infections, as well as in anaphylaxis. Experimentally it has been produced by temporary ischemia, trauma, high fever and prolonged pressure in muscles. The cells appear swollen, with hyaline acidophilic or amphophilic cytoplasm and with a loss of nuclei in the sarcolemma. Probably this degeneration represents the final stage of less severe but progressive lesions of muscle fibers. Although it has been attributed to an excess of lactic acid, this supposition has not been confirmed. Since it tends to appear mainly in muscles associated with respiration, such as the rectus abdominis and the diaphragm, it may contribute to the clinical severity of some infections through deficiencies in the ventilatory mechanics.[88]

Liver cells may show several types of hyaline degenerations. Hyaline globules have been experimentally observed in the cytoplasm of rat liver cells 20 minutes after the rats received 10 per cent of their body weight of warm saline *per os*.[89] These hyaline globules vary in size from very small to larger than the nucleus, are spherical, birefringent, acidophilic and well delimited; most of the time they are intracellular but may be observed within the sinusoid capillaries. Cells containing these globules are otherwise normal; the significance of this change is unknown. Another type of hyaline degeneration in liver cells appears in subjects with a history of chronic and/or acute, prolonged alcoholism, usually associated with Laennec's cirrhosis. It is characterized by the presence of one or several intracytoplasmic, acidophilic masses, usually lobulated and arranged around the nucleus, with diffuse limits and a "smoky" aspect (Fig. 1–20). These bodies are intensely stained with silver and protein dyes, such as Roque's chromotrope; they are known as Mallory's bodies or "alcoholic hyalin," and are apparently the same change described by Costero and Barroso-Moguel[90] with the name of cholechrysocytosis. Preliminary histochemical studies reported by Mallory[91] reveal that they are denatured protein with no neutral fat or carbohydrate fraction and probably with a high histone content; they are somewhat resistant to pepsin digestion but eventually are destroyed so that they no longer stain with aniline blue. For these

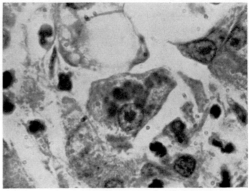

FIG. 1–20.   "Alcoholic hyalin" or Mallory body from a case of cirrhosis of the liver.

reasons it may be suspected that they are related to mitochondria. These bodies have also been observed in experimental cirrhosis produced in monkeys with a protein deficient diet and no alcohol,[92] so the time-honored designation of "alcoholic" may have to be reconsidered; on the other hand, decolored bile may be easily mistaken for them, so care must be exercised in their identification. The severity of the lesion represented by Mallory's bodies has been documented in a study of their prognostic significance; patients with "alcoholic hyalin" survive for a shorter period than those who fail to show this in liver biopsies.[93] Mallory's bodies probably represent the morphologic manifestation of cellular disorganization preceding death, and are caused by coagulation of proteins. They can be considered as the most advanced stage of many other, so far unnamed, pictures of cytoplasmic granulation and clumping which are commonly observed in patients with severe liver failure.

Two other types of intracellular hyaline degeneration are the Councilman bodies of yellow fever and the "hyaline globules" described by Axenfeld and Brass[94] in viral hepatitis. The latter are observed either within the cytoplasm of liver cells or, more frequently, lying free in the sinusoids. They are spherical, well limited, acidophilic and strongly birefringent masses which progressively increase in size until the whole cell is replaced (Fig. 1–21). The presence of these hyaline globules is a good histologic sign of activity in hepatitis and suggests a

viral etiology. Indeed, they should be considered rather as a form of coagulative necrosis and not as a degeneration, but in some cases (especially when the nucleus is preserved) it is difficult to draw the line between these two phenomena.

Less severe forms of intracellular hyalinizations are exemplified by hyaline droplet degeneration of the convoluted tubules of the kidney. In a very complete review of the history and mechanism of this phenomenon, Rather[95] has described hyaline droplets as, ". . . discrete spherical intracytoplasmic bodies . . . eosinophilic, rather refractile, variable in size, although usually smaller than the cell nuclei and [could be] sharply stained by a number of dyes including iron hematoxylin" (Fig. 1–22). The change is also known as athrocytosis (speicherung). Rather believes that hyaline droplet degeneration is not a degeneration but simply the morphologic evidence that structures involved in tubular reabsorption are intact. In support of this view are the interesting experiments of Oliver, et al.,[96, 97] where hyaline droplets are considered as protein adsorbed to mitochondria; these authors contend that the change is only an exaggerated manifestation of a normal process which should be interpreted as evidence for the important role played by the kidney in the intermediary metabolism of protein. From careful histologic and histochemical observation on hyaline droplets experimentally produced in the rat kidney by the injection of egg white, Oliver and his associates have derived the far-reaching the-

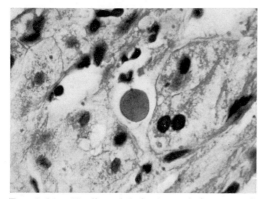

FIG. 1–21. Hyaline globule (coagulative necrosis of liver cell) in viral hepatitis.

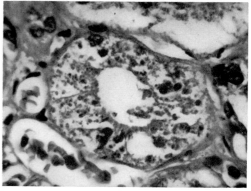

FIG. 1–22. Hyaline droplet degeneration in renal tubular cells in eclampsia.

ory that proteins passing the glomerular filter are in part directly absorbed by the epithelial cells of the proximal convolution of the nephron with no apparent alteration of the cytologic pattern. If, however, the absorptive capacity of these cells is exceeded either by the amount or the nature of the protein, the accessory mechanism of droplet formation is brought into play. Here the mitochondria are involved through a metabolic process.

This process was further elaborated by Kretchmer and Dickerman,[98] who employed homogenization and ultracentrifugation to separate different fractions in cells with hyaline droplet formation. Shifts of enzymatic activity were studied during the formation and evolution of droplets in the proximal convoluted tubule of the rat, with special attention to oxidative enzymes in different cellular fractions. Their results are highly suggestive of the formation of droplets by the incorporation of protein in mitochondria through the intermediary of microsomal particles. Strauss[99] has isolated hyaline droplets produced experimentally and has found that they contain phospholipids and ribonucleic acid, a high concentration of acid phosphatase, but few oxidative enzymes (catalase, succinic dehydrogenase and cytochrome oxidase). Since the droplets are supravitally stained by neutral red, Janus green, methylene blue and other dyes, the conclusion seems logical that they are mitochondria.

Other studies, however, seem to indicate that the composition of hyaline droplets may vary. Telford Govan[100] made histochemical observations of hyaline droplets in the renal epithelium in cases of eclampsia, normal pregnancy and clinical nephritis in pregnant and nonpregnant women, and believes that there is no relationship to proteinuria. He has suggested that the droplets are formed by globulins adsorbed to glycoprotein, probably derived from hormones excreted in large amounts. In this conclusion he is in agreement with similar observations of Lynch.[101] Furthermore, Skelton[102] has studied the presence of hyaline droplets in the cytoplasm of the adrenal cortex of rats treated for variable periods with methylandrostenediol and has suggested that they are formed by glycoprotein; these droplets ap-

peared with equal frequency in cells with abnormal changes and in normal cells. Therefore, Skelton submits that hyaline droplet accumulation is not a degeneration but rather a transient functional modification, and that perhaps it represents the morphologic picture of secretion (or absorption) of excessive amounts of administered hormones.

From the previous paragraphs it should be clear that hyaline degenerations are a heterogeneous group of similar morphologic changes with very different etiology, pathogenesis and functional significance. Advances in cellular pathology will soon make it obsolete and a new grouping will be necessary, perhaps based on a more clear understanding of their mechanism and of their meaning for the life of the cell.

D. Amyloidosis. In a strict sense, amyloidosis is a form of extracellular hyaline de-

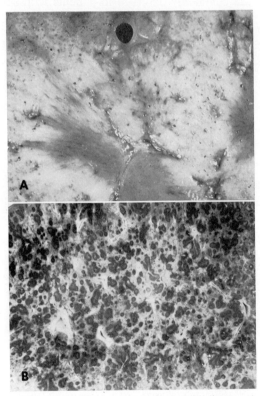

FIG. 1–23. Gross aspect of amyloid disease. *A*, Close-up view of the kidney with amyloidosis, showing glomeruli as tiny raised, gray or black, round bodies. The black color is due to iodine reaction. *B*, Close-up view of the cut surface of the spleen with extensive amyloid deposition.

generation. It is discussed under a separate heading because of its peculiar staining characteristics and its association with certain diseases. Known for many years, it was baptized by Virchow with its present name because of its affinity for iodine, with which it gives a reddish brown color in a fashion similar to starch.

Amyloidosis is characterized by the extracellular deposition of an acidophilic, homogeneous, structureless substance which produces atrophy of neighboring cells. In some special localizations it may give rise to symptoms complicating other diseases and constituting more or less characteristic syndromes.

Amyloid deposition imparts a characteristic gross picture to involved organs. They are enlarged, have an increased or rubbery consistency and on section there may be loss of architecture and plaques or nodules of whitish-gray, translucent material. However, when the deposit is not very extensive the different organs may be normal. Grossly, amyloid may be recognized by the Lugol reaction, originally described by Virchow: in contact with the iodine solution, amyloid deposits turn reddish-brown. This reaction is not constant, and an organ may be riddled with amyloid and still fail to show it; the brown discoloration may be modified by the addition of 1 per cent sulphuric acid, with which it may turn to bluish-purple. The change is more frequently observed in the spleen and kidney (Fig. 1–23). Under the microscope it appears that amyloid substance is exclusively deposited in the extracellular structures, beginning with collagen fibers, subendothelial spaces and smooth muscle fibers. As the amount of amyloid increases, the neighboring cells undergo pressure atrophy and are replaced by the foreign substance (Fig. 1–24). These features are common to all types of amyloidosis. Amyloid substance is acidophilic; after peptic digestion it shows metachromasia

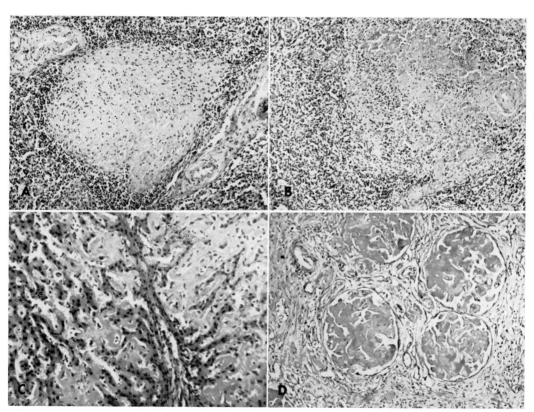

FIG. 1–24. Microscopic aspect of amyloid disease. *A,* Nodular form of splenic amyloidosis. *B,* Diffuse form of splenic amyloidosis. *C,* Amyloidosis of the liver. *D,* Amyloid deposition in renal glomeruli.

with toluidine blue,[103] which may also be demonstrated by staining with high concentrations of the same dye at 70° C.; metachromasia is also present with methyl violet and crystal violet, although the form associated with multiple myeloma is orthochromatic with the latter dye; all types seem to be PAS positive.[104]

Amyloidosis has been classified in four groups[105] as follows: (1) Primary amyloidosis, when there is no other pathologic process associated with the extracellular degeneration. This is very rare and the deposits are mainly found in mesenchymal tissues such as heart, tongue, intestines, skin and lungs.[106] (2) Secondary amyloidosis, the most frequent form, usually accompanies chronic destructive processes such as tuberculosis, osteomyelitis, leprosy, etc. In this type deposits are found in the kidney, spleen, adrenals, liver and intestine; amyloidosis of the kidney may give rise to complicating symptoms (nephrotic syndrome) in 16 per cent of the cases.[107] (3) Localized or tumoral amyloidosis, which involves the skin, tongue, larynx, salivary glands and other tissues. In this form, amyloid is frequently atypical in its staining reactions.[108] (4) Amyloidosis associated with plasma cell myeloma or lymphoma, which occurs in 7 to 18 per cent of the cases of such tumors and is deposited in mesenchymal tissues.[109] This classification into four groups is quite artificial and may be reduced to two, primary and secondary, which is more in keeping with what is actually seen in human material.

A variety of techniques have been used with success to produce amyloidosis in experimental animals. Cattle, horses, rabbits, hamsters, guinea pigs and mice have been reported as capable of developing the disease when given the proper stimulus. The stimulus has consisted of either injection, usually serial, of a variety of substances, or dietary variations, such as cheese supplements or vitamin C deficiency. A reliable technique is the serial injection of sodium caseinate in rabbits.[110] When not very extensive, amyloid has been observed to disappear after the main disease is under control.[111]

The chemical composition of amyloid has been much discussed; it has been mentioned that carbohydrate was considered as an important component because of its reaction with Lugol. Later it was suggested that in cases of extensive bone destruction, chondroitin sulphuric acid was released from the involved skeleton and deposited in the intracellular structures. Hass et al.[112] have shown that there is not one but several varieties of amyloid and that their chemical composition varies according to animal species, localization and inducing stimulus; however, they found that almost all amyloids were formed by a mixture of two slightly different protein fractions and a sulphated polysaccharide. Giles and Calkins[113] analyzed chemically a case of secondary amyloidosis in the liver and found that it contained 82.8 per cent of water; the other components appear in Table 4. In view of their findings, Giles and Calkins concluded that amyloid is a hydrophilic protein mixed with glycoprotein and a polysaccharide; chondroitin sulphuric acid, as such, is not present in amyloid.

The histochemistry of amyloid is also helping in the clarification of its major components. Braunstein and Buerger[114] concluded from their studies that three components were identifiable: protein, carbohydrate (or glycoprotein) and acid mucopolysaccharide, probably of carboxylated nature. Using fluorescent antibody techniques, Vazquez and Dixon suggested that globulin is an important component of amyloid, which probably represents an antigen-antibody precipitate;[115] on the other hand, immunochemical studies of Calkins, et al. tend to deny this hypothesis.[116]

The mechanisms of production and dep-

Table 4. Chemical Composition of Secondary Amyloid

Neutral sugars (glucose and galactose)	1.86
Hexosamine (glucosamine and galactosamine)	1.55
Uronic acid	0.60
Hydroxyproline	1.50
Glycine	3.80
Tyrosine	4.10
Nitrogen	14.20
Phosphorus	0.02
Ashes	3.20

(Data from Giles and Calkins[113])

osition of amyloid are unknown. There are several hypotheses on the origin of the substance, of which three will be considered here. The first postulates that amyloid is the result of an antigen-antibody reaction, and it is supported by the high concentration of gamma globulin observed in amyloid by means of fluorescent antibody[115, 117] and by chemical analysis;[118] furthermore, Wagner[119] studied the serum and amyloid proteins of a patient with primary amyloidosis by means of filter paper electrophoresis and found that in the serum α-2 and β-globulin fractions were elevated. The greater part of amyloid protein was formed by the same globulin fractions, so the conclusion was that, "The hypothesis that amyloid represents the tissue localization of a circulating abnormal protein complex is most attractive." Using casein-induced amyloidosis in rabbits, Giles and Calkins[120] studied the relationship between serum hexosamine, globulins and antibodies, and the deposition of amyloid; they found that in all animals there was an increase in serum hexosamine and all globulin fractions, but no correlation was established with the antibody titer. The second hypothesis on the origin of amyloid considers that it is the tissue deposition of a circulating glycoprotein, present in high concentrations in the serum because of destruction and solubilization of connective tissue.[121] Finally, Teilum[122] has suggested that amyloid is an abnormal secretion of local reticuloendothelial cells, which normally form the serum globulins; under a pathologic stimulus the cells would change the nature of the protein synthesized in their cytoplasm and the abnormal secretion would then be precipitated in tissues. These three hypotheses fail to explain why amyloid is extracellular and why it is deposited in different organs according to the various types.

E. Mucoid and Colloid Degenerations. All the so-called mucoid degenerations are characterized by an increase in mucin, which can be mesenchymal or epithelial in origin. Therefore, it would be more appropriate to consider them as infiltrations. Normally, the organism produces mucus in many epithelial linings, such as the respiratory, digestive or female genital tracts; this mucus is formed by variable proportions of protein and acid mucopolysaccharides. The same components make up the ground substance or intercellular mucoid of connective tissue, except that the polysaccharide varies according to the different areas of the organism. The amount of mucin or mucoid substance can increase, both in epithelium and in connective tissue; in the first place it will be intracellular while in the second it will be interstitial.

Epithelial mucoid degeneration can be inflammatory in nature, as it appears in nasal catarrh, gastritis, chronic colitis or bronchial asthma. In all these cases there is mucus-secreting cell hyperplasia (Fig. 1–25). On the other hand, epithelial neoplasias may also show an exaggerated production of mucus, as in colloid carcinoma of the stomach and colon, and in some carcinomas of the breast. A special case is mucocele of the appendix,[123] a condition resulting from the occlusion of the lumen

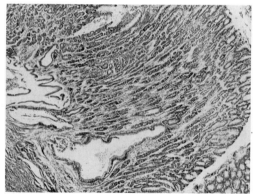

Fig. 1–25. Hypertrophic gastritis illustrating glandular hyperplasia with mucus overproduction. (Tissue courtesy of Dr. Edmundo Rojas.)

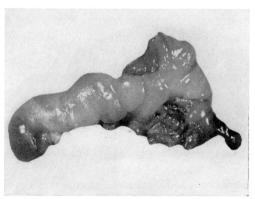

Fig. 1–26. Mucocele of appendix. The organ is distended by mucus.

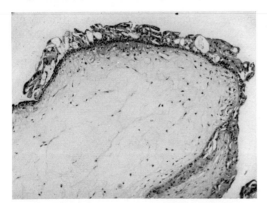

FIG. 1–27. Mucoil degeneration in stroma of hydatidiform mole. The tenuous fibrillary material is basophilic.

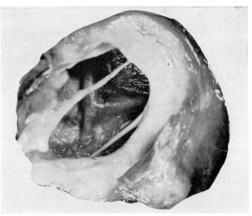

FIG. 1–28. Aneurysmal sac resected in a case of Marfan's syndrome. The cavity is crossed by a connective tissue band connected with the intima without elastic tissue.

and hyperplasia of mucus glands (Fig. 1–26). The distended organ may rupture into the peritoneal cavity and the cells continue their secretory activity, filling the abdomen with a gelatinous, lobulated, yellowish-pink mass. The same condition is also seen in peritoneal metastasis of colloid carcinomas of the stomach or of pseudomucinous cystadenocarcinoma of the ovary. Mixed tumors of salivary gland can show mucinous metaplasia of the stroma, which is also derived from the epithelium; this represents an exception to the intracellular nature of most epithelial mucoid degenerations.

Mesenchymal mucoid degeneration is best exemplified by myxedema, where there is a considerable increase in ground substance in the interstitial spaces; it is also present in the stroma of fibroadenoma of the breast or of chorionic villi in hydatidiform mole (Fig. 1–27). Cystic collections of mucoid material are found in the media of the aorta in Erdheim's disease (idiopathic cystic medionecrosis of the aorta)[124] and in cases of Marfan's syndrome, a hereditary disorder of connective tissues in which there is frequent formation of dissecting or saccular aneurysms[125] (Fig. 1–28). An increase in the amount of interstitial basophilic (hematoxylinic) substance is observed in the heart during acute attacks of rheumatic fever; Lannigan[126] has emphasized the significance of this change in the histologic diagnosis of activity of this disease. The so-called mucinous edema preceding fibrin-

oid necrosis and granuloma formation in collagen diseases is also a form of mucoid degeneration of mesenchymal tissues (see Chapter VI).

Mucoid substances of connective tissues are under hormonal control, at least in certain specialized areas such as the rooster comb, the retro-ocular, retroperitoneal and axillary soft tissues of the guinea pig, the "genital" skin of Macacca and the stroma of the breast. Hormonal stimulation of these areas will produce an increase in the interstitial ground substance, but it is doubtful that such change can be considered degenerative. Mucoid degenerations are mostly reversible processes, but very little is known of the intimate mechanisms of production; the field of their functional effects on cells and tissues is completely unexplored.

Colloid degeneration refers to the accumulation in the thyroid follicles and in the cystic cavities of the pars intermedia of the pituitary gland, of hyaline, eosinophilic material. There seems to be no reason to preserve the term since it serves no defined purpose. Colloid milium, a rare condition of the skin in which collagen fibers undergo marked hyaline degeneration, might be the only true example of such a process.[128]

F. Glycogenic Infiltration. This term refers to the abnormal presence or increase in the amount of intracellular glucogen. This substance is water soluble, so it is necessary to fix the tissues in fluids with an alcoholic basis, in order to avoid loss of glycogen from the cells during the process of preparation of microscopic slides. Glycogenic infiltration appears mainly in three organs, liver, kidney and pancreas. In the liver there is a large amount of intracellular glycogen (from 4 to 14 per cent of the dry weight of the organ, according to the animal species and the metabolic phase) which may be revealed by special stains such as Best's carmine or the PAS technique; most of this glycogen is intracytoplasmic. In certain conditions, such as diabetes mellitus, or even in normal subjects, the nuclei of liver cells appear enlarged and empty, with very clear nuclear membranes; this aspect is due to the accumulation of glycogen, which is lost during histologic manipulations. The cause and meaning of this change is unknown, but Baird and Fisher[129] have been able to produce it experimentally by incubating liver slices in hypotonic media. They claim that vacuolation of nuclei of hepatic cells is the result of an alteration in fluid balance within the liver cell resulting in an increase of water within this structure; the presence of glycogen within the nucleus is incidental and is apparently derived from cytoplasmic glycogen when present in these cells in increased amounts. In cases of poorly controlled diabetes, the kidney may show extensive glycogenic infiltration, especially in the loops of Henle. The tubular cells appear enlarged with well defined limits and empty, clear cytoplasm; the picture is very similar to vegetable cells and there are no nuclear changes. The lesion is known as Aramanni-Ebstein cells [130] and is due to the accumulation of glycogen in the cytoplasm. With the better treatment of diabetes available today the lesion is only rarely observed.

Glycogenic infiltration of the β-cells of the islands of Langerhans has been known since 1901,[131] but because at that time no staining techniques for glycogen were available the change was referred to as "hydropic" degeneration. It is found in variable proportions in diabetic patients (4.5 to 18 per cent) and also in animals with experimental diabetes produced by alloxan, adrenocortical steroids, anterior pituitary extracts and purified growth hormone. Toreson[132] demonstrated that glycogenic infiltration also occurs in the duct epithelium of the pancreas, and Lazarus and Volk[133, 134] have submitted that glycogenic infiltration may not be involved in the pathogenesis of diabetes, but merely be a manifestation of elevated glucose levels in the blood, as the Aramanni-Ebstein cells of the kidney or glycogenic infiltration of the myocardium.

Finally, in certain malignant tumors the cellular cytoplasm may be filled with glycogen, as in carcinoma of the kidney or seminoma of the testis; it is possible that this change might be indicative of a severe modification in the metabolic activities of the cells. So far, however, the little evidence available seems to suggest that glycogenic infiltration is without functional significance.

III. REGRESSIVE DISTURBANCES

A. Necrosis. Necrosis means rapid death of a limited area of the organism and constitutes the final stage of irreversible degenerative processes. The term is usually applied to acute changes since slow death of groups of cells is difficult to observe under the microscope and the result is a decrease in the total number of cells, which is known as atrophy. The latter may be the result of necrosis or of a decrease in the size of the cells. The limits between necrosis and atrophy are made even less clear by the concept of necrobiosis, which is sometimes used to indicate cellular changes accompanying a more or less slow death.

Although the causes of necrosis are naturally many, it is always possible to reduce them to a severe interference with the utilization of oxygen by the cell or to a disruption of cellular structures. It is customary, however, to describe the causes of necrosis as ischemic (anoxic), physical and toxic; some authors separate the bacterial from other toxic substances because microorganisms form a very important group of etiologic agents. Nevertheless, it should be remembered that bacterial toxins causing necrosis will do it through the same mechanisms as inert or toxic substances.

Interference with circulation must be sudden in order to produce necrosis. If blood

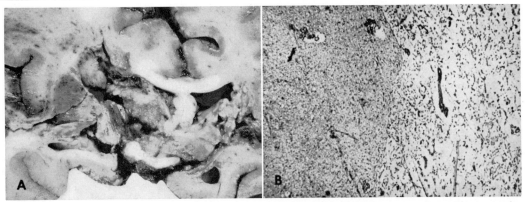

FIG. 1–29. Old cerebral infarct with reabsorption of necrotic tissue and cyst formation. *A,* Gross aspect. *B,* Microscopic picture of the edge of the lesion, showing scavenger cells (microglia) and scarce blood vessels.

flow is slowly decreased the result is not cellular death but atrophy. The most frequent causes of ischemia are thrombosis or embolism, and anoxia secondary to cardiac standstill. The resistance of different cells to oxygen deprivation varies according to the animal species and the involved organ. In general, it can be said that the more differentiated the cells of the tissue the less resistant they are to the lack of oxygen. In man, the central nervous system is the most sensitive organ, while striated muscle and connective tissue will resist anoxia for prolonged periods. Changes in the brain caused by anoxia have been summarized by Krainer,[135] who points out that they are of two types: selective neuronal necrosis and malacia. Vulnerability of different areas of the brain varies with the type of anoxia involved; in anoxic anoxia lesions of the pallidum, corpus Luys and dentate nucleus appear earlier and are more constant, while in stagnant anoxia cortical lesions predominate. Differences of vulnerability have been explained as due to vascular arrangement or to metabolic variations in the different areas of the brain. Experimental studies by Levine[136] suggest that changes in blood supply suffice to explain the variegated distribution of changes. These data refer to a generalized decrease in oxygen involving the entire brain, but when the sudden lack of oxygen is limited to one section of an organ the result is an infarct, i.e., a mass of necrotic tissue. All the components of the involved area die: cells, blood vessels, inter-

cellular substances, etc. The gross and microscopic aspect, the functional significance and the final destiny of an infarct depend on a series of variables, the most important of which may be listed as follows: (1) the organ involved, (2) the size of the occluded vessels, (3) the type of circulation (anastomosed or terminal) of the affected tissue, (4) the status of the arterial vessels and (5) the nature of the obstruction. In the following paragraphs each one of these factors is briefly discussed.

1. *Organ Involved.* It appears obvious that functional disturbances produced by a more or less extensive area of necrosis will vary according to the organ involved. Whatever the site of infarction, all physiologic processes cease abruptly in the necrotic area.

In the brain infarcts usually appear as well limited areas of softening, which in time may be partially reabsorbed leaving cystic cavities filled with a thick, greenish-yellow fluid; under the microscope there is marginal gliosis and accumulation of microglial cells which show enlarged and vacuolated cytoplasm. These cells are scavenger elements in the central nervous system and contain lipids in the cytoplasm, the remnants of ingested myelin (Fig. 1–29). In all other organs infarcts appear as well limited, conical areas of increased consistency, with peripheral basis and the apex directed towards the occluded vessel; some organs show anemic infarcts while in others they are usually hemorrhagic. The latter owe their aspect to the fact that neighboring capillaries are ruptured and the area of necrosis is flooded with blood. Hemorrhagic infarcts are the rule in the lung and spleen. In time, the blood pigments are reabsorbed and the necrotic area becomes pale or yellow (Fig. 1–30); tissue debris is removed and connective tissue proliferates, leaving a depressed scar which deforms the external surface of the organ. This scar may be very prominent, as in the myocardium, where the entire wall may be replaced by fibrous tissue (Fig. 1–31), or it may become a thin and hardly perceptible line, as often happens in the lung, where distention of the neighboring alveoli replaces the lost tissue.

2. *Size of the Occluded Vessel.* The influence of this factor is self-evident. Most of the time, the size of the occluded vessel will correspond to the extension of the necrotic area, but occasionally other factors play an important role, such as the presence of collateral circulation or of disturbances of

blood flow. The latter is frequently seen in the lung, where an infarct is possible only when there is sudden obstruction of a pulmonary artery and congestion of the lesser circulation. In fact, it is not rare to see pulmonary embolism without infarction when there is no slowing of the circulation through the lungs.[137] On the other hand, in cases of severe, chronic heart failure, pulmonary infarcts may appear even without occlusion of pulmonary arteries.

3. *Type of Circulation (Anastomosed or Terminal).* This is a highly important factor and on many occasions it may determine the presence or absence of necrosis after vascular occlusion. The situation in the lung has been discussed in the preceding paragraph; another organ where it plays a very important role is the liver. Blood enters the liver by the hepatic artery and the portal vein; therefore, occlusion of a branch of the hepatic artery will produce necrosis only if

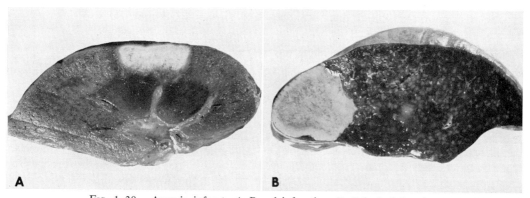

FIG. 1–30. Anemic infarct. *A*, Renal infarction. *B*, Splenic infarction.

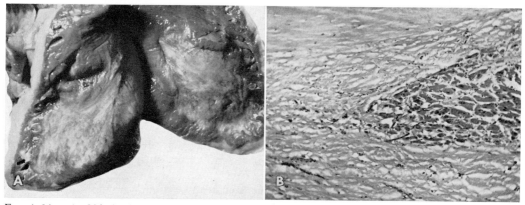

FIG. 1–31. *A*, Old, healed myocardial infarction involving the interventricular septum. *B*, A bundle of myocardial fibers surrounded by scar tissue.

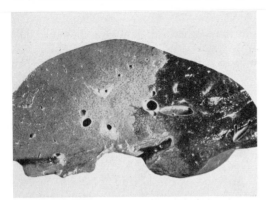

FIG. 1–32.   Red "infarct" of the liver.

the circulation provided by the portal vein is poor, as in heart failure.[138] Even so, anemic infarcts of the liver are extremely rare; the most common form is "red" infarct, which is not a true zone of necrosis since the cells survive (Fig. 1–32). It appears when one of the two sources of blood is closed, with persistence of the circulation through the other; in this case, the intrahepatic distribution of blood distal to the area of occlusion is enhanced by the lack of blood pressure from the closed vessel and an area of congestion supervenes.

Double circulation is not the only type of anatomic distribution of blood vessels influencing the development of infarctions; anastomoses are present in all vascular territories, but in some they are peripheral and capillary in nature (terminal circulation) while in others they occur at different levels (anastomosed circulation). Terminal circulation is present in the myocardium, the spleen and the kidney, and in these organs the sudden occlusion of an arterial blood vessel will be followed by the development of an area of necrosis corresponding to the distribution of the closed segment of the arterial tree. On the other hand, anastomosed circulation is characteristic of the stomach and intestines, and it is well known that in the latter the necrotic zones are usually smaller than the area served by the vessel occluded.

4. *Status of the Arterial Vessels.* The ability of a given vascular territory to expand and develop a collateral circulation after an occlusion will not influence the appearance of infarcts, but it will determine the degree of restitution of blood flow. The nature of the stimulus for the growth of collateral vessels after the interruption of blood flow is not known, but its discovery would be of great help in the treatment of many forms of localized circulatory insufficiency. By means of plastic casts, Liebow[139] has shown that the mediastinal veins enlarge and multiply in cases of extensive destruction of pulmonary parenchyma, thus facilitating the return circulation of bronchial arteries. Rosenberg and Liebow[140] pointed out that collateral circulation may result from two different factors or a combination of both: expansion of preexisting vessels or neoformation of vascular channels in connective tissue. The stimulus for vascular proliferation was considered humoral in nature by Lewis,[141] and mechanical by Holman.[142] Vascular dilatation after occlusion of an artery is of a reflex nature and is influenced by the sympathetic nervous system.

5. *Nature of the Occlusion.* If the occlusion is produced by an embolus, the nature of the impacted material will determine in part the effect of the ischemia. Fat embolism is reabsorbed and the patency of the vessel is reestablished, but septic embolism during subacute bacterial endocarditis adds to the circulatory disturbance the problems of metastatic infection.

Physical agents of necrosis are trauma, temperature, electricity, ionizing radiation and many others. They are very important in forensic pathology and the mechanisms by which they bring about the death of cells and tissues are usually the disruption of anatomic structures, sudden and profound dehydration, or blocking of enzymatic mechanisms.

Necrosis may be produced by many toxic substances which affect living structures at various levels of organization. The effects of toxins depend on three fundamental factors: (a) chemical nature, (b) concentration and (c) tissue involved. The last includes not only the histologic nature, but also the nutritional and metabolic status, which may determine the presence and extension of necrosis. For instance, chloroform attacks liver cells, tetanic toxin the central nervous system and mercuric bichloride the kidney. A most vivid description of the intracellular events occurring after the administration of carbon tetrachloride has been given by Cameron:[143] "Imagine the confusion and chaos throughout the cell that ensues when all kinds of coordinated enzymic systems get out of hand. Little wonder is it that, sooner or later, cell structure begins to crumble as order fails, and that the innumerable interphases now fall into the ways of dead membranes. Deprived of energy supply, the mitochondrial dynamos run down, nuclear function falls into enigmatical confusion and no longer directs the future of the cell according to the primordial law. And so disintegration spreads, with cleavage and disruption of function from structure until the cell collapses and falls victim to its own forces of dismemberment." A detailed analysis of the mechanism of action of several toxic agents of necrosis can be found in Dawkins and Rees' book.[144]

Necrosis may also appear as the result of the absence of some dietary elements. The lack of protein or methionine will produce massive necrosis in the rat liver[145] and thiamine deficiency will induce myocardial necrosis in guinea pigs. Selye[146] has shown that treatment with cortisol acetate and monosodic phosphate followed by immobilization of the experimental animal will lead to massive myocardial infarcts.

A useful classification of necrosis follows the anatomic characteristics of the necrotic material and distinguishes the following types: coagulation, colliquative, caseous, hemorrhagic, fibrinoid and fat necrosis. In coagulation necrosis cells die rapidly, nuclei are distintegrated and cytoplasmic debris fuse forming a yellowish-white firm mass, usually mixed with fibrin. Details of the microscopic architecture may be observed, especially of the stroma, but the parenchymatous elements are completely erased or appear as "ghost" structures (Fig. 1–33). This aspect may be observed in anemic infarcts, in diphtheria, in bacillary dysentery, or in rapidly growing tumors. Colliquative or liquefaction necrosis is found mainly in the central nervous system, where infarcts are soft and become fluid; it is also seen in malignant tumors and in the liver parenchyma, in cases of amebic "abscess" (Fig. 1–34).

Of greater importance because of its frequency throughout the world as well as because of its complexity is caseous necrosis. This form of tissue death occurs mainly in tuberculosis but it may also be seen in syphilis, malignant tumors and some types of infarcts. Although known for a long time, it was first well described by Virchow. In this type of necrosis tissues are transformed into a yellowish-white mass of vari-

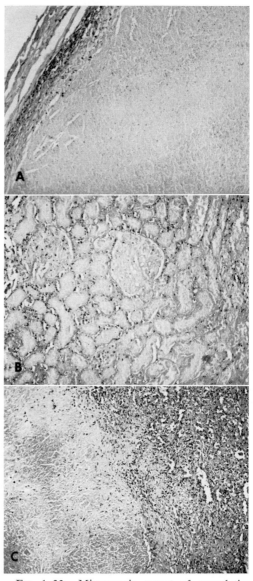

Fig. 1–33. Microscopic aspect of coagulative necrosis. *A,* Caseation in tuberculosis. *B,* Recent renal infarct. *C,* Splenic infarct.

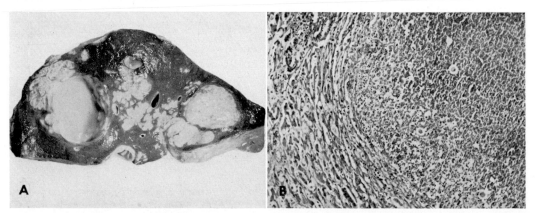

FIG. 1–34.   Colliquative or liquefactive necrosis. *A*, Amebic abscesses of the liver showing different degrees of liquefaction in necrotic areas. *B*, Microscopic picture of one of the preceding abscesses. Notice abundance of polymorphonuclear leukocytes and several amebae.

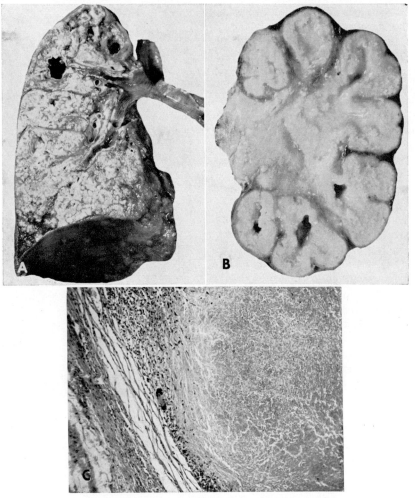

FIG. 1–35.   Caseous necrosis in tuberculosis. *A*, Extensive caseation of lung (caseous bronchopneumonia). *B*, Renal tuberculosis. *C*, Microscopic aspect of caseous necrosis.

able consistency but usually firm, friable, granular and well outlined. It may be very hard (cretaceous) when the calcium content is high or else it may be fluid as in caseous pneumonia (Fig. 1–35). Occasionally the resemblance to certain types of cheese is striking, although the comparison reveals very poor taste. Caseous necrosis represents the most important event in the pathology of tuberculosis; although its mechanism has been intensely explored it is not adequately explained.[147, 148] Apparently, caseous necrosis is death of cells and tissues with incomplete autolysis. All the cells of the organism contain enzymes which carry out their metabolic functions and, while they are confined to the cytoplasm, anabolic processes balance out catabolic reactions; however, when these enzymes are released to the interstitial tissues they continue acting and induce destruction of cells and tissues. In caseous necrosis, enzymatic activity is inhibited either because proteins are destroyed or because of the presence of inhibiting substances blocking their effect. Rich[149] believes that enzymes are primarily derived from macrophages and that the biochemical environment (especially pH changes) of the lesion is not favorable to their activity. Another important problem in tuberculosis is liquefaction of caseous material, which brings about disastrous consequences to the patient. It has been suggested that liquefaction is due to complete digestion of unhydrolyzed proteins by the enzymes of polymorphonuclear leukocytes,[150] or to hypersensitivity, or to increased multiplication

of tubercle bacilli in the lesion, etc. The existence of many hypotheses to explain the same phenomenon indicates that there is no adequate solution.

The flooding of tissues by blood is another cause of necrosis, which is then known as hemorrhagic. However, hemorrhage may also be caused by necrosis of blood vessels. Widespread anastomoses are necessary to observe this phenomenon as it occurs in the lung, where hemorrhagic infarcts are the rule (Fig. 1–36). On the other hand, in organs with closed or terminal circulation infarcts are usually anemic. Invasion of dead tissues by pathogenic germs gives rise to wet gangrene, and when the bacteria are anaerobic gas is produced in the tissues (gaseous gangrene). Bacteria in necrotic areas may be nonpathogenic, and then gangrene will be dry; in these cases the area distal to vascular occlusion undergoes necrosis and dehydration. A dark discoloration is usually present before the infarct is finally eliminated (Fig. 1–37).

Fat necrosis is caused by two main factors: pancreatic digestion and trauma. The former appears in acute pancreatitis and also in conditions with prolonged courses; in these cases, pancreatic secretions escape from the ducts of this organ and come in contact with peripancreatic or abdominal fatty tissues in general. The extensive experimental studies of Panabokké[151] suggest that in pancreatic fat necrosis there is a triple mechanism, characterized as follows: (1) an initiating process, in which the fat-cell membrane is damaged by enzymatic

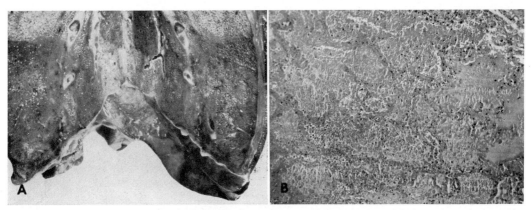

FIG. 1–36. Recent, hemorrhagic infarct of the lung. *A,* Gross aspect of the cut surface; notice embolus in cut vessel near top of picture. *B,* "Ghost" structure in hemorrhagic necrosis of lung parenchyma.

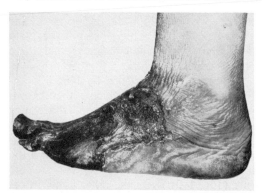

Fig. 1–37. Dry gangrene of ischemic origin in a diabetic patient.

activity, probably amylase, lecithinase, or others, (2) a liberating process, with release of lipase and probably other enzymes from the cytoplasm and (3) self-digestion of cell fat by released lipase. Proteolytic enzymes destroy the cellular cytoplasm and lipase digests neutral fats, releasing fatty acids and glycerol; the latter is reabsorbed and metabolized while the former are combined with sodium, potassium or calcium ions of tissues and form soaps. Later, calcium may precipitate in tissues as the corresponding phosphates or carbonates (Fig. 1–38). Post-traumatic fat necrosis has been described in newborns and in adults, especially in the breast.[151] Trauma breaks the cell membrane and the cytoplasmic lipids come in contact with interstitial tissues, provoking a foreign body reaction with formation of granulomas and many giant cells. Fat necrosis has also been observed without antecedent trauma.

A special type of necrosis that has received much attention in recent years is "fibrinoid" necrosis.[153, 154] It may be seen particularly in two areas: the blood vessel wall and the interstitial tissues. It appears as a loss of structure which is replaced by a hyaline, finely granular or smooth, acidophilic substance, giving positive reactions with fibrin stains (Fig. 1–39). It is quite possible that there may be several kinds of fibrinoid necrosis, and in some of them it seems certain that fibrin forms a very important component. It is one of the characteristic lesions of "collagen" diseases (rheumatic fever, rheumatoid arthritis, disseminated lupus erythematosus, polyarteritis nodosa, scleroderma, etc.), although it has been observed also in atherosclerosis, malignant hypertension, peptic ulcer, thromboangiitis obliterans, serum sickness and other conditions.[155] Experimentally, it has been produced by hypersensitivity, nephroprival hypertension and chronic administration of adrenocortical steroids. There are four main hypotheses on the origin of fibrinoid necrosis: (a) it is necrosis of the smooth muscle of vascular walls;[156] (b) it is a mixture of plasma fibrinogen and tissue elements;[157] (c) it is mainly fibrin;[158] (d) it contains important amounts of gamma globulin.[159] A more detailed discussion of this change is given in Chapter VI.

Morphologic changes in dying cells have been carefully documented.[160] The most important alterations occur in the nucleus, where decrease in size, condensation of chromatic material and increase in stain-

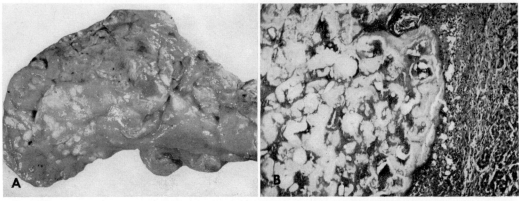

Fig. 1–38. Fat necrosis. *A,* The white, chalky spots near the left portion of the pancreas are characteristic of fat necrosis. *B,* Microscopic aspect with incipient calcification.

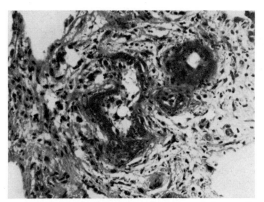

FIG. 1–39. Fibrinoid necrosis of arteriolar walls after radiation for carcinoma of the breast.

ability with basic dyes are known collectively under the name of pyknosis. Fragmentation of nuclear material (karyorrhexis) and progressive disappearance (karyolysis) are probably more advanced stages of the same process. Eventually there appear modifications in the cytoplasmic structures, with loss or drastic changes in tinctorial affinities and finally there is destruction of cell limits with complete obliteration of individual elements. These modifications have been studied cytochemically, and Leuchtenberger[161] and Pollister[162] have commented on the similarity between pyknosis and mitosis with regard to loss of functional activity. Cytophotometric determinations of pyknosis in different materials agree in that nuclear condensation involves at first a loss of protein.[163] Unmasking of charged groups previously made unavailable by the associated nonhistone protein leave chiefly a condensed nucleohistone residue. Loss of desoxyribonucleic acid occurs very probably as a later secondary event, during karyorrhexis or karyolysis.[164]

The exact point at which death of a cell occurs is unknown. Although it is possible at certain stages to say of a cell that it is "alive" or "dead," the transition period between these two stages is as yet ill-defined. It is not known which function or chemical reaction, when lost, is the cause of irreversible damage to structural and metabolic integrity. In a series of studies, King et al.[165–168] have made an extended analysis of several properties of isolated cells in tissue culture and have emerged with an organized scheme describing a typical pattern of cell death. Ehrlich tumor cells were subjected to three different types of injury (incubation in Krebs-Ringer medium, irradiation and treatment with Salyrgan) and several measurements were made, relative to the four major processes of the cell: biosynthesis of enzymes, production of energy, repair and restoration of structural deficiencies and maintenance of a satisfactory ionic

Table 5. Stages of Cell Death

Stage 1
1. Division stops, as the cell fails to undergo mitosis.
2. Deoxyribonucleic acid is lost from the cell nucleus.
3. Protein is lost concurrently with the first two steps, probably from both the nucleus and the cytoplasm.
4. The formation of blebs, granules, and minor changes in the size of the nucleus and cytoplasm occur.

Stage 2
5. Respiration ceases several hours later.
6. Lactic acid production continues for a short time following cessation of respiration.
7. Total dehydrogenase activity is lost, with interruption of complex oxidative and fermentative cycles.
8. Mitochondria decrease in number and increase in size throughout the experiment, but they do not disappear completely with the loss of metabolic functions.

Stage 3
9. Potassium loss from the cell is concurrent with the entrance of sodium and water. Although small variations in these constituents may occur earlier, the terminal changes appear to be associated with the loss of energy production following breakdown of the glycolytic cycle.
10. Trypan blue enters the cell and stains the nucleus and cytoplasm.
11. At a critical point, in a rather narrow range, the cell bursts, releasing large amounts of sodium and water. This results in contraction in size, although a protein framework in the cytoplasm and nucleus remains intact.

Stage 4
12. The denatured protein of the cytoplasm takes up additional amounts of sodium and water. Later, as the protein is dissolved into the surrounding medium, the total content of sodium and water is reduced.
13. The terminal picture is that of a few irregularly stained nuclei embedded in a conglomerate mass of precipitated protein.

(King and associates[167])

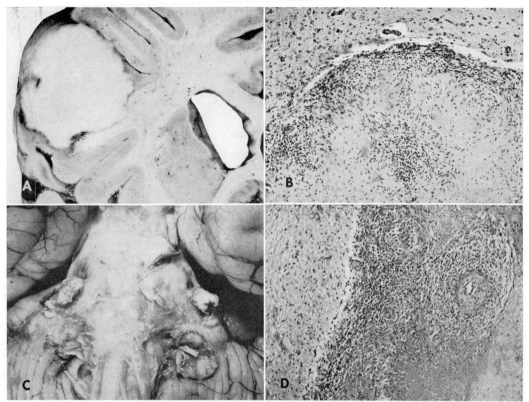

FIG. 1–40. Cerebral tuberculoma and tuberculous meningitis. *A,* A large, solitary tuberculoma in the brain, ruptured into the subarachnoid space. *B,* Microscopic aspect of the same lesion, showing good demarcation from surrounding brain parenchyma. *C,* Fibrous, dense tuberculous meningitis. *D,* Tuberculous exudate in the subarachnoid space with necrosis and vascular lesions.

environment. The results appear in Table 5. It was also observed that nuclear changes occurred some time before there was any demonstrable alteration in mitochondrial structure, plasma membrane structure, amount of ions or water, dehydrogenase activity, respiration or lactic acid production. Probably the most important and unique property of protoplasm is the ability to duplicate its constituents exactly, and the loss of this quality may be the first stage in an irreversible chain leading to cell death.

The final fate of an area of necrosis is elimination from the organism. This can be accomplished in several ways. If destroyed tissues find their way to one of the organic cavities or ducts, they rupture into it. This is especially important with abscesses, which may break into the meninges, the pleural or the abdominal cavities, causing severe complications such as meningitis, empyema or peritonitis. Good examples of this event are tuberculomas of the brain, which may break into the subarachnoid space and produce tuberculous meningitis (Fig. 1–40), or amebic abscess of the liver, which may rupture into the pleural or peritoneal cavities, or even into a hollow viscus in the abdomen. In the first case the collection of necrotic, liquefied liver tissue combined with bacteria will cause very severe disturbances; in the second case, the opening into a hollow viscus may provide a way out for necrotic fluid, although the clinical results are usually not as benign as might be expected. Another way of eliminating necrotic areas from the organism is encapsulation. The surrounding tissues of an infarct will show inflammatory changes with vascular proliferation first and deposition of connective tissue later. The result is the formation of a thick, dense capsule of hyalinized, collagenous fibers which isolate the dead tissues from the rest of the organism. Sometimes necrosis is slowly reabsorbed and replaced by a scar.

B. Autolysis and Putrefaction. Autolysis means digestion of tissues by their own enzymes under aseptic conditions. Therefore, it is necessary for cells to die without inactivation of enzymes. In accidental ingestion of phenic acid, the surface of the gastric mucosa is not autolyzed because phenol will fix the structures, precipitating intracytoplasmic proteins and inactivating enzymes; if the subject dies the deep layers of the gastric mucosa will undergo decomposition, the same as the rest of the organism.

All tissues undergo autolysis but they do it at variable times and with different degrees of intensity, because of the different intracellular concentration of enzymes. Thus, the pancreas and digestive tract are rapidly digested while the brain and connective tissues take more time. Temperature is also important. When cadavers are not refrigerated immediately after death the temperature goes down first in the skin and the subcutaneous tissues but is maintained for variable periods in the deeper parts, which explains in part the rapid autolysis of spleen, kidneys and adrenals.

The morphology of autolyzed cells is sometimes difficult to distinguish from pathologic processes occurring during life. There are excellent studies on this subject,[169–170] which point out the varieties according to tissues and even to the particular area of tissue involved; in the kidney, the picture of autolysis in the proximal convoluted tubule is different from that in the distal convoluted tubule. In the former, cytokaryolysis is observed from the beginning while in the latter there is first acidophilia of the cytoplasm and nuclear pyknosis. In the liver, during the first 20 hours there is a decrease in the intensity of cytoplasmic and nuclear staining and the cellular volume decreases; after this period, there is a new increase in affinity for dyes and finally karyorrhexis and pyknosis appear. This biphasic response has been associated with the glycogen content of the cell, but other factors such as time, temperature and the reserve capacity of the organ are also important.

Histochemical studies of different tissues at variable periods of autolysis have been published by several authors. Among these, Kent[171] observed that in liver, kidney and myocardium of dogs, succinic dehydrogenase and alkaline phosphatase were present and active when incubated at 4° C. up to 144 hours, but when incubation was done at 37° C. the activity diminished in 12 hours; under the latter conditions there was considerable diffusion of enzymes. Smith et al.[172] analyzed seven different enzymes in the rabbit brain at postmortem intervals of 2 to 6 hours; there was no significant deterioration, migration or diffusion of the activities of these enzymes in the period studied with the exception of phosphofructokinase, which proved to be very unstable after only short postmortem intervals. These results are in agreement with the general experience of acceptable postmortem preservation of microscopic structure of brain tissue. Finally, Taft[173] studied the effect of postmortem autolysis in the rat liver on five hydrolytic enzymes, after intervals of up to 6 hours, and found that there is no disappearance of enzymatic activity. Indeed, some of the enzymes actually showed an increase in activity with autolysis, a phenomenon previously studied by Berthet, et al.[174] in acid phosphatase of rat liver; these authors concluded that the enzyme is naturally present in the cells within granules that are osmotic systems surrounded by semipermeable membranes. Disintegration of cytoplasmic structures would release the enzyme protein and facilitate further hydrolysis of surrounding substrate.

Biochemical changes in tissues during autolysis have also been observed in recent years.[175, 176] When the liver is ground immediately after death and small portions are taken for chemical analysis at variable periods the first change observed is in pH, which decreases rapidly because of the release of phosphoric acid from nucleic acids through the effect of phosphatases. Proteolysis is also immediate and may be determined by an increase in trichloroacetic acid soluble material. The speed and extension of proteolysis depend on several factors, among them the tissue pH, since proteolytic enzymes will act better in neutral pH, and the oxygen concentration, which when high will oxidate SH groups of cathepsins and block their action. Dawkins[177] has found that autolytic changes are slower in fetal than in adult liver as judged by the survival of oxidative phosphorylation; this might be expected since fetal liver is rich in glycogen, which is remarkably stable during autolysis. Glycogen stability may be attributed to the low activity of glucose-6-phosphatase. The question arises here as to why normal cells do not undergo autolysis when they contain the same enzymes responsible for this process after death.[178] Although several reasons may be quoted in this respect, the problem is yet to be solved. (a) Many enzymes are not secreted in active form but as zymogens, which require the presence of extracellular factors in order to exert their action; once outside the cells they are activated. Cells with external layers formed by glyco- and mucoproteins are resistant to enzymatic action, so the cellular membrane must be intact for the cells to be safe. (b) The catabolic effects of many intracellular enzymes is balanced in life by the anabolic action of others. When the cell dies, synthetic activities cease entirely and there is a predominance of autolytic or destructive enzymes. (c) Once digestion of the cell is started by its own enzymes it is favored by other factors such as the disappearance of intracytoplasmic osmotic barriers, which uncover previously protected structures and may be a substrate to enzymatic action. This sequence has been characterized by Gallagher, et al.[175] as follows: "When a tissue is deprived of its blood supply, no more exogenous substrate is being supplied to the cells and their store of substrate soon becomes depleted. The level of ATP in the cell drops as it is utilized in numerous reactions in the cell's economy. In the cell under normal conditions of blood supply there exists a state of dynamic equilibrium where synthesis balances breakdown, but if blood-flow is interrupted, synthesis is arrested and such substances as coenzymes are broken down and because of the lack of ATP they cannot be synthesised. Permeability barriers are no longer maintained, ion exchanges occur and calcium enters the cell, which can no longer carry out oxidative phosphorylation; the process has become irreversible and the cell dies. Cathepsins, activated by reduced glutathione, now break down the cell structure by proteolysis."

Cadaveric putrefaction results from the entrance into the circulation of saprophytic bacteria, usually from the digestive tract, and of anaerobic germs of the type of clostridia. Some of these bacteria produce gases, such as hydrogen sulphide and methylmercaptan, which are responsible for the foul smell, and also for the discoloration observed in some organs and tissues (digestive tract and abdominal wall). The discoloration is caused by a combination of gases with blood and tissue pigments. Occasionally, some organs show multiple cavitations which are the result of tissue distention by gases produced by anaerobic bacteria; this is frequently observed in the brain and in the liver.

REFERENCES

1. Cameron, G. R.: New Pathways in Cellular Pathology, London, Edward Arnold, 1956.
2. Davidman, A., and Dolley, D. H.: Cloudy swelling; a process of stimulation, J. Med. Res. 42:515, 1921.
3. Bell, E. T.: Cloudy swelling. A preliminary report, J.A.M.A. 61:455, 1913.
4. Fonnesu, A., and Severi, C.: Nucleic acids in the kidney in cloudy swelling, Brit. J. Exper. Path. 34:341, 1953.
5. Cameron, G. R.: Pathology of the Cell, London, Oliver and Boyd, 1952.
6. Lucké, B., and McCutcheon, M.: Reversible and irreversible swelling of living and of dead cells, Arch. Path. 2:846, 1926.
7. Zollinger, H. U.: Les mitochondries (leur étude à l'aide du microscope à contraste de phases), Rev. hémat. 5:696, 1950.
8. Harman, J. W.: Cytochondrial aspects of cellular pathology, J. Clin. Path. 11:495, 1959.
9. Christie, G. S., and Judah, J. D.: Mechanism of action of carbon tetrachloride on liver, Proc. Roy. Soc. London s.B 142:241, 1954.
10. Aterman, K.: The nature of "watery vacuolation" of the liver cell, Quart. J. Exper. Physiol. 40:272, 1955.
11. Aterman, K.: Observations on the nature of "watery vacuolation," Lab. Invest. 7:577, 1958.
12. Robinson, J. R.: Osmoregulation in surviving slices from the livers of adult rats (with a note on cloudy swelling), Proc. Roy. Soc. London s.B 140:135, 1952.
13. Robinson, J. R.: Metabolism of intracellular water, Physiol. Rev. 40:112, 1952.
14. Dixon, K. C., and McCullagh, G. P.: Protein in dying liver cells, Quart. J. Exper. Physiol. 42. 104, 1957.
15. Dixon, K. C., King, A. J., and Malinin, T.: Protein in dying β-cells of the pancreatic islets, Quart. J. Exper. Physiol. 45:202, 1960.
16. Rigdon, R. H., and Cardwell, E. S.: Renal lesions following the intravenous injection of a hypertonic solution of glucose, Arch. Int. Med. 69: 670, 1952.
17. Kulka, J. P., Pearson, C. M., and Robbins, S. L.:

A distinctive vacuolar nephropathy associated with intestinal disease, Am. J. Path. *26:*349, 1950.

18. Pérez Tamayo, R., and Saenz Ruiz, A.: Lesiones renales consecutivas a la derivación ureteral, Rev. Latinoamer. Anat. Pat. *1:*131, 1957.

19. Relman, A. S., and Schwartz, W. B.: The kidney in potassium depletion, Am. J. Med. *24:*764, 1958.

20. Tauxe, W. N., Wakim, K. G., and Baggenstoss, A. H.: The renal lesions in experimental deficiency of potassium, Am. J. Clin. Path. *28:*221, 1957.

21. Kennedy, G. C., Flear, C.T.G., and Parker, R. A.: Renal disease and secondary potassium depletion in aging rats, Quart. J. Exper. Physiol. *45:*82, 1960.

22. Wachstein, M., and Neisel, E.: Enzymatic staining reactions in the kidneys of potassium-depleted rats, Am. J. Path. *35:*1189, 1959.

23. Smetana, H.: The histopathology of acute nonfatal hepatitis, Bull. New York Acad. Med. *28:* 482, 1952.

24. Doniach, I., and Weinbren, K.: The development of inclusion bodies in the cells of the rat liver after partial hepatectomy, Brit. J. Exper. Path. *33:*499, 1952.

25. Manuelidis, E. E.: Pathological Swelling and Vacuolization of Cells, in Palay, S. L. (ed.): Frontiers in Cytology, New Haven, Yale University Press, 1958.

26. Adams, R. D., Denny-Brown, D., and Pearson, C. M.: Diseases of Muscle. A Study in Pathology, New York, P. B. Hoeber, 1953.

27. Kay, W. W., and Whitehead, R.: Fatty Substances, in Brontë, J. G., and Painter, T. S. (eds.): The Microtomists Vademecum (Bolles-Lee), ed. 10, London, Blakiston's Son, 1937.

28. Deane, H. W.: Intracellular Lipids: Their Detection and Significance, in Palay, S. L. (ed.): Frontiers in Cytology, New Haven, Yale University Press, 1958.

29. Virchow, R.: Reizung and Reizbarkeit, Virchows Arch. path. Anat. *14:*1, 1858.

30. Lebedev: quoted in Lubarsch, O.: Fettdegeneration und Fettinfiltration, Ergebn. allg. Path. *3:* 631, 1897.

31. Dible, J. H., and Gerrard, W. W.: The source of fat in experimentally produced fatty degeneration of the heart, J. Path. & Bact. *46:*77, 1948.

32. Rosenfeld, G.: Fettbildung, Erg. d. Physiol. *1:* 651, 1902; *2:*50, 1903.

33. Lewis, M. R., and Lewis, W. H.: The cultivation of tissues from chick embryos in solutions of NaCl, CaCl$_2$, KCl, and NaHCO$_3$, Anat. Rec. *5:*277, 1911.

34. Lambert, R. A.: The effect of dilution of plasma medium on the growth and fat accumulation of cells in tissue cultures, J. Exper. Med. *19:*398, 1914.

35. Dible, J. H.: Fat mobilization in starvation, J. Path. & Bact. *35:*451, 1932.

36. Dible, J. H.: Is fatty degeneration of the heart muscle a phanerosis? J. Path. & Bact. *39:*197, 1934.

37. Dible, J. H., and Libman, J.: Further observations on fatty mobilization in starvation, J. Path. & Bact. *38:*269, 1934.

38. Dible, J. H., and Popják, G.: The distribution of fatty change in the kidneys and some factors influencing its production, J. Path. & Bact. *53:* 133, 1941.

39. Best, C. H., Hartroft, W. S., Lucas, C. C., and Ridout, J. H.: Effects of dietary protein, lipotropic factors and realimentation on total hepatic lipids and their distribution, Brit. M. J. *1:*1439, 1955.

40. King, D. W., Socolow, E. L., and Bensch, K. G.: The relation between protein synthesis and lipid accumulation in L strain cells and Ehrlich ascites cells, J. Biophys. Biochem. Cytol. *5:*421, 1959.

41. Dixon, K. C.: Fatty deposition, Quart. J. Exper. Physiol. *43:*139, 1958.

42. Elvehjem, C. A.: Amino acid imbalance, Fed. Proc. *15:*965, 1956.

43. Meyer, J. S., and Hartroft, W. S.: Hepatic lipid produced by polyphagia in albino rats. Relationships to dietary choline and casein, Am. J. Path. *36:*365, 1960.

44. Deo, M. G., and Ramalingaswami, V.: Production of periportal fatty infiltration of the liver in the Rhesus monkey by a protein-deficient diet, Lab. Invest. *9:*319, 1960.

45. Rappoport, A. M., Borowy, Z. J., Lougheed, W. M., and Lotto, W. N.: Subdivision of liver lobules into a structural and functional unit: role in hepatic physiology and pathology, Anat. Rec. *119:*11, 1954.

46. Dianzani, M. U., and Scuro, S.: Effects of some inhibitors of oxidative phosphorylation on morphology and enzymic activities of mitochondria, Biochem. J. *62:*205, 1956.

47. Christie, G. S., and Judah, J. D.: Mechanism of action of carbon tetrachloride on liver cells, Proc. Roy. Soc. London s.B *142:*241, 1954.

48. Ennor, A. H.: Oxygen consumption and ketone body production in carbon tetrachloride and phosphorus fatty liver, Australian J. Exper. Biol. & M. Sc. *20:*73, 1942.

49. Dianzani, M. U.: The content of adenosine polyphosphates in fatty livers, Biochem. J. *65:*116, 1957.

50. Friede, R. L.: Inverse histochemical distribution of fat and oxidative enzymes in fatty livers produced by carbon tetrachloride, J. Path. & Bact. *79:*109, 1960.

51. Recknagel, R. O., and Anthony, D. D.: Biochemical changes in carbon tetrachloride fatty liver: separation of fatty changes from mitochondrial degeneration, J. Biol. Chem. *234:*1052, 1959.

52. Calvert, D. N., and Brody, T. M.: Biochemical alteration of liver mitochondria by treatment with carbon tetrachloride *in vitro* and *in vivo,* Fed. Proc. *17:*356, 1958.

53. Popják, G.: The mechanism of parenchymatous degeneration produced by diphtheria toxin, J. Path. & Bact. *60:*75, 1953.

53a. MacDonald, R. A., Schmid, R., and Mallory, G. K.: Regeneration in fatty liver and cirrhosis, Arch. Path. *69:*175, 1960.

54. Graham, R. L.: Sudden death in young adults in association with fatty liver, Bull. Johns Hopkins Hosp. *74:*16, 1944.

55. Spiro, D. M.: The structural basis of proteinuria in man. Electron microscopic studies of renal biopsy specimens from patients with lipid nephrosis, amyloidosis and subacute and chronic glomerulonephritis, Am. J. Path. *35:*47, 1959.

56. Farquhar, M. G.: Review of normal and pathologic glomerular ultrastructure, in Metcoff, J. (ed.): Proc. Tenth Annual Conf. Nephrotic Syndrome, New York, The National Kidney Disease Foundation, 1959.

57. Ober, W. B., and LeCompte, P. M.: Acute fatty metamorphosis of liver associated with pregnancy; distinctive lesion, Am. J. Med. *19:*743, 1955.

58. Hartroft, W. S.: The locus of the beginning of dietary cirrhosis, Tr. 8th Conf. Liver Injury, Macy Foundation, 1950.

59. Hartroft, W. S., and Ridout, J. H.: Pathogenesis of the cirrhosis produced by choline deficiency. Escape of lipid from fatty hepatic cysts into the biliary and vascular systems, Am. J. Path. 27:951, 1951.

60. Fadell, E. J., and Sullivan, B. H.: Fatty liver and fat embolism, U. S. Armed Forces M. J. 8:1, 1957.

61. Hartroft, W. S., and Sellers, E.: The dissolution of fatty cysts in precirrhotic and cirrhotic livers of choline deficient rats treated with lipotropic factors, Am. J. Path. 28:387, 1952.

62. Sepúlveda, B., Rojas, E., and Landa, L.: La etiología de la cirrosis del hígado tipo Laennec. Rev. invest. clín. 4:321, 1952.

63. Chaikoff, I. L., and Connor, C. L.: Production of cirrhosis of the liver of the normal dog by high fat diets, Proc. Soc. Exper. Biol. & Med. 43: 638, 1940.

64. Connor, C. L.: The etiology and pathogenesis of alcoholic cirrhosis of the liver, J.A.M.A. 112: 387, 1939.

65. Hartroft, W. S.: The sequence of pathologic events in the development of experimental fatty liver and cirrhosis, Ann. New York Acad. Sc. 57: 633, 1954.

66. Gilman, J., and Gilbert, C.: Aspects of nutritional liver disease, human and experimental, Ann. New York Acad. Sc. 57:737, 1954.

67. Asboe-Hansen, G.: Hypertrophic scars and keloids. Etiology, pathogenesis, and dermatologic therapy, Dermatologica 120:178, 1960.

68. Herxheimer, G.: Ueber das verhalten der kleinen Gefässe der Milz, Berl. klin. Wchnschr. 54:82, 1917.

69. Moritz, A. R., and Oldt, M. R.: Arteriolar sclerosis in hypertensive and nonhypertensive individuals, Am. J. Path. 13:679, 1937.

70. Bell, E. T.: Pathological Anatomy in Primary Hypertension, in Bell, E. T. (ed.): Symposium on Hypertension, Minneapolis, University of Minnesota Press, 1951.

71. Duguid, J. B., and Anderson, G. S.: Pathogenesis of hyaline arteriosclerosis, J. Path. & Bact. 64:519, 1952.

72. Crawford, T., and Woolf, N.: Hyaline arteriolosclerosis in the spleen: an immuno-histochemical study, J. Path. & Bact. 79:221, 1960.

73. Smith, J. P.: Hyaline arteriolosclerosis of the kidney, J. Path. & Bact. 69:147, 1955.

74. Montgomery, P. O'B., and Muirhead, E. E.: A characterization of hyaline arteriolar sclerosis by histochemical procedures, Am. J. Path. 30:521, 1954.

75. Bell, E. T.: Hyalinization of the islands of Langerhans in nondiabetic individuals, Am. J. Path. 35:801, 1959.

76. Opie, E. L.: The relation of diabetes mellitus to lesions of the pancreas. Hyaline degeneration of the islets of Langerhans, J. Exper. Med. 5:527, 1901.

77. Moschowitz, E.: The pathogenesis of the hyalinization of the islands of Langerhans, Arch. Path. 61:136, 1956.

78. Kimmelstiel, P., and Wilson, C.: Intercapillary lesions in the glomeruli of the kidney, Am. J. Path. 12:83, 1936.

79. Bell, E. T.: Renal Diseases, Philadelphia, Lea and Febiger, 1950.

80. Gellman, D. D., Pirani, C. L., Soothill, J. F., Muehrcke, R. C., and Kark, R. M.: Diabetic nephropathy: a clinical and pathologic study based on renal biopsies, Medicine 38:321, 1959.

81. Laufer, A., and Stein, O.: The exudative lesion in diabetic glomerulosclerosis, Am. J. Clin. Path. 32:56, 1959.

82. Muirhead, E. E., Montgomery, P. O'B., and Booth, E.: The glomerular lesions of diabetes mellitus, Arch. Int. Med. 98:146, 1956.

83. Wilens, S. L., Elster, S. K., and Baker, J. P.: Glomerular lipidosis in intercapillary glomerulosclerosis, Ann. Int. Med. 34:592, 1951.

84. Farquhar, M. G., Hopper, J., and Moon, H. D.: Diabetic glomerulosclerosis: electron and light microscopic studies, Am. J. Path. 35:721, 1959.

85. Fernández de Cicero, M., Montfort, I., and Pérez Tamayo, R.: El tejido conjuntivo del glomérulo renal humano. Estudio bioquímico, Rev. Latinoamer. Anat. Pat. 3:17, 1959.

86. Pearse, A.G.E.: The nature of Russell bodies and Kurloff bodies. Observations on the cytochemistry of plasma cells and reticulum cells, J. Clin. Path. 2:81, 1949.

87. White, R. G.: Observation on the formation and nature of Russell bodies, Brit. J. Exper. Path. 35:365, 1954.

88. Wells, H. G.: Waxy degeneration of the diaphragm. A factor causing death in pneumonia and other conditions, Arch. Path. 4:681, 1927.

89. Balcázar, A., and Pérez Tamayo, R.: Unpublished data.

90. Costero, I., and Barroso-Moguel, R.: Bases morfológicas de las ictericias hepatocelulares, Memorias del I Congreso Mexicano de Medicina, 1947.

91. Mallory, G. K.: Liver diseases associated with chronic alcoholism, Lab. Invest. 9:132, 1960.

92. Wilgram, G. F.: Experimental Laennec type of cirrhosis in monkeys, Ann. Int. Med. 51:1134, 1959.

93. Rice, J. D., Jr., and Yesner, R.: The prognostic significance of so-called Mallory bodies in portal cirrhosis, Arch. Int. Med. 105:99, 1960.

94. Axenfeld, H., and Brass, K.: Klinische und bioptische Untersuchungen über die sogennanten Icterus catarrhalis, Frankfurt Ztschr. Path. 57: 147, 1942.

95. Rather, L. J.: Filtration, resorption and excretion of protein by the kidney, Medicine 31:357, 1952.

96. Oliver, J., MacDowell, M., and Lee, Y. C.: Cellular mechanisms of protein metabolism in the nephron. I. The structural aspects of proteinuria, tubular absorption, droplet formation and the disposal of proteins, J. Exper. Med. 99:589, 1954.

97. Oliver, J., Strauss, W., Kretchmer, N., Lee, Y. C., Dickerman, H. W., and Cherot, F.: The histochemical characteristics of absorption droplets in the nephron, J. Histochem. 3:277, 1955.

98. Kretchmer, N., and Dickerman, H. W.: Cellular mechanism of protein metabolism in the nephron. IV. The partition of succinoxidase and cytochrome oxidase activities in the cells of the proximal convolution of the rat after intraperitoneal injection of egg white, J. Exper. Med. 99:629, 1954.

99. Strauss, W.: Isolation and biochemical properties of droplets from the cells of rat kidney, J. Biol. Chem. 207:745, 1954.

100. Telford Govan, A. D.: Hyaline droplet change in renal epithelium, J. Path. & Bact. 68:642, 1954.

101. Lynch, J. B.: Hyaline droplets in the cervical segment of the proximal convoluted tubule of the human kidney, J. Path. & Bact. 73:539, 1957.

102. Skelton, F. R.: Experimental hypertensive vascular disease in the rat, Arch. Path. 60:190, 1950.

103. Windrum, G. M., and Kramer, H.: Some observations on the histochemical reactions of amyloid, Arch. Path. 63:373, 1957.

104. Larsen, B.: Metachromasia of amyloid with toluidine blue, Acta path. et microbiol. scandinav. *42:*265, 1958.

105. Reiman, H. R., Koucky, R. F., and Eklund, C. M.: Primary amyloidosis limited to tissues of mesenchymal origin, Am. J. Path. *11:*977, 1935.

106. Báez Villaseñor, J., Rojas, E., and Chávez Rivera, I.: Amiloidosis primaria, Rev. invest. clín. *5:*311, 1953.

107. Zuckerbrod, M., Rosenberg, B., and Kayden, H. J.: Renal insufficiency and hypertension associated with secondary amyloidosis, Am. J. Med. *21:* 227, 1956.

108. Bauer, W. H., and Kuzma, J. F.: Solitary "tumors" of atypical amyloid (paraamyloid), Am. J. Clin. Path. *19:*1097, 1949.

109. Báez Villaseñor, J., and Hernández Esquivel, G.: Amiloidosis en los padecimientos hematológicos, Rev. invest. clín. *6:*65, 1954.

110. Cohen, A. S., Calkins, E., and Levene, C. I.: Studies on experimental amyloidosis. I. Analysis of histology and staining reactions of casein-induced amyloidosis in the rabbit, Am. J. Path. *35:*971, 1959.

111. Parkins, R. A., and Bywaters, E. G. L.: Regression of amyloidosis secondary to rheumatoid arthritis, Brit. M. J. *1:*536, 1959.

112. Hass, G. M., Huntington, R., and Krumdieck, N.: Amyloid. III. The properties of amyloid deposits occurring in several species under diverse conditions, Arch. Path. *35:*226, 1953.

113. Giles, R. B., and Calkins, E.: Studies on the composition of secondary amyloid, J. Clin. Invest. *34:*1476, 1955.

114. Braunstein, H., and Buerger, L.: A study of the histochemical and staining characteristics of amyloid, Am. J. Path. *35:*791, 1959.

115. Vázquez, J. J., and Dixon, F. J.: Immunohistochemical analysis of amyloid by the fluorescence technique, J. Exper. Med. *104:*727, 1956.

116. Calkins, E., Cohen, A. S., and Gitlin, D.: Immunochemical determinations of gamma globulin content of amyloid, Fed. Proc. *17:*431, 1958.

117. Vázquez, J. J., and Dixon, F. J.: Studies on the immunohistochemical composition of inflammatory and degenerative lesions, Am. J. Path. *32:* 615, 1956.

118. Wagner, B. M.: Nature of amyloid, Fed. Proc. *17:* 564, 1958.

119. Wagner, B. M.: Histochemical studies of fibrinoid and other abnormal proteins. IV. Protein character of amyloid, Arch. Path. *60:*221, 1955.

120. Giles, R. B., Jr., and Calkins, E.: The relationship of serum hexosamine, globulins and antibodies to experimental amyloidosis, J. Clin. Invest. *37:* 846, 1958.

121. Pirani, C. L.: The pathogenesis of amyloidosis, Lancet *2:*116, 1951.

122. Teilum, G.: Periodic acid-Schiff positive reticuloendothelial cells producing glycoprotein. Functional significance during formation of amyloid, Am. J. Path. *32:*945, 1956.

123. Hilsabeck, J. R., Judd, E. S., Jr., and Woolner, L. B.: Carcinoma of the vermiform appendix, Surg. Clin. North America *31:*995, 1951.

124. Burman, S. O.: Medial degeneration and its relation to dissecting aneurysm, Surg., Gynec. & Obst. (Intntl. Abst.) *110:*1, 1960.

125. McKusick, V. A.: The cardiovascular aspects of Marfan's syndrome, Circulation *11:*321, 1955.

126. Lannigan, R.: The rheumatic process in the left auricular appendage, J. Path. & Bact. *77:*49, 1959.

127. Ihnen, M., and Pérez Tamayo, R.: Breast stroma. Morphologic and histochemical study, Arch. Path. *56:*46, 1953.

128. Guin, J. D., and Seale, E.: Colloid degeneration of the skin (colloid milium), Arch. Dermat. & Syph. *80:*533, 1959.

129. Baird, W. F., and Fisher, E. R.: Observations concerning vacuolation and deposition of glycogen in nuclei of hepatic cells, Lab. Invest. *6:*324, 1957.

130. Ritchie, S., and Waugh, D.: The pathology of Armanni-Ebstein diabetic nephropathy, Am. J. Path. *33:*1035, 1957.

131. Weichselbaum, A., and Stangl, E.: Zur Kenntniss der feineren Veränderungen des Pankreas bei Diabetes Mellitus, Wien. klin. Wchnschr. *14:* 968, 1901.

132. Toreson, E. W.: Glycogen infiltration (so-called hydropic degeneration) in the pancreas in human and experimental diabetes mellitus, Am. J. Path. *27:*327, 1951.

133. Lazarus, S. S., and Volk, B. W.: Studies on the pathogenesis of "hydropic degeneration" of the pancreatic β-cells, Am. J. Path. *33:*600, 1957.

134. Lazarus, S. S., and Volk, B. W.: Glycogen infiltration ("hydropic degeneration") in the pancreas, Arch. Path. *66:*59, 1958.

135. Krainer, L.: Pathological effects of cerebral anoxia, Am. J. Med. *25:*258, 1958.

136. Levine, S.: Anoxic-ischemic encephalopathy in rats, Am. J. Path. *36:*1, 1960.

137. Parker, B. M., and Smith, J. R.: Pulmonary embolism and infarction, Am. J. Med. *24:*402, 1958.

138. Woolling, K. R., Baggenstoss, A. H., and Weir, J. F.: Infarctions of the liver, Gastroenterology *17:*479, 1951.

139. Liebow, A. A.: The bronchopulmonary venous collateral circulation with special reference to emphysema, Am. J. Path. *29:*251, 1953.

140. Rosenberg, M. Z., and Liebow, A. A.: Effects of age, growth hormone, cortisone and other factors in collateral circulation, Arch. Path. *57:*1, 1957.

141. Lewis, T.: Adjustments of blood flow to affected limb in arteriovenous fistula, Clin. Sc. *4:*277, 1940.

142. Holman, E.: Problems in the dynamics of blood flow: conditions controlling collateral circulation in the presence of an arteriovenous fistula following the ligation of an artery, Surgery *26:* 889, 1949.

143. Cameron, G. R.: The exploration of the cell in health and disease, Brit. M. J. *2:*1061, 1954.

144. Dawkins, M. J. R., and Rees, K. R.: A Biochemical Approach to Pathology, London, Edward Arnold, 1959.

145. Goettsch, M.: Dietary methods for induction of necrotic liver degeneration, Ann. New York Acad. Sc. *57:*839, 1954.

146. Selye, H.: Conditioning by cortisol for the production of acute massive myocardial necroses during neuromuscular exertion, Circulation Res. *6:*168, 1958.

147. Canetti, G.: The Tubercle Bacillus, New York, Springer, 1955.

148. Long, E. R.: The Chemistry and Chemotherapy of Tuberculosis, ed. 3, Baltimore, Williams and Wilkins, 1958.

149. Rich, A. R.: The Pathogenesis of Tuberculosis, ed. 2, Springfield, Charles C Thomas, 1950.

150. Tabachnik, J., and Weiss, C.: Mechanism of softening of tubercles. IV. Digestion of caseous tubercles by a proteinase extracted from polymorphonuclear leucocytes. Arch. Path. *61:*76, 1956.

151. Panabokké, R. G.: An experimental study of fat necrosis, J. Path. & Bact. *75:*319, 1958.

152. Adair, F. E., and Munzer, J. T.: Fat necrosis of the female breast, Am. J. Surg. *74:*117, 1947.

153. Pérez Tamayo, R.: Histoquímica de la necrosis fibrinoide, Principia Cardiol. *3:*81, 1956.

154. Movat, H. Z., and More, R. H.: The nature and origin of fibrinoid, Am. J. Clin. Path. *28:*331, 1957.

155. Altschuler, C. H., and Angevine, D. M.: Histochemical studies on the pathogenesis of fibrinoid, Am. J. Path. *25:*1061, 1949.

156. Booth, E., Muirhead, E. E., and Montgomery, P. O'B.: The "fibrinoid" of renal cortical necrosis due to the Shwartzman reaction, Arch. Path. *61:*169, 1956.

157. Schrader, W. H., Jarvis, B. W., and Brunson, J. G.: Studies on the mechanisms of production of fibrinoid lesions by x-ray and Gram-negative endotoxin, Lab. Invest. *8:*996, 1958.

158. Gitlin, D., Craig, J. M., and Janeway, C. A.: Studies on the nature of fibrinoid in the collagen diseases, Am. J. Path. *33:*55, 1957.

159. Vázquez, J. J., and Dixon, F. J.: Immunohistochemical analysis of lesions associated with "fibrinoid" change, Arch. Path. *66:*504, 1958.

160. Ludford, L. J.: Pathological Aspects of Cytology, in Bourne, G. (ed.): Cytology and Cell Physiology, New York, Oxford Press, 1951.

161. Leuchtenberger, C.: A cytochemical study of pyknotic nuclear degeneration, Chromosoma *3:*449, 1950.

162. Pollister, A. W.: Nucleoproteins of the nucleus, Exper. Cell Res., Supp. *2:*59, 1952.

163. Alfert, M.: Changes in the staining capacity of nuclear components during cell degeneration, Biol. Bull. *109:*1, 1955.

164. Godman, G. C.: Pathological changes affecting the nuclear constituents: cytochemical studies, J. Mt. Sinai Hosp. *24:*888, 1957.

165. King, D. W., Paulson, S. R., Hannaford, N. C., and Krebs, A. T.: Cell death. I. The effect of injury on the proteins and deoxyribonucleic acid of Ehrlich tumor cells, Am. J. Path. *35:*369, 1959.

166. King, D. W., Paulson, S. R., Hannaford, N. C., and Krebs, A. T.: Cell death. II. The effect of injury on the enzymatic protein of Ehrlich tumor cells, Am. J. Path. *35:*575, 1959.

167. King, D. W., Paulson, S. R., Puckett, N. L., and Krebs, A. T.: Cell death. III. The effect of injury on water and electrolytes of Ehrlich tumor cells, Am. J. Path. *35:*835, 1959.

168. King, D. W., Paulson, S. R., Puckett, N. L., and Krebs, A. T.: Cell death. IV. The effect of injury on the entrance of vital dye in Ehrlich tumor cells, Am. J. Path. *35:*1067, 1959.

169. Cruickshank, J.: Histological appearances occurring in organs undergoing autolysis, J. Path. & Bact. *16:*167, 1912.

170. More, R. H., and Crowson, C. N.: Glomerulotubular nephrosis correlated with hepatic lesions. I. A morphologic investigation of the changes of progressive autolysis in human, rabbit and rat tissues, Arch. Path. *60:*63, 1955.

171. Kent, S. P.: Effect of postmortem autolysis on certain histochemical reactions, Arch. Path. *64:*17, 1957.

172. Smith, D. E., Robins, E., Eydt, K. M., and Daesch, G. E.: The validation of the quantitative histochemical method for use on postmortem material. I. The effect of time and temperature, Lab. Invest. *6:*447, 1957.

173. Taft, E. B.: Quantitative histochemical observations of postmortem autolysis in rat liver, Lab. Invest. *9:*169, 1959.

174. Berthet, J., *et al.:* Tissue fractionation studies: 2. The nature of the linkage between acid phosphatase and mitochondria in rat-liver tissue, Biochem. J. *50:*182, 1951.

175. Gallagher, C. H., Judah, J. D., and Rees, K. R.: Enzyme changes during liver autolysis, J. Path. & Bact. *72:*247, 1956.

176. Dawkins, M. J. R., Judah, J. D., and Rees, K. R.: Factors influencing the survival of liver cells during autolysis, J. Path. & Bact. *77:*257, 1959.

177. Dawkins, M. J. R.: Autolytic changes in foetal liver, J. Path. & Bact. *79:*289, 1960.

178. Cameron, G. R., and Abraham, E.: Necrosis, Calcification and Autolysis, in Florey, W. W. (ed.): Lectures on General Pathology, ed. 2, Philadelphia, W. B. Saunders Co., 1958.

INFLAMMATION

I. INTRODUCTION

Inflammation is one of the most frequent and important processes encountered in the practice of medicine. It is met by the practicing physician more often than degenerative, neoplastic, congenital or toxic diseases. In some of its protean forms and manifestations, inflammation lurks behind the most important cause of death in the world today: infection. Although considered a defense mechanism, the inflammatory process is also directly responsible for many of the symptoms and complications of numerous diseases as in the following examples: necrosis of the inflammatory exudate causes cavity formation in tuberculosis; a thick, fibrinous inflammatory exudate obstructs the upper respiratory tract in diphtheria; the multiple emboli of subacute bacterial endocarditis are composed of fibrin, bacteria and inflammatory cells. But the great frequency of inflammation is only half of the reason for the prominent place that this process occupies in medicine. The other half is that, partly hidden by the complexity of biochemical, morphologic and functional changes appearing during inflammation, there lies an intriguing example of homeostasis. On first examination, the inflammatory process is just a series of cellular and tissue reactions to injury following a certain basic pattern which repeats itself in many different species; however, a closer and more detailed view reveals that this pattern is another instance of the general tendency of the organism to maintain a constant internal environment. A biologic interpretation of inflammation is easy prey for teleologists, and the previous sentences might be interpreted along those lines. Homeostasis, however, is the result of an automatic, self-determined group of processes that may be analyzed within their own context, without recourse to unscientific explanations. When adequately tempered by an objective attitude, the study of inflammation as a manifestation of homeostasis represents one of the most appropriate introductions to the science of disease. Such is the purpose of the present chapter.

Perhaps the most important aspect of inflammation is that it is a process, not a static change. From the very beginning of the inflammatory reaction to whatever end it may lead (repair of the injured area, necrosis of tissues or death of the organism), it is continuously changing. This change is apparent at any level of organization at which phenomena are observed; there are modifications in the biochemical environment of cells and tissues, profound metabolic disturbances in all participating elements, anatomic lesions depicting degenerations, regressions and proliferative reactions, etc. Furthermore, a localized area of inflammation is almost never without systemic consequences, such as fever, general malaise, leukocytosis or other changes in the peripheral blood count, increased sedimentation rate of erythrocytes, etc. The very essence of inflammation is its changing nature, and this should always be kept in mind when the unity of such a concept is surrendered to the needs of exposition. The inflammatory process must be analyzed to be described, but in this dissection there is danger of overlooking the fact that the resulting parts are meaningless without continuous reference to the whole. The following discussion might be compared to the examination of a series of isolated frames of a moving film, from which not only the intermediary stages must be reconstructed but also the speed and movement of the entire process. Recent advances in technique have provided methods for direct and continuous observation of living structures, so many aspects of inflammation that were previously inferred are now confirmed and refined. Yet, knowledge is almost purely descriptive and at the morphologic level; mechanisms are mostly hypothetical; and

biochemical and functional interrelations are only beginning to be explored. The field of research in inflammation is as active as the process itself, and the use of modern techniques will surely provide a clearer and more coherent picture in the near future.

Inflammation is a local reaction of vascular connective tissues to injury. Changes in parenchymatous cells, which were considered by Virchow as the dominating lesions, have been relegated to a second place and are accepted today as degenerative. All elements integrating vascular connective tissues participate in inflammation; therefore the more complicated this tissue is the more complex will be the picture of the inflammatory process. Obviously, the complexity of inflammation increases as the zoologic scale is climbed. In lower animals without a vascular system, inflammation is represented by phagocytosis. Indeed, it was in a transparent starfish larva that Metchnikoff described the ingestion of particles by cells and conceived their important role in defense.[1] But the emergence of blood vessels and a well defined circulation introduces a radical change in the mechanisms of inflammation, although cells continue to play a preeminent role. It should be added that in species with circulatory systems, inflammation will not appear in avascular areas, such as the cornea, unless it is preceded by vascular proliferation.

The general outline of this chapter is first, to present a description of the inflammatory process; second, to review the mechanisms involved in the different phenomena; third, to examine the biochemical modifications of the area of inflammation and to discuss the influence of different factors; and fourth, to attempt a synthesis of the data discussed within the general frame of homeostasis. Since systemic consequences of inflammation play a very important role in the host-parasite relation, their study is undertaken in Chapter VII.

II. THE VASCULAR PHENOMENA OF ACUTE INFLAMMATION

A. Lewis' "Triple Response." For a long time inflammation was considered a well defined and specific disease entity characterized by four cardinal signs: "calor," "tumor," "rubor" and "dolor" (heat, swelling, redness and pain). A fifth sign, "functio laesa" (loss of function), was added by Galen some time later. It was not until John Hunter (Fig. 2–1) called attention to the unspecificity of the process, that inflammation was recognized as the result of many different causes. But Hunter's contribution went beyond this, and clearly established that the inflammatory process is essentially protective in nature. Further advances in knowledge, ably summarized and beautifully illustrated by Florey,[2] showed that many types of inflammation do not partake of all the "classic" signs and led to a more adequate, microscopic characterization of the process. Many definitions have been attempted, but they portray the personal philosophic inclinations of their authors rather than the objective phenomena. In an international symposium on inflammation published in 1953, with participation of some of the most distinguished investigators in this field, twelve pages are dedicated to defining inflammation without reaching an agreement.[3]

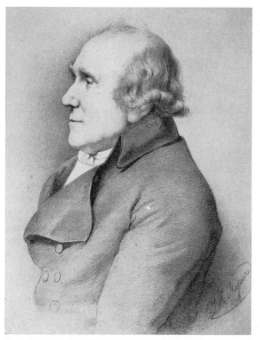

FIG. 2–1. John Hunter. (Courtesy of Cushing Library, Yale University School of Medicine.)

Vascular changes are considered today as the central phenomena of inflammation. When the stimulus is not very intense, they are the only ones observed. Lewis examined the modifications in blood vessels in inflammation in a series of experimental studies which remain as a model of what can be done in research with a minimum of equipment and a maximum of scientific ingenuity and imagination.[4] The following description is quoted from this author:[5]

"If the human skin is stroked firmly with a blunt point, a local reaction of the vessels follows which is visible to the naked eye. . . . A red line appears, marking out with considerable precision the area of skin pressed upon; it begins to appear in from 3 to 18 seconds and is at its height in 30 to 50 seconds. It is at first a red line, shortly acquiring a bluish tinge. The red line is due to dilatation of the capillaries and minute venules of the skin, and this dilatation is brought about by (a) primary dilatation of the vessels themselves, and (b) in part by coincident dilatation of the corresponding terminal arterioles. . . . In a number of subjects in whom the skin is hypersensitive, or in less sensitive skins where the stroke is very heavy, the red line is shortly followed (20–60 seconds after stimulation) by (c) bordering areas of erythema; this flush surrounds the red line, is of brighter red colour and has an irregular margin. . . . Finally, the region of the red line may develop swelling, in the form of a more or less pronounced urticarial wheal, a local oedema. . . . The wheal becomes perceptible within 1 to 3 minutes of the stroke and quickly rises to its height (usually in 3–5 minutes from the stroking); it is at first red. During the red stage the wheal itself, and the surrounding flush, present capillary pulsation. Shortly it pales, as does the surrounding flush, but still remains prominent. It lasts one or many hours."

The intensity of the vascular response varies from one person to another but in all it is essentially the same. It is more violent and easy to appreciate in certain subjects with cutaneous manifestations of allergy (dermographism) (Fig. 2–2). The simple experiment of irritating the skin with a blunt object reproduces four of the classic signs of inflammation, namely, pain, redness, swelling and heat; the last is easy to appreciate if the temperature of the irritated area is compared to that of the neighboring skin. Furthermore, if the irritation is stronger and is made on the skin overlying a joint, the swelling and pain may hinder the movements so that the fifth classic sign of inflammation, "functio laesa," is also present. With those unsophisticated observations

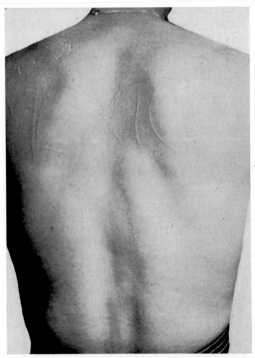

FIG. 2–2. Exaggerated skin response to irritation with a blunt object (dermographism).

Lewis proved experimentally Hunter's idea that inflammation may have many causes. In addition. Lewis made many other observations on the mechanisms of vascular phenomena in inflammation which are summarized below. But a general principle of great significance derived from his work is that vascular phenomena constitute the fundamental core of the inflammatory process, and that many diseases which lack the "classic" signs are still inflammatory in nature. This is true not only of diseases involving organs such as skin and joints, which are easily accessible to physical examination, but also of processes affecting organs and tissues of difficult clinical appreciation, such as the kidney or the endocardium.

B. Microscopic Changes. The relative simplicity of Lewis' "triple response," which reproduces the classic gross signs of inflammation, acquires a striking complexity when observed under the microscope. There are several excellent descriptions of microscopic changes in acute inflammation,[2, 6, 7] based on experimental observations *in vivo*. Methods used have been based on the direct study of blood vessels in thin and trans-

lucent tissues, such as the tongue of the frog, or the mesoappendix or mesentery of the rat. A very simple technique is the Sandison-Clark clear window in the rabbit's ear, which permits repeated and prolonged observations of living tissues throughout the inflammatory process. With these methods, previous accounts of microscopic changes in inflammation based on fixed and stained preparations have been confirmed and extended. The following description is essentially that of Allison and associates,[7] who used clear chambers in the rabbit's ear and a standard injury produced by a microburn, and followed the events with microcinephotography. For the sake of convenience, changes will be described under four separate headings.

1. *Changes in Blood Flow.* Immediately after injury there is a variable but usually short period of ischemia in which arterioles decrease in caliber and may even close completely. But in a few moments blood flow is reestablished throughout the area, there is arteriolar dilation and the circulation increases considerably, not only because of the greater vascular caliber but also because many previously closed capillaries open to the circulation. Arteriolar dilation continues for long periods (up to 24 hours) and the blood flow maintains increased volume and pressure. Furthermore, arteriolar pulsation is transmitted more clearly to capillaries and venules so that the whole area of inflamed tissue can be seen to pulsate. In the immediate neighborhood of injury blood flow undergoes the same changes described but in a short time it slows down until a few hours later it stops completely and the vascular lumen is occupied by a thrombus. For the remainder of the process, circulation is increased in the periphery of the lesion while in the area of injury there is hardly any blood flow at all.

In addition to changes in speed, pressure and volume of blood flow there are modifications in the distribution of circulating elements within arterioles and capillaries. Normally, blood circulates within capillaries in two different streams: one, central or axial, where erythrocytes, leukocytes and platelets are found; and the other, peripheral or marginal, is occupied by plasma.[8] During acute inflammation there is a tendency for these two zones of flow to exchange places, so that cells are displaced towards the periphery and plasma is seen to occupy the axial stream. The redistribution of circulating elements is of great significance for the understanding of other phenomena occurring simultaneously or a short time later.

2. *Changes in Formed Elements of the Blood.* At the same time as pressure, speed and volume of blood flow increase, and the circulating elements are redistributed within the lumen of capillaries, important changes occur in the blood cellular elements. Red cells agglutinate and form "rouleaux," which adhere momentarily to the capillary endothelium. When the lesion is early or of slight intensity, erythrocytes are carried by the blood flow beyond the injured area and lose their "adhesiveness," appearing normal in every respect. But when the lesion is severe or some time has elapsed (2 to 4 hours) the red cells remain adherent to the endothelium and accumulate within the lumen until the circulation is completely interrupted. "Adhesiveness" is also observed in platelets, which become attached to the capillary endothelium. In a similar fashion, leukocytes also appear adherent to the vessel wall; indeed, the phenomenon occurs before and more intensely in these cells than in any other element, and is more apparent in capillaries and venules (Fig. 2–3). Increased "adhesiveness" and sticking of leukocytes to the endothelial cells are not necessarily preceded by vasodilation, since they may be observed in capillaries of normal caliber. Furthermore, leukocytes show no preference for the endothelium; these cells may also stick to each other, thus showing that the change is not limited to the endothelial cell. Finally, if a leukocyte is released from its attachment to the vessel wall and is carried away from the inflamed area by the circulation it will not stick to the walls of undamaged vessels.

Soon after leukocytes begin sticking to the endothelium some of them migrate through the vessel wall into perivascular tissues. This phenomenon is known as diapedesis and is one of the most important mechanisms of accumulation of cells in the injured area. Before passing through the wall of the capillary, the intravascular leukocytes adhere to the inner surface of the endothelium and migrate over it at random. When a suitable spot for penetration is found, the process of diapedesis begins. It takes from 3 to 12 minutes to be completed, and the cell can be seen to move actively until it is deposited on the outside of the capillary[9] (Fig. 2–4). No modifications are perceptible in the vessel wall, although an area of easier penetration is probably created since many leukocytes can follow the first through the same spot. The change in the endothelium is reversible; Clark and Clark[10] observed that occasionally a leukocyte was trapped on its way out of the capillary and even lost part of its cytoplasm, as if restitution of imperviousness of the vessel wall was accompanied by a drastic change in the elasticity of the endothelium. In general, diapedesis parallels the intensity of leukocytic sticking and is first noticed in

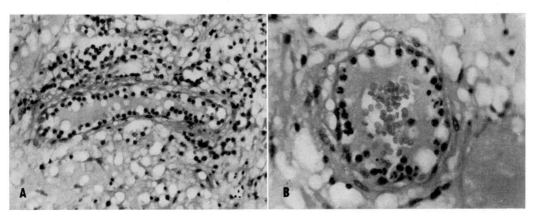

FIG. 2–3. Two instances of margination of leukocytes during acute inflammation. Observe that both capillaries are dilated and in *B* red blood cells are occupying the axial flow.

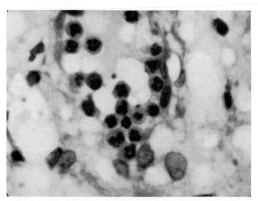

FIG. 2–4. Diapedesis of polymorphonuclear leukocytes in acute inflammation. A group of leukocytes is leaving the capillary lumen through a localized area of the blood vessel.

capillaries near the lesion. In time, however, many of the vessels in the immediate neighborhood of injury become static and the scene of most intense diapedesis moves to the periphery. Leukocytes continue migrating through the walls of capillaries in which blood flow has ceased altogether, although they do it in lesser numbers. This observation is important since it has been argued that hydrostatic pressure is one of the forces driving the leukocytes outside the vessels.

Diapedesis is not limited to leukocytes; red blood cells can also be seen leaving the capillaries and in small collections in the interstitial spaces near the lesion. This phenomenon, however, seems to be purely passive, since it occurs only when stasis and vasodilation have become marked. Some red cells may migrate through the same spots used by leukocytes, but they are few and when the spot "closes" erythrocytes are swept back into the circulation.

3. *Changes in Plasma.* Within the first hour of injury there appear some modifications in plasma that may take different aspects according to the techniques used. Following microtrauma to capillaries in the mesentery of anesthetized rats, Zweifach[11] observed the formation of an intravascular gelatinous precipitate which appeared to impart an increased adhesiveness to the endothelium. In bacteremic states during which leukocytic sticking is a prominent feature, Wood, et al.[12] described microscopic gelatinous "clots" within the capillaries which were not sufficiently extensive to cause throm-

bosis. Allison, *et al.*[7] found numerous intra- and extravascular globular bodies of unknown identity and significance in lesions produced by heat. They were usually of the size of a red blood cell although some were observed to be several times the diameter of a leukocyte. The globules were devoid of any internal structure, and were of variable shape, highly refractile and elastic; they were not stained with fat or protein dyes (Fig. 2–5). These modifications in the physical structure of plasma have been associated with partially polymerized fibrin and considered to be fundamental to an explanation of the sticking of erythrocytes, platelets and leukocytes. They are further discussed below.

4. *Changes in the Capillary Wall.* The walls of the capillaries traversing an area of inflammation are profoundly altered; changes in this structure might well represent the difference between a minimal, self-limited reaction to injury, and a severe and prolonged inflammatory process. Damage to the blood vessel wall may be demonstrated in two different ways, which are probably manifestations of the same basic phenomenon. There is increased adhesiveness of the inner surface of endothelial cells, and the permeability of the capillary wall is increased. It has been shown that the limits of endothelial cells of normal capillaries can be stained by injecting a suspension of fine particles of graphite. With this procedure the endothelial cells are outlined, since the graphite particles will adhere only to the intercellular cement.[13] But when there is

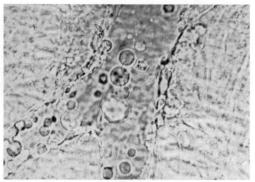

FIG. 2–5. Intravascular "globular bodies" in acute inflammation produced by heat. (Courtesy of Dr. F. Allison, Jr., and the Editor, Journal of Experimental Medicine.)

tissue injury and inflammation, the administration of graphite particles will result in a uniform darkening of all capillary structures under the microscope, because the particles become adherent to the entire inner surface of the endothelium.[6] This suggests that endothelial cells have increased their adhesiveness, a possibility already pointed out by the sticking of leukocytes mentioned in the previous paragraph.

The permeability of capillaries is increased during most of the duration of the inflammatory process, and this has been shown by many different techniques. Since protein molecules cannot directly be observed to migrate through the wall of permeable capillaries, the practical demonstration and measurement of increased capillary permeability depends either on observing the accumulation of fluid exudate or on labeling the proteins in some way. The increase in volume secondary to accumulation of fluid exudate can be measured by plethysmography or other means,[14] but visual estimation appears to be equally accurate.[15] Labeling of proteins can be accomplished by means of dyes such as pontamine blue, Evans blue (T-1824) or trypan blue, which bind themselves firmly and rapidly to plasma albumin[16] and thus provide a method of following the loss of such protein from the vessels into the interstitial tissues[17] (Fig. 2–6). Plasma proteins may also be labeled with radioactive isotopes, especially when the permeability of capillaries near a body cavity is to be measured;[18] the labeled protein is injected intravenously and the rate of passage into an exudate in the body cavity (pleural cavity, peritoneum) is used as a quantitative index of permeability. Using the ear-chamber technique and T-1824 as an indicator, Allison and Lancaster[19] studied the events in capillary permeability after tissue injury produced by a microburn. They observed three stages in the development of increased passage of protein. The first was an immediate but modest leakage of dye-stained plasma; the second was a gradual and transient increase of permeability lasting 3 to 4 hours and subsiding by the sixth hour; the third was slight increase in capillary permeability persisting for the next 24 hours. All visible segments of the vasculature participated, but leakage of dye was more prominent about vessels near an arterial communication and around venules. Studies of inflammation produced by chemical injury[20] or bacterial infections[21] agree with these observations, with differences that they may be due to the animal species and experimental techniques used.

C. Mechanisms of Vascular Changes in Acute Inflammation. The previous examination of microscopic vascular changes in inflammation, which account for Lewis' "triple response," has been merely descriptive. It now seems pertinent to attempt a summary of the mechanisms underlying such changes. However, at the outset it must be said that knowledge of these mechanisms is rudimentary and hypothetical. Many factors must be taken into account, such as the large variety of agents capable of inducing the inflammatory reaction, the orderly sequence of events of which it is composed, the reciprocal influence of some phenomena and the apparent independence of others, and the fact that some types of injury, such as mechanical trauma or burns, add nothing material to the affected tissues. Not all the changes described have received equal attention, so that in the following paragraphs the account will be limited to the mechanisms of vasodilation, modifications in blood flow, diapedesis and increased capillary permeability.

1. *Mechanism of Vasodilation.* In Lewis' "triple response" there are two phases of

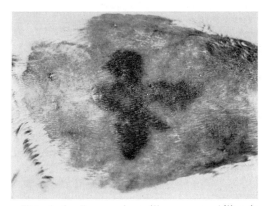

FIG. 2–6. Increased capillary permeability in acute inflammation. The skin of the rabbit was irritated to produce inflammation and some time later an intravenous injection of trypan blue was given. The dye leaks at the area of increased permeability.

vasodilation: the reddening of the irritated area and the appearance of a surrounding zone of erythema. These two different phases correspond to equally different microscopic phenomena: the red line is due to capillary and venular dilation and seems unrelated to the nervous system, while erythema is the result of arteriolar dilation and depends on the integrity of the local nerve structures.

That erythema is produced by arteriolar dilation secondary to peripheral nervous mechanisms was shown by Lewis and Grant in 1924.[22] Skin denervated for longer than 6 to 10 days will fail to show erythema after irritation, while the red line continues to appear each time the skin is irritated. Furthermore, if the test is made on denervated skin before there has been time for degeneration of the nerve fibers distal to the section, there will be erythema. Therefore, it was concluded that in this phase of the triple response a reflex mechanism is involved which is independent of the nervous centers. This mechanism is the axon reflex. The sensory nerves carry the impulse from the irritated area to the bifurcation of the nerve, and from there it is conducted antidromically to the peripheral arteriole, where dilation of the vessel is produced. The proof that this reflex mechanism participates in the vascular changes of inflammation is not only the result of surgical denervation, since arteriolar dilation will also fail to appear when the area to be injured is treated with cocaine,[23] which provokes paralysis of the nerve ends.

In addition to the reflex mechanism, Lewis also demonstrated the presence of a humoral substance or substances which induce vasodilation in arterioles. If the circulation in one arm is stopped by means of an arm band while blood flow in the other arm is left free, irritation of the skin will result in the "triple response" in both; however, in the arm with free circulation it will last for approximately 10 minutes, while in the other it will persist as long as there is no blood flow. When the band is released and circulation is reestablished, the "triple response" disappears in approximately the same 10 minutes. From this observation Lewis concluded that the lesion will liberate a substance or substances capable of inducing arteriolar dilation; while blood flow is prevented this factor or factors continue to act on the blood vessels, but when the circulation is reestablished it is removed by the blood. Since the local injection of histamine faithfully reproduces the gross changes observed with many other types of irritants, Lewis suggested that it was histamine or a very similar substance (H substance) that was released in tissues as a result of injury. More recently, Hilton and Lewis[24] have presented evidence favoring the local formation of vasoactive peptides to account for prolonged arteriolar dilation.

Capillary dilation is brought about by all those substances which increase capillary permeability to protein. In general, a higher concentration is needed to increase permeability than to cause vasodilation, so the possibility exists that increased permeability is a more advanced stage of a reaction whose initial phase is vascular dilation. For this reason, humoral factors involved in changes in vascular caliber and permeability will be discussed together in a later section.

2. Mechanisms of Changes in Blood Flow. There seems to be little doubt that acceleration of blood flow in acute inflammation is caused by arteriolar dilation, and the same is true for increases in blood pressure and circulating volume. However there are other changes requiring analysis, and these are the redistribution of blood flow within the capillary lumen and the progressive slowness of circulation in vessels near the lesion that eventually ends in complete flow stop and thrombosis.

As previously mentioned, blood flows within the normal capillary in two different streams, axial and marginal, which are inverted during inflammation. Fahareus[25] has demonstrated that heavier elements will circulate in the center of the lumen, so that leukocytes occupy the axial stream; however, soon after the onset of inflammation red blood cells adhere to each other forming rouleaux, which are naturally heavier than leukocytes. The latter are thus displaced from the axial stream and circulate in the marginal zone, closer to the endothelial cells.[26] The reason for rouleaux formation (sludged blood) seems to be a change in plasma proteins, although other mechanisms such as changes in electric charges of the cell surface may also be at play.[27] Although forces of these types undoubtedly determine leukocytic margination, Florey[2] believes that it may also be explained by a greater adhesiveness of the leukocyte to the endothelial wall, "much as a fly is caught in flypaper."

Blood stasis develops soon after injury in the capillaries close to the lesion. Red blood cells form rouleaux, stick to the endothelium and form a growing mass which progressively occludes the lumen of the vessel. In order to explain this phenomenon, Landis[28] called attention to the fact that increased permeability of the capillary wall will facilitate the passage of fluids to the interstitial space, with a consequent increase in the viscosity of intracapillary contents. This rise in viscosity is not directly proportional to the amount of fluid lost; it increases at a higher rate as equal volumes of fluid leave the vessel[29] (Fig. 2–7). Greater viscosity will oppose the pumping action of the heart, increasing peripheral resistance. Furthermore, the damaged endothelium is also likely to present a greater resistance to blood flow, and the increase in extravascular tissue pressure due to accumulation of exudate will limit the capacity of blood injection into the dilated capillaries. The sum of all these factors would be a slower blood flow favoring the development of thrombosis.

In spite of the logical coherence of the preceding explanation and of the experimental demonstration that increase in viscosity of plasma is greater than fluid loss, some observations suggest that there may be other factors involved in stasis and thrombus

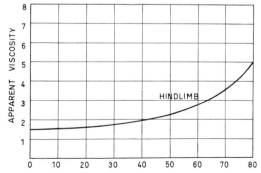

FIG. 2–7. Increase in apparent viscosity of blood with increasing corpuscular concentration. (Redrawn from Whittaker and Winton.[29])

formation in the capillaries of acute inflammation. Allison and Lancaster[19] found that little dye leaked from vessels shown to be static immediately after injury. These capillaries were involved in the lesion, so that perhaps the direct effect of heat caused profound changes in the wall. No time relation for stasis was found, however, in capillaries showing major leakages of dye, since some developed it only after 2 to 3 hours of injury while others continued patent for 4 to 6 hours. If fluid loss was the only explanation for stasis, a more or less simultaneous appearance of this phenomenon could be expected in all vessels involved to the same extent. Therefore, they concluded that enhanced capillary permeability was not the lone factor responsible for stasis.

3. *Mechanism of Diapedesis.* The migration of blood cells through the capillary wall during inflammation has had the attention of many investigators. The presence of polymorphonuclear leukocytes in the interstitial spaces is one of the most telling microscopic signs of inflammation. Diapedesis should not be confused with chemotaxis, a phenomenon to be discussed later, which predicates change in direction of the random cellular movements by the influence of certain substances in the medium. Three factors have been postulated for diapedesis to occur: (a) persistency of blood flow, and therefore of intracapillary hydrostatic pressure, (b) sticking of leukocytes to endothelial cells and (c) weakness of the endothelial lining which permits the passage of formed elements. A variation of the last hypothesis suggests the existence of "pores" in the blood vessel wall.

For a long time it has been accepted that diapedesis requires intravascular hydrostatic pressure, which would act as a force driving the leukocytes out of the capillary; such an idea was based on the observation that when blood flow ceased there was no more diapedesis,[30] and also on the decreased leukocytic migration during the stasis of shock.[31] However, both Zweifach[11] and Allison, *et al.*[7] have seen leukocytes migrate from vessels in which blood flow has stopped altogether. It would seem apparent that hydrostatic pressure is not a prerequisite for leukocytic diapedesis. On the other hand, sticking of leukocytes to the endothelial lining is a necessary step in diapedesis and it has been seen to parallel in general the intensity of migration through the vascular wall.

The mechanisms by which leukocytes acquire "adhesiveness" are not well understood, but several hypotheses have been suggested. First, it has been held that vasodilation is somehow related to leukocytic sticking, perhaps assuming that stretching of the vessel wall would lead to changes in the state of the endothelial lining which in turn might cause leukocytes to become adherent to it. Direct observation of living tissues during acute inflammation has shown that leukocytic sticking frequently occurs in vessels with no increase in caliber, or even in vessels which have become constricted rather than dilated. Second, changes in cellular surface charges have been held responsible for the adhesiveness of leukocytes,[32] but this is purely speculative since no direct measurements have been made of the surface charges of damaged endothelium, which would support the hypothesis. Sawyer's[33] demonstration that aortic endothelium changes from electronegative to electropositive after injury shows this modification to be immediate, whereas sticking of leukocytes is apparent 10 to 15 minutes after injury. Third, some investigators believed that the mechanism of blood clotting was intimately involved in the sticking of leukocytes to the vascular endothelium. This was first suggested by Zweifach,[11] who observed the appearance of an intravascular gelatinous precipitate which appeared to impart an increased adhesiveness to the endothelium and the cellular elements of the blood; the administration of heparin prevented the formation of the gelatinous precipitate and at the same time there was no leukocytic sticking. More recently, Allison and Lancaster,[34] have shown that activation of fibrinolysin *in vivo* by streptokinase did not impair sticking of white blood cells. After several trials, circulating fibrinogen was finally eliminated by injecting infusions of thromboplastin and streptokinase with thrombin; under such circumstances leukocytic sticking following heat injury occurred without reduction. The results indicate that fibrin is apparently not involved in the causation of increased adhesiveness of leukocytes and endothelial cells. These observa-

tions apply to leukocytic sticking, which is only part of the phenomenon of diapedesis. Actual migration through the capillary wall is an active process, in which the leukocyte is seen to move until it is deposited outside the blood vessel. This has suggested to some that leukocytes are attracted by chemotactic substances released in the interstitial tissues by bacteria or injured cells. Most of the substances causing increased capillary permeability will also induce diapedesis, but only of a modest degree. On the other hand, Spector and Storey[35] found that aqueous extracts of uterus from mice previously treated with estrogens cause a migration of leukocytes from skin vessels which is much more striking than that produced by any other agent tested. Acid polysaccharides such as dextran sulphate and chondroitin sulphate on intradermal injection cause a slow but progressive leukocyte migration, which is greatly increased by the presence of fibrinogen in the injection medium; polysaccharides derived from bacteria also share this property. It is not clear to what extent these reactions are due to tissue damage by the injected substances with the resultant development of true inflammation, but Spector[36] believes that tissue components such as chondroitin sulphate after local injury undergo a change which causes them to induce leukocyte diapedesis; this change could be a combination with fibrinogen exuded from capillaries rendered permeable to protein in an earlier stage of the reaction. In summary, the two most important factors in diapedesis seem to be increased adhesiveness of leukocytes and endothelial cells, and the active movements of leukocytes; the mechanisms by which these two phenomena are brought about are still unknown.

4. *Mechanism of Increased Capillary Permeability*. The idea that the capillary wall functions as an inert and semipermeable membrane, at least in relation to the exchange of fluids and electrolytes in tissues, was expressed by Starling,[37] as an alternative hypothesis to Heidenhain's views, who together with other "vitalists" believed that endothelial cells had secretory activities. Starling's hypothesis is discussed in Chapter IX; what is of interest here is that the normal capillary wall is freely permeable to water and electrolytes and only very slightly

permeable to protein. Therefore, increased capillary permeability means an increase in permeability to plasma protein. The capillary wall is a complex formed by several different layers, enumerated by Zweifach[13] as follows: (a) a proteinaceous component, possibly formed by plasma and platelets, adherent to the inner surface of endothelial cells, (b) the endothelial cell proper, (c) in some places, intercellular cement and (d) a pericapillary layer of condensed connective tissue fibers. Theoretically, plasma protein could leave the capillaries through the cytoplasm of endothelial cells or through the intercellular cement. Chambers and Zweifach[38] remarked some time ago that when capillaries are made permeable to protein, the molecules leave the blood vessel at such a rate and for such a long period that it seems unlikely for any cell, however specialized, to survive this dramatic transformation of its internal environment. In addition, it has been shown that intercellular cement becomes sticky and soft, and even sloughs during episodes of increased capillary permeability.[39]

To these objective observations Pappenheimer[40] has added a very pertinent theoretical analysis of the passage of molecules through capillary walls, where the conclusion is reached that proteins leave capillaries through water-filled channels in the vessel wall and that these channels constitute no more than 0.2 per cent of the surface of the capillary. Furthermore, the channels are of uniform diameter, about 40 Å, and may very well lie in the intercellular cement. The structure of this cement is porous and is formed by calcium proteinate with another component of large molecular weight adhering to the proteinate and decreasing the size of the pores; Daniell[41] believed this component to be the blood platelets, but Curran[42] has presented evidence suggesting that the endothelium may continuously synthesize intercellular cement. That the size of the pores postulated by Pappenheimer is greater than the molecular size of proteins, and yet these substances leave the vessel very slowly, can be explained by the concept of "restricted diffusion." This means that there are a series of factors limiting the free passage of proteins to tissues, such as viscous drag between the protein molecule and the walls of the chan-

nel, and steric hindrance, which means that the protein molecule will pass through the pores if it does not impinge first on the margins of the channel. An increase in capillary permeability would be due to the disappearance of factors restricting diffusion, for example, opening of many new channels or alterations in charge at the pores. These modifications in the physical characteristics of the capillary wall may be due to changes in the intercellular cement or to damage to the endothelial cell, which would then be reflected in deficiencies in the intercellular substance; the latter possibility is less likely since capillary permeability increases very rapidly after injury and a metabolic disturbance of the endothelium leading to defective synthesis of intercellular cement would take some time in becoming manifest.

Florey, Poole and Meck[43] have made a detailed analysis of endothelial cement lines with both the light and electron microscope and suggest that cement lines are much thinner than previously considered; still, the average thickness of the intercellular spaces found by these authors is of the order of 0.02μ, which is not in conflict with the previous statements.

The mechanism by which capillary permeability is increased in inflammation has been postulated as humoral. This viewpoint implies that injury releases or activates endogenous substances which are then responsible for the changes in the capillary wall discussed in the previous paragraph. Not only is capillary permeability modified in this fashion, but many of the other different phenomena composing the picture of inflammation are also held to be mediated through humoral factors. Thus, the inflammatory process would be a problem in autopharmacology, and the influence of the exogenous causal agent is considered subsidiary, a form of "trigger" mechanism. These endogenous pharmacologically active substances are discussed in detail in the section on Biochemistry of Inflammation.

III. THE INFLAMMATORY EXUDATE

A. Formation of the Exudate. All cellular and vascular changes described so far

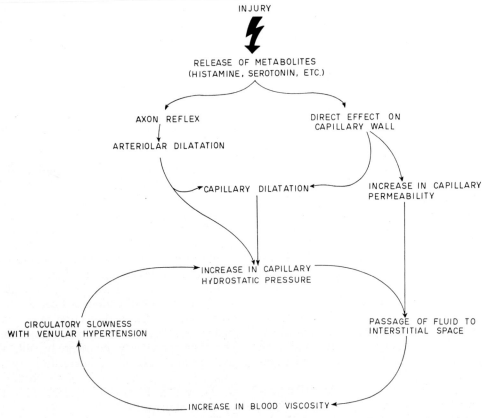

FIG. 2–8. Schematic representation of sequence of events leading to accumulation of exudate in acute inflammation.

concur to the same end, the accumulation of circulating elements, both fluid and formed, in the area of injury. The sequence may be summarized as follows: one effect of injury is the release or activation of metabolites of the type of histamine, which induces capillary dilation and increased permeability. Capillary dilation is also the result of arteriolar dilation with increased flow, secondary to the axon reflex initiated by the injury and/or some chemical mediator. Arteriolar and capillary dilation are accompanied by an increase in hydrostatic pressure, which combined with the increase in capillary permeability drives fluid and proteins out of the blood vessels (capillaries and venules) into the interstitial spaces. The decrease in intravascular fluid increases disproportionately the viscosity of the blood, which together with rouleaux formation and other factors will bring about stasis and eventual thrombosis. In capillaries where no thrombi are seen, partial obstruction of distal venules will increase hydrostatic pressure and favor the leakage of more fluid and proteins. The sequence is represented in Figure 2–8.

Depending on the nature of the causal agent, the intensity of injury, the seat of the process and many other factors, the exudate accumulated in inflammation will show predominance of one or another of the blood elements, and this predominance suggests denominations such as serous, fibrinous pseudomembranous, hemorrhagic and purulent inflammation (Fig. 2–9). Combinations of these elements also occur and when they are prominent mixed names can be used, such as fibrinopurulent inflammation. In the following paragraphs the two main components, fluid and cellular, of the inflammatory exudate are described separately, but it must be remembered that their accumulation is almost simultaneous.

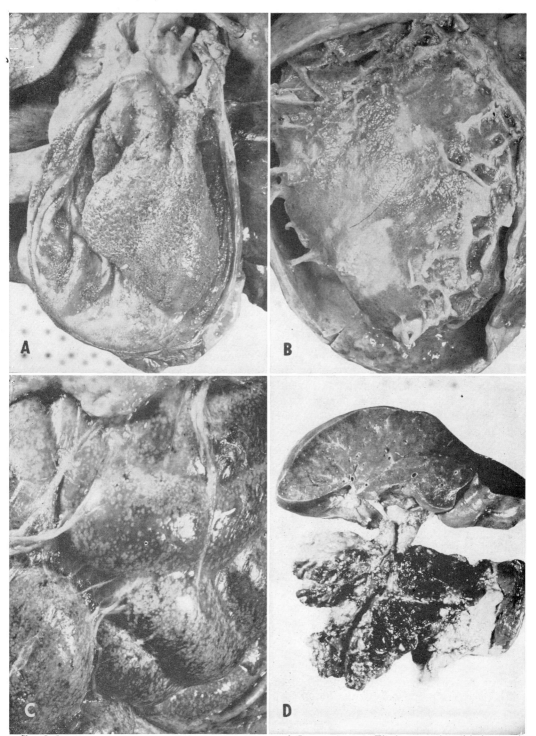

FIG. 2–9. Some gross aspects of the exudate in acute inflammation. *A*, Fibrinous pericarditis in uremia due to acute renal failure. *B*, Purulent pericarditis secondary to pneumococcal pneumonia. *C*, Tuberculous peritonitis. *D*, Hemorrhagic inflammation in acute, necrotizing pancreatitis.

Table 6. Dimensions of Typical Crystalloid and Colloid Plasma Solutes

SUBSTANCE	MOLECULAR WEIGHT	MOLECULAR SIZE (in μ)	
		LENGTH	DIAMETER
Sodium ion	23	0.2	0.2
Chloride ion	35	0.4	0.4
Glucose	180	1.0	0.7
Serum albumin	69,000	15.0	3.8
Serum (gamma) globulin	150,000	32.0	3.6
Fibrinogen	500,000	90.00	3.3

Data from Conn[44]

B. Fluid Component of the Inflammatory Exudate. Blood plasma carries a large number of substances of variable form, size and molecular weight.[44] In Table 6 there is a list of some of them, where it can be appreciated that the composition of the inflammatory exudate will vary according to the degree of increase in capillary permeability. In general, one of the most constant features of fluid accumulated in interstitial spaces is the elevated protein content. In fact, it used to be said that an exudate could be distinguished from a transudate or effusion in that the latter never had more than 2.5 Gm. of albumin per 100 ml. of fluid; this distinction is artificial and there are too many exceptions to use it as a sound guide in the differential diagnosis of exudate from transudate. The high protein concentration of inflammatory exudates is of fundamental importance since it is in this fraction that the greater part of antibodies are contained, and these elements play a very important role in inflammation. Furthermore, fibrinogen is also present and may be transformed into fibrin, creating a barrier to the inflammatory process and blocking the lymphatic capillaries, in addition to its previously mentioned possible role in stimulating diapedesis. The significance of the accumulation of these and other substances in the inflammatory focus is discussed later.

C. Cellular Components of the Inflammatory Exudate. 1. *Cells of the Exudate.* When a microscopic slide of a tissue with acute inflammation is examined, a large number of cells are seen in which polymorphonuclear leukocytes may predominate, although there are many other elements such as macrophages, lymphocytes, plasma cells, mast cells, eosinophils, giant cells, etc. These cells have come to the seat of inflammation from the blood vessels, but some may also correspond to those previously present in the tissue. These two different origins of cells in the exudate are respectively known as hematogenous and histogenous (Fig. 2–10). Many factors determine what types of cells are encountered and which predominate, such as the nature of the etiologic agent, the duration of inflammation, the presence or absence of hypersensitivity, the localization of the process, etc. A detailed description of each one of these cell types would be out of place here, but there are three aspects of their behavior which require special attention; they are chemotaxis, phagocytosis and the sequence of appearance of cells in exudates.

2. *Chemotaxis.* Most of the cells in an inflammatory exudate possess the capacity to move. When the direction of this movement is determined by substances present in the environment the process is known as chemotaxis.[45] If the movements of the cell are directed towards the stimulating substance chemotaxis is positive, and if they are directed away from the stimulus it is negative. When a substance fails to influence the direction of cell movements there is no chemotaxis. This phenomenon does not imply an increase in the speed of displacement; it is only a change in direction. A large number of plants and animals can show chemotaxis,[46] but the interest here is on its influence in inflammation. Chemotaxis, when present, is responsible for the greater concentration of inflammatory cells near the lesion and the causal agent; some hypotheses concerning its possible influence in diapedesis have been mentioned previously.

Many substances and bacteria have been studied in search of chemotactic properties. With few exceptions bacteria will attract polymorphonuclear leukocytes; their power varies with distance and it seems that microorganisms of rapid growth exert their influence at greater distances than those of slow growth, such as *Myco. tuberculosis*. Some bacteria, for instance *Cl. welchii,* produce a toxin which paralyzes leukocytes, a phenomenon incorrectly referred to as negative chemotaxis. Viruses have not been found to influence the direction of cell movements at a distance but a few parasites may do it, such as *P. vivax*. No satisfactory demonstration exists of the alleged positive chemotaxis of injured tissues,[47] although some extracts of inflammatory exudates such as leukotaxine are powerful agents.[48] The property of positive chemotaxis of most bacteria resides in a polysaccharide fraction;

this is true of *B. anthracis, C. diphtheriae, D. pneumoniae, E. coli, Myco. tuberculosis. Sal. typhi, M. pyogenes* var. *albus, Str. pyogenes,* etc. Starch, arabinose and glucosamine are also positive.

Chemotaxis has no influence on the phagocytic capacity of inflammatory cells. Its only role in inflammation is to increase the probabilities of contact between phagocytes and particles, and this is accomplished by

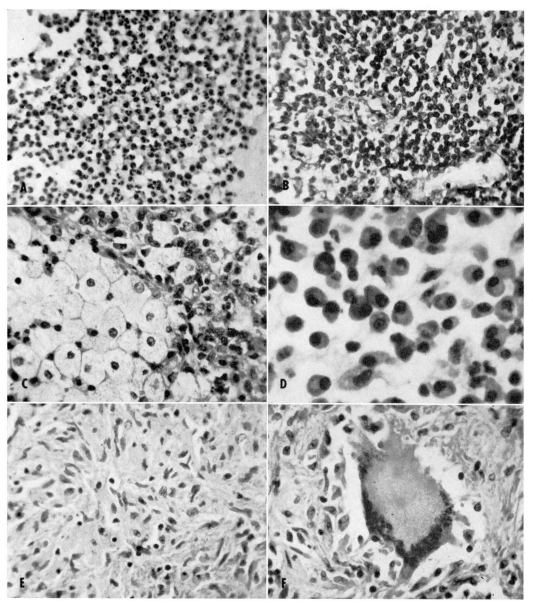

FIG. 2–10. Some types of cells encountered in inflammation. *A,* Polymorphonuclear leukocytes in acute inflammation. *B,* Groups of lymphocytes in chronic inflammation. *C,* Foamy macrophages in chronic pyelonephritis. *D,* Plasma cells. *E,* Epithelioid cells in tuberculosis. *F,* Giant cell in tuberculosis.

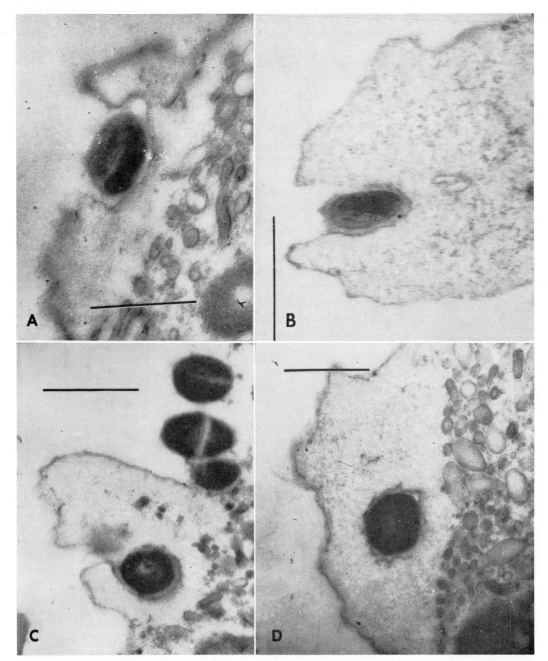

Fig. 2–11.   Electromicrographs of leukocytes ingesting avirulent streptococci. (Courtesy of Dr. Joseph R. Goodman and the Editor, Journal of Bacteriology.)

influencing the cell movements and favoring a greater accumulation of cells in the neighborhood of the stimulating agent. The mechanism by which a substance can modify the cell movements at a distance is not known. McCutcheon[49] has suggested that it may be due to the ability of chemotactic substances to adsorb from the medium the factors stim-

ulating cell migration. A concentration gradient would be created and the cell attracted; the opposite explanation would account for negative chemotaxis.

3. *Phagocytosis.* The capacity to ingest and digest particles is a basic mechanism of nutrition of protozoans and some metazoans; ingestion is also known as phagocy-

tosis, and when it is not of particles but of fluids it is referred to as pinocytosis. As the zoologic scale is climbed and organization becomes more complicated, some organs appear whose function is to prepare nutritive substances for utilization by all cellular elements of the organism. Thus, in a multicellular organism many elements lose (or never show) their capacity to phagocytose. Some cells remain, however, that preserve this ability and play a very important role in inflammation; they are the polymorphonuclear leukocyte and the macrophage. Most of the phagocytic cells present in an inflammatory process are of hematogenous origin; a few macrophages may be derived from the tissue involved, but the evidence in this respect is controversial.[50, 51]

When phagocytosis is observed *in vivo,* the cell comes near the particle, emits a pseudopod surrounding it, and slowly or rapidly the particle is introduced within the cytoplasm where it appears surrounded by a clear vacuole.[52, 53] Contact between cell and particle is essential, as well as a certain adhesiveness which in many cases is due to the presence in the plasma of substances known as opsonins. In the case of bacteria, opsonins may be natural or the organism may form them when in contact with the microorganism. Macrophages will fail to phagocytose bacteria when suspended in a drop of plasma without opsonins; however, Wood[54] has shown in his studies that if the experimental situation is modified by introducing fibrin threads, filter paper or pieces of lung and bronchi, bacteria are trapped between the surface introduced and the phagocyte, and ingestion can occur. This phenomenon was called "surface" phagocytosis and it has been observed *in vivo,* in the subcutaneous tissues.[49] Lerner[55] suggests that the effect is not mechanical but chemical in nature, but even so the idea that phagocytosis may occur in the absence of opsonins is of great interest. How frequently it does occur in infectious diseases in man and how important it is as a defense mechanism remain to be determined. Therefore, there are two general types of phagocytosis. The most frequent form requires the presence of phagocyte, particle and opsonins, while "surface" phagocytosis can occur without opsonins, in which case a physical

obstacle to the displacement of particles is necessary.

Once within the cellular cytoplasm, the fate of the particle will depend mainly on its nature but there are only four possibilities: (a) the particle is digested by the cell; (b) the particle is eliminated from the cell; (c) a type of symbiosis develops in which neither cell nor particle appears to influence the other; and (d) the cell is destroyed by the particle, which regains an interstitial position.

A. DIGESTION. Digestion of the particle by the cell is carried out by intracytoplasmic enzymes. Many of these catalytic proteins have been described in both polymorphonuclear leukocytes and macrophages[56] (Table 7) but not all will participate in the destruc-

Table 7. Enzymes of Phagocytes

ENZYME	LEUKOCYTE	MACROPHAGE
Esterases	+	+
Simple esterase	+	+
Lipase	+	+
Cholinesterase	+	−
Alkaline phosphatase	+	−
Acid phosphatase	+	+
ATP-ase	+	−
Nuclease	+	−
Nucleotidase	+	−
Carbohydrases		
Polysaccharidase	+	
Nucleosidase	+	
Peptidases		
Dipeptidase	+	
Tripeptidase	+	
Proteinases		
Peptic		+
Tryptic	+	
Catheptic	+	
Phosphorylase	+	
Oxidoreductases		
Dehydrogenase	+	
Oxidase	+	+
Hydrases		
Glyoxalase	+	
Beta-glucuronidase	+	
Protein-zinc	+	

(Modified from Suter [56])

tion of the particle since bacteria appear to be unaffected by many proteolytic enzymes.[57] Some enzymes, however, have been directly implicated in digestion of certain bacteria, such as lysozyme and phagocytin. The latter was isolated by Hirsch in 1956[58]

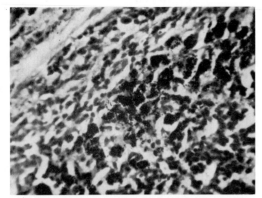

FIG. 2–12. A group of phagocytes with carbon particles in a mediastinal lymph node.

from rabbit leukocytes and found to be a very active globulin against intestinal gram-negative bacilli.[59] Further studies have shown that phagocytin is different from histone B, a protein derived from the thymus which also shows bactericidal properties.[60] Another factor probably playing a role in the destruction of intracytoplasmic bacteria is autolysis of the microorganism brought about by enzymes similar to those responsible for their digestion by cells. Finally, the particle may influence the cell to the degree that some of the enzymatic systems may be reorganized, creating new conditions incompatible with survival of bacteria within the cytoplasm; this may be especially true in chronic infections.

B. EGESTION. Wilson[61] has shown that polymorphonuclear leukocytes will, under certain circumstances, egest particles that were previously phagocytized. In this case, the cells survive both the process of phagocytosis and egestion, so the situation is different from the release of particles after death of the cell.

C. SYMBIOSIS. Symbiosis between particle and cell is of great significance in pathology. Inert substances may be found within the cytoplasm of macrophages for prolonged periods, such as carbon particles in phagocytic cells of pulmonary hilar and mediastinal lymph nodes (anthracosis) (Fig. 2–12). Some bacteria will remain viable within the cellular cytoplasm for some time;[62] in this intracellular situation they are protected by the cellular membrane from the action of both humoral factors such as antibodies and substances introduced in the circulation with

therapeutic aims,[63] such as antibiotics. The microorganism is not only protected, but is also transported by the cell wherever it may go, thus favoring widespread dissemination of the disease. This seems to be the case in tuberculosis,[64] brucellosis[65] and other chronic infections.

D. DESTRUCTION OF THE CELL. Finally, the particle may destroy the phagocyte and regain an interstitial position, for example, when Koch's bacillus is ingested by polymorphonuclear leukocytes during the first stages of tuberculosis or when human leukocytes phagocytize virulent staphylococci, as shown by Rogers and Melly.[66]

Besides those already mentioned there are numerous other factors influencing phagocytosis which may be considered in two groups: factors enhancing the ingestion of particles by cells and factors inhibiting the process; only a few will be discussed (Table 8). Temperature changes have a clear effect

Table 8. Some Factors which Influence Phagocytosis

FACTORS FAVORING PHAGOCYTOSIS	FACTORS INHIBITING PHAGOCYTOSIS
Temperature (37° to 40°)	Temperature ($> 40°$ C)
Mild ionizing radiation	Intense ionizing radiation
Opsonization	Capsular factors
Nervous stimuli	Leukemia
Hormones (ACTH, cortisone)	Acid pH (6.6)
Calcium ions	Z potential
Good nutritional status	Gastric mucin
Anemia (experimental)	

on phagocytosis which increases up to 100 per cent between 38° and 40° C.; higher elevations of temperature will decrease considerably the ingestion of particles. This effect may be due to the general enhancement of metabolism produced by increases in temperature but the problem has not been studied directly; if these *in vitro* observations were to be confirmed *in vivo* they would add greatly to the understanding of the effect of fever in infection. Bacterial opsonization has been mentioned but its importance cannot be exaggerated, especially when considered in relation to capsular factors of microorganisms which inhibit phagocytosis.[67] Such factors have been named aggressins or antiphagins and appear to be different for each type of bacteria. For instance, in streptococcus C it is hyaluronic acid, in streptococcus A it is protein M, in staphylococcus they are leukocidins, which have been shown to be three,[68] in *Past. pestis* it is fraction I, etc. Fortunately most of these factors are antigenic and, therefore, stimulate the production of antibodies by the organism; specific antibodies will neutralize the antiphagocytic effect of capsular factors and phagocytosis will take place. The influence of malnutrition in phagocytosis is of great interest, although according to Schneider,[69] "it has become conspicuous more by reiteration than by demonstration." Much of the published information is very difficult to analyze[70] but it may be stated with confidence that some types of malnutrition favor phagocytosis while others inhibit it.[71] Against all predictions, anemia seems to stimulate the phagocytic activity of macrophagic cells. Berry and Haller[72] observed experimentally that anemic mice would resist better than normal mice the same doses of *Sal. typhimurium* (Fig. 2–13); it would be extremely important to extend these observations to other species with different pathogenic microorganisms. Studies on patients with leukemia have produced contradictory results,[73, 74] but it may be concluded that in general phagocytosis is decreased. Boggs[75] found that in human leukemia the cellular composition of inflammatory exudates was normal in the chronic forms and deficient in leukocytes in the acute type. For more details, the excellent reviews of Mudd and McCutcheon,[76] Berry and Spies[77] and Suter[56] should be consulted.

The intimate mechanisms of phagocytosis seem to depend partly on physical factors. Fenn[78] suggested that ingestion of particles by macrophages was the result of an interplay of surface tensions between phagocyte and particle. Important in this respect are the surface tension between the phagocyte and the medium (S_1), between the particle and the medium (S_2) and the macrophage-particle interphase (S_{1-2}). Ponder[79] reasoned that when phagocyte and particle came in contact, ingestion would occur if:

$$\frac{S_1 - S_{1-2}}{S_2} = 0 \text{ or } > (+1)$$

On the other hand, when the result of the equation is equal to or less than 1 there is no phagocytosis; therefore, phagocytosis is facilitated by decreasing the value of S_2, which is the net result of opsonization, or by increasing S_1 or S_{1-2}, or by any combination of these factors. A further proof of the suggestion that surface tensions are important in determining phagocytosis is the experimental observation of Berry and associates,[80] who showed that substances decreasing surface tension such as detergents increase phagocytosis. This theory is based on a too simplified system; furthermore, recent data suggest that during phagocytosis there are important metabolic modifications in the cell, which should not occur if the entire phenomenon were due only to changes in surface tensions.[81] Stähelin and associates[82-84] found that a dramatic increase in the oxygen uptake rates of polymorphonuclear leukocytes or monocytes occurred while tubercle bacilli were ingested; in a further study from the same laboratory, Sbarra and Karnovsky[85] reported their findings in certain metabolic changes appearing in guinea pig leukocytes during the ingestion of inert particles. Phagocytosis occurred equally well under aerobic and anaerobic conditions, but in aerobiosis leukocytes showed increased lactate production, increased oxygen uptake, increased appearance of C-1 of glucose as CO_2 relative to

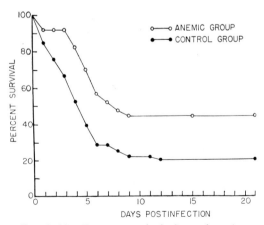

FIG. 2–13. Per cent survival of anemic and normal mice infected with *Sal. typhimurium*. (Courtesy of Dr. J. L. Berry and the Editor, Blood.)

C-6 of glucose; and in anaerobiosis there was a significant increase in the consumption of glycogen and glucose by the cells. Interference with glycolysis by iodacetate and fluoride inhibited phagocytosis, while other poisons such as cyanide and dinitrophenol had no effect on the ingestion of particles. Similar results have been reported by Cohn and Morse,[86] who in addition studied the effect of lipopolysaccharide endotoxin on the phagocytic ability of polymorphonuclear leukocytes; it had been observed that such endotoxins increase the resistance of laboratory animals to bacterial infection, but the mechanism was not clear. Cohn and Morse found that lipopolysaccharide endotoxin changes the cell surface and, of special significance here, increases the rate of glycolysis while there is a definite stimulation to phagocytosis.[87] The effect of lipopolysaccharide endotoxin is more complex than this, however, since it has been shown that it can also increase the opsonization capacity of mouse sera.[88] These data suggest that phagocytosis does require the expenditure of energy, which is derived from the degradation of glucose, and that in addition to surface tension changes, the process involves drastic modifications in cellular metabolism.

4. *Sequence of Appearance of Cells in the Exudate*. In the vast majority of acute inflammations the first cells appearing in the interstitial tissues are polymorphonuclear leukocytes; after a while, macrophages are found in significant numbers, and the last to appear are lymphocytes. This sequence was observed at the turn of the century by Borrel,[89] and ever since it has been the subject of numerous studies. Available information shows that even in inflammatory processes in which usually there is a predominance of macrophages and lymphocytes, such as tuberculosis and typhoid fever, in the very beginning there is a predominance of leukocytes. Menkin[90] has suggested that the sequence is due to local changes in pH; according to this author, inflammation is accompanied by an increase in H^+ ion concentration in tissues, the result of anaerobic glycolysis and accumulation of lactic acid. Since polymorphonuclear leukocytes are unable to survive below a pH of 7.0 while macrophages

resist pH values of pH 6.7 or lower, a decrease in pH will destroy leukocytes leaving only macrophages. In Menkin's own words, "it is a problem of survival of leukocytes at different pH levels and not of mobilization."[91] These ideas have been severely criticized by Steinberg and Dietz,[92] and Harris,[45] but Menkin's data are very suggestive.

Other ideas regarding the mechanism of the sequence of appearance of cells in inflammatory processes are as follows:[45] (a) migration of macrophages occurs late, as a response to substances different from those attracting leukocytes; (b) macrophages are mainly derived from tissues and not from the blood, which implies a slower mobilization of histogenous cells; (c) migration of leukocytes and macrophages is simultaneous, but their respective resistance to the agent causing inflammation is different, so that after death of leukocytes there would be a predominance of macrophages.

It has been mentioned already that there seems to be no difference in chemotaxis of the different phagocytic cells,[93] so the first hypothesis may be discarded. In regard to the second hypothesis, at least during acute inflammation produced experimentally in the rabbit's ear by microburns[7] and in experimental tuberculosis of the same site,[51] tissue macrophages do not participate in the process; rather, all inflammatory cells appear to be derived from the blood vessels. The third hypothesis mentioned is defended by Harris[45] and is based on the intra- or extracellular position of microorganisms causing inflammation. It has been shown that in tuberculosis polymorphonuclear leukocytes appear first and rapidly phagocytize many tubercle bacilli, but in so doing they succumb and leave macrophages in charge of ingesting most bacilli and cellular debris. Within these phagocytes bacilli seem to remain essentially unmodified and the cells are also unaltered. Furthermore, intracellular bacilli will no longer irritate the surrounding tissues so that no greater affluence of polymorphonuclear leukocytes will be induced. The prolonged survival of macrophages, together with the previously mentioned circumstances, would explain the predominance of macrophages in tuberculosis. On the other hand, in pyogenic inflammation bacteria are mainly extracellular, they grow rapidly and produce exotoxins perpetuating tissue damage and the consequent vascular changes with further migration of leukocytes.

Page and Good[94] have added a very interesting observation to this problem; they studied a patient with cyclic neutropenia who at times possessed no circulating neutrophils and at other times had an adequate supply of these cells. Inflammation was induced by applying a drop of streptokinase-streptodornase to the skin (the patient was known to be sensitive to this antigen) and the cellular sequences examined by Rebuck's technique.[95] It was found that when no neutrophils were present in the early stages of inflammation, the further appearance of lymphocytes and macrophages was also lacking. Other experiments were carried out in rabbits made leukopenic with nitrogen mustard with identical results; i.e., the absence of polymorphonuclear leukocytes com-

pletely changed the further development of inflammation. Page and Good concluded that the sequence and time relationship of events in acute inflammation in normal man and animals is a function, in part at least, of the circulating neutrophils.[96] In summary, the sequence of appearance of cells in inflammation may not be purely temporary but selective, with pH changing the characteristics of the causal agents and the nature of the first events determining the predominating types.

The previously mentioned hypotheses refer to polymorphonuclear leukocytes and macrophages or monocytes, but fail to explain the presence and functions of the lymphocyte. These cells show no chemotaxis, are not phagocytic and at present their role in antibody production[97] is still inadequate to explain their unfailing attendance in inflammation. A recent conference on the lymphocyte and lymphocytic

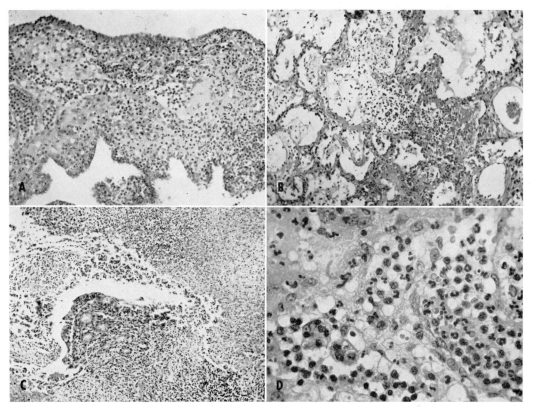

FIG. 2–14. Some types of acute inflammation. *A,* Acute salpingitis with intense edema and vascular congestion. Some polymorphonuclear leukocytes are present in the interstitial tissues. *B,* Acute bronchopneumonia with scarce edema and fibrin deposition in alveoli, vascular congestion and some necrosis of alveolar septa. *C,* Acute necrotizing appendicitis. *D,* Detail of exudate in acute inflammation.

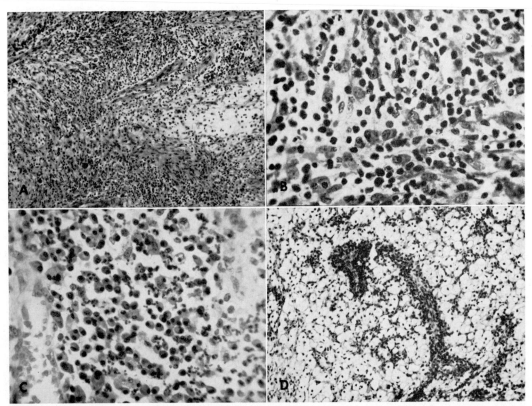

Fig. 2–15. Some types of chronic inflammation. *A*, Proliferation of vascular and connective tissue, edema, and pleomorphic cellular infiltration. *B*, Detail of exudate in chronic inflammation. *C*, Predominance of plasma cells. *D*, Predominance of foamy macrophages (Mikulicz cells) in rhinoscleroma.

tissue[98] has revealed that there is still no adequately documented role for the lymphocyte in inflammation; indeed, the function of this cell remains one of the most challenging mysteries in biology. Costero[99] believes that interstitial lymphocytosis in rheumatic fever and other inflammatory conditions showing accumulations of these cells in areas of tissue atrophy may be explained by the local transformation of histiocytic cells, stimulated by the structural proteins of destroyed cells. Sieracki and Rebuck[100] have summarized their ideas on the role of the lymphocyte in inflammation into four main categories, namely phagocytosis (based on the alleged transformation of lymphocytes in mobile macrophages), antibody production, trephocytic activities and cytopoietic functions. Direct evidence is available only for the participation of lymphocytes in antibody synthesis; the remaining functions are inferred from sequential studies in human skin

windows and skin blister techniques, which fail to provide direct evidence of transformation of lymphocytes into macrophages or other elements.

D. Types of Inflammation. The classification of inflammations according to the macroscopic aspect of the accumulated exudate has been mentioned, but the different resulting types may appear at various times in the same process and have little clinical significance. On the other hand, factors such as the duration of the inflammatory process, the nature of the causal agent, the immune response, etc., will modify the morphologic nature of inflammation. Therefore, in the following discussion a series of different types of inflammation are described with no attention to the gross aspect of the exudate.

1. *Acute, Chronic, Granulomatous and Organized Inflammations.* Acute inflammation is characterized by rapid onset and by

a predominance of vascular changes, such as pronounced vasodilation, edema and leukocytic infiltration (Fig. 2–14). On many occasions the process persists unmodified for several weeks, and then there is a dissociation between the clinical and the pathologic concepts of acute inflammation. Lack of signs of repair is also important, but in this context it should be remembered that a pathologic diagnosis of acute inflammation refers to a morphologic picture and not to clinical duration. There are exceptions to the predominance of polymorphonuclear leukocytes in acute inflammation, such as typhoid fever and certain viral diseases, in which almost from the beginning there is a predominance of macrophages and lymphocytes; exceptions only prove the rule. Sometimes an acute inflammation will be combined with the features of chronic inflammation. In these cases, decisions as to the duration of the process are often difficult.

In chronic inflammation the microscopic picture is a mixture of vascular and exudative changes with those representing repair. In this particular form the effect of the causal agent persists but not with sufficient intensity to destroy all tissues; the irritation is continuous; the vascular response is maintained; the nature of the inflammatory cells changes with predominance of macrophages and lymphocytes; and there is proliferation of fibroblasts with laying down of connective tissue fibers (Fig. 2–15). Chronic inflammation is extremely important in pathology; few diseases escape this manifestation, in greater or lesser degree.

Granulomatous inflammation is easy to describe but difficult to interpret. The pathogenesis of this form of inflammation is incompletely understood. Essentially granulomatous inflammation is a chronic process with a mixture of exudative and reparative changes, but it shows two special character-

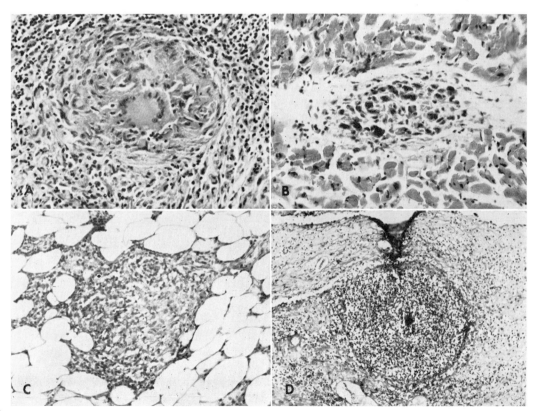

FIG. 2–16. Some types of granulomatous inflammation. *A*, Tuberculous granuloma (Köster's nodule). *B*, Aschoff bodies in acute rheumatic fever. *C*, Granuloma in leprosy. *D*, Granulomatous inflammation in nocardiasis.

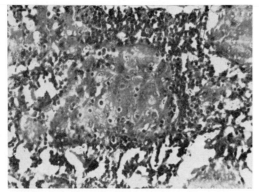

FIG. 2–17. Group of epithelioid cells in sarcoidosis.

istics separating it from other types of inflammation. First, there is a change in the structure of inflammatory cells which results in the formation of elements known as epithelioid and giant cells; and second, the cells become organized as nodules with a morphologic nature peculiar to the causal agent, which facilitates histologic diagnosis. Many of the chronic infectious diseases fall in this category, such as tuberculosis, syphilis, brucellosis, certain mycoses, etc., and other inflammatory processes of uncertain etiology, such as Boeck's sarcoid, rheumatic fever, rheumatoid arthritis, etc. The nodule formed by epithelioid and giant cells is known as a granuloma, and there are some which are highly characteristic such as Köster's nodule in tuberculosis. Aschoff bodies in active rheumatic fever, the gumma of syphilis, the periarticular nodes in rheumatoid arthritis, etc. (Fig. 2–16).[101, 102] Forbus has suggested that granulomatous inflammation is the result of the local response of the reticuloendothelial system and a systemic immune reaction. Metaplasia of local reticuloendothelial cells would be secondary to the predominantly intracellular position of the causative agents, such as *Myco. tuberculosis* or *B. suis*. Generalized hypersensitivity is demonstrated by special skin tests, such as the tuberculin test in tuberculosis and the coccidioidin test in coccidioidomycosis. Epithelioid cells are probably macrophages showing abundant, pale cytoplasm and vesicular nucleus; their name is derived from the fact that there is very little intercellular substance between them, so they sometimes

resemble the malpighian strata but without intercellular bridges (Fig. 2–17). Giant cells vary in size and shape in different inflammations (Fig. 2–18). In brucellosis they are relatively small, with irregular, acidophilic cytoplasm and two or three large, kidney-shaped nuclei with prominent nucleoli. They are very similar to those found in Hodgkin's disease (Reed-Sternberg cells), a type of malignant lymphoma which is not too different histologically from brucellosis. Giant cells in tuberculosis are larger and contain many small, round or oval nuclei forming a peripheral row; their cytoplasm is finely granular, acidophilic and may be vacuolated, with fine filiform prolongations in all directions (Langhans' cells). In Boeck's sarcoid giant cells are similar to Langhans' cells but occasionally they may show various types of cytoplasmic inclusions such as crystalloids, stellate bodies, etc. Foreign body giant cells are very irregular in size, show many nuclei and are usually arranged in the neighborhood of the foreign body; when the size of the foreign body permits, it may be observed within the cytoplasm of the giant cells.

Some granulomatous inflammations are specific; i.e., the observation of the granuloma is sufficient evidence to diagnose the disease, as in the case of Aschoff's nodule in rheumatic fever.[103] This highly characteristic granuloma is found in the cardiac structures (endocardium and myocardium) of patients with rheumatic fever and in no other disease.[104] It represents a histologic sign of activity and until recently it was thought that patients without clinical manifestations of active rheumatic fever did not show Aschoff's nodules in the heart, so it was also considered as a sign of clinical activity. The examination of auricular appendages of commissurotomy patients, however, has shown Aschoff's nodules to be present even when rheumatic fever was quiescent clinically.[105, 106] In view of this finding Aschoff's nodule cannot be considered as an indication of clinical activity, though its specificity for rheumatic fever remains unshaken. Granulomas occurring in diseases of uncertain etiology may not be diagnostic but their presence suggests the disease and, taken together with the entire clinical picture, they serve to confirm the diagnosis. Such is the case in Boeck's sarcoid, where granulomas show no necrosis and although there is confluence of various lesions they usually preserve their outlines;[107] even in cases where the histologic picture is typical, the other manifestations of the disease must be considered before rendering a final opinion as to the nature of the process, in order to avoid embarrassing and often dangerous mistakes. A classic example is tuberculosis, where granulomas are formed by a central area of necrosis surrounded by epithelioid and Langhans' giant cells and with an outer ring of lymphocytes. Although this histologic picture is highly suggestive of tuberculosis it may also occur in other infectious diseases, such as coccidioidomycosis, histoplasmosis and syphilis, as well as in Boeck's sarcoid and tuberculoid leprosy; therefore, it is imperative to search for the etiologic agent with appropriate methods before a final diagnosis is given. These methods may be the adequate staining of the causal agent in tissues, or even better the culture and inoculation of bacteria and fungi, which provide a closer identification of strains and a better idea of drugs to be used in treatment. Weed and Dahlin[108] have published a series of cases where bacteriologic studies gave unexpected results after histologic examination; and Schulz and associates[109] found in a series of 140 cases of granulomatous inflammation of the lung that 14.2 per cent were not caused by tuberculosis. These findings suggest that unless the causal agent is identified, granulomatous inflammation should be diagnosed as such, with suggestions as to the most probable etiology but without dogmatic statements based on the mistaken notion that morphology suffices to determine the cause of disease.

Some authors have thought that granulomatous inflammation is an expression of a

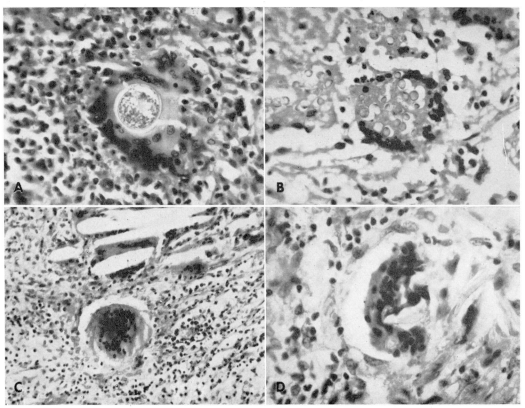

FIG. 2–18. Some types of giant cells in inflammation. *A*, Coccidiodomycosis. *B*, Blastomycosis. *C*, Foreign body (cholesterol crystals) giant cells. *D*, Foreign body (cotton sutures) giant cell.

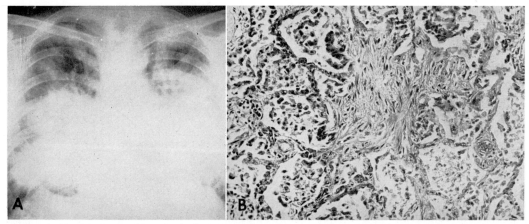

Fig. 2–19.   X-ray and microscopic picture of organizing exudate in pneumonia.

hypersensitive state, and Goddard[110] suggested that anaphylactic granulomas were specific and qualitatively different from a common inflammatory response. In a more conservative vein, Goldgraber and Kirsner state, "It would appear that the presence of granulomas and giant cells should arouse suspicion of a hypersensitivity mechanism,"[111] after 5 of 12 sensitized guinea pigs on the third day after the eliciting injection developed granulomas. There can be no doubt that hypersensitivity is capable of inducing the formation of granulomatous inflammation, but great care must be exercised in generalizing from the effect of a particular etiologic agent to all other possible causes. Inflammation is the local tissue reaction to injury and tissue reactions can produce a limited number of morphologic pictures; certainly no one would believe that the foreign body granuloma of talcum powder is the result of hypersensitivity (see below).

Organizing inflammation is a very interesting phenomenon. Many inflammatory processes, when healed, leave little or no structural changes in the involved tissue. This result is known as *restitutio ad integrum,* and a very good example is lobar pneumococcal pneumonia, where inflammation begins with the outpouring of large amounts of fluid into the alveoli; with further increase in capillary permeability fibrin is also deposited in the air spaces and polymorphonuclear leukocytes appear somewhat later. In this stage the picture is composed of congested capillaries and alveoli filled with edema, fibrin and polymorphonuclear leukocytes, actively engaged in phagocytosis of pneumococci. Death and destruction of leukocytes is accompanied by release of cytoplasmic proteolytic enzymes which digest the fibrin and liquefy the exudate, thus facilitating its elimination through bronchi or lymphatic vessels and the complete restitution of the pulmonary structure. However, when for some reason fibrin is not eliminated it stimulates proliferation of fibroblasts and nomicoplasia of other connective tissue cells, which penetrate within the fibrin plugs, deposit connective fibers and transform them into fibrous nodules. The final stage of this process is known as organizing inflammation (Fig. 2–19). It has been determined by Auerbach and associates[112] that the frequency of organizing pneumonia has increased in recent times, and these authors suggest that the introduction of antibiotics and the prevalence of

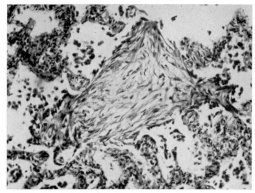

Fig. 2–20.   Masson body in chronic pulmonary inflammation (bronchiectasis).

viral forms of pneumonitis may be partly responsible for it. Antibiotics would interfere with the natural course of the process just described, decreasing the number of leukocytes and inhibiting the enzymatic degradation of fibrin. A less extensive but identical process is represented by Masson bodies,[113] which are small masses of organized connective tissue (Fig. 2–20) found within the alveoli in cases of rheumatic[114] and uremic pneumonia,[115] as well as in many other conditions[116] such as bronchiectasis,

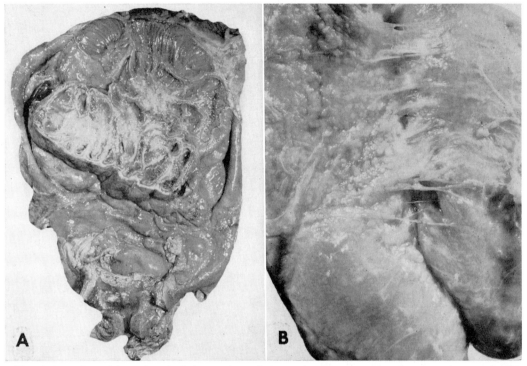

FIG. 2–21. Organizing, chronic inflammation of the peritoneum. *A,* Chronic tuberculous peritonitis with extensive adhesions of intestinal loops. *B,* Detail to show the presence of fibrous bands passing from one loop to another.

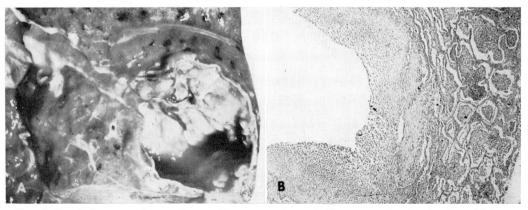

FIG. 2–22. Pulmonary abscess due to *D. pneumoniae* and *K. pneumoniae.* Notice bronchial communication and thin pyogenic membrane. *B,* The wall of the abscess, with inflammation in the surrounding parenchyma.

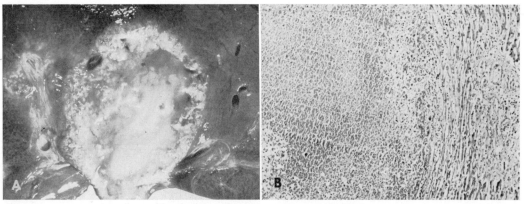

FIG. 2–23.   Amebic abscess of the liver.

emphysema, abscesses, chronic pneumonitis, etc. Organizing inflammation can also occur in other areas of the organism, such as the peritoneal cavity, where the formation of fibrous bands and adhesions may give rise to pictures of intestinal occlusion, or the pericardium, where an old and organized tuberculous inflammation is frequently the cause of constrictive pericarditis (Fig. 2–21).

2. *Abscess*. This is a form of inflammation characterized by extensive necrosis and liquefaction of the exudate, with formation of a cavity filled with a more or less viscous fluid. The wall of the cavity is composed of acute inflammation and several layers of connective tissue in different stages of organization; the inner lining is known as pyogenic membrane, a descriptive name indicating that polymorphonuclear leukocytes and fibrin are the main components (Fig. 2–22). It really is a layer of condensed exudate where the cells are better preserved. The content of the cavity is formed by necrosis and proteolytic digestion of exudate and cells; there usually are abundant polymorphonuclear leukocytes in different stages of regression, which represent the main source of enzymes. The biochemical environment created by necrosis and digestion of cells and fluid is incompatible with the survival of many bacteria and most cells. In some types of abscesses certain substances will accumulate that inhibit the bactericidal or bacteriostatic effect of antibiotics, thus proving a very serious obstacle in adequate treatment; in older lesions, the capsule may

become very thick and poorly vascularized, so that therapeutic elements introduced into the circulation will not reach adequate concentrations for effective action. These aspects are further analyzed in the next section.

If the definition of abscess is strictly applied, the most frequent form of liver "abscess" cannot be considered as such. Invasion of the liver by *E. histolytica* will be followed many times by the presence of one or several localized areas of destruction of liver tissue without formation of exudate (Fig. 2–23).[117] Why necrosis and dissolution of tissue cells should fail to arouse a violent inflammatory process is not known, but even in very early lesions participation of leukocytes with exudate is minimal or nonexistent.[118] A similar situation is also seen in the colon, where amebas induce bland necrosis and lysis of tissues without inflammation; the latter is only present in case of secondary infection.

3. *Allergic Inflammation*. Some aspects of granulomatous inflammation have been discussed. Two different situations may be encountered in which hypersensitivity participates in the causation of inflammatory processes. One, where inflammation is provoked by an antigen-antibody reaction, without additional etiologic agents, as in the Arthus and Shwartzman phenomena, etc.; the other, in which inflammation is the result of an agent which at the same time acts as an antigen, as in many bacterial infections.

When hypersensitivity is the lone factor

responsible for the inflammatory process the result is a very rapid development of edema, indicating immediate onset of increased capillary permeability; besides polymorphonuclear leukocytes, macrophages, and the other elements forming the exudate, there may be abundant eosinophilic leukocytes. Vascular lesions may be prominent, with necrosis of arterioles and extensive thrombosis. In some situations the blood vessels show fibrinoid necrosis, which may also be found in focal areas of connective tissue. According to Goddard,[119] the Arthus phenomenon in rabbits shows vascular changes not present in the guinea pig and characterized by hyperplasia and hypertrophy of the muscle coat in the arterial branches, coupled with the presence of surrounding rings of myoblasts or histiocytes, as well as development of aberrant muscle fibers in the media. In the venules there is endothelial ingrowth leading to valvelike structures and formation of intraluminal septa. Goldgraber and Kirsner[120] induced the Arthus phenomenon in the colon of rabbits and did serial histologic studies over a period of 4 weeks; the results were the same enhanced and stormy inflammatory process in the beginning, and histiocytosis with granuloma formation and eosinophilia in later stages. In several publications, Rössle[121] and other members of his school[122, 123] suggested that inflammation resulting from hypersensitivity was only quantitatively different from the inflammatory process induced by other mechanisms, and coined the terms "hyperergic" and "normergic" to characterize these two different aspects. However, more recent and detailed studies of the Arthus phenomenon[124] and anaphylaxia[125] by More and Movat have shown that, in addition to the explosive nature of the tissue response, there are also some qualitative differences in the type of cells involved, characterized by intense proliferation of macrophages and maturation and proliferation of plasma cells. The pathogenetic sequence suggested by these authors is as follows: the exudative process, progressing to thrombosis, would result from antigen-antibody interaction; the macrophage reaction would be the morphologic counterpart of antigen removal; and the proliferation of plasma cells would repre-

sent the anatomic expression of antibody formation. By means of immunohistochemical techniques, Dixon[126] and others[127] have shown that antigen is deposited in injured areas only after antibody is synthesized, so the first idea proposed by More and Movat seems to be acceptable. Evidence presented by White et al.,[128] and Askonas and White,[129] support the contention that macrophages in hypersensitivity inflammation contain the injected antigen, and there is much information[130] favoring the role of plasma cells as elements responsible for the synthesis of antibodies. In addition, Movat et al.[131] induced mechanical injury by incision, chemical injury by the injection of trypsin and physical damage by the implantation of radon seeds into the flanks of rabbits; all three methods of connective tissue damage resulted in deposition of fibrinoid material without collagen degeneration, but the plasma cell infiltration was not seen. All these data make More and Movat's interpretation very likely. It is quite another thing to accept with them that, "the lesion complex of acute destruction with exudation and granulomatous reaction, particularly when characterized by the presence of plasma cells, is pathognomonic for the tissue response of hypersensitivity."[125] Many inflammatory processes show this picture and yet are known to be caused by other agents, and in several publications Klemperer[132, 133] has warned against a too facile generalization from morphologic observations. These problems are further discussed in Chapter VI, in connection with the so-called "collagen diseases."

IV. BIOCHEMISTRY OF INFLAMMATION

This aspect of inflammation is not new. For a long time mechanisms responsible for most of the changes described in inflammation have been considered as humoral and names were assigned to them, although their existence was purely hypothetical. Thus, substances acting on vascular structures were referred to as "phlogangines," those responsible for degenerative and regressive changes were named "phlogotoxins," and humoral factors influencing growth and repair after injury were known as "phlogotrophins."[134] Since the pioneer efforts of Lewis and Menkin, however, direct experimental analyses of humoral "mediators" in inflammation have provided much information that can replace old terms and primitive ideas, although much remains to be done. On the other hand, the inflammatory process is a microcosmos where a biochemical environment is created that differs greatly from the previously normal conditions and from those persisting in the rest of the organism. These changes are of great significance to understand not only the intimate mechanisms of inflammation itself, but also the biologic meaning of the process in the preservation and maintenance of homeostasis.

A. Humoral Mediators in Inflammation. Chemical mediators have been studied in relation to both local tissue changes and systemic modifications in inflammation. The latter are discussed in connection with the general pathology of the host-parasite relation (Chapter VII) where they play a very important role. In this section some of the data pertaining to substances which increase capillary permeability and which induce pain and necrosis of tissues are presented.

1. *Substances Which Increase Capillary Permeability*. It has been mentioned that Lewis and Grant,[22] as a result of some simple observations, postulated the existence of a humoral factor as the cause of increased capillary permeability in acute, aseptic inflammation. Since the local effects of histamine were identical with those obtained by many other types of irritations, they suggested that it was this chemical or a closely related substance (H substance) that was released in the tissues and induced increased capillary permeability.

Following this suggestion many other observers found that histamine itself is released in tissues after burns,[135] chemical injury, or bacterial infections, as well as in anaphylaxis.[136] The mere presence of histamine, however, does not suffice to conclude that this substance is causing increased vascular permeability; antihistaminics should prevent the appearance of the phenomenon. Evidence obtained in these types of experiments is contradictory, but antihistamine drugs will not always block the effects of endogenous

histamine,[138] and not all antihistaminics are specific in their action. Pyrilamine (mepyramine) maleate in moderate doses does seem to antagonize effectively only histamine, and the urticarial wheals of patients suffering from some types of allergy are abolished completely when treated with this substance.[139] On the other hand, increased permeability of skin capillaries in the Arthus and Shwartzman phenomena,[140] as well as after burns produced in different species including man,[141] is not influenced by the administration of antihistamine drugs; the only type of inflammation due to local tissue injury that has been shown to be inhibited by antihistaminics is the immediate increase in permeability that follows intrapleural injection of turpentine in the pleural cavity of rats. In these experiments, Spector and Willoughby[142] used mepyramine or promethazine and reduced ten times the amount of exudate obtained 30 to 60 minutes after injection of turpentine, as well as obtaining a similar decrease in the quantity of protein-bound trypan blue passing into the pleural cavity from the circulation. Perhaps a more careful study of other experimental situations, taking into account differences among species, types of injury and susceptibility to endogenous histamine, will reveal that this substance plays an important role in the first stages of inflammation. Certainly its wide distribution in the organism, its presence in platelets and tissue mast cells and the apparent ease with which it is liberated would suggest it.

In 1936, Menkin[143] criticized Lewis' suggestion that histamine was responsible for increases in capillary permeability during acute inflammation and instead proposed that the principle was present in inflammatory exudates and could be extracted by means of dialysis, butyl alcohol and acetone. This principle was called "leukotaxine" because it would also attract leukocytes. Leukotaxine is thermostable, can precipitate with certain salts, will not induce contraction of smooth muscle of the guinea pig gut nor hypotension in the cat; and its effect on capillary permeability is not blocked by antihistamine drugs.[91] This work was confirmed by Cullumbine and Rydon,[144] who also were able to prepare a series of peptides capable of inducing leakage of circulating dyes by digesting several proteins with various proteases. Previously, Duthie and Chain[145] had done the same by digesting plasma proteins with trypsin. Spector[146] published a more detailed study of such peptides and showed that capillary activity was shared by those with 8 to 14 amino acids, that less than 5 amino acids in the molecule were incompatible with activity, and that they behaved like cations on electrophoresis. These peptides, however, stimulate the smooth muscle of the intestine of several species and are hypotensive in the cat and dog. Some of these peptides have been extensively studied and are known as bradykinin, kallidin, substance P, substance U, pepsitensin, kinin and angiotensin. That all these substances are capable of altering capillary permeability is a fact confirmed by several authors, but that they play a significant role in inflammation has been questioned by Spector, who studied the activity of pleural exudates in rats obtained from 1 to 24 hours after injury and found little or no activity on capillary permeability. In addition, changes in capillary permeability in the pleura were not accompanied by modifications in the concentration of peptides,[147] but this could be explained if these substances enjoyed only a transient existence in inflamed tissues. More studies are necessary before the exact role of protein fractions in inflammation is understood. Menkin[148] has isolated another factor from acid exudates which is not present in the protein fraction, is dialyzable and has effect only on capillary permeability, since it fails to attract leukocytes; the name proposed for this factor is "exudin."

Recently, Rowley and Benditt[149] have suggested that serotonin, also known as 5-hydroxytryptamine or enteramine, may be responsible for increased capillary permeability in inflammation. Since it has been shown that serotonin is present in large amounts in mast cells, release of this substance should be accompanied by degranulation of tissue mast cells, a fact observed by Benditt, et al.[150] with the use of some histamine liberators such as compound 48/80, dextran, ovomucoid and testicular extract. Furthermore, the capillary effect of serotonin is abolished by dibenamine and by 2-bromolysergic acid diethylamine bitar-

trate, which are specific antagonists of serotonin.[151] These observations, however, are applicable almost only to the rat, which is weakly responsive to histamine but very sensitive to serotonin; furthermore, it has been tested only on the skin.[152] Whether it plays a more general role in inflammation remains to be established. Another factor that may be important in capillary permeability is relaxin, a substance of uncertain nature that induces relaxation of the pelvic ligaments as occurs in pregnancy.[153] Storey[154] has suggested that the relaxation effect is due in part to increased capillary permeability in the ligaments with resulting edema and unwinding of collagen spirals. It has been mentioned that Spector and Storey[35] have obtained a factor from estrogen-treated uteri of ovariectomized mice, which will increase leakage of dye when injected in the subcutaneous tissues. It is doubtful that these observations will have any application to the problem of inflammation other than to suggest the possible nature of other active compounds.

Perhaps one of the most important recent contributions in this field is the discovery by Miles, Wilhelm and their colleagues, that guinea pig,[155-157] rat and rabbit[158] and human serum[159] acquire, on dilution, the property of increasing capillary permeability when tested in the skin of guinea pigs. Fractionation with ether also activated this factor, and certain sulphated dextrans and soy bean trypsin inhibitor prevented activation of the serum by dilution. This nondialyzable substance is present in the α-2-globulin fraction of the serum and is antagonized by an inhibitor present in the α-1-globulin fraction of serum. In the rat the inactive precursor of the permeability factor can be separated from the blood and activated by incubation with isolated lung mitochondria.[160] It has been suggested that the active factor is a protease, mainly because of its inactivation with soy bean trypsin inhibitor, but no direct proof of enzymatic action is available. Spector reasons that it is possible for activated globulins to provide a substrate for tissue or plasma proteases or other enzymes which then split off peptides responsible for the altered capillary permeability. The best study of the effect of globulin fractions on capillary permeability has been presented by Spector,[147] who showed that in rats there was a simultaneous development of both leakage of labeled plasma albumin into the pleura and the ability of the globulin fraction of the exudate to induce leakage of dye in the rat skin. As the permeability of pleural capillaries returned to normal, the globulin fraction of the exudate ceased to be active on the skin capillaries and there was an increase in the specific inhibitor in the plasma. Salicylate and diisopropyl-fluorophosphonate inhibited the development of increased permeability and this observation is of interest since it has been shown that these two substances prevent activation of the globulins. Further characterization of the chemical mediators of this phase of inflammation has been presented by Spector and Willoughby, who found that a number of antiesterases (diisopropyl-fluorophosphonate, quinine, quinidine, chloroquine, caffeine and salicylate) inhibit increased capillary permeability following thermal injury or intrapleural injection of turpentine.

2. *Chemical Mediation of Pain.* It is apparent that most of the pain felt during acute inflammation is due to tissue distention by edema and accumulation of exudate. In addition, direct involvement of nerve fibers by the inflammatory process may also play a role, especially after burns or trauma. On the other hand, some observations suggest that, at least in part, pain may also result from the action of chemical substances released or activated by tissue injury. Armstrong and associates[162] isolated from certain inflammatory exudates a pain-producing substance resembling bradykinin, which is released when the plasma is brought in contact with glass and shows a definite incubation period. Serotonin is also capable of producing intense pain when injected intradermally or when applied to a blister base.[163] Moulton and his colleagues[164] have found that minute quantities of the nucleoside xanthosine and of its base xanthine can cause intense pain on intradermal injection. Other active peptides may also be involved in the causation of pain during the acute inflammatory process.

3. *Tissue Necrosis.* Menkin[153] isolated a factor from the euglobulin fraction of exudates which on intradermal injection may produce swelling and necrosis. Microscopically there is acute inflammation and lymphatic blockade; one of the earliest changes is swelling of collagenous bundles. The factor was called "necrosin" and the effect thought to be due to proteolytic activity. There can be no doubt that during inflammation many substances are formed which are toxic in high degree; it is quite another thing to accept that the same type of substance is always formed and that it is responsible for necrosis in inflammation. The concept of necrosin, however, served to call attention to the fact that at the same time as certain phenomena were occurring in inflammation, which could be interpreted as defensive in nature, others were also taking place that went against the organism itself. It is of interest that these toxic, aggressive substances are endogenous in nature, probably the result of proteolysis with formation of active peptides.

4. *Origin and Release of Chemical Mediators in Inflammation.* The presence of humoral substances in the local reaction of connective tissue to injury is well documented and their possible role in determining some of the changes has been discussed. It is of interest, however, to inquire about the origin and release of these factors, since it is well known that they do not exist in active form in normal tissues. Histamine is widely distributed throughout the tissues of animals and plants[166] and shows great variations in concentrations in different species and tissues. One of the major storehouses of histamine in the body is the mast cells;[167] this substance is also present in platelets,[168] although the concentration varies with the species considered. The release of histamine is accomplished by a series of exogenous substances such as proteolytic enzymes, detergents, lysolecithin, snake venom, dextran, ovomucoid and bile salts.[169] In addition, other basic substances of known chemical structure can induce the release of histamine, the best known being compound 48/80. The intimate mechanism of release of histamine from mast cells is not known, although it has been suggested that compound 48/80 may act by removing the inhibitor of a naturally occurring enzyme in the surface of the cell, which in turn attacks the cell membrane and releases histamine.[170]

A somewhat different problem is posed by anaphylaxis, where it has been shown that there is increase of histamine in the blood. Ungar[171] suggested that activation of proteolytic enzymes such as fibrinolysin was responsible for histamine release, but the careful experiments of McIntire[172] have shown that soy bean trypsin inhibitor and antifibrinolysin do not inhibit anaphylactic release in the rabbit, and that streptokinase activates rabbit blood protease without causing histamine release. Dale[173] has suggested that antigen-antibody reactions alter cellular permeability and it is possible that such a phenomenon could lead to release of histamine from platelets and mast cells; indeed, anaphylaxis is known to induce degranulation of mast cells with apparent dissolution of the cell membrane.[174]

Menkin's leukotaxine and the many other peptides which increase capillary permeability have no known depot in the normal organism; indeed, they appear to be formed only during inflammation, as a result of proteolysis.[175] It is also possible that peptides exist bound to some other tissue constituent by an amide linkage and require the severance of only one bond to become activated. Spector[176] suggests that peptides are probably formed by activation of specific enzyme substrate systems, rather than from a general destruction of tissues and resultant proteolysis.

Serotonin is widely distributed throughout the organism;[177] the highest concentrations are found in the brain, platelets, mast cells, gastrointestinal tract and lungs. It is released by some of the histamine liberators such as compound 48/80, Propamidine and morphine, although species differences are prominent; dextran, ovomucoid and testicular extract are also active.[178] An endogenous factor in kidney and gastric mucosa of the dog has been described by Toh,[179] which is capable of releasing serotonin from platelets. In anaphylaxis there is an increase of serotonin in the plasma, which seems derived from platelets, but the intimate mechanism of this action is unknown. The origin and activation of plasma globulins have been mentioned above.

Menkin[180] has suggested an all-embracing concept of biochemical mechanisms in inflammation, with the injured cell as the potential source of all chemical mediators identified so far. In addition, this author has used the technique of differential centrifugation on exudative material and on the homogenates of inflamed tissue in order to substantiate his theory.[181] Leukotaxine was found primarily in "mitochondrial" and "microsomal" fractions of alkaline exudates, and in the corresponding fractions of inflamed tissue homogenate when the exudate is at an alkaline pH. Exudin was found only in the supernatant after centrifugation to obtain mitochondrial-microsomal fractions and in the nuclear fraction.

5. *An Integrated Theory on the Mechanisms of Inflammation.* As an example of the possible integration of the concepts previously described in this section, McGovern's theory[182] on the mechanism of inflammation will be summarized. This is intended only to show that the many pieces of the puzzle can readily fit into a scheme, the heuristic value of which is openly recognized. There are other hypotheses in the literature,[183] equally suggestive and equally speculative.

According to McGovern, mast cells play a central role in the early stages of inflammation. In response to injury, they secrete histamine, a permeability factor (serotonin?) and heparin. Histamine increases the local blood supply, and the permeability factor alters the consistency of the cement film upon the endothelial surface of the capillaries. Capillary permeability is thereby increased and fluid passes to the surrounding tissues. Heparin bears a negative electrical charge and is normally held in solution in the endothelial cement film, thus constituting an electrostatic barrier which repels the negatively charged leukocytes. With severe injury, however, the mast cells become exhausted, and if the endothelium is damaged so that it cannot restore an adequate cement film, leukocytes accumulate on the intimal surface. When the liberated heparin has become dissipated, the tissues become positively charged and leukocytes, attracted by the positive charge, migrate from the capillaries, there being no electrically charged cement barrier to their passage. This hypothesis pays no attention to circulating factors, as Robb-Smith's does,[183] but they can be easily brought into action without essential modifications. Furthermore, the continuation of the process, the development of chronic inflammation and of inflammatory reactions in organs and tissues without mast cells are not explained. This is undoubtedly due to the precariousness of knowledge on the intimate changes in inflammation; most of what is known is related to morphologic lesions, but it is not beyond reason to suppose that finer techniques may reveal subtle but important changes in other levels of organization which would make the picture clearer. Some of these changes are examined in the following paragraphs.

B. Biochemical Changes in Inflamed Tissues. The inflammatory reaction is accompanied by a series of biochemical changes in the injured tissues. The significance of these modifications in the chemical environment can be appreciated from three different angles: first, the morphologic nature of the lesion is profoundly influenced; second, in inflammatory processes caused by biologic agents the fate of the causal organism is determined to a great extent by the surrounding biochemical characteristics; and third, the mechanism of action of many substances used therapeutically is blocked or inhibited by some chemical substances accumulated in the inflammatory focus. A most useful summary of many aspects of these problems has been published by Dubos in his monograph: *"Biochemical Determinants of Microbial Disease."*[184]

One of the most important local chemical changes in inflammation is a decrease in oxygen consumption with increase in CO_2;[185] many of the subsequent modifications in the biochemistry of the inflammatory focus seem to depend on the relative anaerobiosis created by injury. Local tissue anoxia is probably the result of vascular damage and blocking of lymphatic vessels by fibrin and proteins; furthermore, it is not difficult to imagine that with tissue injury the same depression in oxygen consumption occurs as with the generalized metabolic response to injury (see Chapter X). If this is the case, decreased supply of oxygen would only be part of the explanation, the other being cellular inability to use it. Cells are provided with two different mechanisms for the obtainment of the energy necessary for metabolism. The most frequently used is

glycogen oxidation to CO_2 and H_2O, and the other is anaerobic degradation of glycogen to lactic and pyruvic acids. The latter compounds cannot be used in Krebs' cycle and accumulate in the organism. When the chemical composition of an exudate of several hours' duration is examined intense glycolysis, lactic acid accumulation, decrease in pH and O_2 and increase in CO_2 are found.[172] Additional changes in inorganic compounds, potassium and magnesium, are analyzed by Menkin.[91]

Parallel to the changes mentioned above there is accumulation of certain substances in the inflammatory focus which will play a very important role in the ultimate fate of the causal agent, especially when the latter is of biologic nature. In pneumococcal pneumonia large amounts of long chain fatty acids accumulate in the consolidated lung which are bactericidal for pneumococci.[186] This effect is enhanced in an acid environment, which is present in this condition in the lung. In addition to long chain fatty acids, autolytic enzymes released from destroyed cells act on proteins and produce other compounds such as peptides and organic acids, which in turn have a marked bacteriostatic effect. Lactic acid is also bacteriostatic and even bactericidal, and this effect is exaggerated with increased partial tensions of CO_2, as well as in anaerobiosis.[187] On the other hand, certain dicarboxylic and ketonic acids favor the growth of many bacterial strains and may even replace CO_2 as a growth factor; furthermore, they also antagonize the effect of lactic acid and other substances.[188] It is clear that accumulation of these acid substances is detrimental to the host and may counteract the bacteriostatic or bactericidal action of peptides and organic acids.

A clear example of the previous situation is the fate of tubercle bacilli within a focus of caseous necrosis. For the purpose of this discussion, pulmonary changes in tuberculosis may be considered in two groups: open lesions, which are communicated with the environment through a bronchus, and closed lesions, completely surrounded by a capsule of connective tissue and without communication with the surrounding environment. The number of viable tubercle bacilli found in open lesions is usually greater than in closed areas of caseous necrosis;[189] in the latter, survival is made improbable by the acid pH and the presence of bacteriostatic, long chain fatty acids. That these substances are not the only ones responsible for the loss of viability of tubercle bacilli is demonstrated by the fact that caseous material mixed with albumin is an excellent growth medium for these bacteria *in vitro*. Therefore, it must be accepted that the entire physicochemical environment of the closed lesion includes other circumstances that make life impossible for bacilli.

Perhaps of greater significance is the failure of therapeutic drugs conditioned by chemical changes in tissues. Certain drugs which are powerfully bacteriostatic *in vitro* against tubercle bacilli and effective *in vivo* against other bacterial infections are of no value in the treatment of human tuberculosis; for instance, sulfonamides and chloramphenicol. Furthermore, although it is relatively simple to stop the evolution of tuberculosis with streptomycin, nicotinic acid isoniazid and para-aminosalicylic acid, it is very difficult, even with prolonged treatments, to sterilize necrotic lesions.[189] A partial explanation is the intracellular phase of tuberculosis, since streptomycin at least fails to penetrate inside the cell and is therefore effective only against extracellular organisms.[190] Another important factor is the biochemical environment within the lesion, since both streptomycin and sulfonamides are without effect in the acid pH prevailing in necrosis. In addition, certain substances accumulate in the caseous lesions which block the activity of antibiotics, such as nucleic acids which inhibit streptomycin, para-aminobenzoic acid which antagonizes the effect of para-aminosalicylic acid, and ketonic acids and pyridoxal which limit the activity of nicotinic acid isoniazid.[191] The net result is that, even when antibiotics can penetrate within a necrotic lesion, their effect will be inhibited by the presence of the aforementioned substances and medical treatment will not succeed in sterilizing the lesion. The emergence of bacterial resistance to antibiotics is also influenced by the biochemical conditions of the inflammatory focus. Theoretically the administration of two or more combined drugs should prevent the emergence of bacterial resistance, since

in accordance with the genetic hypothesis the probability of bacteria becoming resistant to two or more drugs simultaneously is infinitely small.[192] However, laboratory tests are performed in simple media, under controlled conditions and insuring close contact between antibiotics and bacteria. In inflammation, on the other hand, the environment is variable from one moment to the next and it contains variable amounts of inhibiting substances. When a necrotic lesion contains sufficient para-aminobenzoic acid and the patient receives nicotinic acid isoniazid and para-aminosalicylic acid, the blocking effect of para-aminobenzoic acid may accelerate the emergence of resistance to isoniazid, which then acts as if it had been administered alone. These instances referring to tuberculosis are also applicable to other infections, especially those with an intracellular phase and extensive necrosis[193] (see Chapter VII).

V. ENDOCRINE CONTROL OF INFLAMMATION

Several aspects of the inflammatory response are regulated or influenced by the endocrine system. It is important, however, to separate those effects belonging to acute inflammation proper from the influence of hormones on the processes of repair and regeneration; the latter are discussed in Chapters III and VI, while here reference will be made only to endocrine influences on increased capillary permeability and phagocytosis.

In 1940, Menkin[194] found that adrenal cortex extracts were capable of inhibiting the increase in capillary permeability induced by acute inflammation or the injection of leukotaxine; later, the same author pointed out that compound E or cortisone had a similar effect.[195] These two observations served as the basis for numerous other studies on the influence of the endocrine system, and especially of adrenocortical hormones, on inflammation. Selye[196] separated hormones into "phlogistic" and "antiphlogistic" according to their ability to enhance or inhibit the inflammatory response as observed with the "granuloma pouch" technique. In this method, a bleb of air is introduced into the subcutaneous tissue of the dorsum of the rat and a cavity is created where different substances may be deposited; since the wall of the cavity shows inflammation, whatever changes are observed in the inner layer may be considered as the local effect of the substances used.[197] This and other techniques have shown that cortisone has an inhibitory effect on increased capillary permeability, and that this effect is blocked by desoxycorticosterone, somatotropin and aldosterone. Direct observation of the effect of cortisone on acute inflammation by means of a clear chamber in the rabbit's ear revealed that vasodilation and adherence of leukocytes to the vascular endothelium were decreased.[198] Since these two changes precede the accumulation of both fluid and cells in the surrounding interstitial tissues, the end result was strikingly different from that obtained without the hormone. Fewer leukocytes, little hemorrhage and edema and only slight vasodilation in the periphery of the lesion were the most conspicuous differences. In slower types of inflammation, such as tuberculosis and serum sickness,[199] as well as in acute reactions to microtrauma in the rat's mesoappendix[11] and to thermal injury in the hamster's cheek pouch,[200] the same results have been observed. The mechanism of action of cortisone in acute inflammation has been postulated as a protective effect of the endothelium to injury; evidence that it inhibits chemical mediators is at present limited to histamine and leukotaxine.

It has been said that cortisone inhibits phagocytosis, but the evidence is contradictory. With reference to ingestion of particles by free, wandering cells in the inflammatory focus it seems that this hormone has no influence on the actual process of phagocytosis. Gell and Hinde[201] found that cortisone decreases cellular motility, perhaps because of changes in interstitial fluids, and that this would account for the lesser number of phagocytic cells found. Once the particle is ingested, intracellular digestion is slower under the effect of cortisone.[202] Detailed studies of Spain,[203, 204] Duke-Elder and Ashton,[205] Dougherty and Schneebeli[206] and others have shown that the suppressing ef-

fect of cortisone is observed in many animal species including man, and with almost any type of causal agent. An interesting observation is that of Lattes and associates,[207] who found that bacterial infection would inhibit the effect of cortisone in inflammation.

Few other hormones have been studied in this context. Perhaps the only other observation is that of Menkin with ACTH.[208] This author found that exudin, the permeability factor obtained from acid exudates, was inhibited by corticotrophin, and that this effect was direct since it also appeared in adrenalectomized animals.

VI. BIOLOGY OF INFLAMMATION

Reference to some of the definitions of inflammation proposed by different authors reveals that there are two general tendencies: one, to consider inflammation as an essentially protective process, serving the organism as a local defense mechanism; the other tendency is purely descriptive and avoids finalist interpretations. An instance of the first tendency is Payling Wright's definition:[209] "Inflammation is the process by means of which cells and exudate accumulate in irritated tissues and usually tend to protect them from further injury." An example of a purely descriptive definition is Moore's:[210] "Inflammation is the sum total of the changes in the tissues of the animal organism in response to an injurious agent, including the local reaction and the repair of the injury." The main difference in the two tendencies represented by these definitions of inflammation is that the first emphasizes the protective role of the process, while Moore continues by adding, "If the inflammatory reaction is adequate, it minimizes the effect of the injurious agent, destroys the injurious agent, and restores the part to as near normal structure and function as possible. If it is not adequate, there are extensive destruction of tissue, invasion of the body and somatic death."

The foregoing indicates that, although not included in some definitions, the concept of inflammation as a local defense mechanism is implied by most authors. This is only natural, since the apparent final result of the process is the accumulation of exudate in the injured area, and both fluid and cellular elements of the exudate play a very important role in the defense of the organism. The fluid component dilutes the causal agent, thus lowering its concentration in tissues and decreasing its capacity to produce injury. Furthermore, antibodies are present in the fluid and they act by antagonizing the effect of toxins and by favoring phagocytosis. Another role of the fluid component of the exudate is the blocking of lymphatic vessels, and therefore of drainage, of the inflammatory focus. Menkin has suggested that fibrin deposited in tissues and in the lumen of the lymphatic capillaries may act as a filter, hindering spreading and lymphatic dissemination of the causal agent of inflammation.[211] This would be of special significance in inflammatory processes due to bacterial infections. It has been observed, however, that events following the entrance of microorganisms in tissues are determined by what happens during the first 4 to 6 hours,[212] and fibrin clots blocking the lumen of lymphatic vessels appear much later. This was demonstrated by Bangham and associates,[213] who found that intraperitoneal injection of radioactive particles in animals with turpentine peritonitis was followed by rapid accumulation of radioactive material in draining lymph nodes, and that the effect was unmodified for 24 hours; after this period there was a fall in the movement of particles from the peritoneum to the lymph nodes, but by that time the animals were comatose and in severe shock. Young, working with experimental staphylococcus infection in the hamster cheek pouch, found that within 5 hours of infection bacteria were recovered from all outlying areas of the pouches; between 24 and 48 hours there was a sharp decrease of bacteria outside the site of inoculation, and at the end of 3 days the infection was adequately localized to the cheek pouch. Localization was not due to a "walling off" process but probably to delayed inability of bacteria to survive away from the area of inflammation.[214] Cells in the exudate are responsible for phagocytosis, of great significance in local defense.

The protective role of inflammation, so prominent in cases of bacterial infection, becomes less apparent when all other inanimate causal agents are considered. Against these, antibodies and phagocytosis have little or no effect, and they appear as part of a misfired reaction of the organism. Nevertheless, even in these cases inflammation may be taken as part of a general protective reaction, since it acts as a stimulus for repair of damaged tissues. Carrel[215] observed some years ago that open wounds protected with fascia remained indolent for periods of up to two weeks, but when slight irritants were applied healing was immediately started; Schilling and associates[216] have shown that the *in vitro* growth of guinea pig fibroblasts obtained during the early stages of inflammation is similar to that of fibrosarcomas or embryonal tissues; Savlov and Dunphy[217] relate that cortisone inhibition of healing is not present when the hormone is administered two or three days after wounding, implying that inflammation is well developed by that time and can stimulate repair. In a recent review on wound healing, Edwards and Dunphy[218] state that, "These observations suggest a close and possibly causal relation between acute inflammation and subsequent connective tissue proliferation." Therefore, it seems permissible to suppose that, besides its local protective effect, inflammation also acts as a stimulus for tissue repair, contributing in this way to the well-being of the entire organism.

But there are many cases where inflammation is detrimental to the individual. Intracellular parasites which are not destroyed by phagocytic cells represent a potential danger, not only because of the possibility of destruction of the cell with release of the microorganism but also because the cell may be carried away from the local area of inflammation, helping bacterial dissemination. Throughout the period that the microorganism remains within the cellular cytoplasm it is protected from the effect of antibodies and antibiotics. It has also been mentioned that within the inflammatory focus substances may accumulate that inhibit the effect of therapeutic drugs. In some special fields, the battle may be won by inflammation but at a very high price, as it occurs in the eye or in the inner ear, where loss of function is the usual result. Examples of these unhappy results of inflammation could be multiplied, but the foregoing should suffice to show that there are many instances where the wisdom of Nature seems to have failed. But the apparent paradox of a protective mechanism causing an injury worse than the one expected from the effect of the causal agent is resolved when inflammation is considered from a more general viewpoint.

There is no "purpose" in inflammation. To describe it as a defense mechanism is to ignore the largest group of conditions in which it occurs and to concentrate on inflammation caused by infection. And even here the protective role of the inflammatory process has been found to be at fault in many cases. It is not necessary to postulate that inflammation is defensive since it adds nothing to the understanding of the process, but it cannot be denied that on some occasions the results of inflammation are favorable to the individual. Perhaps a more useful description of this process would be as a disturbance of local homeostasis. A characteristic of living organisms is their tendency to maintain a constant internal environment, and the integration of all mechanisms contributing to this constancy is known as homeostasis. Inflammation, the local reaction of tissues to injury, represents a drastic modification of the internal environment of a limited area of the organism: vasodilation, changes in blood flow, phagocytosis, release of chemical mediators and all other phenomena are self-regulated and automatic.[219] Nothing really new is added to the tissues except the injury, no specially created mechanisms come into play. The result is simply an area of enhanced physiologic activity where stimuli and responses are sequentially integrated as in normal tissues. That this physiologic activity will result in the extravascular accumulation of exudate is just an accident, a coincidence blindly working sometimes in favor of the host, sometimes in favor of the parasite, itself not knowing which. The accident may be happy, the coincidence may be useful, and then inflammation is considered protective; on the other hand, the accident may be useless and the coincidence detrimental, and then inflammation fails as a defense mechanism. But these are considerations dealing mostly with the individual; when the inflammatory process is envisaged at the species level, a less stringent interpretation is possible. In this respect, it is better to quote the elegant words of Dubos:[184]

"Even though inflammation frequently has unfavorable effects on the individual, it helps in overcoming infection probably more often than it enhances disease. If its results could be expressed statistically, inflammation would be found in all likelihood to have survival value for the species. In infectious diseases, just as in other physiological and pathological processes, the wisdom of the body is not concerned with the well-being of one individual at a given time, but expresses itself rather in reactions which permit the collectivity—the species or the group—to function, survive, and reproduce itself in a given environment. The importance of inflammation as a protective mechanism against microbial diseases can be measured only on the evolutionary scale."

REFERENCES

1. Hirsch, J. G.: Immunity to infectious diseases: review of some concepts of Metchnikoff, Bact. Rev. *23:*48, 1959.
2. Florey, H. W.: Inflammation, in Florey, H. W. (ed.): General Pathology, ed. 2, Philadelphia, W. B. Saunders, 1958.
3. Jasmin, G., and Robert, A. (eds.): The Mechanism of Inflammation. An International Symposium, Montreal, Acta, 1953.
4. Lewis, T.: The Blood Vessels of the Human Skin and their Responses, London, Shaw and Sons, 1927.
5. Lewis, T.: Vascular reactions of the skin to injury. I. Reaction to stroking; urticaria factitia, Heart *11:*120, 1924.
6. Zweifach, B. W.: Circulatory Changes in the Peripheral Vascular Bed Following Local Injury, in Jasmin, G., and Robert, A. (eds.): The Mechanism of Inflammation. An International Symposium, Montreal, Acta, 1953.
7. Allison, F. J., Jr., Smith, M. R., and Wood, W. B., Jr.: Studies on the pathogenesis of acute inflammation. I. The inflammatory reaction to thermal injury as observed in the rabbit ear chamber, J. Exper. Med. *102:*655, 1955.
8. Bayliss, L. E.: The axial drift of the red cells when blood flows in a narrow tube, J. Physiol. *149:* 593, 1960.
9. Clark, E. R., Clark, E. L., and Rex, R. O.: Observations on changes in blood vascular endothelium in the living animal, Am. J. Anat. *57:* 385, 1935.
10. Clark, E. R., and Clark, E. L.: Observations on the polymorphonuclear leukocytes in the living animal, Am. J. Anat. *59:*123, 1936.
11. Zweifach, B. W.: The exchange of materials between blood vessels and lymph compartments, in Ragan, C. (ed.): Tr. 5th Conf. Connective Tissues, Josiah Macy Jr. Foundation, 1954.
12. Wood, W. B., Jr., Smith, M. R., Perry, W. D., and Berry, J. W.: Studies on the cellular immunology of acute bacteriemia. I. Intravascular leukocytic reaction and surface phagocytosis, J. Exper. Med. *94:*521, 1951.
13. Zweifach, B. W.: Structural makeup of capillary wall, Ann. New York Acad. Sc. *61:*670, 1955.

14. Cerletti, A., and Rothlin, E.: The pharmacological basis of calcium-antihistamine combination, Internat. Arch. Allergy 6:230, 1955.
15. Parrat, J. R., and West, G. B.: Release of 5-hydroxytryptamine and histamine from tissues of the rat, J. Physiol. 137:179, 1957.
16. Rawson, R. A.: The binding of T-1824 and structurally related diazo dyes by the plasma proteins, Am. J. Physiol. 138:708, 1943.
17. Miles, A. A., and Miles, E. M.: Vascular reactions to histamine, histamine liberator and leukotaxine in the skin of guinea pigs, J. Physiol. 118: 228, 1952.
18. Spector, W. G.: The mediation of altered capillary permeability in acute inflammation, J. Path. & Bact. 72:367, 1956.
19. Allison, F., Jr., and Lancaster, M. G.: Studies on the pathogenesis of acute inflammation. I. Changes of endothelial permeability in rabbit ear-chambers injured by heat, Brit. J. Exper. Path. 40:324, 1959.
20. Rigdon, R. H.: A study of capillary permeability and inflammation in the skin of rabbits given adrenalin, Arch. Surg. 41:96, 1940.
21. Burke, J. F., and Miles, A. A.: The sequence of vascular events in early infective inflammation, J. Path. & Bact. 76:1, 1958.
22. Lewis, T., and Grant, R. T.: Vascular reaction of the skin to injury. II. The liberation of histamine-like substance in injured skin; the underlying cause of factitious urticaria and of wheals produced by burning; and observations upon the nervous control of skin reactions, Heart 11: 209, 1924.
23. Krogh, A.: Studies on the capillary motor mechanism. I. The reaction to stimuli and the innervation of the blood vessels in the tongue of the frog, J. Physiol. 53:399, 1920.
24. Hilton, S. M., and Lewis, G. P.: The mechanism of the functional hyperemia in submandibular salivary gland, J. Physiol. 129:253, 1955.
25. Fahraeus, R.: The influence of the rouleau formation of the erythrocytes on the rheology of the blood, Acta med. scandinav. 161:151, 1958.
26. Vejlens, G.: Distribution of leukocytes in vascular system, Acta path. et microbiol. scandinav. Supp. 33:1, 1938.
27. Lutz, B. R.: Intravascular agglutination of the formed elements of the blood, Physiol. Rev. 31: 107, 1951.
28. Landis, E. M.: Micro-injection studies of capillary permeability. I. Factors in the production of capillary stasis, Am. J. Physiol. 81:124, 1927.
29. Whittaker, S. R. F., and Winton, F. R.: The apparent viscosity of blood flowing in the isolated hind limb of the dog, and its variations with corpuscular concentration, J. Physiol. 78:339, 1933.
30. Cohnheim, J.: Inflammation, in Lectures on General Pathology, London, The New Sydenham Society, 1889.
31. Miles, A. A., and Niven, J. S. F.: The enhancement of infection during shock produced by bacterial toxins and other agents, Brit. J. Exper. Path. 36:71, 1955.
32. Abramson, H. A.: The electrical charge of the blood cells of the horse and its relation to the inflammatory process, Cold Spring Harbor Symp. Quant. Biol. 1:92, 1933.
33. Sawyer, P. N., and Pate, J. W.: Bio-electric phenomena as an etiologic factor in intravascular thrombosis, Am. J. Physiol. 175:103, 1953.
34. Allison, F., Jr., and Lancaster, M. G.: Studies on the pathogenesis of acute inflammation. II. The relationship of fibrinogen and fibrin to the leu-

kocytic sticking reaction in ear chambers of rabbits injured by heat, J. Exper. Med. 111:45, 1960.
35. Spector, W. G., and Storey, E.: A factor in estrogen-treated uterus causing leukocyte emigration, J. Path. & Bact. 75:383, 1958.
36. Spector, W. G.: Endogenous Mechanisms in the Acute Inflammatory Reaction, in Collins, D. H. (ed.): Modern Trends in Pathology, London, Butterworth, 1959.
37. Starling, E. H.: On the absorption of fluids from the connective tissue spaces, J. Physiol. 19:312, 1896.
38. Chambers, R., and Zweifach, B. W.: Intercellular cement and capillary permeability, Physiol. Rev. 27:436, 1947.
39. Chambers, R., and Zweifach, B. W.: Capillary endothelial cement in relation to permeability, J. Cell. & Comp. Physiol. 15:255, 1940.
40. Pappenheimer, J. R.: Passage of molecules through capillary walls, Physiol. Rev. 33:387, 1916.
41. Danielli, J. F.: Capillary permeability and oedema in the perfused frog, J. Physiol. 98:109, 1940.
42. Curran, R. C.: The elaboration of mucopolysaccharides by vascular endothelium, J. Path. & Bact. 74:347, 1957.
43. Florey, H. W., Poole, J. C. F., and Meek, G. A.: Endothelial cells and "cement" lines, J. Path. & Bact. 77:625, 1959.
44. Cohn, E. J.: Chemical, physiological and immunological properties and clinical uses of blood derivatives, Experientia 3:125, 1947.
45. Harris, H.: Role of chemotaxis in inflammation, Physiol. Rev. 34:529, 1954.
46. McCutcheon, M.: Chemotaxis in leukocytes, Physiol. Rev. 26:319, 1946.
47. Moon, V. H., Grand, C. G., and Tershakovec, G. A.: Dynamics of inflammation and repair. IV. Chemotactic substances in normal tissues, Arch. Path. 57:44, 1954.
48. Menkin, V.: Studies on inflammation. XIV. Isolation of the factor concerned with increased capillary permeability in injury, J. Exper. Med. 67:129, 1938.
49. McCutcheon, M.: Chemotaxis and locomotion of leukocytes, Ann. New York Acad. Sc. 59:941, 1955.
50. Tompkins, E. H., and Grillo, M. A.: Factor favoring phagocytosis by reticulo-endothelial cells early in inflammation, Am. J. Path. 29:217, 1953.
51. Dodson, L. F., Sanders, A. G., and Florey, H. W.: Observations on tuberculous lesions in a transparent chamber in the rabbit's ear, Brit. J. Exper. Path. 35:338, 1954.
52. Goodman, J. R., and Moore, R.: Electron microscopic study of phagocytosis of staphylococcus by human leukocytes, J. Bact. 71:547, 1956.
53. Goodman, J. R., Moore, R. E., and Baker, R. F.: Electron microscopic study of phagocytosis of staphylococcus by human leukocytes. II. Virulent and non-virulent staphylococci, J. Bact. 72: 736, 1956.
54. Wood, W. B., Jr.: Studies on the cellular immunology of acute bacterial infections, Harvey Lect. 47:72, 1951.
55. Lerner, E. M.: Phagocytosis of bacteria in the absence of antibody and the effect of physical surface. A reinvestigation of "surface phagocytosis," J. Exper. Med. 104:233, 1956.
56. Suter, E.: Interaction between phagocytes and pathogenic microorganisms, Bact. Rev. 20:94, 1956.
57. Salton, M. J. R.: Cell structure and the enzymic lysis of bacteria, J. Gen. Microbiol. 9:512, 1953.
58. Hirsch, J. G.: Phagocytin: a bacterial substance

from polymorphonuclear leukocytes, J. Exper. Med. *103*:589, 1956.

59. Hirsch, J. G.: Studies on the bactericidal action of phagocytin, J. Exper. Med. *103*:613, 1956.

60. Hirsch, J. G.: Further studies on preparation and properties of phagocytin, J. Exper. Med. *111*:323, 1960.

61. Wilson, A. T.: The egestion of phagocytized particles by leukocytes, J. Exper. Med. *98*:305, 1953.

62. Tompsett, R.: Protection of pathogenic staphylococci by phagocytes, Tr. A. Am. Phys. *69*:84, 1956.

63. Shaffer, J. M., Kucera, C. J., and Spink, W. W.: The protection of intracellular Brucella against therapeutic agents and the bactericidal action of serum, J. Exper. Med. *97*:77, 1953.

64. Mackaness, G. B.: The action of drugs on intracellular tubercle bacilli, J. Path. & Bact. *64*:429, 1952.

65. Magoffin, R. L., and Spink, W. W.: The protection of intracellular Brucella against streptomycin alone and in combination with other antibiotics, J. Lab. & Clin. Med. *36*:959, 1950.

66. Rogers, D. E., and Melly, A. M.: Further observations on the behavior of staphylococci within human leukocytes, J. Exper. Med. *111*:533, 1960.

67. Hirsch, J. G., and Church, A. B.: Studies of phagocytosis of group A streptococci by polymorphonuclear leukocytes in vitro, J. Exper. Med. *111*:309, 1960.

68. Gladstone, G. P., and van Heyningen, W. E.: Staphylococcal leucocidins, Brit. J. Exper. Path. *38*:123, 1957.

69. Schneider, H. A.: Nutrition and resistance to infection, Vitamins & Hormones *4*:35, 1946.

70. Chandler, A. C.: Interrelations between nutrition and infectious disease in the tropics, Am. J. Trop. Med. *6*:195, 1957.

71. Minor, R. W. (ed.): Nutrition in infections, Ann. New York Acad. Sc. *63*:175, 1955.

72. Berry, L. J., and Haller, E. C.: The influence of anemia on phagocytic function in rats, Blood, Suppl. *1*:108, 1947.

73. Strumia, M., and Boerner, F.: Phagocytic activity of circulating cells in the various types of leukemias, Am. J. Path. *13*:335, 1937.

74. Silver, R. T., Beal, G. A., Schneiderman, M. A., and McCullough, N. B.: The role of the mature neutrophil in bacterial infections in acute leukemia, Blood *12*:814, 1957.

75. Boggs, D. R.: The cellular composition of inflammatory exudates in human leukemia, Blood *15*:466, 1960.

76. Mudd, S., McCutcheon, M., and Lucké, B.: Phagocytosis, Physiol. Rev. *14*:210, 1934.

77. Berry, L. J., and Spies, T. D.: Phagocytosis, Medicine *28*:239, 1949.

78. Fenn, W. O.: The adhesiveness of leukocytes to solid surfaces, J. Gen. Physiol. *5*:143, 1922.

79. Ponder, E.: The influence of surface charge and of cytoplasmic viscosity on the phagocytosis of a particle, J. Gen. Physiol. *11*:757, 1927–28.

80. Berry, L. J., Starr, L. W., and Haller, E. C.: The effect of surface active agents on phagocytosis, J. Bact. *57*:603, 1949.

81. Karnovsky, M. L., and Sbarra, A. J.: Metabolic changes accompanying the ingestion of particulate matter by cells, Am. J. Clin. Nutrition *8*:147, 1960.

82. Stäehlin, H., Suter, E., and Karnovsky, M. L.: Studies on the interaction between phagocytes and tubercle bacilli. I. Observations on the metabolism of guinea pig leukocytes and the influence of phagocytosis, J. Exper. Med. *104*:121, 1956.

83. Stäehlin, H., Karnovsky, M. L., and Suter, E.: Studies on the interaction between phagocytes and tubercle bacilli. II. The action of phagocytes upon C14-labelled tubercle bacilli, J. Exper. Med. *104*:137, 1956.

84. Stäehlin, H., Karnovsky, M. L., Farnham, A. E., and Suter, E.: Studies on the interaction between phagocytes and tubercle bacilli. III. Some metabolic effects in guinea pigs associated with infection with tubercle bacilli, J. Exper. Med. *105*:265, 1957.

85. Sbarra, A. J., and Karnovsky, M. L.: The biochemical basis of phagocytosis. I. Metabolic changes during the ingestion of particles by polymorphonuclear leukocytes, J. Biol. Chem. *234*:1355, 1959.

86. Cohn, Z. A., and Morse, S. I.: Functional and metabolic properties of polymorphonuclear leucocytes. I. Observations on the requirements and consequences of particle ingestion, J. Exper. Med. *111*:667, 1960.

87. Cohn, Z. A., and Morse, S. I.: Functional and metabolic properties of polymorphonuclear leucocytes. II. The influence of a lipopolysaccharide endotoxin, J. Exper. Med. *111*:689, 1960.

88. Whitby, J. L., and Rowley, D.: The role of macrophages in the elimination of bacteria from the mouse peritoneum, Brit. J. Exper. Path. *40*:358, 1959.

89. Borrel, A.: Tuberculose pulmonaire expérimentale. Étude anatomo-pathologique du processus obtenu par injéction veineuse, Ann. Inst. Pasteur *7*:593, 1893.

90. Menkin, V., and Warner, C. R.: Studies on inflammation. XIII. Carbohydrate metabolism, local acidosis and the cytological picture in inflammation, Am. J. Path. *13*:25, 1937.

91. Menkin, V.: Biochemical Mechanisms in Inflammation, Springfield, Charles C Thomas, 1956.

92. Steinberg, B., and Dietz, A.: Inflammation of serous surfaces. Hydrogen ion concentration in relation to cell type, Arch. Path. *25*:777, 1938.

93. Harris, H.: Chemotaxis of monocytes, Brit. J. Exper. Path. *34*:276, 1953.

94. Page, A. R., and Good, R. A.: A clinical and experimental study of the function of neutrophils in the inflammatory response, Am. J. Path. *34*:645, 1958.

95. Rebuck, J. W., Smith, R. W., and Margulis, R. R.: The modification of leukocytic function in human windows by ACTH, Gastroenterology *19*:644, 1951.

96. Carlisle, J. W., and Good, R. A.: The inflammatory cycle, Am. J. Dis. Child. *99*:193, 1960.

97. Roberts, J. C., Jr.: Role of the Lymphocyte in Antibody Formation, in Rebuck, J. W. (ed.): The Lymphocyte and Lymphocytic Tissue, New York, Paul B. Hoeber, 1960.

98. Rebuck, J. W. (ed.): The Lymphocyte and Lymphocytic Tissue, New York, Paul B. Hoeber, 1960.

99. Costero, I.: Linfocitosis intersticial en el reumatismo y en otros procesos inflammatorios, Arch. Inst. cardiol. México *26*:471, 1946.

100. Sicracki, J. C., and Rebuck, J. W.: Role of the Lymphocyte in Inflammation, in Rebuck, J. W. (ed.): The Lymphocyte and Lymphocytic Tissue, New York, Paul B. Hoeber, 1960.

101. Forbus, W. D.: Granulomatous Inflammation, Springfield, Charles C Thomas, 1950.

102. Forbus, W. D.: Granulomatous inflammation; a clinical and pathological challenge, Am. J. Clin. Path. *25*:927, 1955.

103. Clark, R. M., and Anderson, W.: Rheumatic activity in auricular appendages removed at mitral valvoplasty, Am. J. Path. *31:*809, 1955.

104. Saphir, O.: The Aschoff nodule, Am. J. Clin. Path. *31:*534, 1959.

105. Tedeschi, G. C., Wagner, B. M., and Pani, K. C.: Studies in rheumatic fever. I. The clinical significance of the Aschoff body based on morphologic observations, Arch. Path. *60:*408, 1955.

106. Lannigan, R.: The rheumatic process in the left auricular appendage, J. Path. & Bact. *77:*49, 1959.

107. Longcope, W. T., and Freiman, D. G.: A study of sarcoidosis, Medicine *31:*1, 1952.

108. Weed, L. A., and Dahlin, D. C.: Bacteriologic examination of tissues removed for biopsy, Am. J. Clin. Path. *20:*116, 1950.

109. Schulz, D. M., Tucker, E. B., and McLoughlin, P. T.: Observations on the laboratory diagnosis of granulomatous inflammation of the lung, Am. J. Clin. Path. *29:*28, 1958.

110. Goddard, J. W.: Granuloma, a characteristic "qualitative" change in focal anaphylactic inflammation, Am. J. Path. *23:*943, 1947.

111. Goldgraber, M. B., and Kirsner, J. B.: Granulomatous lesions, an expression of a hypersensitive state: an experimental study, Arch. Path. *66:*618, 1958.

112. Auerbach, S. H., Mims, O. M., and Goodpasture, E. W.: Pulmonary fibrosis secondary to pneumonia, Am. J. Path. *28:*69, 1952.

113. Masson, P., Riopelle, J. L., and Martin, P.: Poumon rhumatismale, Ann. d'anat. Path. *14:*359, 1937.

114. Cuéllar, A., and Pérez Tamayo, R.: Estudio anatomoclínico de la neumonitis reumática, Arch. Inst. cardiol. México *21:*594, 1951.

115. Hopps, H. C., and Wissler, R. W.: Uremic pneumonitis, Am. J. Path. *31:*261, 1955.

116. Herbut, P. A., and Manges, W. E.: The Masson body in rheumatic pneumonia, Am. J. Path. *21:*741, 1945.

117. Biagi, F. F., Villa Treviño, S., Navarrete, F., and Grácia, P.: Amibiasis hepática incipiente, Rev. Latinoamer. Anat. Pat. *1:*163, 1957.

118. Brandt, H., and Alonso, P.: Pathology of amebic abscess of the liver. In preparation.

119. Goddard, J. W.: Vascular changes in the Arthus phenomenon, Arch. Path. *66:*384, 1958.

120. Goldgraber, M. B., and Kirsner, J. B.: The Arthus phenomenon in the colon of rabbits, Arch. Path. *67:*556, 1957.

121. Rössle, R.: Die geweblichen Ausserungen der Allergie, Wien. klin. Wchnschr. *45:*609, 648, 1932.

122. Gerlach, W.: Studien über hyperergische Entzündung, Virchows Arch. path. Anat. *247:*294, 1923.

123. Frölich, A.: Ueber lokale gewebliche Anaphylaxie, Ztschr. Immunitätsforsch. *20:*476, 1913–14.

124. More, R. H., and Movat, H. Z.: Cellular and intercellular changes in the Arthus phenomenon, Arch. Path. *67:*679, 1959.

125. More, R. H., and Movat, H. Z.: Character and significance of the cellular response in the collagen diseases and experimental hypersensitivity, Lab. Invest. *8:*873, 1959.

126. Dixon, F. J., Vázquez, J. J., Weigle, W. O., and Cochrane, C. G.: Pathogenesis of serum sickness, Arch. Path. *65:*18, 1958.

127. Mellors, R. C., Ortega, L. G., and Holman, H. R.: Role of gammaglobulins in pathogenesis of renal lesions in systemic lupus erythematosus and chronic membranous glomerulonephritis with an observation on the lupus erythematosus cell reaction, J. Exper. Med. *106:*191, 1957.

128. White, R. G., Coons, A. H., and Connolly, J. M.: Studies on antibody production. III. The alum granuloma, J. Exper. Med. *102:*73, 1955.

129. Askonas, B. A., and White, R. G.: Sites of antibody production in the guinea pig: the relation between in vitro synthesis of anti-ovalbumin and -globulin, and distribution of antibody-containing plasma cells, Brit. J. Exper. Path. *37:*61, 1956.

130. Coons, A. H., Leduc, E. H., and Connolly, J. M.: Studies on antibody production. I. A method for the histochemical demonstration of specific antibody and its application to a study of the hyperimmune rabbit, J. Exper. Med. *102:*49, 1955.

131. Movat, H. Z., More, R. H., and Wolochow, D.: Cellular and intercellular changes after mechanical or radiation injury of connective tissue, Brit. J. Exper. Path. *41:*97, 1960.

132. Klemperer, P.: The concept of collagen diseases, Am. J. Path. *26:*505, 1950.

133. Klemperer, P.: Diseases of the collagen system, Bull. New York Acad. Med. *23:*581, 1947.

134. Costero, I.: Tratado de Anatomía Patológica, Atlante, México, 1948.

135. Rosenthal, S. R., Samet, C., Winzler, R. J., and Shkolnik, S.: Substances released from the skin following thermal injury. I. Histamine and proteins, J. Clin. Invest. *36:*38, 1957.

136. Zon, L., Ceder, E. T., and Crigler, C.: Presence of histamine in inflammatory lesions, Arch. Path. *33:*452, 1942.

137. Adam, H. M.: Excretion of histamine in human urine, Quart. J. Exper. Physiol. *35:*281, 1950.

138. Hunter, R. B., and Dunlop, D. M.: A review of anti-histamine drugs, Quart. J. Med. *17:*271, 1948.

139. Bain, W. A.: Quantitative comparison of histamine antagonists in man, Proc. Roy. Soc. Med. *42:*615, 1949.

140. Brocklehurst, W. E., Humphrey, J. H., and Perry, W. L. M.: The role of histamine in cutaneous antigen-antibody reactions in the rat, J. Physiol. *129:*305, 1955.

141. Weeks, R. E., and Gunner, R. M.: Effect of tripelennamine HCl on acute inflammation, Arch. Path. *48:*148, 1949.

142. Spector, W. G., and Willoughby, D. A.: The demonstration of the role of mediators in turpentine pleurisy in rats by experimental suppression of the inflammatory changes, J. Path. & Bact. *77:*1, 1959.

143. Menkin, V.: Studies in inflammation. XII. Mechanism of increased capillary permeability. A critique of the histamine hypothesis, J. Exper. Med. *64:*485, 1936.

144. Cullumbine, H., and Rydon, H. N.: A study of the formation, properties and partial purification of leucotaxine, Brit. J. Exper. Path. *27:*33, 1946.

145. Duthie, E. S., and Chain, E.: A polypeptide responsible for some of the phenomena of acute inflammation, Brit. J. Exper. Path. *20:*417, 1939.

146. Spector, W. G.: The role of some higher peptides in inflammation, J. Path. & Bact. *63:*93, 1951.

147. Spector, W. G.: The mediation of altered capillary permeability in acute inflammation, J. Path. & Bact. *72:*367, 1956.

148. Menkin, V.: Further studies on mechanism of increased capillary permeability in inflammation with the aid of cortisone and ACTH, Proc. Soc. Exper. Biol. & Med. *77:*592, 1951.

149. Rowley, D. A., and Benditt, E. P.: 5-Hydroxytryptamine and histamine as mediators of the vascular injury produced by agents which damage mast cells in rats, J. Exper. Med. *103:*399, 1956.

150. Benditt, E. P., Wong, A. L., Arase, M., and Roeper, E.: 5-Hydroxytryptamine in tissue mast cells, Proc. Soc. Exper. Biol. & Med. *90:*303, 1955.

151. Parrat, J. R., and West, G. B.: 5-Hydroxytryptamine in tissue mast cells, J. Physiol. *137:*169, 1957.

152. Sparrow, E. M., and Wilhelm, D. L.: Species differences in susceptibility to capillary permeability factors. Histamine, 5-hydroxytryptamine and compound 48/80, J. Physiol. *137:*51, 1957.

153. Abramovitz, A. A., Money, W. L., Zarrow, M. X., Talmage, R. U. N., Kleinholz, L. H., and Hisaw, F. L.: Preparation, biological assay and properties of relaxin. Endocrinology *34:*103, 1944.

154. Storey, E.: Relaxation in the pubic symphysis of the mouse during pregnancy and after relaxin administration, with special reference to the behaviour of collagen, J. Path. & Bact. *74:*147, 1957.

155. Miles, A. A., and Wilhelm, D. L.: Enzyme-like globulins from serum reproducing the vascular phenomena of inflammation. I. An activable permeability factor and its inhibitor in guinea-pig serum, Brit. J. Exper. Path. *36:*71, 1955.

156. Wilhelm, D. L., Miles, A. A., and McKay, M. E.: Enzyme-like globulins from serum reproducing the vascular phenomena of inflammation. II. Isolation and properties of the permeability factor and its inhibitor, Brit. J. Exper. Path. *36:*82, 1955.

157. Wilhelm, D. L., Mill, P. J., and Miles, A. A.: Enzyme-like globulins from serum reproducing the vascular phenomena of inflammation. III. Further observations on the permeability factor and its inhibitor in guinea-pig serum, Brit. J. Exper. Path. *38:*446, 1957.

158. Wilhelm, D. L., Mill, P. J., Sparrow, E. M., McKay, M. E., and Miles, A. A.: Enzyme-like globulins from serum reproducing the vascular phenomena of inflammation. IV. Activable permeability factor and its inhibitor in the serum of the rat and the rabbit, Brit. J. Exper. Path. *39:*228, 1959.

159. Elder, J. M., and Miles, A. A.: Enzyme-like globulins from serum reproducing the vascular phenomena of inflammation. V. Activable permeability factor in human serum, Brit. J. Exper. Path. *39:*335, 1958.

160. Spector, W. G.: Activation of a globulin system controlling capillary permeability in inflammation, J. Path. & Bact. *74:*67, 1957.

161. Spector, W. G., and Willoughby, D. A.: The suppression by anti-esterases of increased capillary permeability in acute inflammation, J. Path. & Bact. *79:*21, 1960.

162. Armstrong, D., Jepson, J. B., Keele, C. A., and Stewart, J. W.: Pain-producing substance in human inflammatory exudates and plasma, J. Physiol. *135:*350, 1957.

163. Spector, W. G., and Willoughby, D. A.: Experimental suppression of increased capillary permeability in thermal burns in rats, Nature *182:*949, 1958.

164. Moulton, R., Spector, W. G., and Willoughby, D. A.: Histamine release and pain produced by xanthosine and related compounds, Brit. J. Pharmacol. *12:*365, 1957.

165. Menkin, V.: Chemical basis of injury in inflammation, Arch. Path. *36:*269, 1943.

166. Feldberg, W.: Distribution of histamine in the body, in Ciba Foundation Symposium on Histamine, London, J. & A. Churchill, 1956.

167. Fulton, G. P., Maynard, F. L., Riley, J. F., and West, G. B.: Humoral aspects of tissue mast cells, Physiol. Rev. *37:*221, 1957.

168. Humphrey, J. H., and Jaques, R.: The histamine and 5-hydroxytryptamine content of platelets and leukocytes in various species, J. Physiol. *124:*305, 1954.

169. Paton, W. D. M.: Histamine release by compounds of simple chemical structure, Pharmacol. Rev. *9:*269, 1957.

170. Uvnäs, B.: The mechanism of histamine liberation, J. Pharmacol. *10:*1, 1958.

171. Ungar, G.: Mechanism of histamine release, in Ciba Foundation Symposium on Histamine, London, J. & A. Churchill, 1956.

172. McIntire, F. C.: Mechanism of histamine release, in Ciba Foundation Symposium on Histamine, London, J. & A. Churchill, 1956.

173. Dale, H. H.: Antihistamine substances, Brit. M. J. *2:*281, 1948.

174. Riley, J. F.: The Mast Cells, Edinburgh and London, E. & S. Livingstone, 1959.

175. Menkin, V.: Biochemical mechanism in inflammation, Brit. M. J. *1:*1521, 1960.

176. Spector, W. G.: Substances which affect capillary permeability, Pharmacol. Rev. *10:*475, 1958.

177. Erspamer, V.: The distribution of 5-hydroxytryptamine, in Ciba Foundation Symposium on Hypertension, Humoral and Neurogenic Factors, London, J. & A. Churchill, 1954.

178. Page, I.: Serotonin (5-hydroxytryptamine); the last four years, Physiol. Rev. *38:*277, 1958.

179. Toh, C. C.: The presence of a hydroxytryptamine (serotonin) liberator in the gastrointestinal tract, J. Physiol. *138:*488, 1957.

180. Menkin, V.: Biology of inflammation, Science *123:*527, 1956.

181. Menkin, V.: Chemical mediators in relation to cytologic constituents in inflammation, Am. J. Path. *34:*921, 1958.

182. McGovern, V. J.: The mechanism of inflammation, J. Path. & Bact. *73:*99, 1957.

183. Robb-Smith, A. H. T.: Some aspects of inflammation and infection, Lancet *1:*699, 1957.

184. Dubos, R. J.: Biochemical Determinants of Microbial Disease, Cambridge, Harvard University Press, 1954.

185. Frunder, H.: Der Stoffwechsel des entzundeten und geschadigten Gewebes, in Jasmin, G., and Robert, A. (eds.): The Mechanism of Inflammation. An International Symposium, Montreal, Acta, 1953.

186. Kelleg, W. W., Scadron, E. N., and Shiners, B. M.: Hydrogen ion concentration in exudates of pneumococcus infection, J. Exper. Med. *67:*659, 1938.

187. Dubos, R. J.: Effect of the composition of the gaseous and aqueous environment on the survival of tubercle bacilli *in vitro,* J. Exper. Med. *97:*357, 1953.

188. Dubos, R. J.: Effect of ketone bodies and other metabolites on the survival and multiplication of staphylococci and tubercle bacilli, J. Exper. Med. *98:*145, 1953.

189. Bojalil, L. F., and Coria, R.: Recovery of tubercle bacilli from resected pulmonary tuberculous lesions with the use of four different media, Acta tuberc. scandinav. *34:*260, 1957.

189a. Bastarrachea, F., and Cicero, R.: Viabilidad y resistencia del bacilo tuberculoso en las lesiones pulmonares, Rev. Latinoamer. Microbiol. *1:*171, 1958.

190. Mackaness, G. B., and Smith, N.: The bactericidal action of isoniazid, streptomycin and ter-

ramycin on extracellular and intracellular tubercle bacilli, Am. Rev. Tuberc. *67:*322, 1953.

191. Long, E. R.: The Chemistry and Chemotherapy of Tuberculosis, ed. 3, Baltimore, Williams and Wilkins, 1958.

192. Finland, M.: Emergence of antibiotic-resistant bacteria, New Eng. J. Med. *253:*909, 1019, 1955.

193. McDermott, W.: The Nature of the Lesion and the Response to Antimicrobial Therapy, in McLeod, C. M. (ed.): Evaluation of Chemotherapeutic Agents, New York, Columbia University Press, 1949.

194. Menkin, V.: Effect of adrenal cortex extract on capillary permeability, Am. J. Physiol. *129:*691, 1940.

195. Menkin, V.. Effects of cortisone on the mechanism of increased capillary permeability to trypan blue in inflammation, Am. J. Physiol. *166:*509, 1951.

196. Selye, H.: The Part of Inflammation in the Local Adaptation Syndrome, in Jasmin, G., and Robert, A. (eds.): The Mechanism of Inflammation. An International Symposium, Montreal, Acta, 1953.

197. Selye, H.: Use of "granuloma pouch" technic in the study of antiphlogistic corticoids, Proc. Soc. Exper. Biol. & Med. *82:*328, 1953.

198. Allison, F., Jr., Smith, M. R., and Wood, W. B., Jr.: Studies on the pathogenesis of acute inflammation. II. The action of cortisone on the inflammatory response to thermal injury, J. Exper. Med. *102:*669, 1955.

199. Ebert, R. H., and Barclay, W. R.: Changes in connective tissue reaction induced by cortisone, Ann. Int. Med. *37:*506, 1952.

200. Shulman, M. H., Fulton, G. P., and Moront, G. P.: Effect of cortisone on the healing of localized burns in the hamster cheek pouch, New Eng. J. Med. *251:*257, 1954.

201. Gell, P. G. H., and Hinde, I. T.: The effect of cortisone on macrophage activity in mice, Brit. J. Exper. Path. *33:*273, 1953.

202. Clawson, B. J., and Nerenberg, S. T.: Effect of large doses of cortisone upon ability of reticuloendothelial cells to phagocytose streptococci, J. Lab. & Clin. Med. *42:*746, 1953.

203. Spain, D. M., Molomut, N., and Haber, A.: Studies of the cortisone effects on the inflammatory response. I. Alterations of the histo-

pathology of chemically induced inflammation, J. Lab. & Clin. Med. *39:*383, 1952.

204. Spain, D. M., Molomut, N., and Haber, A.: Biological studies on cortisone in mice, Science *112:*335, 1950.

205. Duke-Elder, S., and Ashton, N.: Action of cortisone on tissue reactions of inflammation and repair with special reference to the eye, Brit. J. Ophth. *35:*695, 1951.

206. Dougherty, T. F., and Schneebeli, G. L.: Role of cortisone in regulation of inflammation, Proc. Soc. Exper. Biol. & Med. *75:*854, 1950.

207. Lattes, R., Martin, J. R., and Ragan, C.: Suppression of cortisone effect on repair in the presence of local bacterial infection, Am. J. Path. *30:*901, 1954.

208. Menkin, V.: Modern views on inflammation, Internat. Arch. Allergy *4:*131, 1953.

209. Payling Wright, G.: An Introduction to Pathology, ed. 2, London, Longmans Green, 1954.

210. Moore, R. A.: A Textbook of Pathology, ed. 2, Philadelphia, W. B. Saunders, 1951.

211. Menkin, V.: The significance of lymphatic blockade in immunity, Ann. New York Acad. Sc. *46:*789, 1946.

212. Miles, A. A.: The sequence of vascular events in early infective inflammation, J. Path. & Bact. *76:*1, 1958.

213. Bangham, A. D., Magee, P. M., and Osborn, S. B.: The effect of inflammation and other factors on the movement of radioactive glass particles from the peritoneal cavity, Brit. J. Exper. Path. *33:*1, 1953.

214. Young, G.: Experimental staphylococcus infection in the hamster cheek pouch: The process of localization, J. Exper. Med. *99:*299, 1954.

215. Carrel, A.: Cicatrization of wounds. XII. Factors initiating regeneration, J. Exper. Med. *34:*425, 1921.

216. Schilling, J. A., Favata, B. V., and Radanovitch, M.: Studies of fibroplasia in wound healing, Surg. Gynec. & Obst. *96:*143, 1953.

217. Savlov, E. D., and Dunphy, J. E.: Healing of disrupted and resutured wounds, Surgery *36:*362, 1954.

218. Edwards, L. C., and Dunphy, J. E.: Wound healing, New Eng. J. Med. *259:*224, 1958.

219. Cameron, R. G.: The chemical mediation in inflammation, Rev. Latinoamer. Anat. Pat. *3:*5, 1959.

CHAPTER III

REPAIR, REGENERATION

AND TISSUE TRANSPLANTATION

I. INTRODUCTION

In the previous chapter some aspects of the local, unspecific reaction of connective tissues to injury were reviewed. It was mentioned that cell death and disintegration are frequently seen during inflammation, and that they probably play an important role in starting the entire sequence of events. Following tissue injury, and therefore almost simultaneous with the inception of the inflammatory process, another group of phenomena develops, the final result of which will be the restitution of continuity in the injured area. In fact, this group of phenomena is difficult to separate from the inflammatory reaction, and many authors consider inflammation and repair together. That this is not done here is both because it makes description easier, and also because some details of the reparative process differ according to the type of injured tissue. Furthermore, parenchymatous organs such as the liver or kidney, epithelial surfaces such as the skin or the gastrointestinal mucosa, are regenerated following stimuli and mechanisms probably different from those involved in repair of mesenchymatous organs such as bone, blood and connective tissue. In addition, with extensive loss of substance the organism may require outside help to accomplish an adequate restitution, and for this purpose different types of tissue transplants have been developed. Tissue transplantation has opened a fascinating new field of research, which so far has contributed much to the understanding of many apparently unrelated phenomena, besides giving promise of finding means of alleviating pathologic conditions which are presently incurable. For these reasons repair, regeneration and tissue transplantation are separately discussed in this chapter.

Connective tissue is widely disseminated throughout the organism, so that few areas are devoid of it. Tissue injury will almost invariably affect a section of connective tissue, with or without involvement of epithelial elements. In cases where the lesion is small or destruction of parenchyma is minimal, the speed of repair of connective tissue will be beneficial for the organism as a whole since healing is accomplished quite rapidly. But when the lesion includes major portions of epithelial elements, such as skin or parenchymatous organs, rapid proliferation of connective tissues will have the detrimental effect of occupying the space destined to the slower growing epithelial cells. Anatomic integrity may be regained but function will be defective, as the connective tissue cells are incapable of substituting highly differentiated and specialized epithelial elements. This disadvantage of healing in parenchymatous organs has found a picturesque expression in the words of Mac-Crae:[1]

"The parenchymatous cell is the professional man in a community, specially trained, not to be replaced but by one of his own class, impressionable by even slight external stimuli, not prone to be physically hardy, not overgiven to reproduction. The supporting cell, on the other hand, is its laboring-class brother, not trained in any high special task, whose supportive work can be replaced by any kind of tissue, even scar tissue, not readily impressionable even by powerful external stimuli, physically strong, and ready in reproduction. These two cells lie side by side in the kidney, exposed to the same toxic influences, but reacting to them each in its own way. A toxin strong enough seriously to damage the high-class cell is only strong enough to irritate the low-class cell to reproduction. When the high-class cell is killed by toxin, in the absence of regeneration by the remaining tubular cells, it leaves no one of its kind in its stead, and its place is occupied, but its function is not performed, by the progeny of its laboring-class brother."

Injury is accompanied by profound changes both at the local and systemic levels. The latter are discussed in detail in Chapter X, while the former are presented in this section. The term regeneration is used when specialized cells proliferate and reestablish the anatomic integrity of a parenchymatous organ or epithelial surface. Repair is synonymous with healing by scar formation, which is only proliferation of connective tissues. Both phenomena are treated separately in the following pages, and at the end a summary of some general principles of tissue transplantation is given.

II. REPAIR

As soon as a lesion is produced in loose connective tissue (the process is similar in different forms of connective tissues, so the loose, areolar type will be used throughout this description) a series of phenomena develop which will result in two different situations. One, inflammation, will lead to the extravascular accumulation of fluid and cells; the other, repair, will continue until anatomic continuity has been reestablished. There is a great deal of overlapping in time of these two different processes, and it has been mentioned that chronic inflammation may be recognized not only by the peculiarities of the exudate, but also by the prolonged coexistence of inflammatory and reparative processes. But time overlapping is no reason to lump together two entirely different phenomena; at most, it only forces an arbitrary decision as to the moment when they depart from each other. Keeping in mind the final results of these two processes, the decision is not difficult to make; repair begins with mobilization of tissue cells which do not participate in phagocytosis but in the laying down of connective tissue.

Before entering a discussion of the different stages in wound healing, a further consideration is necessary. Repair may be normal, or else it may acquire pathologic features. Normal wound healing is *sine qua non* for surgery; without tissue repair the surgeon would find it impossible to cut, dissect and resect. It can even be said that without wound healing surgery would not only be impossible but needless, since life is difficult to conceive under these circumstances. Furthermore, wound healing may be defective or exuberant in response to many different factors, some well known, some only guessed at, many probably unknown. Normal and pathologic wound healing are

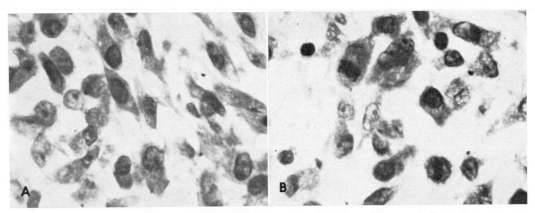

FIG. 3–1. Young fibroblasts proliferating a few hours after infliction of a wound. In B there are two normal mitotic figures.

separately considered in the following paragraphs.

A. Normal Wound Healing. 1. *The Two Types of Normal Wound Healing.* When an aseptic wound is produced without loss of substance and the margins of the wound are placed in contact again, the process of healing that takes place is known as "healing by first intention;" this is what happens with the vast majority of surgical incisions. On the other hand, a loss of substance introduces several modifications in the process of repair, which is then referred to as "healing by second intention" or "by granulation." These modifications are only quantitative, however, so the sequence of phenomena is presented using healing by first intention as an example and the differences will be noted as they arise.

2. *Sequence of Phenomena in Wound Healing.* The first studies of wound healing were carried out on fixed sections of tissues obtained at different stages of the process. Thus, the basis of present day knowledge was established, and more recent developments such as *in vivo* observation, tensile strength, histochemistry and microchemistry, have only added details to the fundamental core of accumulated facts. For the sake of convenience, wound healing may be described in three separate sections: (a) cellular activity, (b) vascular proliferation and, (c) deposit of intercellular substances. It must be remembered, however, that all these phenomena are intimately related, both causally as well as in time.

a. CELLULAR ACTIVITY. The decision has been made to consider the beginning of repair as simultaneous with the mobilization of tissue cells which do not participate in phagocytosis. At this time, leukocytes and macrophages are observed "clearing" the injured area of hemorrhage and necrotic debris; there is edema with accumulation of many plasmatic substances, and the blood vessels are dilated. Lying free in the tissue spaces, and mainly in the immediate neighborhood of capillaries, undifferentiated connective tissue cells known as histiocytes can be seen in normal tissues; these are the first cells to become activated and their participation marks the beginning of healing. Histiocytes show ameboid movements in the direction of the lesion, which they reach a short time before there is vascular proliferation; they move at an average speed of 0.2 μ in 24 hours. With neoformation of capillaries many more histiocytes penetrate the area of injury. They are round or pyriform with abundant, acidophilic cytoplasm and a round, intensely basophilic and homogeneous nucleus. Their phagocytic capacity may be demonstrated by introducing carbon particles or a dye in a clear chamber in the rabbit's ear; the cells can be seen to ingest these particles.[2] In addition, they show intense mitotic activity and even abnormal, bizarre shapes which may be mistaken by the unaware for a malignant tumor (Fig. 3–1). They are, however, nothing but young fibroblasts penetrating the injured area and in an early stage of activity.

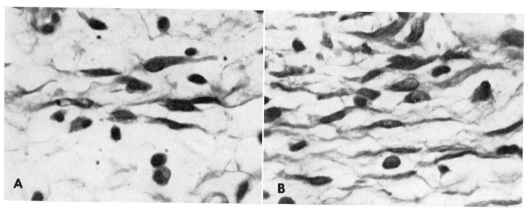

FIG. 3–2. Early polarization of fibroblasts, showing continuity of cytoplasm with fine, wavy fibrils. Extracellular fibers are more abundant in *B*.

The controversy over the origin of these cells, in which some authors claimed that they derived from undifferentiated histiocytes[3] while others postulated that fibroblasts could originate only from other fibroblasts,[4] has been solved by Costero with his concept of nomicoplasia.[5] According to this author, most if not all connective tissue cells have the inherent capacity to lay down fibers, whatever their quiescent morphology may be, and this capacity is fatefully developed upon stimulation. Therefore, it is of little significance to argue what the origin of fiber-producing cells is when the common final end of many connective tissue elements is the formation of fibers (*see* Chapter IV). In the early stages of mobilization, histiocytes and/or fibroblasts present the morphology just described for two or three days after injury, and then many elements adopt a more or less well defined star-shape, with very fine protoplasmic prolongations, granular cytoplasm and pale nucleus. At this stage fibroblastic cells are still irregular in distribution but are more numerous around blood vessels; the protoplasmic prolongations may be stained now with silver and are therefore known as argyrophilic. They form a relatively dense and fine network around the cell body, which becomes looser in the interstitial spaces (Fig. 3–2). From approximately the fourth day on, fibroblasts become bipolar cells, with less abundant, elongated cytoplasm, very fine intracytoplasmic fibrils and spindle-shaped, darker nuclei with pointed ends. These cells are arranged per-

pendicular to blood vessels; their protoplasmic prolongations are only condensations of intracellular fibrils and extend for longer distances. They not only take silver stains avidly, but may be revealed by aniline dyes such as Mallory's aniline blue, Van Gieson's stain or Masson's trichromic mixture. At this time, fibroblasts have changed not only their morphologic nature, but also their functional activity and are actively engaged in laying down interstitial fibrils (Fig. 3–3). From then on, and as time elapses, cells become less and less conspicuous and are replaced by fibers, so that at the end of 8 to 10 days the cellular cytoplasm is much smaller and elongated, the nucleus is also reduced in size and hyperchromatic, and fewer elements are visible between the fully

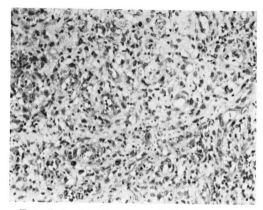

FIG. 3–3. Proliferation of blood vessels in wound healing, with many ovoid or pyriform fibroblasts arranged mainly near capillaries.

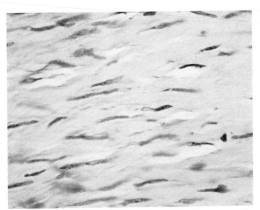

FIG. 3–4. Fibrocytes in an old scar. These cells are probably inactive.

developed collagen bundles (Fig. 3–4). This is the third and final stage of their morphologic and functional evolution, in which they remain for an unknown but probably long period. When this stage is reached the cells are known as fibrocytes; their metabolic functions and role in the maintenance of connective tissues remain to be disclosed. It has been shown, however, that fibrocytes may be awakened again to activity by means of certain stimuli,[6] so that they cannot be considered as "old" but only as quiescent.

In summary, cellular activity during wound healing goes through three different stages in which morphologic and functional changes are parallel. The first stage is one of mobilization and proliferation; the second is characterized by the laying down of fibers, and the third by apparent inactivity. The functional meaning of these three morphologic aspects is discussed in connection with the deposit of intercellular substances. Throughout this period other cells are present in the area of repair, such as leukocytes, macrophages and lymphocytes, but they seem to play no role in healing.

b. VASCULAR PROLIFERATION. This phenomenon may be studied in the clear chamber of the rabbit's ear, as has been done by Clark and Clark,[7] Pullinger and Florey[8] and others.[9] It is one of the most spectacular events of repair, remaining conspicuous for several days until it regresses almost completely; a scar is usually less vascularized than normal tissues. The first vascular buds appear two or three days after injury, originating from preexisting vessels close to the lesion as solid prolongations made up of endothelial cells. They grow towards the area of injury by means of mitoses and cytoplasmic elongation at a speed comparable to that of fibroblasts. Capillary buds show a fine prolongation in the free end, similar to a ship's fender-beam;[10] as this structure grows a lumen develops in the proximal portion, where red cells and leukocytes can be seen animated by pulsating movements synchronous with the heart beat. The vascular sproutings anastomose with each other and form arches at different levels between the lesion and the periphery; blood can be seen circulating through these arches sometimes in one direction, sometimes in the opposite. Not all capillary buds acquire a permanent circulation since many are reabsorbed and others never complete an anastomosis, but those with a definitive circulation differentiate into arterioles, capillaries and venules. Apparently, this differentiation depends on the distance of the bud from the parent arteriole, since it probably requires the presence of contractile elements, which are derived from vessels of greater caliber than capillaries. At the time of maximal development of vascular proliferation the area of repair has more blood vessels than any other in the organism (Fig. 3–5); when there is loss of substance the neoformed capillaries bulge on the surface of the lesion and can be seen grossly as small, reddish granulations, so the term "granulation tissue" is justified. In large wounds the presence of granulation tissue is a good sign since it indicates that the organism is capable of repairing the defect through vigorous proliferation. Plastic sur-

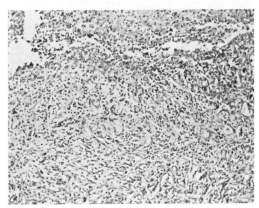

FIG. 3–5. Granulation tissue with abundant vascular proliferation.

geons prefer to place their grafts on healthy granulation tissue since transplants will "take" better than when vascular proliferation is poor. The neoformed vessels are more permeable to plasma proteins than normal capillaries and also have a greater diameter; with passage of time their structure becomes indistinguishable from that of permanent blood vessels. In cases of chronic inflammation, where there is coexistence of vascular proliferation with signs of activity of the inflammatory process, endothelial cells may form solid clumps or nests and since their structure and organization are rather atypical, they may be mistaken for malignant tumors (Fig. 3–6); this is especially true of the small nodules formed at times in the external orifice of the female urethra, known as "caruncle."[11] Larger masses of inflammatory tissue with prominent vascular neoformation are known as "pyogenic granulomas;"[12] they are nothing but exuberant repair of small injuries with exaggerated proliferation of granulation tissue, and are especially frequent in the oral mucosa (Fig. 3–7).

After approximately the sixth day of injury, proliferated vessels tend to decrease in size and number, and at the end of 8 to 10 days there are only scarce and narrow capillaries between the collagen bundles. Weeks or months later the scar will show the characteristic whitish color, indicating the lack of blood vessels, which can be confirmed on microscopic examination, where capillaries are difficult to find between the

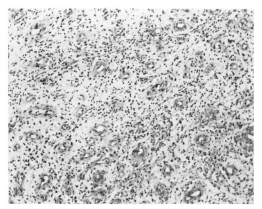

Fig. 3–7. Pyogenic granuloma.

dense, hyalinized bands of extracellular fibers. The causes of this involution are unknown and very little has been done to unravel them; this is all the more striking in view of the prominence of the phenomenon of vascular involution in wound healing. To say that capillaries are pressed out of existence by the developing collagen bundles is equal to accepting that blood vessels kindly leave their seats to the growing connective tissue; both opinions are purely speculative and fail to explain the extraordinary regression of newly formed capillaries. Williams[13] believes that the metabolic activity of a tissue determines the degree of its vascularization, which may be a reasonable explanation for the abundant vasculature of granulation tissue and the disappearance of most of the vessels as the scar matures; these studies, however, have yet to be done.

c. DEPOSIT OF INTERCELLULAR SUBSTANCES. Both cellular activity and vascular proliferation have a transient existence in wound healing. It is not the same with the deposit of intercellular substances (no doubt partly secondary to cellular activity) which will provide the scar with its main characteristic, tensile strength. After all, the desired result of wound healing is repair of damage with restitution of as many of the properties of normal tissues as possible, and one of the essential features of connective tissue is tensile strength. During the first stages of repair, a few hours after injury, the interstitial spaces show edema, which is the manifestation of increased capillary permeability. All structures appear sepa-

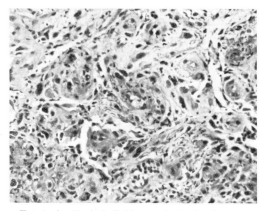

FIG. 3–6. Endothelial hyperplasia showing some hyperchromatism and atypical nuclei. This aspect is not rare and should not be mistaken for a tumor.

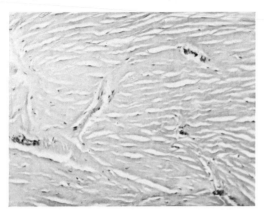

FIG. 3–8. Old scar with hyalinization of collagen fibers, scarce cells and few blood vessels.

rated by a thin, structureless material, faintly stained with eosin and other protein dyes, and more or less invaded by scavenger cells. This edema increases in the following two or three days, during which it acquires a fundamental property revealed by metachromatic dyes and microchemical analysis, which is a progressively increased concentration of acid mucopolysaccharides.[14] These compounds (*see* Chapter VI) form a very important part of the mucoproteins of connective tissue ground substance. In the beginning, metachromasia is apparent in the immediate neighborhood of capillaries, but later it becomes generalized.[15] Four to 6 days after injury the highest concentrations are reached, and from then on they decrease until at the end of 10 to 12 days the wound is found to have normal or even lower concentrations of these substances. Together with acid mucopolysaccharides other substances accumulate in the interstitial space (see below) which will enter into the composition of collagen, so the nature and significance of this "wound fluid," formerly characterized only as edema, are now beginning to be understood.

From the fourth day of injury the protoplasmic prolongations of fibroblasts become apparent as very fine fibrils in the intercellular space, where they may be revealed by special histologic techniques.[16] Approximately 2 days later many fibrils are seen to be independent of cells and to become arranged perpendicular to the capillaries; the same disposition is adopted by fibroblasts, so that both cells and fibers form a field of structures arranged in parallel fashion which is traversed by capillary vessels at right angles with them. The barely visible fibrils grow both in length and in diameter, the latter increase in size being unexplained so far. Some authors believe that fusion of thin fibers accounts for progressive thickening, while others postulate that fibrils serve as templates for the precipitation of soluble precursors synthesized by the cells.[17] Whatever the mechanism, this increase in thickness of fibers is accompanied by changes in their tinctorial affinities, since they become acidophilic and stain red with van Gieson's mixture. Furthermore, their straight course is changed for a more undulating and longitudinally striated structure, which is characteristic of mature collagen bundles. At the end of 10 to 12 days, with completion of healing, the intercellular substance is made up of fully developed, abundant collagen fibers, with few and narrow blood vessels and small fibrocytes scattered in between (Fig. 3–8). The sequence of cellular, vascular and interstitial changes in wound healing by first intention, is summarized in Table 9.

d. CONTRACTION. This interesting phenomenon occurs when there is loss of epithelium, especially in the skin. More than one process is involved in the repair of these wounds; "epidermization" is the term applied to the growth and migration of epithelium from the wound edge across the newly formed bed of the wound. It is a form of regeneration and will be discussed in the following section of this chapter. On the other hand, contraction of the wound means the approximation of the original skin edges and from the standpoint of the area to be covered is more important than epidermization in the closing of a defect in tissue. Billingham and Russell[18] produced large (35 to 40 sq. cm.) wounds in rabbits and observed that after two days contraction is already proceeding at its maximum rate, declines exponentially with the passage of time and after 45 days, when the area of the wound is approximately 2 sq. cm., the rate of contraction is nearly zero. Two main postulates have been suggested to explain the nature of wound contraction. One holds that the phenomenon is due to shrinkage of some constituent of the wound bed, the other contends that movement of the

Table 9. Chronologic Sequence of Events in Wound Healing

DAYS AFTER WOUNDING	CELLULAR ACTIVITY	VASCULAR CHANGES	DEPOSITION OF INTERCELLULAR SUBSTANCES
2	Phagocytosis of blood, tissue debris, etc. Proliferation and mobilization of histiocytes and fibroblasts	Dilation of marginal capillaries and arterioles	Edema with perivascular metachromatic material
4	Multiplication of acid mucopolysaccharide-producing fibroblasts Bipolar fibroblasts with fine argyrophilic prolongations	Proliferation of capillary buds with neoformation of abundant capillaries	Increasing edema with more generalized deposition of acid mucopolysaccharides Appearance of free amino acids such as glycine and proline
6	Transformation of all fibroblasts into bipolar cells in active fibrogenesis, arranged perpendicular to capillaries	Maximum of capillary proliferation reached	Begins the disappearance of edema and acid mucopolysaccharides Appearance of fine argyrophylic fibrils with tendency to arrange perpendicular to capillaries
8	Fibroblasts decrease in size and number, their prolongations are less abundant and appear continuous with intercellular fibers	Number and caliber of blood vessels decrease	Fusion of argyrophylic fibers which become thick acidophilic collagen bundles
	Most fibroblasts appear as fibrocytes	Few and narrow capillaries	Abundant collagen

skin edge across the defect (possibly under the influence of pulsion forces generated in the surrounding skin) can explain the decrease in size of the wound. Grillo, Watts and Gross[19, 20] have shown that the rate of contraction in guinea pig wounds is independent of the concentration of collagen, hexosamine, tyrosine, water or total weight of granulation tissue, and that complete excision of the wound contents has no effect on contraction; on the other hand, excision of the wound edge will markedly inhibit the phenomenon. These authors concluded that contraction depended upon a narrow band of tissue 1 or 2 mm. in width at the edge of the wound. The extensive study of Cuthbertson[21] revealed, however, that the contracting force was exerted by factors within the wounded area. In the initial stages the scab was responsible for an early contraction probably due to rapid dehydration; after the first 4 days there was further contraction, probably related to decreased capillary permeability and dehydration of the wound bed. In addition, contraction was different in young and old animals, since the latter have less skin mobility.

Contraction should be distinguished from the pathologic process of wound contrac-

ture, which is the end result of scarring and produces deformities of the joint or soft tissue masses involved by the scar. Contracture takes place much later than contraction and its significance is inversely proportional to the adequacy of healing; in full-thickness burns contraction is limited and scar formation is excessive, with contracture becoming a major problem.

e. CHEMISTRY OF WOUND HEALING. It is held that wound healing recapitulates the events of connective tissue growth. With some reservations this idea is accepted here, so the reader is referred to Chapter VI for a more detailed discussion of the chemistry and metabolism of connective tissues. Some specific aspects related to wound healing, however, may be mentioned here. Gillman and Penn[22] saw that after injury and disposal of tissue debris, and immediately before fibroblastic proliferation, a clear fluid different from the exudate accumulated in the lesion. This "wound fluid" has been obtained for sequential chemical analyses by means of a subcutaneously implanted tantalum wire cylinder,[23, 24] or a plastic sponge.[25] The results of chemical analysis reveal an early accumulation of hexosamine, largely derived from plasma glycoproteins; wound fluid is rich in gamma globulins but poor in total protein, lipoproteins, cholesterol, phospholipids, etc. Albumin and chlorides occur in the fluid at plasma concentrations; sodium, potassium, calcium and phosphorus are lower. Indeed, osmotic pressure of the fluid is 17 milliosmols lower than that of plasma, a surprising finding in view of the 7 days allowed for equilibration before sampling. Amino acids are also found, especially glycine, lysine and proline, and this is especially interesting since they will form part of the collagen molecule. Before collagen fibrils become visible in the wound some soluble collagen-like proteins can be found, such as procollagen and tropocollagen. Orekhovitch[26] claims that these proteins have properties similar to collagen isolated from sources other than regenerating wound tissue, but Williamson and Fromm[27] have shown that their content of methionine and cystine is greater per gram of nitrogen. In the earlier stages of healing, proteins with more methionine than cystine are recovered, but later the proportion of cystine increases in the protein molecule. Tensile strength is parallel to the amount of cystine found in the healing wound, in spite of the fact that collagen has no cystine; perhaps cystine-rich proteins are being produced in the wound tissue at approximately the same rate as collagen.[28] Regenerating wound tissue has been shown to incorporate sulphate ions at a very high rate,[29, 30] mainly into the mucopolysaccharides of the ground substance.[31] A proteolytic enzyme has been shown to be present in wound tissue by several investigators[32, 33] as well as a high concentration of phosphatase activity.[34] The origin and functions of these enzymes are unknown.

3. *Normal Pattern of Wound Healing.* Several interpretations of the sequence of events described so far have been offered, two of which will be mentioned. Howes and associates[32] considered that the process of wound healing could be conceived in three separate stages: the exudative or lag phase, the fibroplastic stage and the maturation stage. The lag phase is coincident with reaction to injury, onset of necrosis and exudate accumulation; a coagulum is formed of blood, serum and lymph that serves as a scaffolding to unite temporarily the edges of the wound. The cells observed belong to inflammation, and although there is vascular proliferation, the newly formed capillaries have yet to bridge the gap of the wound. It was considered that during this stage the tissues were deterred from proliferation and repair by the shock of injury.[36] The second or fibroplastic stage covers from the third or fourth day to the twelfth to fourteenth days and is characterized by a progressive increase in tensile strength, caused by deposition of collagen fibers. The third stage or maturation varies according to the tissue involved; in subcutaneous connective tissues it takes only a few days or weeks, while in bones it may take years. This interpretation of the sequence of events in wound healing has been widely accepted since it follows rather well the morphology of each stage.

However, newer knowledge requires a different concept, since now the so-called lag phase cannot be considered as passive as the name implies. In 1956, Dunphy and associates[37] began a series of studies of wound healing with a combination of histologic, histochemical, biochemical and tensile strength techniques which led them to propose a different pattern of wound healing (Fig. 3–9). This pattern consists of two different stages. The first is a productive or substrate phase, which begins shortly after wounding and lasts for about 5 days; during this period mucopolysaccharides and soluble protein precursors of collagen, the building blocks of repair, are produced. The second stage is a collagen phase, in which normal collagen fibers are formed; this begins about the fifth day and lasts until completion of healing. In this concept there is no lag phase to wound healing, and normal tensile strength is a function of collagen formation, not of fibroblastic multiplication as formerly postulated. Dunphy's work has the merit of abandoning a passive first stage for an active and preparatory period, with intense accumulation of building materials for the second stage. In this high metabolic rate both cells and capillaries participate, since some of these materials are deposited by the cells while others are derived from the blood. In addition, this concept is extremely useful because it permits a better appreciation of the mechanism of action of many factors that influence wound healing.

Furthermore, the welding together of chemical composition, anatomical structure and functional meaning represents a more integrated concept of healing, which will surely open new fields of research.

4. *Some Factors Influencing Healing.* A series of factors have been observed to influence healing in experimental animals; not all of them, however, are significant in clinical medicine. In Table 10 they are separated into local and general factors. Additional details may be found in the excellent review by Arey.[38]

a. LOCAL FACTORS IN WOUND HEALING. One of the most important local factors in wound healing is the type of agent causing the lesion. The surgeon's scalpel produces a clean, aseptic wound with ideal conditions for the rapid and efficient growth of connective tissues. On the other hand, a blunt injury with irregular tissue necrosis will

present a more difficult problem for the organism. Burns often heal poorly or not at all, especially when they are deep, since most of the elements involved in repair are destroyed by heat. An operative wound with

Table 10. Factors Influencing Wound Healing

LOCAL FACTORS	GENERAL FACTORS
1. Type of wounding agent (scalpel, contusion, etc.)	1. Age
	2. Temperature
	3. Ultraviolet light
2. Infection	4. Ionizing radiation
3. Size of wound	5. Generalized infection
4. Temperature	6. Nutritional status
5. Ionizing radiation	a. Proteins (methionine)
6. Local stimuli (cartilage powder, tissue tension, etc.)	b. Vitamin C
	7. Hormones
	a. Corticoids
	b. ACTH
	c. Thyroxin
	d. Estrogens
	e. Growth hormone

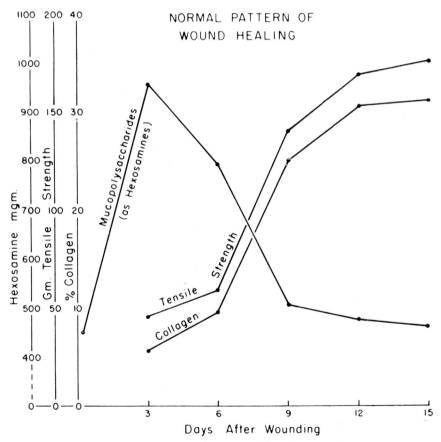

FIG. 3–9. The normal pattern of wound healing as established by chemical, histochemical, histologic and tensile strength studies. (Courtesy of Dr. J. E. Dunphy and the Editor, New England Journal of Medicine.)

traumatic damage caused by rough handling of tissues, prolonged pressure and tearing action of retractors, mass ligatures with large necrotic portions of tissue distal to the ligature, etc., will not heal well.[39] Hematomas interfere with normal wound healing by preventing apposition of the walls of the wound and also serve as good culture medium for the growth of bacteria; the same is true of collections of serosanguineous fluid separating the wound. Foreign bodies, aside from sutures, may also delay the process of healing; a special case is the talcum granuloma, which may enter the wound not only from the outside of the gloves but also from frequent puncture of a finger of the glove. Talcum (hydrous magnesium silicate) mixed with sweat produces an inflammatory reaction in tissues which delays or even inhibits adequate healing; it may be recognized in tissues by its double refractibility with polarized light. Temperature was found by Ebeling to influence the healing of wounds in alligators.[40] But by far the most important cause of healing delay is infection; many of the factors previously mentioned are important not only in themselves, but also in that they facilitate wound infection. The mechanism by which bacteria prevent connective tissue growth is not known; it has been said that microorganisms attack elements responsible for healing as they are formed, or that "an infection in a wound diverts some of the body forces—capillary buds, leukocytes, fibroblasts, tissue fluids, enzymes, etc.—which should go toward healing the wound, in the direction of repelling an even more dangerous trauma to the body, the secondary infection."[39]

Some time ago, Lecomte du Noüy[41] developed a mathematical formula expressing the speed of healing as a function of the size of the wound, the age of the subject, etc., but this formula has found no application in human patients. For some time it was thought that ionizing radiation had a double effect on wound healing, depending on the dose range; it is known now, however, that small doses will have no influence on it,[42] while large doses will result in delay or even complete inhibition.[43] Following the report of Lattes and colleagues,[44] that powdered cartilage would block the inhibiting effect of cortisone on wound healing, Prud-den and associates[45, 46] studied the effect of the same product on the normal healing of rats. They found that powdered cartilage will accelerate the first stages of healing, determined both by tensile strength and by histologic examinations.

Of all the local factors mentioned that influence wound healing, infection and tissue destruction are the most important from a clinical standpoint; temperature, size, ionizing radiation, etc., play a minimal (if any) role in the healing of wounds in human subjects. No local factors have been found that accelerate in a practical way the healing of a wound in a well nourished, otherwise healthy patient.

b. GENERAL FACTORS IN WOUND HEALING. It is a fact that age is an important factor in the speed of healing, and this has been shown to be true both in experimental animals and in human subjects; the effect of age, however, is hardly perceptible in clinical work except in the very old, and here vascular difficulties may also be involved. Ultraviolet light has also been shown to accelerate the rate of healing, but again the effect is minimal and of no practical use. Whole body radiation has the same results as local, small doses stimulate the healing of wounds slightly, while large doses inhibit it.[47] A generalized infection will make wound healing slower. It has been mentioned that poor peripheral circulation is usually accompanied by deficient growth of connective tissues, both because of local nutritional disturbances and because of the effect of temperature. For example, the skin temperature in the feet is several degrees lower than that of the abdomen or trunk, and wounds in the abdomen heal faster than those in the lower extremities.

In malnourished patients with hypoproteinemia wound healing is delayed and the frequency of fusion of surgical incisions is greater than in well nourished subjects.[48] Two factors appear important in this respect, proteins and vitamin C. Experimentally, animals fed a protein-deficient diet will take longer to heal a skin wound, but if methionine is added without increasing the caloric value of the diet, wound healing will become normal. Histologic studies show a delay in fibroblastic proliferation and collagen deposition with a longer period of edema and persistence of metachromatic material in the interstitial spaces[15] (Fig. 3–10). Chemical determinations confirm that healing is detained at the end of the first or substrate phase; addition of methionine to the diet results in a rapid onset of the second or collagen phase[49] (Fig. 3–11).

Further studies h is transformed i it is utilized by exact influence synthesis is not l important for th into insoluble

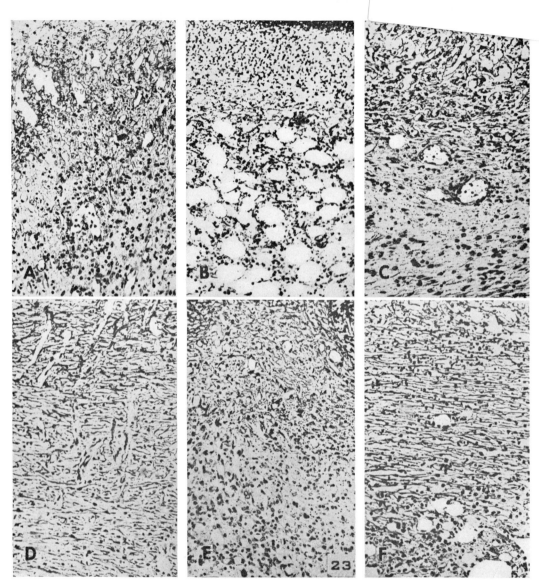

FIG. 3–10. Influence of methionine in wound healing. *A*, Control group 4 days after wounding. Early capillary proliferation with numerous immature fibroblasts. *B*, Microscopic aspect of 4-day-old wound in a rat given a non-protein diet. *C*, Capillary proliferation in a 4-day-old wound in a rat given a non-protein diet supplemented with methionine. *D*, Normal group, 10 days after wounding, showing a well organized scar with few capillaries. *E*, Wound healing in rats fed a protein-free diet, 10 days after injury. The area of reaction is thin. There are some inflammatory cells and numerous capillaries. There is no arrangement of fibroblasts. *F*, There is essentially normal wound healing (compare with *D*) in rats fed a non-protein diet supplemented with methionine. (Courtesy of the Editor, American Journal of Pathology.)

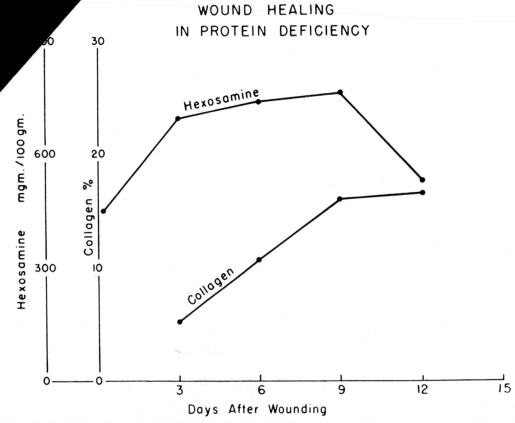

FIG. 3–11. Effect of protein deficiency on the normal pattern of wound healing. (Courtesy of Dr. J. E. Dunphy and the Editor, Annals of Surgery.)

vitamin will be reflected in failure of wound healing. Histologic studies in experimental animals have shown that fibroblasts proliferate but there is no deposition of interstitial fibers;[51] in addition, a predominance of edema and metachromatic material is seen,[52] and it has been claimed that abnormal mucopolysaccharides are deposited.[53] Wound healing in human volunteers with controlled vitamin C deficiency has been studied by Crandon et al.,[54] it took more than 4 months to induce scurvy in man, but at that time the healing of a skin wound was grossly defective and no vascular proliferation was seen at the end of 10 days. Addition of vitamin C to the diet resulted in normal wound healing in 10 days. Histochemical and microchemical determinations by Dunphy, et al.,[55] in experimental animals revealed that the normal pattern of wound healing is disrupted in that it fails to continue after the first or substrate phase. Addition of vitamin C to the diet brings about a prompt decrease in hexosamines and the rise in collagen begins (Fig. 3–12). Human scurvy is extremely rare and these studies are of more use in determining the role of ascorbic acid in the metabolism of connective tissues. Another interesting line of research in wound healing has developed from the discovery of Ponsetti and Baird[56] that feeding of Lathyrus odoratus seeds induces widespread lesions in the connective tissues of rats, with formation of dissecting aneurysm of the aorta and scoliosis. The active principle in the seeds is β-amino-aceto-nitrile.[57] Enzinger and Warner[58] studied the effect of this substance, and of amino-propio-nitrile and β-mercapto-ethyl-amine in wound healing and found that the result was similar to that obtained in scurvy; however, the administration of ascorbic acid had no influence on this form of abnormal wound healing. The mechanism of action of these substances is at present unknown.

Hormonal influences on connective tissues are reflected in wound healing.[59, 60] It is of interest that most contributions in this field deal with the production of abnormalities that lead to defective repair. Hypophysectomy[61] and anterior pituitary extract in doses sufficient to accelerate somatic growth[62] have failed to produce differences in the rate of development of tensile strength and the time required for closure of skin wounds; on the other hand, bovine growth hormone produced an 8.8 per cent increase in tensile strength in rat wounds.[63] Cortisone inhibits wound healing,[64] and so does ACTH, but the effect of the latter is abolished by adrenalectomy.[65] Some authors have failed to observe the inhibiting effect of cortisone on wound healing,[66] while others suggest that this effect may even be reversed by strong irritation,[67] ischemia or infection.[68] The suppressive action of cortisone on connective tissue proliferation is observed both with parenterally administered steroid as well as when the application is local;[69] when cortisone is injected, however, it must be used some days in advance of wounding in order to have any effect. Scarpelli and associates found that oxygen consumption by granulation tissue obtained from rabbits previously treated with cortisone was reduced several times.[70] Histochemical studies have suggested that acid mucopolysaccharides are not produced in normal amounts,[71] and Layton found that synthesis of chondroitin sulphate was diminished *in vitro* by hydrocortisone[72] and *in vivo* by cortisone.[73] The last studies were confirmed by Schiller and Dorfman in the rat,[74] and in addition they found that formation of hyaluronic acid was also decreased. Pernokas and associates[75] used the polyvinyl sponge to study collagen formation under the effect of cortisone and found it depressed. It should not be surprising, therefore, that tensile strength of skin wounds is markedly depressed by cortisone

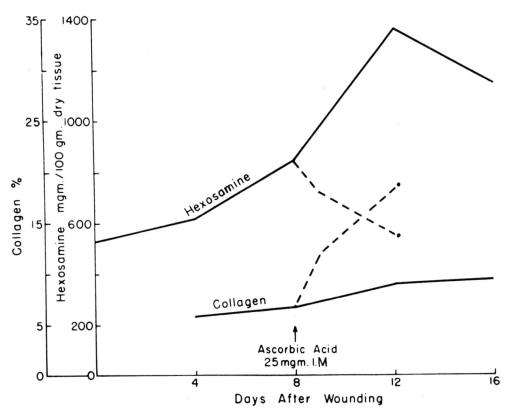

WOUND HEALING PATTERN IN SCORBUTIC ANIMALS

FIG. 3–12.   Effect of vitamin C deficiency on the normal pattern of wound healing in guinea pigs. (Courtesy of Dr. J. E. Dunphy and the Editor, Annals of Surgery.)

in several animal species.[76] According to Billingham and Russell,[18] contraction of the wound is reduced to about half its normal rate in rabbits treated with cortisone, an effect shared by adrenalectomy. Desoxycorticosterone, on the contrary, seems to enhance formation of granulation tissue in rats and guinea pigs, as reported by Taubenhaus and Amromin[77] and Pirani, et al.[78]

Estrogens administered systemically in large doses appear to have a definite inhibitory effect on the formation of granulation tissue; in contrast with cortisone, the local application of estrogens is without effect on wound healing. Taubenhaus[79] has found that simultaneous administration of pituitary growth hormone and estrogens will result in blocking of the depressive effect of the latter. A similar situation has been found with androgens, but adrenalectomy eliminates the suppressive action of testosterone on proliferation of connective tissue.[80] Thyroidectomized rats have been reported to show inhibition of healing by histologic observations,[81] but they have also been found to develop normal tensile strength in surgical wounds.[82] Animals treated with thyroxine show a deficient sulphate uptake in a healing wound, and also a slower gain in tensile strength.[83] All these observations on endocrine influence in wound healing have little or no counterpart in clinical experience, but they are of interest in the biology of connective tissues (*see* Chapter VI).

5. *Stimulus for Wound Healing.* What causes repair after injury? Some considerations of the stimulus for capillary growth, increased capillary permeability and other phenomena of inflammation which may participate in the initiation of the healing process have been made. It is of interest to inquire into the nature of the stimulus for proliferation of connective tissue, which is the essence of repair. It is wise to remember that this is no disorderly proliferation; on the contrary, cellular multiplication precedes interstitial deposit of ground substance and collagen fibers, with a definite orientation and for a certain period, after which the process stops and the scar "matures." Any suggestion as to the nature of the stimulus or stimuli involved in wound healing must take into account the basic facts that there is tissue growth, and that this growth proceeds in an orderly fashion.[84] At the outset it must be said that the nature of the factor or factors responsible for wound healing is unknown. Many years ago, Carrel[85] observed that extracts of chick embryos stimulated the growth of fibroblasts in tissue cultures, while extracts of adult animals produced the opposite effect. The factor in extracts of chick embryos responsible for stimulation was found to be an unstable and thermolabile protein which completely lost activity when broken down to aminoacids, but preserved part of it in some polypeptides. More recently, Kutsky and Harris[86] analyzed cellular fractions of chick embryos and found that growth stimulating factors are present in nucleoproteins, mitochondria, microsomes and in the soluble, dialyzed fraction of embryonal cells; additional work on this problem has been published by Maganini, et al.,[87] who believe that growth promoting factors in chick embryos are complex nucleoproteins of high molecular weights or dissociated derivatives of lower molecular weight that react positively with Folin's reagent and exhibit an absorption maximum at about 2560 Angstrom units. As a further hypothesis, Carrel suggested that injured tissues will produce substances stimulating connective tissue growth, and when the latter has been completed a state of equilibrium is reached with the plasma; these substances were held to result from cell breakdown or injury by Loofbourow, et al.[88] Direct examination of this possibility has been published by Edwards, et al.,[89] who used tissue extracts of homogenized chick embryos, autologous spleen and autologous post-traumatic granulation tissue with Tyrode's solution. Ivalon sponges were filled with such extracts and implanted in the subcutaneous tissue of rabbits; a definite stimulation of connective tissue growth was observed, characterized by increased number of fibroblasts and increased rate of maturation of collagenous fibrils in the sponges containing tissue extracts.

B. Abnormal Wound Healing. There are two general types of abnormal wound healing. One occurs when there is depression of connective tissue proliferation, and the other is the result of the opposite process; i.e., an exaggerated growth of capillaries and abundant deposit of intercellular substances, which overshoots the needs created by injury. An additional type of defective healing of wounds appears with "fusion" of surgical incisions, which are observed in obese individuals with long, usually traumatized and infected wounds; this last type, however, is really not due to disturbances in the mechanism of repair but to certain conditions (some of them described above) which interfere with an otherwise healthy process.[90]

Churchill[91] considers two types of abnormal scars due to excessive production of connective tissue. One is the product of repetitive insults which bring about "stormy healing," a term used by Stearns[9] in reference to multiple episodes of fibroblastic proliferation due to repeated injuries; this is known as "hypertrophic" scar.[92] The other type of abnormal healing would be caused by a local immunologic response to displaced protein of endogenous origin, and is the same as "keloid." These ideas are supported by the studies of Glücksman,[93] Solomons[94] and others,[95] who found frequent foreign bodies within keloids. The foreign bodies were exogenous or endogenous in origin, the latter being displaced hair follicles and other keratinized inclusions in the dermis. Both hypertrophied and keloid scars are the result of excessive proliferation of connective tissue which fails to be reabsorbed at the end of healing. Grossly they appear as elevated, reddish and shiny lobulations of firm tissue, covered by atrophic epithelium without skin appendages. Under the microscope, collagen fibers are not only abundant and hyalinized but also thicker than normal (Fig. 3–13); frequently, there

are changes in their affinity for certain dyes, such as Van Gieson's mixture or aniline blue. Cells are scarce and blood vessels may be prominent.[96] Endocrine influences have been suspected in the production of keloids since they do not appear in castrates and are more frequent in young women.

III. REGENERATION

In 1740, a poorly paid tutor of the children of the Comte de Bentinck, a Swiss by the name of Abraham Trembley, became interested in some slender organisms living in the ponds of the count's garden. Because of their green color they seemed to be plants, but when Trembley saw them swallow tiny crustaceans he was inclined to consider them as animals. To solve this riddle he made use of a favorite test of that time, based on the belief that plants survive when cut into multiple fragments whereas animals succumb. It came as a great surprise to this scientist that the different fragments of the hydra were able to regenerate mutilations at great speed and that soon they were transformed into complete, although smaller, hydras.[96]

Spallanzani, the great anatomist of the seventeenth century, observed that *Triton vulgaris* would regenerate tail or legs after amputation. After many studies of this and other animals, Spallanzani summarized the problem as follows:[97]

"But if these species [frogs] are able to renew their legs when young, why should they not do the same when farther advanced? . . . Are the wonderful reproductions hitherto mentioned [in newts] only to be ascribed to the effect of water, in which these animals were kept? This is contradicted in the instance of the salamander, whose parts were reproduced even on dry ground. But if the above-mentioned animals, either aquatic or amphibian, recover their legs when kept on dry ground, how comes it to pass that other land animals, such as are accounted perfect, and are better known to us, are not endued with the same power? It is to be hoped that they may acquire them by some useful dispositions? And should the flattering expectation of obtaining this advantage for ourselves be considered entirely as chimerical?"

These types of regeneration, and others that could be mentioned in lower animals,

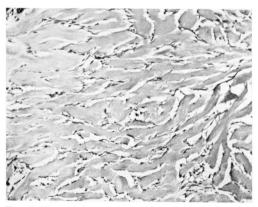

FIG. 3–13. Old scar with thickening and hyalinization of collagen bundles (keloid).

are characterized not only by growth of the amputated portion but also by the differentiation of cells in various types according to tissues regenerated and by the harmonic organization of the entire process. Indeed, the capacity for self-reduplication is the fundamental difference between the inert and the living worlds; the only reason to accept viruses as alive is their ability to multiply, which means protein synthesis. Regeneration is, therefore, a basic property of living organisms. But what is almost unrestricted ability to regenerate lost parts in lower animals becomes more and more limited as the zoologic scale is climbed, so that at the level of *Homo sapiens* only tissues (and not all) preserve this property. Cells can still multiply but organizers are weak or nonexistent. Willis[98] considers that regeneration of whole limbs and other complex parts seen in the amphibia are a resumption of embryonic growth, and that in less spectacular fashion the regeneration of mammalian tissues conforms to the same principle. Many interesting details on regeneration in fish, amphibia and reptiles can be found in Willis' excellent monograph "The Borderland of Embryology and Pathology," together with a full bibliography, and an extensive treatment of this subject from a biologic standpoint which has been published by Needham.[99]

Regeneration occurs in three situations, different in appearance but identical in nature, which are better characterized as physiologic, compensatory and pathologic regenerations. Physiologic regeneration is seen in tissues where there is a continuous loss of cellular elements, such as skin, blood and testes; this form of regeneration is also known as renewal and has been analyzed by Leblond and Walker.[100] Compensatory regeneration appears in paired organs such as kidneys or adrenals, when there is loss of one of the organs of the pair; as it is usually accomplished through cellular multiplication, the term "compensatory hyperplasia" is also used. Pathologic regeneration is the type usually referred to in discussions of these phenomena and is present when there is sudden loss of epithelial tissues; in this case, cells proliferate and increase in size until the total mass of normal functioning protoplasm has been attained again. In the three types of regeneration the final goal of the organism is the restitution of a given mass of specialized protoplasm, and this is accomplished by cellular proliferation and/or increase in size of the cells, as well as by organized reconstruction of the architecture of the involved tissue. The latter process is better exemplified by the normal liver after experimental partial hepatectomy, a phenomenon which will be described in some detail. What is of interest now is that liver cells multiply rapidly and replace the lack of functioning cytoplasm and the structure of liver tissue as well, to the extent that it is impossible to distinguish microscopically between a regenerated and a normal, control liver.

A. Classification of Tissues. At the turn of the century, Bizzozero[101] distinguished three types of tissues in the adult organism according to the number of mitoses usually present: (1) labile cells, with mitotic activity throughout the life of the individual, (2) stable cells, with occasional but rare mitoses and (3) permanent cells, which never show mitoses. This classification of tissues referred to their regenerating ability; tissues composed of labile cells retained to a great extent their capacity to regenerate, while those tissues formed by permanent cells were completely unable to reconstitute themselves after a loss of substance, or did it to a very limited degree. In a more quantitative fashion, Leblond and Walker[100] have postulated that mitoses are a measure of tissue renewal or physiologic regeneration; thus, rat tissues showing between 0.8 and 1.5 per cent of the cells in mitoses at a given moment are not regenerating but only keeping pace with the animal growth, while more than 1.5 per cent of mitoses is indicative of renewal. It is feasible to consider Bizzozero's three groups of tissues in the light of Leblond and Walker's observations, and the results are identical lists, as shown in Table 11. Nevertheless, it is the *potential* capacity to regenerate and not the actual manifestation of mitotic activity in normal organs that is the main factor involved in determining what the tissue will do when the total mass of functioning protoplasm is decreased; this can be appreciated from the fact that the liver is a stable tissue with no more than 1.5 mitoses per cent. (Actually,

Table 11.	Classification of Tissues	
LABILE (>1.5 mitoses)	STABLE (0.8–1.5 mitoses)	PERMANENT (0 mitoses)
†Epidermis	†Liver	Nervous system
†Mucosa	Kidney	Striated muscle
digestive	Endocrine glands	Adrenal
respiratory	Thyroid	medulla
urinary	Pituitary	Sensory organs
genital	Adrenal cortex	Ear
Hemopoietic	Exocrine glands	Eye
organs	Pancreas	
†Bone marrow	Salivary	
Lymph nodes	Prostate	
Spleen	Bone	
	Cartilage	

† Tissues with great regenerative capacity (Bizzozero; Leblond and Walker)

this is a very high count; other authors believe that liver cells show 1 mitotic figure for every 10,000 to 20,000 cells.[102]) The same can be said of thyroid and bone. This potential capacity for regeneration is manifested to different degrees under pathologic conditions, some of which are briefly summarized in the following paragraphs.

B. Regeneration of Some Special Tissues. Regeneration has been mainly studied in the liver and the peripheral nervous system, but there are data pertaining to other tissues.

1. Glandular and Lining Epithelium. All surface epithelia show great regenerating capacity, including those of glandular structure. It is commonly observed that in skin wounds with loss of substance regeneration of epithelium occurs through proliferation of epithelial elements from the margins of the wound, which bridge the gap by growing on top of granulation tissue. The process involves two different mechanisms. There is flattening and elongation of epithelial elements in the margins of the lesion, which extend their cytoplasm on the connective tissue bed, forming a very thin membrane. The membrane moves slowly in the opposite direction to its origin, not by ameboid movements since cells remain attached to each other, but probably because of increase in the amount of cytoplasm and redistribution in space; decrease in volume is coterminous with increase in extension. This sliding of epithelial cells on the raw surface of the wound requires softening of the complex anchoring of epithelium to connective tissue

with actual detachment of the epithelial lining, a process observed in amphibians by Weiss and Ferris.[103] This anchoring is represented by an extremely thin, structureless membrane which undergoes changes suggesting a transition from gel to sol state. The other mechanism responsible for epithelial displacement is cell proliferation, which is apparent slightly behind the advancing edge and continues until the defect is closed.[104] As long as the surface of the wound is not covered completely by an epithelial lining, the growing membrane is one or two cells thick, but when surface regeneration is completed the epithelial membrane grows in depth until a more or less normal thickness is achieved. Rete pegs, however, are seldom as deep as in normal skin and sometimes are not formed at all. When the tissue loss includes skin adnexae such as hairs or sweat glands they fail to regenerate, but if the injury is superficial the remaining elements are capable of reconstituting these structures. A scab is no obstacle for epithelial regeneration, which occurs underneath; for unknown reasons the growth of epithelium inhibits proliferation of granulation tissues and avoids the development of retractile scars. Therefore, when tissue destruction is extensive surgeons are prone to help rapid epithelialization by placing skin autografts on the raw granulation tissue, from which cells grow in all directions and the defect is covered more rapidly.

Mucosal surfaces regenerate better than skin epithelium, since the latter reproduces only polystratified layers and is unable to differentiate into hair and glandular appendages; on the other hand, mucosae regenerate most of the lost structures. Wilhelm[105] has published an experimental study of epithelial regeneration in the trachea of the rat, with results similar to those obtained in the gastrointestinal mucosa. The following figures give an idea of the speed of the process. A wound 2 mm. in width is completely covered by mucosa in 36 to 48 hours; ciliated elements appear in 10 to 14 days; goblet cells appear in 12 to 14 days, and differentiation is completed in approximately 6 weeks. Florey and Harding[106] examined the regenerating mechanism of an experimentally produced lesion in the duo-

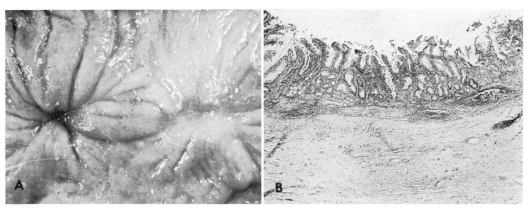

FIG. 3–14. Healed peptic ulcer. *A,* Gross aspect of the gastric mucosa with two peptic ulcers; the one on the left is active, the one on the right has been healed with epithelial growth. *B,* Microscopic aspect of the healed gastric ulcer, showing thin mucosa with few glands lying on dense fibrous tissue with chronic inflammation.

denal mucosa of the cat, where villi, crypts of Lieberkühn and Brunner glands are normally present; immediately after injury the defect is filled with a blood clot which proceeds to organization through the process of healing described in the previous section. However, 24 hours later mitoses were observed in the neighboring crypts and Brunner glands; a thin layer of epithelial elements derived from the former advances on top of the surface of granulation tissue. As in the skin, these epithelial cells show no mitoses. When the entire defect has been covered by mucosa, finger-like prolongations penetrate downwards and form new crypts, while epithelial foldings grow upwards and become villi. Ciliated and mucus cells are present, and sometimes even elements similar to those observed in the gastric mucosa can be seen also. A similar process operates in the healing of peptic ulcerations in man, but the area may be recognized often by the retraction of connective tissue formed at the base of the ulcer, replacing muscularis mucosae and part of the muscular layers, and because the mucosal foldings radiate from the area of healing and are less deep than normal. Microscopic examination shows regenerated epithelium with glands resembling either gastric or, more often, intestinal mucosa (Fig. 3–14). In actively regenerating gastric epithelium some of the cells may have atypical features suggestive of neoplasia;[107] in other cases, repeated episodes of peptic digestion and regeneration may leave islands of epithelium within connective tissue in the margins of the ulcer, which may be mistaken for a malignant tumor.[108] Stewart[109] described a group of such cases and called attention to their benign nature. In idiopathic ulcerative colitis there are recurrent losses of mucosal lining with regeneration, sometimes forming bridges over denuded areas;[110] these redundant, polypoid masses of regenerated epithelium have been held responsible for the increased frequency of carcinoma of the large intestine in this condition,[111] which occurs in 10 to 20 per cent of patients, depending on the chronicity of the disease.[112, 113]

Two organs with continuous or cyclic regeneration are the testes and the endometrium. During the reproductive period, normal women regenerate the glands and the stroma of the endometrium every 28 days, and this regeneration stems from the deeper portions of the glands which are not lost during menstruation since they are found in the basal or reticular area. During the first 14 days of the menstrual cycle mitoses are abundant in glands and stroma, and the former increase in number, size and tortuosity; during the following 14 days glandular secretion, pseudodecidual reaction and edema of the stroma appear in successive stages under the influence of progesterone secreted by the corpus luteum (Fig. 3–15). This sequence is so exact that it permits the dating of the menstrual cycle in endometrial biopsies,[114] a method widely

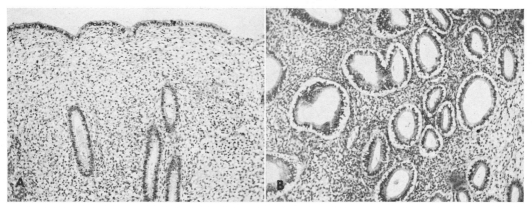

FIG. 3–15. Hormonal control of endometrial regeneration. *A*, Estrogenic influence with proliferation of glands and stroma. *B*, Progestational influence, with secretion accumulated in the basal portion of glandular cells.

used in clinical studies. Endometrial biopsy is also a most useful technique for the diagnosis of abnormalities in the endocrine balance responsible for the changing morphologic nature of stroma and mucosal lining.

2. *Liver.* The study of liver regeneration began in 1890 when Ponfick[115] showed that it was possible to remove several lobes of this organ from rabbits and observe the growth of the remainder until the normal weight of the liver was restored. In 1931, Higgins and Anderson[116] published a long series of experiments in rats and standardized the technique of partial hepatectomy, which can be done in this animal with relative ease since each one of the 5 lobes has an independent vascular and biliary pedicle. Cameron[117] has formulated a series of "fundamental theorems of liver behavior," some of which are as follows: no part of the liver is essential for the complete and normal functioning of the organ; it is of little significance where and how frequently the liver is sectioned, regeneration will be adequate from the remaining fragment as long as this portion suffices for maintenance of minimal liver function; the regenerating unit of the liver is smaller than the lobule as long as adequate circulation and excretory systems are maintained; the regenerating unit of the liver is independent from the nervous system. These postulates are basic both to physiology and pathology of the liver and serve as a frame of reference for the interpretation of many data.

In the rat, the usual experiment consists of removal of the two left and the middle lobes of the liver (the rat liver has 5 lobules), which constitute approximately 65 per cent of the total liver weight. If a series of animals is so treated and representative groups are sacrificed at succeeding intervals, liver weight will serve to measure regeneration quantitatively; furthermore, microscopic examination and chemical composition of the growing lobes will help to integrate the picture, which may be completed with enzymatic determinations. There have been studies of regeneration of many elements at different levels of organization in the liver which permit a comprehensive understanding of the process;[118] data combined from various studies of this sort appear in Figure 3–16.

One of the most striking results is the speed of liver regeneration. In 48 hours over 40 per cent of the weight removed has been recovered and in 6 days some animals may even show a liver weight greater than calculated from the amount resected, which is probably the result of water accumulation inside regenerating cells. This rate of growth is greater than that of any malignant tumor, greater than the normal embryo; in fact, no tissue, normal or abnormal, grows as fast as the regenerating liver. This finding contrasts with the normal occurrence of no more than 1 mitosis per 10,000 to 20,000 liver cells, a fact already mentioned; regenerating liver often shows 5 or more mitoses per high power field (Fig. 3–17).

Many factors have been studied from the standpoint of their influence in regeneration

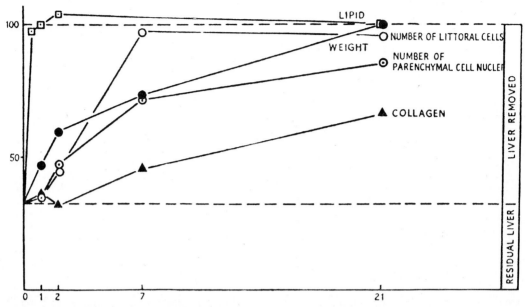

FIG. 3–16.   Regeneration of several parameters in rat liver after partial hepatectomy. (Courtesy Dr. R. D. Harkness and the Editor, British Medical Bulletin.)

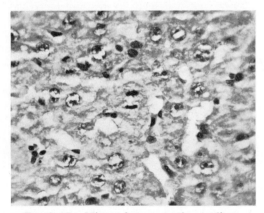

FIG. 3–17.   Mitoses in regenerating rat liver.

special interest is the influence of cirrhosis in regeneration of the liver; earlier workers pointed out the fact that fatty liver and cirrhosis produced by dietary and toxic means were opposed to adequate hepatic regeneration,[123] but more recent studies suggest that the liver is not only capable of

of the liver. It has been said that a vitamin-deficient, low caloric diet decreases hepatic regeneration;[119] if the data obtained in such experiments are corrected for the expected weight of the liver, calculated from body weight loss and not from the amount removed, it can be seen that lack of food has no influence on liver regeneration[120] (Fig. 3–18). Ferguson, et al. described some time ago that experimental bile duct obstruction would depress regeneration of the liver,[121] but the careful studies of Weinbren have shown that this is not the case.[122] A rat infected during partial hepatectomy will regenerate the liver parenchyma poorly. Of

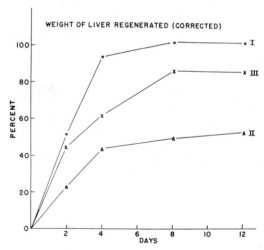

FIG. 3–18.   Per cent of liver regenerated after partial hepatectomy in control (I), cortisone-treated (II) and underfed rats (III). Differences between controls and underfed rats are not statistically significant once the liver weight regenerated has been corrected for body weight loss. (Courtesy of the Editor, Archives of Pathology.)

rebuilding a substantial amount of functional protoplasm,[124] but also that an otherwise irreversible cirrhosis will disappear during regeneration stimulated by partial hepatectomy.[125] Perhaps the most important factor in liver regeneration is blood flow. Portal circulation has been extensively studied as a factor influencing liver regeneration, and Mann[126] has published an excellent review of the subject. In summary, it can be stated that a decrease of the portal blood flow, produced by means of stenosis, ligature, Eck fistula (anastomosis of the portal vein to the inferior vena cava), etc., will inhibit regeneration of the liver. Mann is inclined to think that this effect results from a quantitative decrease in blood flow, and Child, et al.,[127] and Fisher and colleagues[128] agree. Reduction of the portal blood flow should be no less than 70 per cent to be effective.[129]

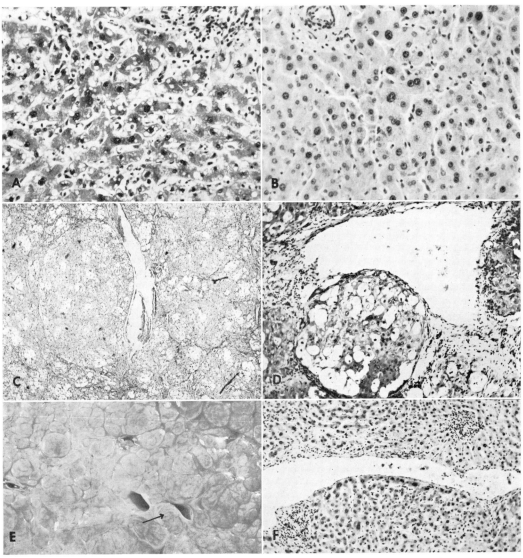

FIG. 3–19. Regeneration of liver cells. *A*, Binucleated and hyperchromatic liver cells in recovery from hepatitis. Notice fine droplet fatty deposition. *B*, Another aspect of regenerating liver cells. *C*, Nodular regeneration in experimental cirrhosis produced with CCl₄ in rats. Compression of a hepatic vein. *D*, A small regenerating nodule of liver parenchyma compressing another vein. *E*, Cut surface of post-necrotic cirrhosis in man. The arrow points out a regenerating nodule partially compressing a vein. *F*, Microscopic picture of the same case.

On the other hand, hepatic artery blood flow can be completely interrupted without affecting experimental regeneration of the liver in the rat.[130]

Liver regeneration plays a very important role in the prognosis and pathogenesis of some of the most frequent diseases of this organ, such as viral hepatitis and the different types of cirrhosis. Frequently, the patient's life will depend on the ability of the liver to regenerate the dead cells; in other cases, regeneration will contribute to the distortion of the parenchyma and of the vascular tree, and this will result in poor intrahepatic circulation and probably in portal hypertension[131] (Fig. 3–19).

3. *Nervous System.* Regeneration in the central nervous system is almost always contemplated with pessimism, since adult nerve cells have lost their capacity to multiply. Inability to undergo mitosis, however, is also observed in the striated muscle, but this structure is still capable of regeneration. An extensive analysis of this problem with reference to many experimental studies has been published by Windle.[132] The point at issue is essentially axonal regeneration, which has been found to occur in three different situations: (a) in young mammals, where some undifferentiated neuroblasts are still present, a gap may be jumped by axons derived from these cells;[133] (b) in adults, axonal regeneration is frequently observed in severed prolongations of central or peripheral neurons; (c) the growth of newly formed axons from uninjured cells close to a lesion has been demonstrated by Liu and Chambers.[134] There are some data suggestive of a beneficial effect of pyrogens in this form of axonal regeneration.[135]

The regenerative capacity of peripheral nerves is great, as long as a series of fundamental conditions are fulfilled. Immediately after section a degenerative process sets in involving the entire distal portion and a part of the proximal portion of the nerve; the process is known as wallerian degeneration (in honor of Waller, who gave the first and most detailed description of this phenomenon). Wallerian degeneration is fragmentation and disintegration of the axon, plus degeneration of myelin; macrophages appear which phagocytose the axon and myelin debris and can be observed as fat-laden cells,

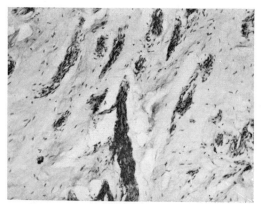

FIG. 3–20. Amputation neuroma. Dense connective tissue with irregular nerve bundles.

together with Schwann cells which are also macrophagic and participate in the "clearing" of the lesion.[136] After elimination of tissue debris regeneration can proceed, but not before Schwann cells of both cut ends of the nerve have reestablished the continuity of the tubes, which are probably formed by the cellular cytoplasm.[137] While these preparations are in process the axon in the proximal end of the severed nerve starts growing as a result of ameboid extension. The required increase in axoplasm for this growth is the result of protein synthetic activity in the nerve cell body; the protein thus formed is passed distally to the fiber tip in a continual proximodistal axoplasmic flow.[138] Nerve fibers grow at an average speed of 3 to 4 mm. per day, within the tubes formed by Schwann cells. Therefore, if neurilemmal elements have been able to bridge the gap produced by injury, continuity will be reestablished and functions recovered, but if the growing axoplasm meets an obstacle in its way, such as a band of connective tissue, regeneration will not be possible. Instead, a disorganized mass of neurofibrils is formed, usually known as amputation neuroma although mutilation is not necessary for its occurrence (Fig. 3–20). Regeneration of neurofibrils is not influenced by electric stimulation, exercise or ionizing radiation, nor does the age or vascularization of the injured area appear to play any role in the process. The review by Guth[139] should be consulted for further details.

4. *Blood.* In the same way as surface epithelia, hemopoietic organs are continuously renewing blood. The average life of a

red blood cell is 100 to 120 days, that of polymorphonuclear leukocytes is 6 to 10 days and of lymphocytes probably as long as 100 days; in the normal subject, however, the numbers of these elements are maintained in the peripheral blood within very narrow limits of variation. Bone marrow and lymphopoietic organs show continuous mitotic activity, accompanied by maturation and release of blood cells. Blood loss is followed by an increase in the speed of production of formed elements and when hemorrhage is abundant these cells enter the circulation in a state of immature development. When blood loss is continuous the bone marrow shows hyperplasia, which disappears with return to normality. The stimulus for this regeneration is discussed below.

C. Stimulus for Regeneration. As in the case of wound healing, studies on regeneration have suggested that the stimulus is humoral in nature and, in parallel with "wound hormones," "regeneration hormones" have been postulated. Another point of view is that decrease in the total mass of functioning cytoplasm creates a state of functional deficit which would represent the true stimulus for regeneration. Finally, it has also been proposed that the predominant stimulus is the circulation of blood and that tissues regenerate not because of the reconstitution of parenchyma, but because of the missing blood vessels, required to provide an adequate vascular bed. Each one of these hypotheses is examined in the following paragraphs.

1. *Humoral Hypothesis of Regeneration.* At present, the humoral hypothesis of regeneration is perhaps the best supported of the three that will be discussed here. Data are mainly derived from studies in embryos, in the liver, in peripheral nerves and in the formed elements of the blood. Weiss[140] postulated that regeneration is ruled by the general principle of active maintenance of the total mass of each organic system in a state of equilibrium, and that the necessary stimuli are specific chemical substances released for each cell type. In support of this concept Weiss relates that if small fragments of liver are placed in the extraembryonal area of a chick embryo, the liver of the embryo grows to a size greater than normal; furthermore, the injection of liver or kidney cellular debris into embryonal blood will result in an increase of mitoses in the homologous organ. Working with the outer orbital gland of the rat, Voutilainen, *et al.*[141] observed that if the duct is ligated and the gland is injured, mitoses increase in the gland and also in the contralateral gland; the same author found that when suspensions of the skin of newborn rats are injected intraperitoneally into 2 to 3 month-old rats, mitotic stimulation of the epidermis occurs, and that when this phenomenon is tested during wound healing the time of epithelization is decreased by almost one-third. Basleer[142] showed that the mitotic rate of one wound is lower than that of two wounds, which suggests the presence of humoral mechanisms acting at a distance.

An increase in the number of mitoses in rat liver cells was obtained by McJunkin and Breuhaus[143] after injecting normal animals with liver extracts in different stages of autolysis; no mention is made, however, of any search for mitoses in other organs. Wenneker and Sussmann,[144] and Bucher and her colleagues[145] published simultaneously the results of experiments in parabiotic rats; in this work, partial hepatectomy is performed on one member of the pair and both the weight and the number of mitoses increase in the liver of the other animal. In view of their results, these two groups of authors suggested the existence of humoral factors stimulating liver growth. On the other hand, Glinos and Gey[146] showed that immediately after partial hepatectomy there is a decrease in plasma proteins and that if this plasma is added to a culture of fibroblasts there is an increase in the number of mitoses. Plasma obtained from an animal after completion of liver regeneration fails to induce this mitotic stimulation. Glinos and Gey believe that normal plasma contains a growth-inhibiting factor for the liver produced by this same organ and present in the proteins; a removal of part of the liver would cause a decrease in the amount of the inhibiting substance and cells would then multiply, increasing in number until adequate amounts of the factor are again synthesized and cellular multiplication stops.[147] A report by Hurowitz and Studer lends support to the hypothesis of a humoral factor in liver regeneration. Using paired, parabiotically united white rats they compared the effects of the mitotic impulse, induced by partial hepatectomy, on the healthy partner with those of the partner which had previously received carbon tetrachloride to induce liver damage. These authors found that while 62 per cent of their undamaged rats showed an increase in mitoses, only 17 per cent of those injured with CCl_4 were capable of reacting to the humoral factor produced by the regenerating liver of the partner.

In the case of regeneration of the nervous system, data are somewhat contradictory. Cajal[149] was the first in suggesting that axonal growth was directed towards the distal end of the severed nerve by chemical substances produced by Schwann cells. This theory was known as "neurotropism"; *in vitro* studies of Weiss and Taylor,[150] however, have shown that nerve fibers fail to grow preferentially towards degenerating nervous tissue, without showing preference for any area. Other observers have not seen nerve fibers grow faster *in vivo* in innervated autografts with wallerian degeneration than in autografts without nerve disintegration. What does appear to influence the direction of axonal growth is the physical structure of the environment, such as fibrin bands or inert cotton threads. In their discussion of neurotropism, Weiss and Taylor remark, "Cajal says . . .: 'As for the theory of neurotropism, far from being for me a dogma, it is simply a working hypothesis which I am willing to correct or even abandon in the presence of better explanations.' We feel the time has come to abandon it. 'Contact guidance' affords a better explanation." It has been suggested that Schwann cells are influenced by the degenerating axon through chemical mechanisms, since mitotic activity is only observed near the area of neurofibril disintegration; i.e., along the distal end of the nerve and in a small part of the proximal end, near the cut section. Furthermore, proliferation of Schwann cells is not immediate but takes a few days in appearing, suggesting that some time is necessary for this substance to accumulate during axonal destruction. This idea has been tested in tissue cultures, with positive results,[151] but so far this is only a temporal

coexistence and the nature of the hypothetical substance released during nerve disintegration remains unknown.

The only case where there is definitive proof of a humoral mechanism in regeneration is the bone marrow; in animals with blood loss due to hemorrhage both plasma and urine contain a substance which, when injected into normal animals, causes hyperplasia of the bone marrow with release of mature elements to the peripheral circulation. This substance is known as "erythropoietin" or "hemopoietin," and its properties have been determined by several groups of investigators.[152] The first observation, made in 1906, was that the injection of anemic rabbit plasma into normal rabbits was accompanied by an elevation in the number of formed elements in the blood of the test animal.[153] In spite of this experiment the attention of investigators was deviated to the influence of oxygen in the bone marrow; it was considered that anoxia was the most important factor in the regulation of hemopoiesis. However, direct measurements by Grant and Root[154] in dogs with hemorrhages of 30 per cent of blood volume revealed no anoxia in the bone marrow; similar results were obtained by Berk and associates[155] in human subjects with anemia or polycythemia vera. Furthermore, Thomas[156] described that anoxia inhibits the synthesis of heme in tissue cultures of bone marrow. A decisive experiment was that of Reissman,[157] who placed one member of a parabiotic pair of rats in a special chamber under conditions of anoxia and observed hyperplasia of bone marrow in both animals; thus, a humoral factor was suggested as responsible for regeneration of blood loss. Many other publications, recently summarized by Gordon,[158] have provided a growing picture of erythropoietin; some of the features are as follows: (a) erythropoietin induces erythoblastic proliferation instead of accelerating maturation; (b) it is present in the protein-free fraction of boiled and acidified plasma; (c) it is not species specific nor antigenic; (d) it is organic in nature; (e) it is not produced by hemopoietic action of lymphoid organs and tissues; (f) the kidney seems to play an important role in its formation; (g) thyroid, gonads and adrenals have been eliminated as possible sources of erythropoietin. The pituitary plays some role in the synthesis of erythropoietin, but the hypophysectomized animal still has some activity in the plasma; (h) there are increased amounts of erythropoietin in the plasma of anemic and polycythemic patients. Theoretical and clinical implications of erythropoietin are many and very great, but here it is of interest only as a demonstrated humoral mechanism in regeneration.

2. *Functional Hypothesis of Regeneration.* This hypothesis is based mainly on studies of regeneration of endocrine glands and may be expressed as follows: a decrease in the total mass of functioning cytoplasm is accompanied by a simultaneous decrease in its specific function, so the persisting elements are forced to increase their activity. Together with enhanced function there is an increase in cellular metabolism, with predominance of anabolic over catabolic phenomena, which results in a greater intracytoplasmic concentration of metabolites and, therefore, more water will pass into the cell. The increase in volume implies a reduction in the exchange surface between cell and surrounding medium, a condition stimulating mitosis.[159] As an example of this sequence Gray's experiments on regeneration of the thyroid may be quoted;[160] this author removed part of the thyroid gland in a group of rats that 10 days later showed an average of 2284 mitoses per slide. A similar group received thyroid extract during the 10 day period following partial thyroidectomy, and upon microscopic examination the remaining gland showed only 45 mitoses per slide. In this case, replacement of function by exogenous thyroid delayed regenera-

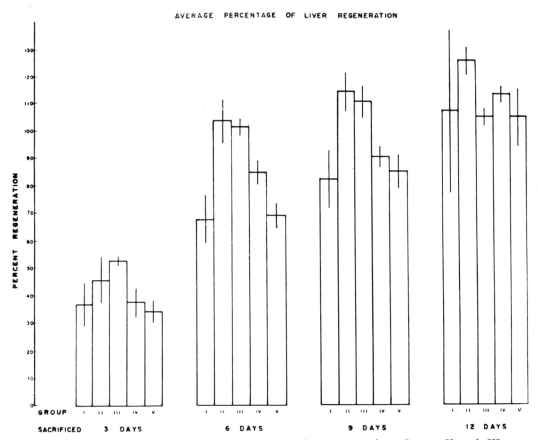

FIG. 3–21. Effect of splenectomy on experimental liver regeneration. Groups II and III were splenectomized and show higher per cent regeneration than other groups at days 6 and 9. (Courtesy of the Editor, Laboratory Investigation.)

tion of the organ. A similar experiment was published by Cameron[161] using pancreas as the effector tissue and insulin to replace the endocrine function after partial pancreatectomy; the result was that only the exocrine portion was regenerated since the function of the islands of Langerhans had been replaced. The functional hypothesis of regeneration has been invoked for the liver, but in this case no important deficiency in hepatic functions has been demonstrated.[162] An experiment related by Weiss[140] may be pertinent in this respect. Wayne Ferris cauterized the metanephros in one side of 12 to 13 day developing chick embryos, when the metanephros is inactive because the mesonephros is still functioning. Two days after the operation mitoses in the metanephros of the opposite site were counted and found to be 70 per cent more numerous than in intact embryos. Furthermore, mitotic increase was limited to the renal epithelium since the supporting connective tissue showed no enhanced proliferation. Weiss' hypothesis on the formation of organ specific, complementary compounds has been mentioned above.

3. *Circulatory Hypothesis of Regeneration.* Mann[126] believes that liver regeneration is secondary to the need of vascular channels for portal blood circulation. The idea is based on results obtained in liver regeneration in dogs with Eck fistula. Other workers, especially Child and associates,[127] have shown that with complete inversion of liver circulation by means of terminal anastomoses between the portal vein and the vena cava, regeneration of the liver returns to almost normal figures. These experiments have not excluded the possibility that the blood is simply acting as a vehicle for some substances regulating liver regeneration; furthermore, Weinbren has shown that liver tissue in the rat is capable of regenerating in the complete absence of the portal blood supply.[163] The liver undergoes atrophy after deviation of its portal blood supply,[164] but this atrophied liver shows conspicuous restoration when stimulated by partial hepatectomy. Finally, splenectomy accelerates the rate of regeneration of the rat liver[165] and there are data suggestive of a humoral and not a circulatory mechanism in this effect, since it does not depend on the amount of

splenic tissue nor on its location in the vascular system[166] (Fig. 3–21).

IV. TISSUE TRANSPLANTATION

As much as the organism is capable of repair and regeneration of its own tissues, this can only be accomplished within certain limits which frequently fall short of the actual needs. It is then necessary to make use of transplants, of which the most commonly performed type is blood transfusion. Extensive wounds, burns involving 15 per cent or more of the body surface, surgical procedures necessitating removal of large areas of tissue or small but highly specialized regions with poor regenerating abilities, all require immediate and expert attention in order to help the organism regenerate epithelium to avoid infection, massive losses of fluid and electrolytes, and/or defective and unsightly scars. These are not the only problems requiring tissue transplantation; sometimes it is also necessary to replace an organ which cannot regenerate, such as the cornea, or a blood vessel with an aneurysmatic dilation, or a trachea destroyed by trauma, or a bone eroded by osteomyelitis. These instances are mentioned because in all of them both experimental and clinical transplants have been attempted, frequently with success, sometimes with failure.

It is easy to imagine the immense benefits that could be derived from the systematic success of surgical treatment by means of tissue transplantation in the cases mentioned, but the possibilities go still further. Vascular surgery has advanced to the point where transplantations of whole organs are entirely feasible from a technical standpoint, and this might be used when disease has destroyed an organ beyond any possibility of regeneration, as the kidney in chronic glomerulonephritis. Indeed, this has been done in a certain number of cases fulfilling a series of conditions (so far *sine qua non*) which will be mentioned below. But the same could be done when rheumatic fever has hardened and deformed the heart valves, or atherosclerosis has caused coronary occlusion and myocardial infarction, or cirrhosis has transformed the liver into a distorted and fibrotic organ (Fig. 3–22). Whole organs for transplantation could be obtained from voluntary donors, when they are paired, such as adrenals or kidneys.

Banks could be established with organs obtained from healthy subjects killed in accidents, much as is done now with cartilage, bone, blood vessels and cornea. Ten years ago these ideas might have been considered

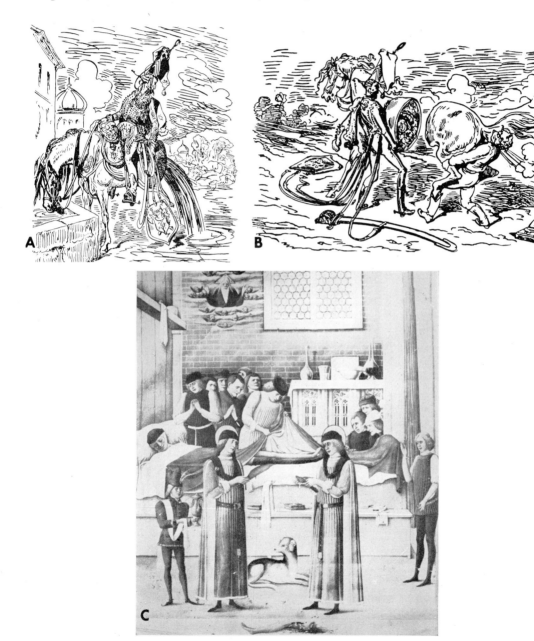

FIG. 3–22.   Two legendary instances of tissue transplantation. *A,* The notorious Baron von Münchhausen, at the end of a fierce battle, realizes that his horse has lost the posterior half. *B,* Having located the lost part, the Baron is assisted to replace it *in situ.* (This is an instance of an autologous orthotopic graft.) *C,* The miracle of St. Cosmas and St. Damian, from a miniature attributed to Mantegna. A man with leg ulcers fell asleep while praying for health; in his sleep the saintly surgeons amputated the sick leg and replaced it by that of a Moor who was going to be buried. (This is an instance of a homologous graft.)

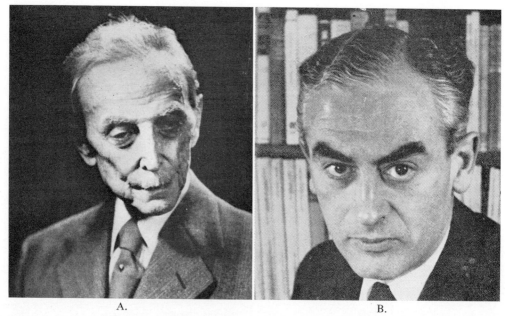

A.   B.

FIG. 3–23.   A, Leo Loeb (1869–1959). B, P. B. Medawar.

infantile; it will be of interest to see what happens in ten more years.[167] Intensive research in this field has shown that the main problems are no longer surgical but immunologic. In the following paragraphs some of the knowledge in this field is summarized, but the literature is extensive and grows very rapidly; those especially interested should consult Peer's book,[168] the symposia published by the New York Academy of Science,[169–171] and recent reviews by Brent,[172] Jacobs, et al.,[173] and Medawar.[174]

A. General Principles of Tissue Transplantation. 1. *Types.* There are three general types of tissue transplantation: (a) An autotransplant is a tissue fragment displaced from its normal position in the same subject. When the bed receiving the graft is adequate, and care is exercised to avoid infection, this form of transplant is usually successful, although large areas of tissue require preservation of their own vascularity until the blood vessels of the bed have grown into the graft. (b) A homotransplant is the displacement of tissue from a donor to a recipient of the same species. (c) The transfer from a donor of one species to a recipient of another species is known as heterotransplant.

The fate of the latter two types of transplants is quite different from the first or autotransplant. Except under extremely rare

conditions, homo- and heterotransplants undergo necrosis and are eliminated or rejected from the recipient after a short period during which they appear normal.[175] Embryonal or neoplastic tissues may "take" when grafted in animals of the same or even different species, but this is an experimental situation revealing interesting aspects of the biology of tissue transplantations, of little practical application so far.

2. *Mechanism of Tissue Transplant Rejection.* Several theories have been suggested to explain the systematic rejection of homo- and heterotransplants, such as the blood group incompatibility theory, which held that rejection resulted from differences in the blood groups of donor and recipient. Some cases were published of persistence of homografts in subjects with similar or identical blood groups; however, the experience of many workers showed these concepts false and they have been abandoned.[176] Another theory, expressed by one of the most distinguished investigators in this field, Leo Loeb (Fig. 3–23, A), may be labeled as "individuality differentials." This author believed that each individual had a series of unique properties and that when his tissues came in contact with those of another individual such "differentials" would enter in conflict and the graft would be treated as a

foreign body. It is not easy to do justice to this theory, since its author never expressed it in more concrete terms, but there is no doubt that it served as the foundation of more recent concepts and those interested should consult Loeb's book "The Biological Basis of Individuality."[177]

In 1944, P. B. Medawar (Fig. 3–23, *B*), from the Zoology and Comparative Anatomy department of University College in London, began to work on this problem, and he and his associates by means of a series of ingenious and careful experiments have established the general nature of the rejection of transplants. From their many and very important observations the immunologic theory of transplant rejection has emerged, which holds that homo- or heterografts act as antigens in the recipient and that their elimination is caused by an antigen-antibody reaction. Some of the most relevant observations supporting this theory are as follows:

a. A homotransplant is not rejected immediately after it has been received by the host; several days elapse, which depend on various factors such as the size of the graft, the number of previous grafts, the animal species, the tissue transplanted, etc. During these days the homograft behaves in a way similar to an autograft; it shows good preservation of structure and becomes vascularized. Suddenly, however, the aspect of the graft changes, it becomes dark and hard, there is thrombosis of blood vessels and the circulation ceases; the tissue undergoes necrosis and if it is a fragment of skin it sloughs off and is eliminated. This first period of well-being of the graft suggests that the host requires some time to synthesize antibodies, but when they are formed the transplant is rejected.[178]

b. After elimination of the first homograft, a second transplant from the same donor is rejected much faster, which can be explained through the "anamnesic" response of an organism previously sensitized with antigen. This phenomenon is known as the "second set" rejection.[179]

c. Tissue homotransplants placed in an avascular bed, such as the anterior chamber of the eye, the cornea or cartilage, survive as long as blood vessels fail to reach them, but when this happens they are rejected in the same way as the others.[180] This observation suggests that there is a substance or substances in the circulation which must reach the transplant before it can be eliminated.

d. If the recipient has agammaglobulinemia (a rare, congenital or acquired disturbance consisting of an inability to form gamma globulins), homotransplants survive as if they were autotransplants.[181] It has been shown that the greater part of antibodies are present in plasma gamma globulins.

e. If the recipients are pretreated with cortisone or given whole body radiation,[182] homotransplants take much longer before they are rejected. It has been determined that cortisone and radiation depress antibody synthesis.

f. When a suspension of epithelial cells from the donor is injected into the recipient some days before grafting, the homotransplant is rapidly rejected. This interesting observation has been interpreted as sensitization of the host by the cells, which would be a variant of the "second set" phenomenon mentioned above.[183]

g. If a suspension of any type of cells from the donor (except red blood cells) is injected into the recipient *in utero* or immediately after birth, homotransplants made when the recipient has grown are not eliminated. This is the phenomenon of "acquired tolerance," one of the most interesting discoveries of Medawar and his group,[184, 185] which should be distinguished from Felton's "immunological paralysis,"[186] a phenomenon observed with massive doses of antigen in adult animals which is described in Chapter VIII.

These and many other data lend strong support to the hypothesis of an immune response as the mechanism of homo- and heterotransplant rejection. Therefore, it is well to inquire into some aspects of this immune response, which seems to be peculiar in many respects. The *nature of the antigen* appears well established since Medawar's demonstration that it is individual specific but not tissue specific,[187] that it is contained in any nucleated cell[188] (with Barret's observation against this[189]), that cells must be viable to preserve intact the ability for inducing homotransplant sensitivity or acquired tolerance,[190] and that this ability resides in the nucleus. Furthermore, Billingham, et al.[191] found that isolated nuclei were one-fifth to one-tenth as potent as intact, viable cells in the capacity to induce homograft sensitivity, and that the incubation of nuclei isolated from spleen cells with ribonuclease had no effect upon their antigenicity; however, when incubation was carried out with desoxyribonuclease antigenicity was lost. For these and other reasons Billingham, et al.[191] suggested that antigens concerned in the induction of homograft sensitivity could be desoxyribonucleoproteins possessing antigenic and genetic specificity. More recently, however, purified preparations of desoxyribonucleic acid obtained from spleen, thymus and liver have been injected into mice in the hope of inducing homograft sensitivity but the results have been negative.[192, 193]

The *nature of the antibody* has been extensively studied and it has been shown that a homotransplant will induce the appearance of humoral and cellular antibodies, both of which appear to play some role in homograft rejection. The participation of humoral antibodies has been difficult to establish, mainly because of technical reasons. Nevertheless, the fact that subjects with agammaglobulinemia fail to reject skin homografts, although they are capable of developing delayed immune responses,[181] suggests that some humoral factor related to gamma globulin is involved in rejection. Billingham and Sparrow[194] found that incubation of dissociated epidermal cells with immune serum from a rabbit sensitized against the same cells prevented their growth when returned to the donor's bed; a similar experiment has been carried out by Mitchison using mouse leukemia cells.[195] At least four different kinds of antibody activity have been found in isoimmune serum: erythrocyte agglutination, leukocyte agglutination, tumor-neutralizing effect and cytotoxic effect. The latter appears to be the type more probably associated with homograft rejection, since *in vitro* it will destroy cells responsible for its formation or other elements with identical genetic structure.[195a] The role of cellular antibodies has been established by Algire et al.,[196] who devised a diffusion chamber which permits free passage of extracellular fluids but is impermeable to cells of the recipient; when a tissue graft is placed within the chamber and this is introduced into the host the graft will survive for periods of up to 4 to 6 months, as long as the cells of the recipient are prevented from coming in contact with the graft. Similar results were obtained by Woodruff.[197] These and other data suggest that homograft rejection is carried out by a combination of humoral and cellular antibodies, neither of which is capable of destroying foreign tissues by themselves. The situation might be compared to opsonization in phagocytosis, and indeed the similarity may be more than superficial.

If cellular antibodies are involved in the homograft rejection, the *nature of the immune response* may be considered as akin to delayed hypersensitivity. There are many similarities between the two phenomena[198] (homograft sensitivity and delayed hypersensitivity) but there are also some differences, such as the cytotoxicity of antigen for explanted cells observed in delayed hypersensitivity[199] and absent in homograft sensitivity, and the fact that cellular transfer of the latter can be accomplished only by cells obtained from the draining lymph nodes and occasionally from the spleen, whereas delayed hypersensitivity may be transferred by any cells from the immunized subject.[200] For these and other reasons, Thomas[201] has suggested that homograft rejection may be mediated by an immune mechanism peculiar to itself that has no counterpart in conventional immunology. Such a mechanism has been developed by Lawrence[202] under the name of the "(Self + X) hypothesis" and may be summarized as follows. Microorganisms responsible for most intense and durable types of delayed hypersensitivity exhibit a preference for intracellular habitat, where they may survive for prolonged periods and even reproduce themselves without killing the cells concerned. It is possible that such scavenger cells, which before being parasitized were recognized by the organism as (self), upon dying with the intracytoplasmic microorganism and being phagocytized by the reticuloendothelial system are considered as complexes such as (self + bacteria). This event, partially out of the ordinary for the reticuloendothelial cells, may evoke a modification of the mechanism postulated for recognition and destruction of mutant cells. "A modified response of this type may be unique of itself or may perhaps vary in intensity from that evoked by overtly foreign tissue cells in homograft sensitivity. However, it may be of the same general nature as the response to unmistakably foreign cells and utilize similar, if not the same, pathways of effector mechanism by which the latter are eradicated by the host." Cells of the leukocytic series would be sensitized to the antigen (self + X), thus developing a highly reactive site specifically directed against all (self + X) tissues. This stimulating speculation is summarized in Figure 3–24, taken from Lawrence.

3. *Compatibility and Incompatibility.* Working with tumor transplantations, Greene[203] has pointed out that tissue compatibility is not due exclusively to its antigenic capacity but also to the conditions of the transplant, the recipient and the bed. In his own words, ". . . the status of a tissue varies with development and may be embryonic or cancerous as well as adult. Further, the body of the recipient, extending beneath the subcutaneous space, contains areas of differentiation such as the brain and the eye, whose special attributes provide the tissue with more suitable conditions for growth but do not confer an independence of the constitutional factors determining the reaction of transplantation." Greene has successfully transplanted many different types of tissues to various sites of the same animal, of other animals of the same species and even to other species. Other important factors are the capacity of the transplant to induce formation of stroma in the host, which favors survival of the graft, and the ability of the recipient to form supporting stroma in contact with the transplant, which also favors survival. When dealing with tissues with a limited ability to induce proliferation of stroma it is possible to make the grafts "take" by accompanying them with fragments of embryonal lung or other tissues, which favor the development of connective tissue. The host may also be conditioned by the administration of cortisone or by total body radiation. Greene's important contribution to tumor transplantation is discussed in Chapter V.

B. Some Practical Uses of Tissue Transplantation. Recent studies of tissue transplantation have served a triple purpose. First, they have revealed a series of basic facts in general biology, immunology and cancerology which otherwise would have remained ignored. Some of them have been mentioned before and others will be described in Chapter VIII. It must be emphasized that this is probably the most important aspect of this field of research, although the glamour of practicality has yet to be bestowed on it. Second, a rather limited use of tissue transplantation may be made in the diagnosis of undifferentiated tumors. The third purpose is the application of new knowledge to the treatment of some pathologic conditions.

1. *Tumor Diagnosis by Tissue Transplantation.* In an instructive paper entitled, "The microscope or the guinea pig?" Greene[204] relates one case of a highly undifferentiated tumor diagnosed differently by several excellent microscopists; heterotransplantation in the guinea pig was tried and

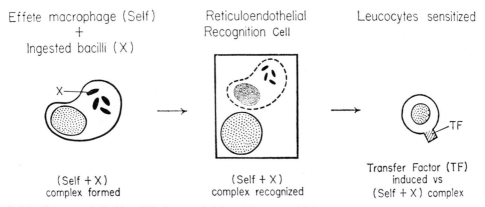

Effete macrophage (Self)
+
Ingested bacilli (X)

Reticuloendothelial
Recognition Cell

Leucocytes sensitized

(Self + X)
complex formed

(Self + X)
complex recognized

Transfer Factor (TF)
induced vs
(Self + X) complex

FIG. 3–24. Lawrence's "self + X" theory of delayed hypersensitivity, exemplified by tubercle bacilli (X) and macrophage (self). (Courtesy of Dr. H. B. Lawrence and the Editor, Physiological Reviews.)

achieved, and the microscopic sections of the growing transplant revealed better differentiated structures that were simpler to interpret. There is no doubt that behavior is more basic than morphology; actually, what the pathologist tries to do with the microscope is to predict behavior from a given morphologic picture. But when behavior may be observed directly and not inferred, the pathologist is one step closer to the real nature of phenomena. The obvious limitations of tissue transplant as a diagnostic technique are that not all tumors "take," that the method is more laborious and time consuming than microscopic analysis and that very few tumors represent a real diagnostic problem to an experienced pathologist. For these reasons, the answer to Greene's dilemma is an emphatic "the microscope," with the qualification that it may be necessary to use additional techniques to establish a satisfactory diagnosis of a given tumor, which include histochemistry, tissue cultures and, of course, tissue transplantation. Many important things have been learned about the biology of malignant tumors through transplantation, and some of them are summarized in Chapter V.

2. *Tissue Transplantation in Treatment.* There are two general uses of transplants in treatment: that which takes advantage not of the physiologic activity of tissues, but of their physical properties, such as transparency in the cornea, rigidity in bone, elasticity in blood vessels; the other represents the substitution of living tissues or entire organs for others irreversibly damaged by disease, in the hope of replacing not only form but also function. The second form is the goal of many investigators and their work has shown that once the difficulties of surgical technique have been solved, the only remaining barrier is the immune response of the host. The summary of some recent attempts to effect living tissue homotransplants will serve to review the present status of the problem confronting those engaged in this type of work.

Although preceded by other publications of attempts to perform kidney homotransplantation both experimental and human,[205] the case published by Michon, *et al.*,[206] in 1953 is a clear example of the difficulties involved in tissue transplantation. A 16 year old carpenter without significant previous history of disease fell from a third floor and was taken to the hospital, where radiologic studies revealed multiple fractures in the pelvic bones; a few hours later an emergency right lumbotomy was performed because of hemorrhagic shock and the presence of lumbar hematoma. The surgeon found an enlarged kidney surrounded by abundant blood clots and decided that nephrectomy was the only way to stop bleeding caused by rupture of the renal pedicle. The operation was performed and the patient did well in the immediate postoperative period; as he failed to void any urine a catheter was passed into the bladder and only a few drops of bloody fluid were obtained. After 48 hours of complete and persistent anuria the patient was moved to another service where it was found that he had congenital absence of the opposite kidney. After 7 days of total anuria, a blood chemistry showed 430 mg./100 ml. of urea, 7 mEq./1. of potassium and profound anemia; it was considered that the only hope of survival was a kidney homotransplant. Although *a priori* it was accepted that chances of success were remote, the special circumstances of the case and the mother's insistence in giving one kidney decided the surgeons to carry out the operation. The kidney was ischemic for 55 minutes before completion of the transplant, which was placed in the pelvis, and for the following 3 hours only a few drops of a reddish fluid came out of the ureter. However, the output increased after this period and rapidly established a rate of 1 drop per second of transparent urine. For the following 21 days the kidney functioned rather well, putting out an average of 1500 ml. of urine per day; azotemia decreased to almost normal figures and there was no more hematuria. Suddenly, however, and without any preceding symptoms, the kidney stopped functioning entirely and definitely at the end of 21 days. The patient was reoperated and the blood vessels and ureter were found to be unaffected; all treatment was useless and the patient died 11 days after the second anuria, 40 days after nephrectomy of the single kidney (Fig. 3–25).

This case is of interest because several

special features were present that had not been observed in previous instances and which support the idea that homotransplants are rejected by an immune response. First, the patient was young and healthy, without vascular lesions or chronic renal disease; second, blood groups were very similar between donor and recipient, which made untenable the opinion that they played a significant role in rejection; third, no local complications such as infection, ureteral necrosis, etc., were present. In a more recent publication referring to 9 cases, Hume, et al.[207] observed that 5 of the 9 transplants never functioned and the remaining 4 secreted urine for periods varying from 37 to 180 days. The difference in duration with Michon's case is probably due to the fact that the patient was a young and healthy boy without previous renal disease, whereas the other 9 cases were all chronic renal patients with disturbances in the plasma proteins

and, therefore, in their immune response. Simonsen[208] and others [209] have called attention to the fact that subjects with chronic renal failure tolerate homografts for longer periods and have suggested that this may be due to a defect in the synthesis of antibody, but Stoloff, et al.[210] studied a group of 14 patients with chronic glomerulonephritis and found that uremia is not accompanied by a delay in the formation of antibodies. This interesting aspect of tissue homotransplantation awaits further studies. Another group of cases in which homotransplants are tolerated for longer periods than usual are Hodgkin's disease[211] and other types of lymphomas.[212] This has been associated with the peculiar inability of such patients to give adequate skin sensitization reactions, but the problem is far from being solved.

A strong confirmation of the idea that homograft rejection is caused by an immunologic mechanism is the result of studies

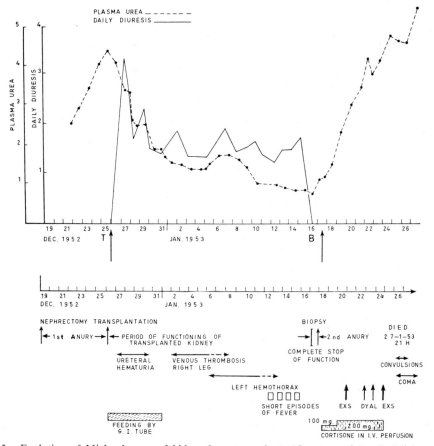

FIG. 3–25. Evolution of Michon's case of kidney homotransplant. (Courtesy of Dr. L. Michon and the Editor, Presse Médicale.)

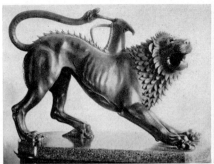

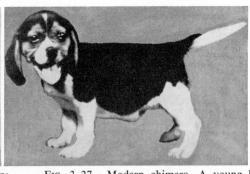

FIG. 3–26. Classic chimera. Etruscan bronze in the Archeological Museum of Florence, 5th century A.D.

FIG. 3–27. Modern chimera. A young beagle five weeks afer 800 r of total-body irradiation and a marrow transplant from a sister. (Courtesy of Dr. J. W. Ferrebee and the Editor, Annals of Internal Medicine.)

of identical twins. Murray and associates have published 7 such cases in which one of the identical twins had chronic glomerulonephritis while the other had normal kidneys;[213] in one of their observations a young man had manifestations of advanced renal atrophy and malignant hypertension. Kidney homotransplantation was carried out in the pelvis with almost immediate establishment of normal function; since the patient continued to have severe hypertension the diseased kidneys were removed in successive operations and the result was complete remission of hypertension.[214] This patient is enjoying normal life 5 years after the transplant; it must be mentioned that before carrying out the procedure Murray and associates assured themselves that they were dealing with identical twins by different tests, including crossed skin homotransplants which were studied both grossly and microscopically. In a strict biologic sense these cases cannot be considered as real homotransplants but rather as autotransplants, since identical twins have the same genetic constitution, and therefore the proteins of the donor are the same as those of the recipient;[25] this is the explanation for the lack of immune response and for the success of the "homotransplant" (isograft).

As the only serious problem in homotransplantation seems to be the recipient's immune response, suggestions have been made to solve it and create true "chimeras." In classic Greek mythology, Chimera (Fig. 3–26) was an animal with a lion's head, a goat's body and a snake's tail, a combination slightly more bizarre than

needed at present. These chimeras exist in cattle and some isolated instances have been described in man,[216] where there is coexistence of theoretically incompatible blood groups; furthermore, they have been produced in laboratory animals by means of acquired tolerance or conditioning of the host with cortisone and/or whole body irradiation. In all these cases homografts are seen to "take" perfectly well. In adult animals autologous or homologous bone marrow transfusion, after treatment with nitrogen mustard or whole body radiation destructive of most or all the bone marrow cells, may be life saving and at the same time creates a real chimera[217] (Fig. 3–27). The effect of chemotherapy or radiation is to inhibit the immune response but it also eliminates the bone marrow; transfused bone marrow repopulates the depleted marrow spaces[218] but fails to provide the animal with a new apparatus for the synthesis of antibodies. Skin homotransplants taken from the bone marrow donor will survive in the recipient since they have the same genetic constitution and will not act as antigens. These chimeras, however, have been desribed by Ferrebee and Thomas as "immunologic cripples," comparable to subjects with agammaglobulinemia and highly susceptible to later death from intercurrent infections. Although autopsies reveal a repopulated marrow, the architecture of the lymph nodes is markedly abnormal, with absence of germinal follicles and striking acellularity.[220] In order to avoid this complication, lymphoid cells obtained mainly from the spleen have been added to the infusion in both mice and dogs, with better results than when only bone marrow is utilized.[221] Should the problem of restoring a radiated subject with both an immunologic apparatus and a sufficient bone marrow population be solved, there is still another unfortunate result of the production of tolerance. This is the so-called "runt disease" or "homologous disease." It has been observed that mice made tolerant of skin grafts by neonatal injection of living spleen cells may fail to grow, develop diarrhea and die in 4 to 6 weeks after birth. There is ample evidence that such deaths are due to a "graft-against-host" reaction;[222] the injected cells, which by their continued presence as living, active, immunologically potent tissues have produced tolerance, by the same token are able to react against the foreign antigen of the host and result in its death.[223] Ferrebee[224] has suggested that prevention of this reaction might be possible by the use of immunologically immature hemopoietic tissue, such as can be obtained from embryo or neonatal donors, and there is some evidence that this is indeed the case.[225, 226]

Faced with problems related to delivering simultaneous, uniform irradiation to the human body comparable to that achieved in mice,[227] the collection, preservation and storage of adequate amounts of bone marrow and lymphoid cells of autologous or embryonal origin,[228] infection and "homologous disease," etc., it is small wonder that the application of these experimental observations to human material has met with failure. Whole body radiation and homologous bone marrow transfusion has been used in the treatment of some cases of leukemia[224] and other bone marrow disorders,[230] with acute leukemia treated by Thomas, et al;[231] in one case of leukemia the patient received 450 r of total body radiation and an infusion of cadaver bone marrow of identical blood type which had been stored for one month. Although the patient lost his graft, marrow function returned; however, he died 8 months later not of leukemia, but of a yeast infection (Fig. 3–28). Others have attempted to solve the problems of homologous disease by treating the postirradiation hematopoietic depression by the infusion of stored autogenous bone marrow obtained before whole body radiation, both in experimental animals[232] and in human cases.[233, 234] This technique permits rapid administration of intensive irradiation to wide areas without fear of hematopoietic depression or immunologic reactions as occurs with homologous transplants. At least one patient with uremia has been irradiated, given marrow and had a kidney transplant; the result, however, was rejection of the graft. Many of the practical problems in the use of tissue transplantation in humans by means of radiation-induced tolerance are summarized as follows by Merrill.[235]

"The clinical application of radiation-induced tolerance appears difficult because of the radiation dosage consideration. In low dose ranges the recipient destroys grafted tissue. In the middle dosage range rejection may occur as well as the graft vs. host reaction. In the high dose range the graft vs. host reaction plus radiation damage is a formidable complication. The use of x-ray dosages in the lower range plus specific lympholytic agents in closely related donor recipient pairs such as mother and son may possibly produce successful grafts. Since histocompatibility seems not to be an all-or-none phenomenon, this appears to be a promising possibility. Finally, the indication that tissue tolerated for long periods of time by use of any of the techniques mentioned above may live in a functional symbiosis with the host in spite of lack of induction of true histocompatibility seems to offer some hope for the eventual clinical solution of the homograft problem."

A different type of problem is encountered with the homotransplantation of endocrine tissues, which may function for prolonged or indefinite periods in the host without actual vessel-to-vessel connection. Merwin and Hill[236] showed conclusively that tissues normally rejected by a host would survive as long as vascularization failed to take place, a fact pointed out previously by Medawar.[180] It is also true that no endocrine deficiency state is a matter of life and death, so the methods used to overcome homograft rejection cannot be as life-endangering as total body radiation of the host. For these reasons, several workers have used Algire's millipore diffusion chamber technique[196] to achieve successful homotransplantation of endocrine tissues. Adrenal glands have been successfully homotransplanted in millipore chambers in rats but not in dogs.[238] Parathyroid glands seem to be poor antigens for the homotransplant rejection, since they

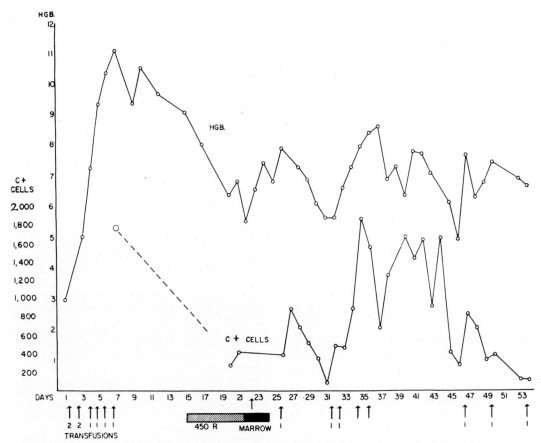

FIG. 3–28. Hematologic course of a patient with leukemia who was given 450 r of total body radiation over an 8-day period, followed by intravenous infusion of cadaver bone marrow stored for one month. C+ cells (donor cells) provided more than half the circulating erythrocytes from the thirty-fifth to the forty-third day. (Courtesy of Dr. E. D. Thomas and the Editor, New England Journal of Medicine.)

may be accepted without any millipore chamber between different strains of rats.[239] On the other hand, parathyroidectomized animals supported with calcium during the immediate postoperative period survive indefinitely and permit a gradual withdrawal of calcium support, so at the end of some months they are thoroughly adapted to hypocalcemia.[237] This complicates interpretation of homograft experiments, which so far have been unsuccessful;[240] limited experience in six human cases has resulted in failure of survival of the graft, except in one case in which viable cells were present in the chamber some 4 months after transplant, but there were no signs of functional activity.[237] Similar results have been obtained with thyroid homografts in man.[241] Ovarian transplantation has been attempted

in patients with Turner's syndrome by Castellanos and Sturgis[242] using approximately 2 Gm. of tissue from normal donors; the longest survival, judged by vaginal smears and urinary levels of follicle-stimulating hormone, was 5 to 6 months. The main problems involved in this technique are the diffusion of oxygen and metabolites through the millipore membrane, which seems to be slower than across biologic membranes, and the development of a capsule of connective tissue around the chamber, with further limitation of free exchange.[243]

REFERENCES

1. MacCrae, J.: quoted in Boyd, W.: Pathology for the Physician, ed. 6, Philadelphia, Lea and Febiger, 1958.
2. Florey, H.: Healing, in Florey, H. (ed.): General Pathology, ed. 2, Philadelphia, W. B. Saunders, 1958.

3. Allgöwer, M.: Cellular Basis of Wound Repair, Springfield, Charles C Thomas, 1956.
4. McDonald, R. A.: Origin of fibroblasts in experimental healing wounds: autorradiographic studies using tritiated thymidine, Surgery 46: 376, 1959.
5. Costero, I.: Caracterización del sistema fibroblástico. I. Bases doctrinarias, Arch. Inst. cardiol. México 24:237, 1954.
6. Barroso-Moguel, R.: Reacción fibroblástica experimental en el peritoneo, Prensa méd. México 23:321, 1958.
7. Clark, E. R., and Clark, E. L.: Further observations on living lymphatic vessels in the transparent chamber in the rabbit's ear—their relation to the tissue spaces, Am. J. Anat. 52:273, 1933.
8. Pullinger, B. D., and Florey, H. W.: Proliferation of lymphatics in inflammation, J. Path. & Bact. 45:157, 1937.
9. Stearns, M. L.: Studies on development of connective tissue in transparent chambers of rabbit's ear, Am. J. Anat. 66:133; 67:55, 1940.
10. Sandison, J. C.: Observations on the growth of blood vessels as seen in the transparent chamber introduced into the rabbit's ear, Am. J. Anat. 41:475, 1928.
11. Marshall, F. C., Uson, A. C., and Melicow, M. M.: Neoplasms and caruncles of the female urethra, Surg. Gynec. & Obst. 110:723, 1960.
12. Kerr, D. A.: Granuloma pyogenicum, Oral Surg. 4:158, 1951.
13. Williams, R. G.: Vascularity of normal and neoplastic grafts in vivo, Cancer Res. 11:139, 1951.
14. Taylor, H. E., and Saunders, A. M.: The association of metachromatic ground substance with fibroblastic activity in granulation tissue, Am. J. Path. 33:525, 1957.
15. Pérez Tamayo, R., and Ihnen, M.: Effect of methionine in experimental wound healing. A morphologic study, Am. J. Path. 29:233, 1953.
16. Wasserman, F.: Fibrillogenesis in regenerating rat tendon, with special reference to growth and composition of collagenous fibril, Am. J. Anat. 94:399, 1954.
17. Jackson, D. S.: Some biochemical aspects of fibrogenesis and wound healing, New Eng. J. Med. 259:814, 1958.
18. Billingham, R. E., and Russel, P. S.: Studies on wound healing with special reference to the phenomenon of contracture in experimental wounds in rabbit's skin, Ann. Surg. 144:961, 1956.
19. Grillo, H. G., Watts, G. T., and Gross, J.: Studies in wound healing. I. Contraction and the wound contents, Ann. Surg. 148:145, 1958.
20. Watts, G. T., Grillo, H. G., and Gross, J.: Studies on wound healing. II. Role of granulation tissue in contraction, Ann. Surg. 148:153, 1958.
21. Cuthbertson, A. M.: Contraction of full thickness skin wounds in the rat, Surg. Gynec. & Obst. 108:421, 1959.
22. Gillman, T., and Pann, J.: Studies on repair of cutaneous wounds, Med. Proc. 2:121, 1956.
23. Schilling, J. A., and Milch, L. E.: Fractional analysis of experimental wound fluid, Proc. Soc. Exper. Biol. & Med. 89:189, 1955.
24. White, B. N., Shetlar, M. R., Shurley, H. M., and Schilling, J. A.: Wound healing: investigation of proteins, glycoproteins, and lipids in experimental wound fluid in the dog, Proc. Soc. Exper. Biol. & Med. 101:353, 1959.
25. Edwards, L. C., Pernokas, L. N., and Dunphy, J. E.: The use of a plastic sponge to sample re-

generating tissue in healing wound, Surg. Gynec. & Obst. 105:303, 1957.
26. Orekhovitch, V. N., and Shpikiter, V. O.: Procollagens as Biological Precursors of Collagen and the Physico-chemical Nature of these Proteins, in Tunbridge, R. E. (ed.): Connective Tissue. A Symposium, Springfield, Charles C Thomas, 1957.
27. Williamson, M. B., and From, H. J.: The incorporation of sulfur aminoacids into the proteins of regenerating wound tissue, J. Biol. Chem. 212:705, 1955.
28. Williamson, M. B. (ed.): The Healing of Wounds, New York, McGraw-Hill, 1957.
29. Layton, L. L.: In vitro sulfate fixation by granulation tissue and injured muscle tissue from healing wounds, Proc. Soc. Exper. Biol. & Med. 73:570, 1950.
30. Upton, A. C., and Odell, T. T., Jr.: Utilization of S^{-35}-labeled sulphate in scorbutic guinea pigs: uptake in healing wounds, megakaryocytes and blood platelets, Arch. Path. 62:194, 1956.
31. Kodicek, E., and Loewi, G.: The uptake of (S^{-35}) sulphate by mucopolysaccharides of granulation tissue, Proc. Roy. Soc. London s.B 144: 100, 1955.
32. Ungar, G., and Damgaard, E.: Protein breakdown in thermal injury, Proc. Soc. Exper. Biol. & Med. 87:378, 1954.
33. Howes, E. L., Armitage, C. M., and Mondl, I.: Enzymes in the healing wound, Surg. Forum 6:54, 1956.
34. French, J. E., and Benditt, E. P.: Observations on localization of alkaline phosphatase in healing wounds, Arch. Path. 57:352, 1954.
35. Howes, E. L., Sooy, J. W., and Harvey, S. C.: The healing of wounds as determined by their tensile strength. J.A.M.A. 92:42, 1929.
36. Whipple, A. O.: The critical latent or lag period in the healing of wounds, Ann. Surg. 112:481, 1940.
37. Dunphy, J. E., and Udupa, K. N.: Chemical and histochemical sequences in the normal healing of wounds, New Eng. J. Med. 253:847, 1955.
38. Arey, L. B.: Wound healing, Physiol. Rev. 16:327, 1936.
39. Harkins, H. N.: Wound Healing, in Allen, J. G., Harkins, H. N., Moyer, C. A., and Rhoads, J. E. (eds.): Surgery, Principles and Practice, Philadelphia, J. B. Lippincott, 1957.
40. Ebeling, A. H.: Cicatrization of wounds. XIII. The temperature coefficient, J. Exper. Med. 35: 657, 1922.
41. Lecomte du Noüy, P.: Cicatrization of wounds. X. A general equation for the law of cicatrization of surface wounds, J. Exper. Med. 29:329, 1919.
42. Pohle, E. A., Ritchie, G., and Moir, W. M.: Studies of effect of roentgen rays on healing of wounds. III. Histological changes in skin wounds in rats following postoperative radiation with very small and moderate doses, Radiology 52:707, 1949.
43. Nickson, J. J., Lawrence, W., Jr., Rachwalsky, I., and Tyree, E.: Roentgen rays and wound healing. II. Fractional irradiation, an experimental study, Surgery 34:859, 1953.
44. Lattes, R., Martin, J. R., Meyer, K., and Ragan, C.: Effect of cartilage and other tissue suspensions on reparative processes of cortisone-treated animals, Am. J. Path. 32:979, 1956.
45. Prudden, J. F., Nishihara, G., and Baker, L.: The acceleration of wound healing with cartilage—I., Surg. Gynec. & Obst. 105:283, 1957.
46. Paulette, R. E., and Prudden, J. F.: Studies on the

acceleration of wound healing with cartilage. II. Histologic observations, Surg. Gynec. & Obst. *108:*406, 1958.

47. Raventos, A.: Wound healing and mortality after total body exposure to ionizing radiation, Proc. Soc. Exper. Biol. & Med. *87:*165, 1954.

48. Thompson, W. D., Ravdin, I. S., and Frank, I. L.: Effect of hypoproteinemia on wound disruption, Arch. Surg. *36:*500, 1938.

49. Udupa, K. N., Woessner, J. F., and Dunphy, J. E.: The effect of methionine on the production of mucopolysaccharides and collagen in healing wounds of protein depleted animals, Surg. Gynec. & Obst. *102:*639, 1956.

50. Robertson, W. van B., Hiwett, J., and Herman, C.: The relation of ascorbic acid to the conversion of proline to hydroxyproline in the synthesis of collagen in the carrageenin granuloma, J. Biol. Chem. *234:*105, 1959.

51. Wolbach, S.: Controlled formation of collagen and reticulum: a study of the source of intercellular substances in recovery from experimental scorbutus, Am. J. Path. *9:*689, 1933.

52. Stein, O., and Wolman, M.: A histochemical study of wound healing in scorbutic guinea pigs, Brit. J. Exper. Path. *39:*418, 1958.

53. Bradfield, J. R. G., and Kodicek, F.: Abnormal mucopolysaccharide and "precollagen" in vitamin C deficient skin wounds, Biochem. J. *49:* XVII, 1951.

54. Crandon, J. H., Lund, C. C., and Dill, D. B.: Experimental human scurvy, New Eng. J. Med. *233:*353, 1940.

55. Dunphy, J. E., Udupa, K. N., and Edwards, L. C.: Wound healing. A new perspective with particular reference to ascorbic acid deficiency, Ann. Surg. *144:*304, 1956.

56. Ponsetti, I. V., and Baird, W. A.: Scoliosis and dissecting aneurysm of the aorta in rats fed with *Lathyrus odoratus* seeds, Am. J. Path. *28:* 1059, 1952.

57. Dupuy, H. P., and Lee, J. G.: The isolation of a material capable of producing experimental lathyrism, J. Am. Pharm. A. *43:*61, 1954.

58. Enzinger, F. M., and Warner, E. D.: Wound healing in experimental lathyrism, Lab. Invest. *6:* 251, 1957.

59. Asboe-Hansen, G.: Hormonal effects on connective tissue, Physiol. Rev. *38:*446, 1958.

60. Asboe-Hansen, G.: Endocrine control of connective tissue, Am. J. Med. *26:*470, 1959.

61. Mueller, C. B., and Graham, E. A.: Influence of hypophysectomy on epithelization of wounds and on fibroplasia, Arch. Surg. *45:*534, 1942.

62. Cuthbertson, D. P., Shaw, G. P., and Young, F. G.: Anterior pituitary gland and protein metabolism. III. Influence of anterior pituitary extract on rate of wound healing, J. Endocrinol. *2:*475, 1941.

63. Prudden, J. F., Nishihara, G., and Ocampo, L.: Studies on growth hormone. III. The effect on wound tensile strength of marked post-operative anabolism induced with growth hormone, Surg. Gynec. & Obst. *107:*481, 1958.

64. Ragan, C., Howes, E. L., Plotz, C. M., Meyer, K., and Blunt, J. W.: Effect of cortisone on production of granulation tissue in the rabbit, Proc. Soc. Exper. Biol. & Med. *72:*718, 1949.

65. Chassin, J. L., McDougall, H. A., Stahl, W., McKay, M., and Localio, S. A.: Effect of adrenalectomy on wound healing in normal and in stressed rats, Proc. Soc. Exper. Biol. & Med. *86:*446, 1954.

66. Lattes, R., Blunt, J. W., Jr., Rose, H. M., Jesson,

R. A., Vaillancourt, de G., and Ragan C.: Lack of cortisone effect in early stages of inflammation and repair, Am. J. Path. *29:*1, 1953.

67. Selye, H.: Part of Inflammation in Local Adaptation Syndrome, in Jasmin, G., and Robert, A. (eds.): The Mechanism of Inflammation. An International Symposium, Montreal, Acta, 1953.

68. Lattes, R., Martin, J. R., and Ragan, C.: Suppression of cortisone effect on repair in presence of local bacterial infection, Am. J. Path. *30:*901, 1954.

69. Baker, B. L., and Whitaker, W. L.: Interference with wound healing by local action of adrenocortical steroids, Endocrinology *46:*544, 1950.

70. Scarpelli, D. G., Knouff, R. A., and Angerer, C. A.: Cortisone and oxygen consumption of granulation tissue from rabbit, Proc. Soc. Exper. Biol. & Med. *84:*94, 1953.

71. Persson, B. H.: Studies on the connective tissue ground substance; histochemical features of ground substance mucopolysaccharides; organization of ground substance in ascorbic acid deficiency and its modifications by action of cortisone, Acta Soc. Med. Upsalien. Suppl. 2, *58:*3, 1953.

72. Layton, L. L.: Effect of cortisone upon chondroitin sulphate synthesis by animal tissues, Proc. Soc. Exper. Biol. & Med. *76:*596, 1951.

73. Layton, L. L.: Cortisone inhibition of mucopolysaccharide synthesis in intact rat, Arch. Biochem. *32:*224, 1951.

74. Schiller, S., and Dorfman, A.: Metabolism of mucopolysaccharides in animals; effect of cortisone and hydrocortisone on rat skin, Endocrinology *60:*376, 1957.

75. Pernokas, L. N., Edwards, L. C., and Dunphy, J. E.: Hormonal influence on healing wounds: effect of adrenalectomy and cortisone on quantity and collagen content of granulation tissue, Surg. Forum *8:*74, 1958.

76. Alrich, E. M., Carter, J. P., and Lehman, E. P.: Effect of ACTH and cortisone on wound healing: an experimental study, Ann. Surg. *133:*783, 1951.

77. Taubenhaus, M., and Amromin, G. D.: Influence of steroid hormones on granulation tissue, Endocrinology *44:*359, 1949.

78. Pirani, C. L., Stepto, R. C., and Sutherland, K.: Desoxycorticosterone acetate and wound healing, J. Exper. Med. *93:*217, 1951.

79. Taubenhaus, M.: Hormonal Influences on Granulation Tissue Formation, in Williamson, M. B. (ed.): The Healing of Wounds, New York, McGraw-Hill, 1957.

80. Ducommun, S., Ducommun, P., and Salgado, E.: Etude du mécanisme d'action de la testostérone sur le tissu de granulation, Rev. Can. Biol. *11:* 300, 1952.

81. Taubenhaus, M., and Amromin, G. D.: The effects of the hypophysis, thyroid, sex steroids and the adrenal cortex upon granulation tissue, J. Lab. & Clin. Med. *36:*7, 1950.

82. Moltke, E.: Wound healing influenced by thyroxine and thyrotrophic hormone: tensiometric study, Proc. Soc. Exper. Biol. & Med. *88:*596, 1955.

83. Moltke, E.: Uptake of [35]-S-sulphate by healing wounds: effect of thyroxine and of ascorbic acid deficiency, Acta endocrinol. *25:*179, 1957.

84. Hunt, A.: Wound healing, Proc. Roy. Soc. Med. *53:*41, 1960.

85. Carrel, A.: Tissue culture and cell physiology, Physiol. Rev. *4:*1, 1924.

86. Kutsky, R. J., and Harris, M.: Growth promoting

agents in cell fractions of chick embryos, J. Cell. & Comp. Physiol. *43:*193, 1954.

87. Maganini, H., Hass, G. M., Schweitzer, A. W., and Wallace, B.: Factors in chick embryo extracts that stimulate fibroblasts to grow in tissue culture, Lab. Invest. *9:*239, 1960.

88. Loofbourow, J. R., Dwyer, C. M., and Cronin, A. G.: Proliferation-promoting intercellular hormones. II. Evidence for their production by living cells as a response to injury, Biochem. J. *35:*603, 1941.

89. Edwards, R. H., Sarmenta, S. S., and Hass, G.: Stimulation of granulation tissue growth by tissue extracts, Arch. Path. *69:*286, 1960.

90. Hardy, J. D.: Pathophysiology in Surgery, Baltimore, Williams and Wilkins, 1958.

91. Churchill, E. D.: in Patterson, W. B. (ed.): Wound Healing and Tissue Repair, Chicago, University of Chicago Press, 1956.

92. Mowlem, R.: Hypertrophic scars, Brit. J. Plast. Surg. *4:*113, 1951.

93. Glücksman, A.: Local factors in the histogenesis of hypertrophic scars, Brit. J. Plast. Surg. *4:* 88, 1951.

94. Solomons, B.: Keloids and their treatment, Practitioner *168:*465, 1952.

95. Levitt, W. M.: Radiotherapy in the prevention and treatment of hypertrophic scars, Brit. J. Plast. Surg. *4:*104, 1951.

96. Asboe-Hansen, G.: Hypertrophic scars and keloids. Etiology, pathogenesis, and dermatologic therapy, Dermatologica *120:*178, 1960.

96a. Berrill, N. J.: The indestructible hydra, Scient. Amer. *197:*118, 1957.

97. Singer, M.: The regeneration of body parts, Scient. Amer. *199:*79, 1958.

98. Willis, R. A.: The Borderland of Embryology and Pathology, London, Butterworth, 1958.

99. Needham, A. E.: Regeneration and Growth, in Nowinski, W. W. (ed.): Fundamental Aspects of Normal and Malignant Growth, New York, Elsevier Publishing, 1960.

100. Leblond, C. P., and Walker, B. E.: Renewal of cell populations, Physiol. Rev. *36:*255, 1956.

101. Bizzozero, G.: Growth and regeneration of the organism, Brit. M. J. *1:*728, 1894.

102. Weinbren, K.: Regeneration of the liver, Gastroenterology *37:*657, 1959.

103. Weiss, P., and Ferris, W.: The basement lamella of amphibian skin: its reconstruction after wounding, J. Biophys. & Biochem. Cytol. Suppl. *2:*275, 1956.

104. Bullough, W. S., and Lawrence, E. B.: Energy relations of epidermal mitotic activity adjacent to small wounds, Brit. J. Exper. Path. *38:*278, 1957.

105. Wilhelm, D. L.: Regeneration of tracheal epithelium, J. Path. & Bact. *65:*543, 1953.

106. Florey, H. W., and Harding, H. E.: The healing of artificial defects of the duodenal mucosa, J. Path. & Bact. *40:*211, 1935.

107. Dible, J. H.: Gastric ulcer and gastric carcinoma: an inquiry into their relationship, Brit. J. Surg. *12:*666, 1925.

108. Klein, S. H.: Malignant degeneration of chronic benign gastric ulcer, Surg. Clin. North Am. *27:*289, 1947.

109. Stewart, M. J.: Cancer of the stomach: some pathologic considerations. Brit. J. Radiol. *20:* 505, 1947.

110. Dukes, C. E., and Mummery-Lockhart, H. E.: Practical points in the pathology and surgical treatment of ulcerative colitis. A critical review, Brit. J. Surg. *45:*25, 1957.

111. Goldgraber, M. B., Humphreys, E. M., Kirsner, J. B., and Palmer, W. L.: Carcinoma and ulcerative colitis, Gastroenterology *34:*809, 1958.

112. Counsell, P. B., and Dukes, C. E.: The association of chronic ulcerative colitis and carcinoma of the rectum and colon, Brit. J. Surg. *39:*485, 1952.

113. Hickey, R. C., and Tidrick, R. T.: Cancer in patients with ulcerative colitis, Cancer *11:*35, 1958.

114. Hertig, A. T.: Diagnosing the endometrial biopsy, in Engle, E. T. (ed.): Proceedings of the Conference on Diagnosis in Sterility, 1945.

115. Ponfick, E.: Experimentelle Beitrage zur Pathologie der Leber. Virchows Arch. path. Anat. *118:* 209, 1889.

116. Higgins, G. M., and Anderson, R. M.: Experimental pathology of the liver. I. Restoration of the liver of the white rat following partial surgical removal, Arch. Path. *12:*186, 1931.

117. Cameron, G. R.: Normal and Pathological Patterns in the Liver, in Studies in Pathology Presented to Peter MacCallum, New York, Cambridge University Press, 1950.

118. Harkness, R. D.: Regeneration of liver, Brit. Med. Bull. *113:*87, 1957.

119. Brues, A. M., Drury, D. R., and Brues, M. C.: A quantitative study of cell growth in regenerating liver, Arch. Path. *22:*658, 1936.

120. Pérez Tamayo, R., Murphy, W., and Ihnen, M.: Effect of cortisone and partial starvation on liver regeneration, Arch. Path. *56:*629, 1953.

121. Ferguson, C. C., Rogers, C. S., and Vars, H. M.: Liver regeneration in the presence of common bile duct obstruction, Am. J. Physiol. *159:*343, 1949.

122. Weinbren, K.: The effect of bile duct obstruction on regeneration of the rat's liver, Brit. J. Exper. Path. *34:*280, 1953.

123. Cameron, G. R., and Karunaratne, W. A.: Carbon tetrachloride cirrhosis in relation to liver regeneration, J. Path. & Bact. *42:*1, 1936.

124. MacDonald, R. A., Schmid, R., and Mallory, G. K.: Regeneration in fatty liver and cirrhosis, Arch. Path. *69:*175, 1960.

125. Islami, A. H., Pack, G. T., and Hubbard, J. C.: Regenerative hyperplasia of the cirrhotic liver following partial hepatectomy, Cancer *14:*687, 1958.

126. Mann, F. C.: Restoration and pathologic reactions of the liver, J. Mt. Sinai Hosp. *11:*65, 1944.

127. Child, C. G., *et al:* Liver regeneration following portocaval transposition in dogs, Ann. Surg. *138:*600, 1953.

128. Fisher, B., Russ, C., and Bluestone, C.: Composition of regenerated dog liver following partial hepatectomy and total arterialization, Am. J. Physiol. *181:*203, 1955.

129. Grindlay, J. H., and Bollman, J. L.: Regeneration of the liver in the dog after partial hepatectomy, Surg. Gynec. & Obst. *94:*491, 1952.

130. Wiles, C. E., Schenk, W. G., and Lindenberg, J.: Influence of hepatic artery ligation on regeneration of liver tissue in the rat, Arch. Surg. *64:* 783, 1952.

131. Baggenstoss, A. H.: Significance of nodular regeneration in cirrhosis of the liver, Am. J. Clin. Path. *25:*936, 1955.

132. Windle, W. F. (ed.): Regeneration in the Central Nervous System, Springfield, Charles C Thomas, 1955.

133. Windle, W. F.: Regeneration of axons in the vertebrate central nervous system, Physiol. Rev. *36:* 427, 1956.

134. Liu, C. N., and Chambers, W. W.: Intraspinal sprouting elicited from intact spinal sensory neurons by adjacent posterior root section, Am. J. Physiol. *183*:640, 1955.

135. Littrell, J. L., Bunnell, D., Agnew, W. F., Smart, J. O., and Windle, W. F.: Effects of a bacterial pyrogen on hind-limb function in spinal cats, Anat. Rec. *115*:342, 1953.

136. Weddell, G., and Glees, P.: Early stages in degeneration of cutaneous nerve fibers, J. Anat. *76*: 65, 1941.

137. Holmes, W., and Young, J. Z.: Nerve regeneration after immediate and delayed suture, J. Anat. *77*: 63, 1942.

138. Hydén, H.: Protein metabolism in the nerve cell during growth and function, Acta physiol. scandinav. Suppl. 17, *6*:1, 1943.

139. Guth, L.: Regeneration in the mammalian peripheral nervous system, Physiol. Rev. *36*:441, 1956.

140. Weiss, P.: Specificity in Growth Control, in Butler, E. G. (ed.): Biological Specificity and Growth, Princeton, Princeton University Press, 1955.

141. Voutilainen, A., Hopsu, V. K., and Teir, H.: Effects of intraperitoneal injections of normal and x-ray irradiated outer orbital gland tissue on the mitotic activity in this organ in young rats, Acta path. et microbiol. scandinav. *45*:49, 1959.

142. Basleer, R.: Effects á distance d'un foyer cutané de nécrose et régénération sur les mitoses de l'épiderme de cobaye, Compt. rend. Soc. Biol. *147*:916, 1953.

143. McJunkin, F. A., and Breuhaus, H. C.: Homologous liver as a stimulus to hepatic regeneration, Arch. Path. *12*:900, 1931.

144. Wenneker, A., and Sussmann, N.: Regeneration of liver tissue following partial hepatectomy in parabiotic rats, Proc. Soc. Exper. Biol. & Med. *76*:683, 1951.

145. Bucher, N. L. R., Scott, J. F., and Aub, J. C.: Regeneration of the liver in parabiotic rats, Cancer Res. *11*:457, 1951.

146. Glinos, A. D., and Gey, G. O.: Humoral factors involved in the induction of regeneration of the liver in the rat, Proc. Soc. Exper. Biol. & Med. *80*:421, 1952.

147. Glinos, A. D.: The Mechanism of Liver Growth and Regeneration, in McElroy, W. D., and Glass, B. (eds.): The Chemical Basis of Development, Baltimore, Johns Hopkins Press, 1958.

148. Hurowitz, R. B., and Studer, A.: Effect of partial hepatectomy on mitosis rate in CCl_4-induced liver damage of parabiotic rats, Arch. Path. *69*:511, 1960.

149. Cajal, S. R.: Degeneration and Regeneration of the Nervous System, London, Oxford University Press, 1928.

150. Weiss, P., and Taylor, A. C.: Further experimental evidence against "neurotropism" in nerve regeneration, J. Exper. Zool. *95*:233, 1944.

151. Weiss, P.: Experiments on cell and axon orientation *in vitro;* the role of colloidal exudates in tissue organization, J. Exper. Zool. *100*:353, 1945.

152. Gurney, C. W., Jacobson, L. O., and Goldwasser, E.: The physiologic and clinical significance of erythropoietin, Ann. Int. Med. *49*:363, 1958.

153. Carnot, P., and Deflandre, C.: Sur l'activité hemopoietique du serum, Compt. rend. Acad. d. Sc. *143*:384, 1906.

154. Grant, W. C., and Root, W. S.: The relation of oxygen in bone marrow blood to posthemorrhagic erythropoiesis, Am. J. Physiol. *150*:618, 1947.

155. Berk, L., Burchenal, J. H., Wood, T., and Castle, W. B.: Oxygen saturation of sternal marrow blood with special reference to pathogenesis of polycythemia vera, Proc. Soc. Exper. Biol. & Med. *69*:316, 1948.

156. Thomas, E. D.: *In vitro* studies of erythropoiesis. II. The effect of anoxia on heme synthesis, Blood *10*:612, 1955.

157. Reissman, K. R.: Studies on the mechanism of erythropoietic stimulation in parabiotic rats during hypoxia, Blood *5*:372, 1950.

158. Gordon, A. S.: Hemopoietine, Physiol. Rev. *39*:1, 1959.

159. Payling Wright, G.: An Introduction to Pathology, ed. 2, London, J. & A. Churchill, 1957.

160. Gray, S. H.: The effect of potassium iodide, thyroid extract and anterior pituitary extract upon regeneration and early compensatory hypertrophy of the thyroid gland, Am. J. Path. *5*: 415, 1929.

161. Cameron, G. R.: Regeneration of the pancreas, J. Path. & Bact. *30*:713, 1927.

162. Weinbren, K., and Billing, B. H.: Hepatic clearance of bilirubin as an index of cellular function in the regenerating rat liver, Brit. J. Exper. Path. *37*:199, 1956.

163. Weinbren, K.: The portal blood supply and regeneration of the rat liver, Brit. J. Exper. Path. *36*:583, 1955.

164. Rous, P., and Larimore, L. D.: Relation of the portal blood to liver maintenance, J. Exper. Med. *31*:609, 1920.

165. Higgins, G. M., and Priestley, J. T.: Experimental pathology of the liver in the white rat after partial removal and splenectomy, Arch. Path. *12*:186, 1931.

166. Pérez Tamayo, R., and Romero, R.: Role of the spleen in regeneration of the liver, Lab. Invest. *7*:248, 1958.

167. Ferrebee, J. W., and Merrill, J. P.: Spare parts; a review with a forward look, Surgery *41*:503, 1957.

168. Peer, L. A.: Transplantation of Tissues, Baltimore, Williams and Wilkins, 1955.

169. The Relation of Immunology to Tissue Homotransplantation, Ann. New York Acad. Sc. *59*: 277, 1955.

170. Second Tissue Homotransplantation Conference, Ann. New York Acad. Sc. *64*:735, 1957.

171. Third Tissue Homotransplantation Conference, Ann. New York Acad. Sc. *73*:539, 1958.

172. Brent, L.: Tissue transplantation immunity, Progr. Allergy *5*:271, 1958.

173. Jacob, S. W., Gowing, D., and Dunphy, J. E.: Transplantation of tissues, Am. J. Surg. *98*:55, 1959.

174. Medawar, P. B.: Reactions to Homologous Tissue Antigens in Relation to Hypersensitivity, in Lawrence, H. S. (ed.): Cellular and Humoral Aspects of the Hypersensitive States, New York, Hoeber-Harper, 1959.

175. Rappaport, F. T., and Converse, J. M.: The immune response to multiple-set skin homografts: an experimental study in man, Ann. Surg. *147*: 273, 1958.

176. Rogers, B. O.: The genetics of skin homotransplantation in the human, Ann. New York Acad. Sc. *64*:741, 1957.

177. Loeb, L.: The Biologic Basis of Individuality, Springfield, Charles C Thomas, 1945.

178. Medawar, P. B.: The behaviour and fate of skin autografts and skin homografts in rabbits, J. Anat. *77*:176, 1944.

179. Medawar, P. B.: A second study of the behaviour

and fate of skin homografts in rabbits, J. Anat. *79:*157, 1945.

180. Medawar, P. B.: Immunity to homologous grafted skin. III. The fate of skin homografts transplanted to the brain, to the subcutaneous tissue and to the anterior chamber of the eye, Brit. J. Exper. Path. *29:*58, 1948.

181. Good, R. A., Varco, R. L., Aust, J. B., and Zak, S. J.: Transplantation studies in patients with agammaglobulinemia. Ann. New York Acad. Sc. *64:*882, 1957.

182. Taliaferro, W. H.: Modification of the immune response by radiation and cortisone, Ann. New York Acad. Sc. *69:*745, 1957.

183. Billingham, R. E., and Sparrow, E. M.: The effect of prior intravenous injections of dissociated epidermal cells and blood on the survival of skin homografts in rabbits, J. Embryol. & Exper. Morphol. *3:*265, 1955.

184. Billingham, R. E., Brent, L., and Medawar, P. B.: "Actively acquired tolerance" of foreign cells, Nature *172:*603, 1953.

185. Billingham, R. E., and Brent, L.: Acquired tolerance of foreign cells in newborn animals, Proc. Roy. Soc. London s.B *146:*78, 1956.

186. Felton, L.: The significance of antigen in animal tissue. J. Immunol. *60:*383, 1949.

187. Medawar, P. B.: Immunity to homologous grafted skin. II. The relationship between the antigens of blood and skin, Brit. J. Exper. Path. *27:*15, 1946.

188. Billingham, R. E., Brent, L., and Medawar, P. B.: Quantitative studies on tissue transplantation immunity. III. Actively acquired tolerance, Philosph. Trans. Roy. Soc. *239 B:* 357,1956.

189. Barret, M. K.: The erythrocyte-borne antigen in tumor immunity. Ann. New York Acad. Sc. *73:*767, 1958.

190. Billingham, R. E., Brent, L., and Medawar, P. B.: Quantitative studies on tissue transplantation immunity. II. The origin, strength and duration of actively and adoptively acquired immunity, Proc. Roy. Soc. London s.B *143:*58, 1954.

191. Billingham, R. E., Brent, L., and Medawar, P. B.: The antigenic stimulus in transplantation immunity, Nature *178:*514, 1956.

192. Haskova, V., and Hrubesova, M.: Part played by deoxyribonucleic acid in transplantation immunity, Nature *182:*61, 1958.

193. Medawar, P. B.: Part played by deoxyribonucleic acid in transplantation immunity, Nature *182:* 62, 1958.

194. Billingham, R. E., and Sparrow, E. M.: Studies on the nature of immunity to homologous grafted skin, with special reference to the use of pure epidermal grafts, J. Exper. Biol. *31:*16, 1954.

195. Mitchison, N. A., and Dube, O. L.: Studies on the immunological response to foreign tumor transplants in the mouse. II. The relation between hemagglutinating antibody and graft resistance in the normal mouse and mice pretreated with tissue preparations, J. Exper. Med. *102:*179, 1955.

195a. Stetson, C. A., and Jensen, E.: Humoral aspects of the immune response to homografts. Ann. New York Acad. Sci. *87:*249, 1960.

196. Algire, G. H., Weaver, J. M., and Prehn, R. T.: Studies on tissue homotransplantation in mice, using diffusion-chamber methods, Ann. New York Acad. Sc. *64:*1009, 1957.

197. Woodruff, M. F. A.: Cellular and humoral factors in the immunity to skin homografts: experiments with a porous membrane. Ann. New York Acad. Sci. *64:*1014, 1957.

198. Lawrence, H. S.: Similarities between homograft rejection and tuberculin-type allergy: a review of recent experimental findings, Ann. New York Acad. Sc. *64:*826, 1957.

199. Rich, A. R., and Lewis, M. R.: The nature of allergy in tuberculosis as revealed by tissue culture studies, Bull. Johns Hopkins Hosp. *50:* 115, 1932.

200. Mitchison, N. A.: Studies on the immunological response to foreign tumor transplants in the mouse. I. The role of lymph node cells in conferring immunity by adoptive transfer, J. Exper. Med. *102:*157, 1955.

201. Thomas, L.: Discussion of Medawar, P. B., in Lawrence, H. S. (ed.): Cellular and Humoral Aspects of the Hypersensitive States, New York, Hoeber-Harper, 1959.

202. Lawrence, H. S.: Homograft sensitivity, Physiol. Rev. *39:*811, 1959.

203. Greene, H. S. N.: Compatibility and Noncompatibility in Tissue Transplantation, in Butler, E. G. (ed.): Biological Specificity and Growth, Princeton, Princeton University Press, 1955.

204. Greene, H. S. N.: The microscope or the guinea pig? Yale J. Biol. & Med. *18:*239, 1946.

205. Servelle, M., Soulié, P., Rougeulle, J., Delhaye, G., and Touche, M.: La greffe du rein, Rev. chir. Paris *70:*186, 1951.

206. Michon, L., *et al.:* Une tentative de transplantation rénale chez l'homme: aspects medicaux et biologique, Presse méd. *61:*1419, 1953.

207. Hume, D. M., Merrill, J. P., Miller, B. F., and Thorn, G. W.: Experiences with renal homotransplantation in the human: report of nine cases, J. Clin. Invest. *34:*327, 1955.

208. Simonsen, M.: Biological incompatibility in kidney transplantation in dogs. II. Serological investigations, Acta path. et microbiol. scandinav. *32:*36, 1953.

209. Dammin, G. J., Couch, N. P., and Murray, J. E.: Prolonged survival of skin homografts in uremic patients, Ann. New York Acad. Sc. *64:*967, 1957.

210. Stoloff, I. L. Stout, R., Myerson, R. M., and Havens, W. P., Jr.: Production of antibody in patients with uremia, New Eng. J. Med. *259:* 320, 1958.

211. Kelly, W., Good, R. A., and Varco, R. L.: Anergy and skin homograft survival in Hodgkin's disease, Surg. Gynec. & Obst. *107:*565, 1958.

212. Green, I., and Corso, P. F.: A study of skin homografting in patients with lymphoma, Blood *14:* 235, 1959.

213. Murray, J. E., Merrill, J. P., and Harrison, J. H.: Kidney transplantation between seven pairs of identical twins, Ann. Surg. *148:*343, 1958.

214. Merrill, J. P., Murray, J. E., Harrison, J. H., and Guild, W. R.: Successful homotransplantation of the human kidney between identical twins, J.A.M.A. *160:*277, 1956.

215. Rogers, B. O.: The problems of homografts, Plast. & Reconstruct. Surg. *5:*269, 1950.

216. Owen, R. D.: Growth inhibition by analogues of pantothenic acid. II. α-and β-substituted pantothenic acids and related compounds, Science *102:*400, 1945.

217. Main, J. M., and Prehn, R. T.: Successful skin homografts after the administration of high dosage x-radiation and homologous bone marrow, J. Nat. Cancer Inst. *15:*1023, 1955.

218. Nowall, P. C., Cole, L. J., Roan, P. L., and Habermeyer, J. G.: Distribution and in situ growth pattern of injected rat marrow in x-irradiated mice, J. Nat. Cancer Inst. *18:*127, 1957.

219. Ferrebee, J. W., and Thomas, E. D.: Radiation injury and marrow replacement: factors affecting survival of the host and the homograft, Ann. Int. Med. 49:987, 1958.

220. Thomas, E. D., Ashley, C. A., Lochte, H. L., Jr., Jaretzki, A., III. Sahler, O. D., and Ferrebee, J. W.: Homografts of bone marrow in dogs after lethal total-body radiation, Blood 14:720, 1959.

221. Uphoff, D. E.: Preclusion of secondary phase of irradiation syndrome by inoculation of fetal hematopoietic tissue following lethal total-body x-radiation, J. Nat. Cancer Inst. 20:625, 1958.

222. Billingham, R. E.: Studies on the reaction of injected homologous lymphoid tissue cells against the host, Ann. New York Acad. Sc. 73:782, 1958.

223. Porter, K. A.: Runt disease and tolerance in rabbits, Nature 185:789, 1960.

224. Ferrebee, J. W.: "Spare parts," New Eng. J. Med. 257:524, 1957.

225. Cole, L. J.: Prevention of late deaths in x-irradiated mice by injected hematopoietic cells from homologous newborn donors, Am. J. Physiol. 196:441, 1959.

226. Porter, K. A.: Use of foetal hemopoietic tissue to prevent late deaths in rabbit radiation chimeras, Brit. J. Exper. Path. 40:273, 1959.

227. Thomas, E. D., Lochte, H. L., Jr., and Ferrebee, J. W.: Irradiation of the entire body and marrow transplantation; some observations and comments, Blood 14:1, 1959.

228. Ferrebee, J. W., Atkins, L., Lochte, H. L., Jr., MacFarland, R. B., Jones, A. R., Dammin, G. J., and Thomas, E. D.: The collection, storage and preparation of viable cadaver marrow for intravenous use, Blood 14:140, 1959.

229. Haurani, F. I., Repplinger, E., and Tocantins, L. M.: Attempts at transplantation of human bone marrow in patients with acute leukemia and other marrow depletion disorders, Am. J. Med. 28:794, 1960.

230. Bridges, J. B., Bridges, J. M., Edelstyn, G. J. A., Lyons, A. R., and Nelson, M. G.: Toxic marrow failure treated by a homograft of fetal hemopoietic tissue, Lancet 1:629, 1960.

231. Thomas, D. E., Lochte, H. L., Jr., Lu, W. C., and Ferrebee, J. W.: Intravenous infusion of bone marrow in patients receiving radiation and chemotherapy, New Eng. J. Med. 257:491, 1957.

232. Mannick, J. A., Lochte, H. L., Ashley, C. A., Thomas, E. D., and Ferrebee, J. W.: Autografts of bone marrow in dogs after lethal total-body radiation, Blood. 15:255, 1960.

233. Kurnick, N. B., Feder, B. H., Montano, A., Gerdes, J. C., and Nakamura, R.: Some observations on the treatment of postirradiation hematopoietic depression in man by the infusion of stored autogenous bone marrow, Ann. Int. Med. 51: 1204, 1959.

234. McGovern, J. J., Jr., Russell, P., Atkins, L., and Webster, E. W.: Treatment of terminal leukemic relapse by total-body irradiation and intravenous infusion of stored autologous bone marrow obtained during remission, New Eng. J. Med. 260: 675, 1959.

235. Merrill, J. P.: Transplantation of normal tissues, Physiol. Rev. 39:860, 1959.

236. Merwin, R. A., and Hill, E. L.: Fate of vascularized and non-vascularized subcutaneous homografts in mice, J. Nat. Cancer Inst. 14:819, 1954.

237. Brooks, J. R., and Hill, G. J.: Current status of endocrine homografts using the millipore diffusion chamber technic, Am. J. Surg. 99:588, 1960.

238. Egdahl, R. H., Roller, F. D., and Varco, R. L.: Survival and function of adrenal cortex and skin in Millipore chambers, Transplant. Bull. 4:146, 1957.

239. Russell, P. S., and Gittes, R. D.: Parathyroid transplants in rats. A comparison of their survival time with that of skin grafts, J. Exper. Med. 109:571, 1959.

240. Swan, H., and Hallin, R. W.: Studies in endocrine tissue homotransplantation in dogs utilizing Millipore membrane diffusion chambers, Surg. Forum 9:628, 1958.

241. Brooks, J. R., Priaro, J. C., and De'Scoville, A.: Endocrine tissue homotransplantation using the Millipore membrane. Surg. Forum 9:633, 1958.

242. Castellanos, H., and Sturgis, S. H.: Ovarian homograft survival within Millipore filter chambers in monkey, Obst. & Gynec. 12:603, 1958.

243. Potter, J. F., and Haverback, C. Z.: Homotransplantation of endocrine tissues in a diffusion chamber, Ann. Surg. 151:460, 1960.

CHAPTER IV

DISTURBANCES OF GROWTH

AND DIFFERENTIATION OF TISSUES

I. INTRODUCTION

Problems related to growth and differention of isolated cells and multicellular organisms occupy a prominent place in modern biology. In the last decades and by means of physicochemical, biochemical, genetic, ultramicroscopic and many other techniques, biologists have accumulated an impressive array of facts, the meaning of which in medicine is only beginning to be understood. Nevertheless, the explanation of many pathologic processes of great significance, such as congenital malformations and neoplasia, lies precisely there, in the laws regulating the amount of living cytoplasm and the integration of different types of specialized protoplasm in a given organism. A mere baconian accumulation of facts cannot serve all the needs of understanding; it is imperative to have ". . . a more precise description and more penetrating analysis of the data in a more rigorous conceptual frame of reference. This need calls for a firmer

trend away from obscurant verbalisms toward objective scientific formulations of the problems involved. We cannot hope to develop a better understanding of the phenomena of growth, differentiation, organization, induction, control, harmony, and so on, unless we first obtain a realistic picture of just what factual content these various labels cover."[1]

The term "growth" refers to an increase in the mass of protoplasm, which in multicellular organisms means proliferation of cells of a given type. Mitotic division is the main mechanism for increasing living protoplasm; laws regulating the dimensions of members of a species, the size of organs of the individual and of each cell, operate through mitosis.[2] It must be added, however, that the volume of individual cells is also subject to considerable variations, which probably depend on the same factors as multiplication by mitotic division. But growth is just increase in the mass of living protoplasm, without separation into different morphologic and functional types; the emergence of different cell types from an identical precursor is known as "differentiation." Both processes of growth and differentiation are closely integrated and together determine the extent of possible physiologic development for the organism. In effect, the greater the differentiation the more varied and complex will be the functions developed and the finer the skill in performance. This would be impossible, however, without a concomitant increase in the number of functioning elements. The mutual dependence of growth and differentiation is also seen in pathologic situations, where disturbances in one are usually accompanied by changes in the other. A rather coarse example is the lack of development of one kidney, where absence of growth is paralleled by lack of function; in this case, compensation is achieved by an increase in size of the homolateral kidney. But this increase in size is no mere multiplication of cells; in addition, they are organized to carry out the extra load of work imposed by functional deficiency.

According to Rusch,[3] all cellular functions may be divided into two chief categories: first, the function of reduplication, and second, all other functions not primarily concerned with cellular multiplication. These two groups of functions are both mutually dependent and competitive, the latter in respect to the cellular nutrients required for their synthesis. Further elaboration of these ideas leads to the following general concepts of normal growth and differentiation:

"1. Normal primordial cells contain many potential mechanisms which ultimately determine differentiation. These mechanisms become functionally active when the constituents attain certain quantitative levels.
2. During the process of growth and differentiation, each living cell acquires or maintains certain biochemical processes or metabolic patterns in common, but in addition each cell type has special characteristic deviations from the general pattern, resulting from variations in its enzyme make up.
3. The specific cell pattern results from the deletion of some of the original complement of mechanisms and from the concomitant increase in other functions. These losses and increases occur in a sequence which serves a useful function and is beneficial to the general economy of the organism.
4. In normal cells, the competing processes for reduplication and for special function alternate in dominance until the final stage of maturation is reached. Then the pattern for reduplication is irrevocably lost in some cells."

An interesting facet of these ideas is that differentiation is not entirely irreversible in most cells, and that loss of specialized functions may be accompanied by gain in reduplication potential. That this is not always

so, however, will be apparent in the next chapter, devoted to the general pathology of tumors. Here it is convenient to emphasize that most elements in the organism are able to carry out their functions without achieving a net synthesis of cell protein, and that when this occurs there is increase in living cytoplasm; i.e., growth. Therefore, growth may be equated with the number and size of cells, while differentiation represents the variety of functions performed by different elements.

A quantitative estimate of growth may be obtained by an analysis of various parameters, such as weight, height, direct measurement of cell size and volume, cell counts, number of mitoses, etc. Differentiation, being the functional spectrum of cells, may be assessed by testing various physiologic mechanisms such as respiration, enzymatic activity, water metabolism, etc. Ordinarily, however, the morphologist distinguishes between different cell types on the basis of structure; i.e., the assumption is made that similarity in morphology is equivalent to similarity in chemistry and function. This assumption has an obvious practical use and in many instances it has proved to be exact, since morphologic features can be considered as visual expressions of physiologic mechanisms. Anatomic techniques, however, are only beginning to approach the level of biochemical and functional explorations, and in many instances they lag behind in discriminative analysis. The result is that two cells with similar structure may show important physiologic differences or, as shown by Harris and Jahnz with the macrophage and the HeLa cell,[4] there are elements with great morphologic dissimilarity that may have identical metabolic pathways for the synthesis of protein and other functions.

It is outside the scope of this book to discuss the several issues raised by the preceding paragraphs, such as the mechanism of mitosis, protein synthesis or the induction of differentiation. Space is not the only reason: the gap between those biologic concepts and disturbances in growth and differentiation has yet to be bridged by something more than highly theoretical (and stimulating) speculations. Needham's[5] and Willis'[6] monographs are suggested for further reading in this field, a true no-man's land in pathology.

II. DISTURBANCES OF GROWTH

There are two general types of growth disturbances: those characterized by an increase in living cytoplasm and those with less protoplasm than normal. The total amount of functioning cytoplasm may be modified according to three different mechanisms: (a) decrease or increase in the number of cells of a given tissue, (b) a change in size of the elements constituting an organ, without modifications in the actual number of cells and (c) a combination of the two preceding processes. Furthermore, the normal number of cells in a given organ may have been achieved during development, to decrease later as the result of pathologic processes; or else there may be partial or complete failure of development of the organ. Each one of these disturbances of growth is known by different names, introduced in pathology long before the true nature of the disturbance was known, so the etymologic meaning is not always representative of the mechanism of production. Some of the most commonly used terms and their meaning appear in Table 13.

The macroscopic diagnosis of growth disturbances is usually based on deviations from standard weights and measures of organs, which are subject to multiple influences such as age, body weight, height, sex, nutrition, sedentary or active life, etc. Therefore, such deviations as may be found should be referred to average values of many determinations obtained from accidentally dead subjects who had been in good health. Several tables of standard averages of weights and measures of normal subjects are extant;[7, 8, 9, 10] Table 14 gives the values currently used at the Pathology Unit of the National University of Mexico Medical School.

A. Aplasia, Agenesia and Hypoplasia. These terms designate congenital lack or insufficient development of tissues or organs. Agenesis is absolute absence of tissue;

Table 13. Disturbances of Growth

Agenesis	Complete absence of growth of an organ or tissue
Aplasia	Congenital disturbance in which there exist only primitive and usually small structures representative of an organ or tissue (anlage)
Hypoplasia	Congenital disturbance occurring during embryonal development of an organ or tissue, resulting in a smaller, and usually deformed, structure which may or may not function.
Atrophy	Decrease in size and/or number of cells of an organ or tissue after it has achieved normal size.
Hyperplasia	Increase in the number of cells
Hypertrophy	Increase in the size of cells

Table 14. Normal Weights and Measures for Organs

Brain	1250–1400 Gm.
Pineal gland	140– 170 mg.
Pituitary gland	600– 650 mg.
Thyroid gland	30– 40 Gm.
Parathyroid glands (4)	115– 130 mg.
Thymus	19– 23 Gm.
Right lung	375– 550 Gm.
Left lung	325– 450 Gm.
Heart	250– 300 Gm.
Tricuspid valve	12 cm.
Pulmonary valve	8.5 cm.
Mitral valve	10 cm.
Aortic valve	7.5 cm.
Circumference of aorta:	
at 5 cm.	8 cm.
at 10 cm.	7 cm.
Mean thickness of right ventricle	0.2– 0.3 cm.
Inflow chamber of right ventricle	10 cm.
Outflow chamber of right ventricle	12 cm.
Mean thickness of left ventricle	0.8– 1.0 cm.
Inflow chamber of left ventricle	8 cm.
Outflow chamber of left ventricle	10 cm.
Liver	1500–1700 Gm.
Circumference of portal vein	3– 3.5 cm.
Circumference of splenic vein	2– 2.5 cm.
Spleen	125–1175 Gm
Pancreas	90– 110 Gm.
Adrenals (2)	12– 14 Gm.
Right kidney	140– 160 Gm.
Left kidney	140– 160 Gm.
Mean thickness of renal cortex	6– 7 mm.
Mean thickness of renal medulla	14– 16 mm..
Ovaries (2)	16– 24 Gm.
Testes (2)	17– 27 Gm.
Prostate	14– 16 Gm.

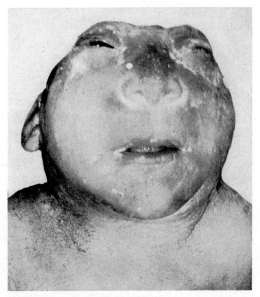

FIG. 4–1. Lack of development of cranial bones and most intracranial contents in anencephalus monster.

aplasia implies the presence of undeveloped "anlage," and hypoplasia means incomplete growth of an organ. Common usage, however, has imposed denominations such as "aplastic anemia," which is the result of bone marrow destruction and therefore is an acquired lesion. Another term also used, although for specific conditions, is atresia, a synonym for agenesis, commonly used as tricuspid valve atresia and bile duct atresia.

Many cases of aplasia are incompatible with life, such as anencephalia, where there is complete absence of the cranial vault bones and of most of the brain (Fig. 4–1); some basal ganglia may be found adherent to the base of the skull.[11] In other cases, a deformity is produced but life is not made impossible, as with phocomelia, where there is aplasia of some bones of the extremities. A typical example is bilateral renal agenesis,[12, 13] where both kidney anlages are present but have failed to develop. The face of the child is usually characteristic: the eyes are widely separated; there is a thick fold in the inner canthus of both eyes, snub nose, receding chin and low insertion of ears. It is of interest that in some rare cases such facial features have been unilateral, coinciding with congenital absence of the kidney in the same side.[14] Lack of development of half of the diaphragm will result in herniation into the thoracic cavity of abdominal organs, a condition frequently incompatible with life.[15] Congenital absence of the biliary ducts, which may involve both intra- and extrahepatic components, is characterized by intense jaundice developing soon after birth and may lead to biliary cirrhosis; in some cases careful dissection of the hilar elements in the liver will demonstrate a fibrous cord replacing the choledochus[16] (Fig. 4–2). Asplenia, or congenital absence of the spleen, may be accompanied by other malformations such as pulmonary isomerism and cardiovascular anomalies;[17] this peculiar combination of disturbances has been beautifully illustrated by Brandt and Liebow[18] (Fig. 4–3).

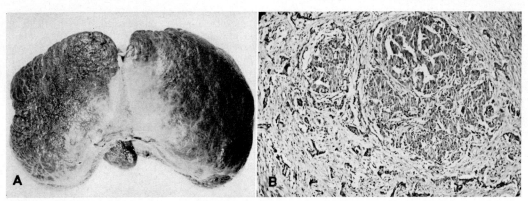

FIG. 4–2. Biliary cirrhosis in congenital atresia of extrahepatic bile ducts. *A,* Gross aspect of the liver at 7 months of life. *B,* Microscopic picture in congenital biliary cirrhosis. Observe proliferation of bile ducts in connective tissue bands. (Courtesy of Dr. Maximiliano Salas.)

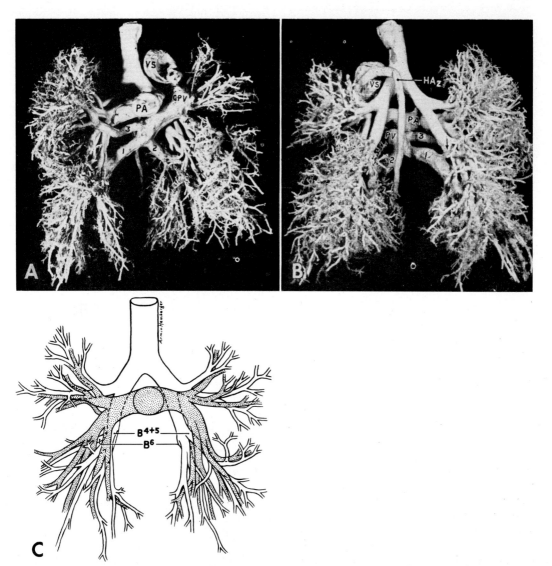

Fig. 4–3. Bronchovascular cast in a case of pulmonary isomerism, asplenia and other congenital anomalies. *A,* Anterior view. The common venous sinus (VS) is seen above the left main bronchus. This communicates anteriorly with the left superior vena cava. It receives the common pulmonary vein (CPV). The latter is formed by the confluence of the following: *1,* right lower lobe plus right middle lobe vein; *2,* left lower lobe vein; *3,* right upper lobe vein; *4,* left middle lobe vein and several small branches from the left upper lobe (PA = pulmonary artery).

B, Posterior view demonstrating the symmetry of the bronchial tree. The upper lobe bronchi arise at the same distance from the carina. Both are epiarterial. The right lower lobe vein is seen to receive a separate superior segmental branch (arrow). Other veins labeled as in *A.* The common venous sinus receives on its posterior aspect a vein occupying the position and subserving the function of the hemiazygos (HAz).

C, Drawing of bronchial tree and pulmonary arteries as shown in the anterior view of the cast. Symmetrical origins of the bilaterally epiarterial upper lobe bronchi are shown, as is the presence of the left middle lobe, which is a mirror image of the right. These are indicated as B^{4-5}. On each side of the middle lobe a bronchus arises just above the superior segmental bronchus (B^6). On the right a branch ascends from the interlobar part of the pulmonary artery to supply the posterior segment of the upper lobe. Otherwise the vessels are symmetrical. (Courtesy of Drs. Herman Brandt and Averill A. Liebow, and the Editor, Laboratory Investigation.)

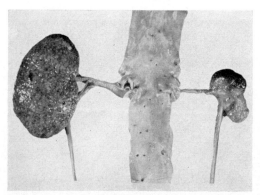

FIG. 4–4.   Atrophy of both kidneys, more severe in the left, in a case of chronic pyelonephritis.

Hypoplasia requires the presence of the underdeveloped organ, as occurs in uterine hypoplasia, a relatively frequent cause of sterility, or in renal hypoplasia, which when unilateral is accompanied by hypertrophy of the other kidney; the differential histologic diagnosis between a congenital hypoplastic kidney and an atrophic pyelonephritis may be very difficult or impossible[19] (Fig. 4–4).

The causes of all these types of growth disturbances are not known with certainty,[20] but there can be no doubt that "organizers" are involved; these are mechanisms regulating growth and differentiation, probably chemical in nature. Primary, secondary and other types of organizers have been described, as well as inductors, which stimulate formation of groups of differentiated cells.[6]

B. Atrophy. Atrophy is a decrease in amount of living cytoplasm after it has achieved normal development. It may be due to a loss in the number of cells, to decrease in size of each of many elements making up an organ, or to a combination of both processes. Cellular loss is the result of death and reabsorption of cells, which may develop slowly or very rapidly; in the latter case, atrophy will be secondary to necrosis. An instance of slowly developing atrophy due to decrease in the number of cells is the progressive disappearance of lymphoid tissue throughout the organism with increasing age. Whereas in children and young adults lymphoid tissue is prominent in the tonsils, pharynx, gastrointestinal tract, etc., in older individuals these collections of lymphoid cells are much decreased in size and number of elements, and even the spleen may be considerably atrophic. On the other hand, sudden atrophy is exemplified by the so-called "acute yellow atrophy" of the liver, appearing in pregnant women, usually during the third trimester of gestation. In these cases there is rapid onset of severe liver failure usually ending in death a few days later, and on autopsy the liver weight may be decreased to half or less than normal. In many cases the cause is acute viral hepatitis and atrophy is due to extensive and irregular areas of necrosis with reabsorption of tissue debris and collapse of the reticular stroma (Fig. 4–5). Most cases of atrophy, however, belong to the slowly developing type, where decrease of living cytoplasm is generalized and involves most of the cells; a prominent exception is

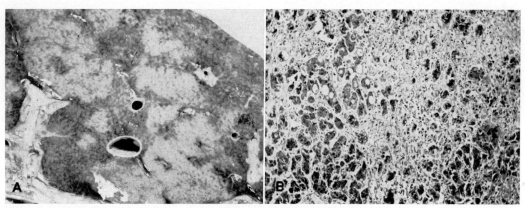

FIG. 4–5.   Acute yellow atrophy of the liver in pregnancy. *A*, Large and irregular areas of soft liver parenchyma with yellow discoloration. *B*, The microscopic picture is characterized by necrosis of liver cells with little inflammatory response.

represented by some types of pressure atrophy.

The normal amount of living cytoplasm depends on three general factors: nutrition, hormonal balance and cellular work. It is not surprising that nutrition should partly determine the weight of organs, since food is the basic material required by the cell to renew its constituents as well as a source of energy to carry out metabolic reactions. In the absence of an external source of energy the cell will use its own material in energy metabolism; the obvious consequence of such autophagy is a decrease in size of the cytoplasm. Furthermore, interference with the utilization of oxygen, be it by anoxic, anoxemic or histotoxic anoxia, will impair respiration and the intermediary metabolism of many compounds. The result is a predominance of catabolic over anabolic processes, synthetic mechanisms will decrease to a lower level where equilibrium is again achieved between oxygen supply and intermediary metabolism, and the cell will have become smaller. Classic forms of atrophy mediated through lack of nutrition (food and/or oxygen) are known as nutritional, ischemic, senile and pressure atrophy; some instances of each are mentioned in the following paragraphs.

Chronic malnutrition will cause generalized atrophy of almost all organs, but not to the same degree nor with the same speed. Very complete studies on the effect of fasting on the weight of different organs in the rat have been published by Jackson,[21] and Addis, et al.[22] Both showed that while the brain maintains almost identical weight the liver and digestive tract decrease in size faster than the animal, and the kidneys are in an intermediary position. No adequate explanation exists for this phenomenon, but it is believed that the extent to which a given organ loses weight during fasting depends on the amount of reserve cytoplasm and the level of energy metabolism of different tissues; the participation of hormones is also suspected. A clinical counterpart of experimental fasting is seen in anorexia nervosa, a form of psychopathic ailment in which patients refuse all food, becoming true living skeletons.[23] Hyperthyroidism, by increasing the metabolic rate, also leads to important losses in body weight. The cachexia of cancer patients is usually the result of mechanical interference with organs of the digestive tract, although psychologic and other mechanisms of more obscure nature are also important.[24] During the Second World War, the caloric value of food given in concentration camps was well below minimum and many inmates reached extreme degrees of malnutrition; the name "mussulman" was applied to these living ghosts, partly because of the state of mental torpor caused by organic atrophy.[25]

Ischemic and pressure atrophy have a similar pathogenesis, since pressure results in vascular collapse and ischemia. When circulatory occlusion is sudden and complete, and the organ involved has no adequate collateral circulation, the result is necrosis (p. 39). However, if decrease in circulation is slow and progressive, and collateral circulation is hindered by previous vascular disease such as atherosclerosis, it will lead to atrophy. The same phenomenon is observed with the effect of pressure on tissues, often exerted between bony structures and a hard object, as in the case of bedsores developing in patients confined to bed for prolonged periods;[26] many of these subjects, however, suffer from severe diseases and malnutrition, which make the pathogenesis somewhat more complicated. Pressure atrophy ends with necrosis and sloughing off of ischemic tissues, thus giving rise to decubitus ulcers, frequently seen in the sacrum, hips and ankles. Atherosclerosis may cause atrophy of muscular masses, especially in the lower extremities. Senile atrophy is probably the result of a combination of nutritional, circulatory and endocrine factors, in which most organs decrease in size, and may even give rise to clinical manifestations, especially when atrophy is pronounced in the brain. Some cases of senile dementia are nothing else but manifestations of cortical atrophy in the brain.

Another important cause of atrophy is disuse. Apparently, the function of a given organ is one of the factors determining its size, so decrease in function for prolonged periods will bring about a decrease in volume. This is observed in the muscles of patients kept at rest for some time, be it bed rest or the immobilization of an extremity because of bone fracture. In either case the total muscular mass will decrease in size and there will also be a loss of strength. Muscular atrophy in poliomyelitis, although determined largely by disuse, is also secondary to loss of innervation; the "trophic" influence of the motor neuron is absent, whatever that influence may be.[27] Physical therapy and exercise are used in the treatment of paralysis caused by poliomyelitis in order to keep the muscle in good condition while innervation is regenerated, and sometimes recovery may be excellent; for this reason, neurogenic atrophy is difficult to accept as an isolated mechanism of decrease in living cytoplasm. Prolonged immobilization is usually complicated by decalcification of bones and the calcium salts may form calculi in the renal pelves; it is doubtful, however, that decalcification of the skeleton can be considered as a form of disuse atrophy[28] since it involves no loss of living cytoplasm. Finally, artificial or exogenous replacement of the function of an organ induces atrophy, a phenomenon clearly seen in the endocrine glands. Sokoloff, *et al.*[29] showed that prolonged administration of cortisone was accompanied by decrease in size of the adrenals; replacement of thyroid secretion with thyroxin results in atrophy of the thyroid; chronic insulin administration brings about decrease in number and size of islands of Langerhans, etc. In all these cases the loss of active cytoplasm is probably the result of lack of function of the cell.

Endocrine glands are important regulators of the size of organs, and this can be confirmed in several different instances of atrophy caused by endocrine disturbances. Destruction of the pituitary gland by embolism, thrombosis or other mechanisms of ischemia, as frequently seen after delivery (Simmonds' disease or Sheehan's syndrome)[30] or associated with eclampsia, bilateral renal cortical necrosis and other manifestations of generalized Shwartzman reaction,[31] eventually leads to the picture of pituitary cachexia, in which all organs are much decreased in size. The pathogenesis of this form of atrophy is complex because at the same time as hormonal influences decrease there is also a marked loss of appetite with consequent malnutrition and an in-

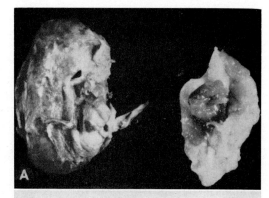
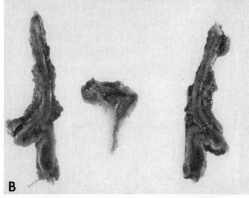

FIG. 4–6. Pituitary gland (*A*) and adrenal (*B*) of a case of Sheehan's disease. Normal sized organs are also shown for comparison. (Courtesy of Dr. Miguel Schulz.)

vincible asthenia which limits movements (Fig. 4–6). But the area where the endocrine influence is better observed is in the group of glands formed by the pituitary and its satellites, thyroid, adrenals and gonads. Here, destruction of the anterior lobe of the pituitary gland abolishes secretion of tropic hormones and the target glands undergo atrophy. Indeed, endocrine atrophy is a form of disuse atrophy.

Exocrine glands undergo atrophy when the excretory duct is obstructed. When a stone or a tumor occludes the duct of Wirsung in the pancreas, acini dilate, acinar cells decrease in size and eventually disappear, so the organ becomes a mass of adipose tissue in which well preserved islands of Langerhans can be observed (Fig. 4–7); the pathogenesis of this type of atrophy is combined, since there is disuse, pressure and often chronic inflammation.

Within certain limits, atrophy is a reversible process; cessation of the causes may be followed by regeneration and recovery of the normal amount of living cytoplasm.[32] Limits are determined by age, nature of the process, duration and the extent of connective tissue proliferation. In young patients or experimental animals regeneration is rapid and the functional results may be excellent, but when atrophy is caused by chronic inflammation with extensive deposits of connective tissue, regeneration is scarce and functional recovery poor. Prolonged atrophy, even when unaccompanied by inflammatory changes, is usually followed by an increase in interstitial fibrous tissue which limits functional recovery.

The consequences of atrophy are easy to imagine. The most important one is decrease in functional capacity, which is quite apparent in muscles, glands and brain. In other cases it increases the frequency of severe infections which may end the patient's life, as in decubitus ulcers. Although the causes of atrophy are multiple and in most cases several factors operate simultaneously, perhaps in last analysis the intimate mechanism of slow loss of living cytoplasm is the same when expressed in biochemical terms. Bradley[33] postulated that tissue anoxia favors the activity of catabolic enzymes, which are more effective at acid pH, so there is a predominance of cytoplasmic destruction over synthesis (*see* Chapter I).

C. Hyperplasia and Hypertrophy. Hyperplasia is the increase in the number of cells constituting a tissue, and hypertrophy is the increase in the size of cells. Both terms are quite specific and should be used with the mentioned connotation, although hypertrophy was introduced in pathologic nomenclature before the microscopic era to indicate increase in size without reference to mechanism and usage has sanctioned terms such as prostatic hypertrophy (which is hyperplasia) and hypertrophic cirrhosis (which is neither hypertrophy nor hyperplasia); in opposition to atrophy, hyperplasia and hypertrophy represent a greater amount of living cytoplasm and, with limitations mentioned below, they often determine increased functional capacity.

The total mass of functioning protoplasm may increase in response to two general types of causes: exaggerated hormonal stimulus and greater functional demands. Other mechanisms may also exist, humoral or of unknown nature, which also participate in this process. Endocrine control of the size of organs and tissues is best represented by somatotropin or growth hormone, described by Evans in 1935.[34] This hormone is secreted by the acidophilic (oligogranular) cells of the anterior lobe of the pituitary gland.[35] In addition to other metabolic effects, growth hormone is responsible for height and, above all, size and weight of the organism as a whole, and of individual organs. Its influence is seen in pathology when a functional tumor is formed by acidophilic cells in the pituitary gland (Fig. 4–8). When this tumor appears before puberty, the result is pituitary gigantism; when the onset of exaggerated secretion of growth hormone occurs after puberty, the picture of acromegaly is produced. Pituitary gigantism is characterized by the extraordinary height of the patients, who retain juvenile somatic features. The acidophilic adenoma may produce signs and symptoms of compression in the neighboring structures, such as visual disturbances, and many patients die at an early age because of hemorrhage and necrosis in the tumor, which may be disproportionately large. In acromegaly there is exaggerated growth of facial and distal bones but height is not increased since epiphyseal growth plates are closed;[36] many organs increase tremendously in size, the heart having weighed 1250 Gm.

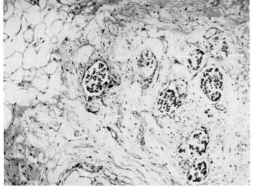

FIG. 4–7. Atrophy of the exocrine portion of the pancreas in occlusion of the pancreatic duct. Only islet tissue remains embedded in loose and fatty connective tissue.

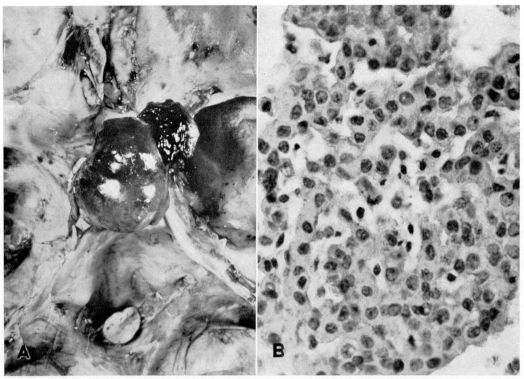

FIG. 4–8. Acidophilic adenoma of pituitary gland. *A*, Gross aspect of the tumor *in situ* after removal of brain. The hemorrhagic area near the anterior surface corresponds to the site of biopsy. *B*, A group of acidophilic cells in a tumor causing acromegaly.

in one case. In acromegaly the living cytoplasm increases mainly through hypertrophy.

Other hormones capable of producing localized hyperplasia and/or hypertrophy are sex hormones. Estrogens induce mammary hyperplasia in males and females, and endometrial hyperplasia in females; androgens produce enlargement of the clitoris. The latter phenomenon is very complex since hyperplasia involves all histologic elements of the organ, in the same way as testicular interstitial cells can induce increase in size of male genital organs (precocious pseudopuberty). Another instance of the multiple effect of hormones in tissues is nodular hyperplasia of the prostate, where some of the nodules are formed by proliferation of glandular elements while others only show smooth muscle and fibrous tissue[37] (Fig. 4–9). Hormones act on effector or target organs which are not necessarily formed by a homogeneous cell population. The intimate mechanism of hormonal control of cell size and number is not known.

Probably one of the most important causes of hyperplasia and/or hypertrophy is increased functional demand. Compensatory hyperplasia is not abnormal. When one kidney is removed the other increases in size by multiplication of tubular cells and enlargement of glomeruli, but this is normal regeneration;[38] furthermore, in this case it has yet to be shown that the stimulus for regeneration is increased work and not a humoral mechanism (*see* Chapter III). The concept should be limited to cases where exaggerated functional demands result in an increase of living cytoplasm beyond the normal amount. The best examples are found in smooth and striated muscles including myocardium, since in these cases the cause and effect relationship is more clear. Other instances only show that an increase in the size and number of cells may be accompanied by excessive functioning, such as thyroid hyperplasia, which produces hyperthyroidism, or adrenal cortex hyperplasia, which results in Cushing's syndrome. In these cases hyperplasia is probably the result of abnormal pituitary stimuli or other less well known mechanisms.

An obstacle in the pylorus or duodenum hampering the free transit of food towards

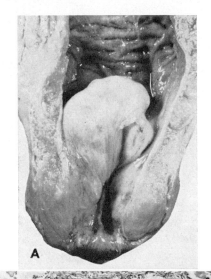

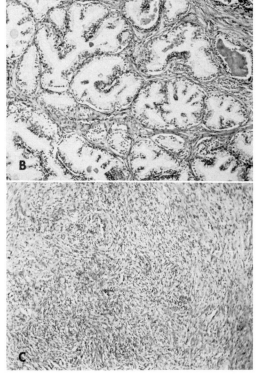

the lower portions of the intestine is followed by dilation of the stomach and thickening of the wall, especially the muscular layers, which develop as a response to the increased pressure necessary to pass the occlusion. A similar change is observed when the obstacle is lower, as in chronic subocclusion of the ileum by a scar or peritoneal adhesion; the wall of the proximal segment of intestine is thickened, sometimes measuring up to 2 cm., and this is the result of smooth muscle hyperplasia. Hypertrophy of striated muscles is well known to all sportsmen. Continuous exercise will bring about an increase in the amount of muscular cytoplasm. This is clearly seen by comparing muscles used more frequently than others in different forms of sport; the active arm of some tennis players, for example, is stronger and thicker than the other.

Cardiac muscle hypertrophy is a very interesting problem. Increased functional demand is obviously a stimulus for it, as witnessed by left ventricular hypertrophy in patients with arterial hypertension, or by right ventricular hypertrophy when there is hypertension of the lesser circulation (Fig. 4–10). But other factors must also be at play since left ventricular hypertrophy may show two different types. One, known as concentric hypertrophy, is characterized by thickening of the wall with little or no dilation, so the net result is a decrease in the capacity of the ventricular cavity. This form is particularly frequent in cases of renal hypertension, such as chronic glomerulonephritis or bilateral polycystic disease of

FIG. 4–9. Nodular hyperplasia of the prostate. *A,* Enlargement of the middle lobe of the prostate showing good encapsulation, muscular hypertrophy and trabeculation of bladder wall. *B,* Glandular hyperplasia. *C,* Stromal hyperplasia.

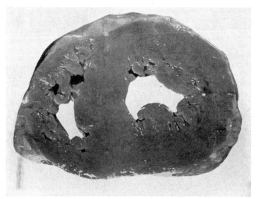

FIG. 4–10. Concentric hypertrophy of the left ventricle in a case of chronic glomerulonephritis.

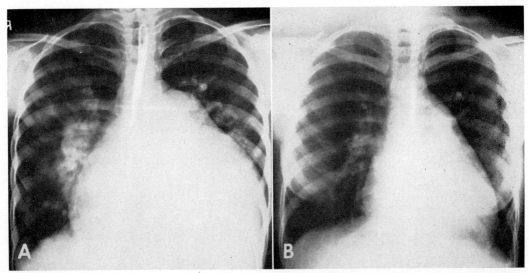

FIG. 4–11. Regression of cardiac hypertrophy in a 12 year old child with interatrial communication and rheumatic endocarditis. *A,* Chest x-ray before operation, showing enlargement of the heart and pulmonary hilar congestion. *B,* Chest x-ray 8 months after surgical closure of the interatrial communication. (Courtesy of Dr. Bernardo Castro Villagrana and the Editor, Postgraduate Medicine.)

the kidneys. The other type of ventricular hypertrophy appears as thickening of the wall with large dilation and is known as eccentric hypertrophy. The most classic example is seen in aortic lesions, especially insufficiency.

Cabrera[39] has attempted an explanation for these two different forms of left ventricular hypertrophy, based on hemodynamic considerations. According to this author, renal hypertension imposes a systolic extra load on the ventricle without increase in diastolic volume, so the initial dilation of the ventricular cavity is soon overcome by hypertrophy, whereas aortic insufficiency results in increased diastolic volume without systolic hypertension, thereby producing mainly dilation. This interesting speculation deserves experimental analysis.

When hypertrophy of the left ventricle is measured without including papillary muscles, the wall seldom if ever is more than 20 mm. in thickness; apparently, this limit is imposed by the vascular supply of the myocardium. But hemodynamic factors are not the only influences (other than increased work) that determine cardiac hypertrophy; for many years Raab[40, 41] has called attention to the presence of high concentrations of catecholamines in hypertrophic hearts. The same author showed that hypertrophy

of the heart will not appear in adrenalectomized animals, even in the presence of high intraventricular hypertension, and that the administration of catecholamines to such animals will restore the capacity of the myocardium to undergo hypertrophy. Furthermore, normotensive animals will develop cardiac hypertrophy with the administration of catecholamines without influence on peripheral vascular resistance. Recently, Barnard[42] showed that prolonged anoxia will be accompanied by left ventricular hypertrophy in guinea pigs and rabbits, and Paplanus, *et al.*[43] were able to induce cardiac hypertrophy in dogs with anemia caused by repeated bleeding. Norman and McBroom[44] obtained cardiac hypertrophy in rats with phenylhydrazine anemia, and more recently Norman and Coers[45] showed that coronary artery ligation in rats will result in myocardial infarction and hypertrophy. Evidence for a relationship between occlusive coronary artery disease and cardiac hypertrophy in man has been summarized by Connolly and Littmann.[46] The mechanism of these forms of hypertrophy is not known.

It has been mentioned that an increase in the amount of living cytoplasm is accompanied by greater functional efficiency, and this is particularly true of the heart. The process, however, has an upper limit determined by unknown factors, and when this threshold is passed functional capacity will rapidly decrease. It has been suggested that blood vessels do not participate in hypertrophy and that as soon as they are unable to supply the greater needs of material for synthesis of cytoplasm, the process stops. Karsner, *et al.*[47] and Roberts and Wearn[48] showed that the normal ratio of myocardial fibers to capillaries is 1:1, and that this ratio is the same even in extreme degrees of hypertrophy. It is apparent, therefore, that the failure of blood vessels to keep up with increasing metabolic demands of a larger mass of active cytoplasm is a good reason for the upper limit of hypertrophy, but this leaves unsolved the mechanism for decrease in functional efficiency. Hypertrophy occurs at the expense of the reserve capacity of cells, which means that the additional amount of work hypertrophic cells can carry out at a given moment is decreased progressively, until in basal conditions they are working at a maximum of capacity; when this maximum is surpassed there will be insufficiency. These concepts are accepted for the myocardium and they probably apply to other forms of hypertrophy as well, but they stand in urgent need of experimental analysis. Perhaps the reason for insufficiency is a combination of factors, among which lack of vascular proliferation, decrease in reserve capacity and increase in functional demand probably play important roles.

As with atrophy, hypertrophy is usually reversible upon cessation of the causal stimulus. A clear demonstration has been presented by Cooley, *et al.*[49] in a case of atrial septal defect and rheumatic myocarditis; the septal defect was closed surgically and in 8 months there was a striking decrease in size of the cardiac shadow; obviously this is not all caused by regression of hypertrophy, but it serves to illustrate the point. It has been said that muscular hypertrophy is secondary to distention of the fibers, and that this elongation is an indispensable prerequisite for increase in size to occur; other factors, however, may be involved, such as anoxia and humoral mechanisms, so it would seem wiser to look for the cause of hypertrophy at the level of cellular metabolism.[50]

III. DISTURBANCES IN DIFFERENTIATION

A multicellular organism is composed of groups of cells differing both in morphology and function. In the beginning the organism starts as a single cell, which is considered as totipotential; i.e., it has the ability to multiply and produce all cell types which eventually form an adult individual. This ability is preserved for only a very short period, extending to the first hours of embryologic development, and can be observed experimentally by separating the cells, which will proceed to form as many organisms as there are cells. Soon, however, the experiment will not result in complete organisms, one for each cell, but only in more or less complex groups of elements, so that the cells are no longer considered as totipotential but only as multi- or pluripotential. At this moment the cells have become differentiated, which means that a normally irreversible change has been produced and their future development has been narrowed. In the adult, fully developed individual, few cells remain in a state of relative undifferentiation, such as the histiocytes of connective tissue or the primitive elements of the bone marrow. On the other hand, in certain pathologic conditions or under the influence of hormones many adult cells can show their hidden capacity to change into a different form of tissue. The transformation of an adult or completely differentiated tissue into another type of adult or differentiated tissue is known as *metaplasia*. Literally, this word means "change of form" and is a clear expression of the change involved. A different form of tissue transformation, where cells appear less differentiated than normal, is known as *anaplasia,* a very important phenomenon in the pathology of tumors. Another, less frequently employed term indicates that normal cells have changed their organization adopting the form of a more elaborate or differentiated tissue; this is *prosoplasia*. Finally, it has been mentioned that many different connective tissue cells, when maintained in tissue culture for prolonged periods or stimulated *in vivo* by several means, change their morphology and become fibroblasts, with fully developed capacity to deposit intercellular fibers. This

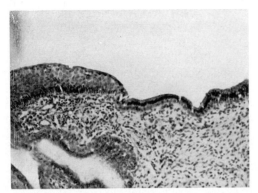

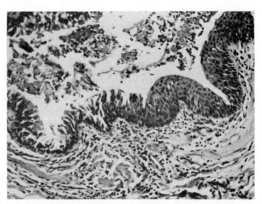

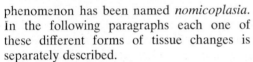

FIG. 4–12. Epidermoid metaplasia of endocervical epithelium in chronic cervicitis.

FIG. 4–13. Epidermoid metaplasia of bronchial epithelium in chronic bronchitis.

phenomenon has been named *nomicoplasia*. In the following paragraphs each one of these different forms of tissue changes is separately described.

A. Metaplasia. Metaplasia is encountered in very different situations which on first examination appear to have little or nothing in common; perhaps the only two acceptable general statements are that metaplasia is more frequent in tissues undergoing active proliferation than in those of a more quiescent nature, and that metaplasia is almost always an abnormal phenomenon.[51] There are almost no physiologic types of metaplasia (see below).

Chronic inflammation is a frequent cause of metaplasia, both in epithelial and connective tissues. A common form is known as leukoplakia, which is the transformation of surface, nonkeratinizing epithelium into a multistratified, keratinizing epithelium (Fig. 4–12). Almost any surface epithelium may develop this form of metaplasia; multistratified epithelium such as in the exocervix, monostratified epithelium as in the endocervix, transitional epithelium as in the urinary bladder, etc. In all these areas metaplasia is usually epidermoid in character; i.e., there is a tendency of the resulting tissue to resemble skin epithelium, but the similarity is only superficial. In rare occasions not only a stratum granulosum and a keratin layer are present, but also sweat and sebaceous glands and hair follicles, as in the case mentioned by Willis.[6] In these cases there is a complication of structure, so the term prosoplasia may be applicable. A very clear example of epidermoid metaplasia occurs in

the epithelial lining of bronchi draining tuberculous cavities in the lung; the frequency of such change has increased since the introduction of more effective antibiotics and chemotherapeutic agents in the treatment of this disease.[52, 53] The usual sequence begins with destruction of the normal bronchial epithelium, followed by regeneration which appears in the form of polystratified layers and grows right into the cavity where it may cover a part or all the inner surface (Fig. 4–13). This probably represents a handicap for closed healing of tuberculous cavities. Recent studies by Auerbach, *et al.*,[54] Valentine[55] and many others[56] have shown that chronic smokers have a higher incidence of epidermoid metaplasia in trachea and bronchi. At the same time, it should be recalled that chronic inflammation of the bronchial tree is frequently accompanied by epidermoid metaplasia, and since chronic smokers are very prone to have long-standing bronchial inflammation, the probability exists that tobacco increases the frequency of bronchial metaplasia by a nonspecific mechanism and not as the result of any specific substance (*see* Chapter V).

Epidermoid metaplasia may be observed in the excretory ducts of the pancreas and for some time it was considered as a possible cause of pancreatitis, after Rich and Duff[57] found it in 54 per cent of their 26 autopsy cases. Since then, however, it has been seen in the pancreas of many subjects without acute pancreatitis, and the change is focal and involves very small ducts. Chronic thyroiditis may also show small areas of epidermoid metaplasia. The mucosa of the

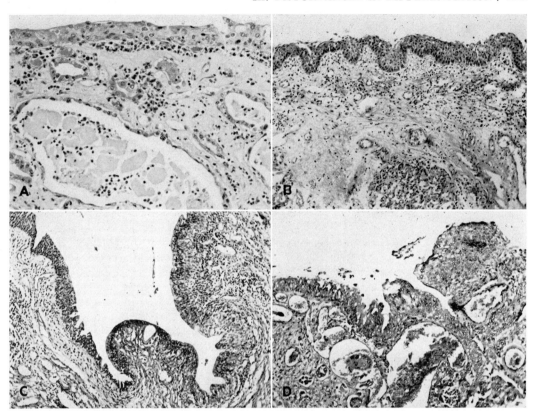

FIG. 4–14. Epidermoid metaplasia in various organs. *A,* In lining epithelium of renal pelvis. *B,* In lining epithelium of bronchus. *C,* In urethra. *D,* In the neighborhood of epidermoid carcinoma of urinary bladder.

urinary tract is especially prone to develop metaplasia, which may be very extensive and involve the entire renal pelvis, particularly when there is chronic pyelitis and stone formation; the urinary bladder may also show focal areas of leukoplakia. These forms of metaplasia are almost always associated with chronic inflammation, which is also the case in the uterine cervix, where epidermoid metaplasia of the surface epithelium and the endocervical glands is an almost obligate change in chronic cervicitis. In the cervix metaplasia may give rise to confusion with other changes, such as pregnancy modifications or carcinoma *in situ;*[58] in this respect it should be recalled that the endocervical epithelial lining is of mesodermal origin.

Metaplasia may be induced experimentally by means of estrogenic hormones, a situation studied in detail by Fluhmann.[59] Vitamin A deficiency may also bring about epidermoid metaplasia of many glandular ducts;[60] of special interest is the extensive metaplasia found in bronchiectatic cavities of the lungs of old rats, which is probably due to a combination of inflammatory and nutritional factors and which may closely resemble a malignant epithelial tumor.[61] This confusion is also of historical interest, since it may account for the pulmonary metastasis found by Fibiger in his animals inoculated with *Gongylonema neoplasticum* (*see* Chapter V).

Some epithelial tumors may show metaplasia, as in the case of adenocarcinoma of the endometrium and occasionally of the ovary, which for this reason are called "adenoacanthoma" (Fig. 4–15); both glandular and epidermoid elements may appear in metastatic nodules, and some cases may even show intercellular bridges. Another frequent area of neoplastic metaplasia is the urinary bladder, where a transitional cell carcinoma may show focal or extensive epidermoid transformation, with keratin forma-

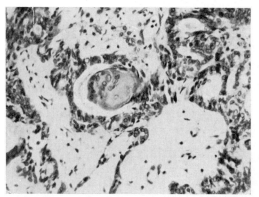

FIG. 4–15. Epidermoid metaplasia in adenocarcinoma (adenocanthoma).

tion and intercellular bridges. In some cases multiple sections of an epidermoid carcinoma of the urinary bladder fail to reveal transitional cells, and since epidermoid metaplasia (leukoplakia) of the bladder is frequent, the assumption is made that the tumor arose from metaplastic epithelium.

Metaplasia is not only epidermoid; it may also be glandular. The renal pelvis can show glandular metaplasia, of which two extraordinary cases have been published;[62] a similar situation may appear in the urinary bladder. Endometriosis (endometrial glands and stroma in ectopic situations such as peritoneum, ovary, intestinal loops or even stomach) has been alternatively considered as metaplastic[63] or secondary to autotransplants of uterine mucosa[64] (Fig. 4–16). A relatively frequent form of metaplasia is the presence of pseudodecidual or decidual reaction in the peritoneal or subperitoneal layers of tubes, ovaries and even appendix; this can also be seen in the connective tissue of the cervix, especially in pregnancy, and is reversible after delivery (Fig. 4–17).

Metaplasia is not limited to epithelial structures; connective tissues also may change from one type to another. The tendency of old scars and necrotic areas to un-

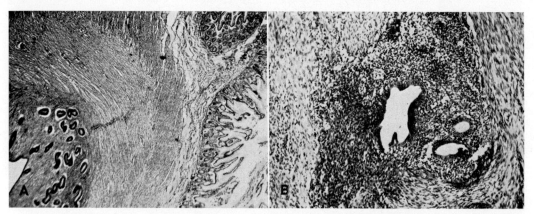

FIG. 4–16. Endometriosis. *A,* In wall of intestine. *B,* In fallopian tube.

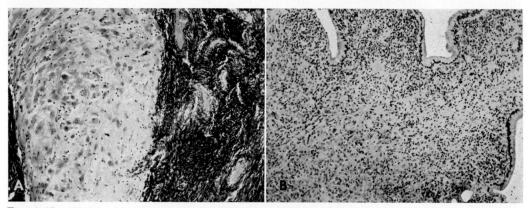

FIG. 4–17. Ectopic decidual reaction, a form of metaplasia. *A,* In ovarian stroma. *B,* In stroma of endocervix.

dergo calcification, ossification and even development of bone marrow is notorious. Huggins[65] showed that bladder epithelium autotransplanted to the anterior abdominal wall of the dog would induce osseous metaplasia in the surrounding connective tissue. The best instances of connective tissue metaplasia, however, are seen in mesenchymal tumors. Chondrosarcomas and fibrosarcomas frequently show osseous metaplasia; liposarcomas and osteosarcomas reveal fibrous metaplasia, etc. (Fig. 4–18). Failure to recognize these changes as different morphologic aspects of the same cell type has given rise to a confusing and useless nomenclature (*see* Chapter V).

Myeloid metaplasia is mainly seen in lymph nodes, spleen and liver in cases where the bone marrow has been destroyed by some pathologic process, which may be toxic or neoplastic;[66] in these cases, undifferentiated cells of the reticuloendothelial system resume their fetal function and produce blood cells. This is a clear instance of prosoplasia, and its mechanism, as in all other examples, is not known.[67]

B. Anaplasia. When an adult, differentiated tissue acquires the organization of a less well differentiated tissue, the change is known as anaplasia. This term is used almost exclusively in tumors, but here it will be briefly discussed since it represents an important disturbance in differentiation. Although not the first author to notice the similarities of some malignant cells to embryonal elements, von Hansemann deserves the credit for having developed and baptized this concept. In 1890, von Hansemann[68] wrote, "The aim of the development of the germ is the greater indifferentiation of one cell (the mature unfertilized ovum). In some stage of this process there must be a de-differentiation, in contrast with differentiation, since there is no doubt that the immature ovum represents in some epoch a well characterized somatic epithelial ele-

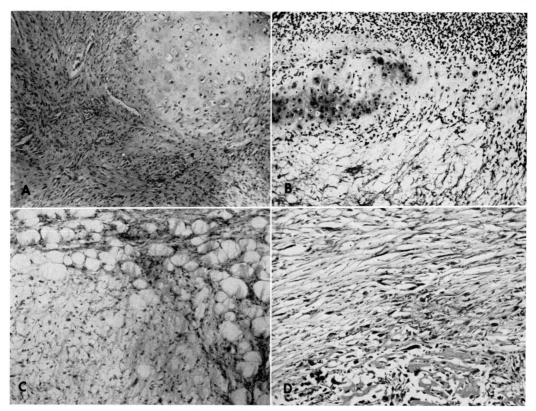

Fig. 4–18. Metaplasia in connective tissue tumors. *A,* Chondroid metaplasia in fibrosarcoma. *B,* chondroid and myxoid metaplasia in osteogenic sarcoma. *C,* Myxoid metaplasia in liposarcoma. *D,* Fibrous (spindle-cell) metaplasia in osteogenic sarcoma.

ment. If we wished a term for each of these two processes, differentiation and de-differentiation, one might be called prosoplasia (advance in form) and the other anaplasia (delay in form). The development of the mature ovum from the somatic cell, as well as the development of the malignant cell from the matrix tissue, occurs through anaplasia, i.e., de-differentiation and increased capacity for independent life." Hansemann studied anaplasia in relation to tumors and found that high degrees of de-differentiation were correlated with a greater tendency to give metastasis. The concepts and terminology of Hansemann were not ignored and soon there appeared opponents such as Ribbert, who remarked that, ". . . such words, taken from an ancient language, can easily assume dogmatic character. A definitive opinion is affixed to them . . . and, what is even worse, they are used as explanations of the very phenomena from which they are deducted. One not only says that cancer cells are anaplastic, but anaplasia is taken as the basis of malignancy."

In spite of that and many other criticisms, the idea that cancer cells are undifferentiated has not only been widely accepted but has received experimental support, especially with the development of tissue culture techniques and biochemical analysis of tumors. Immunologic and biochemical studies have shown that tumor cells resemble other neoplastic elements more closely than cells of the tissue of origin. Besides its theoretical usefulness, the concept of anaplasia served to develop a method which pretended to "predict" the behavior of a particular tumor from the histologic degree of anaplasia. This aspect is more thoroughly discussed in Chapter V; here, it will suffice to state that morphologic criteria of anaplasia are not universal, each school or even each pathologist has developed his own, and many times cells are declared anaplastic because they "look anaplastic." This type of reasoning appears when opinions are based on "experience" and not on objective data, and the only sound criticism is that unverbalized experience cannot be communicated; furthermore, it reveals the most primitive stage of knowledge, when almost everything except the existence of the prob-

lem is ignored, and this cannot even be adequately expressed.

C. Nomicoplasia. This concept was mentioned in Chapter III, in reference to the origin of fibroblasts during the first stages of healing. It originated in a long series of careful studies of tissue cultures, experimental and human material dealing with the connective tissues, by Costero, *et al.*[69, 70] According to this author, "All connective tissue cells not completely differentiated tend to become fibroblasts. This can be observed in many pathologic processes (especially in wound healing) in all connective tissue tumors (especially in endotheliomas) and in the normal connective tissue (especially during the spontaneous involution of organs). The transformation of connective tissue cells into fibroblasts is a particular form of metaplasia, which is not progressive as prosoplasia nor regressive as anaplasia, and not even necessarily pathologic; it is the expression of laws ruling the evolution of tissues, and for this reason we have designated it with the name of nomicoplasia. The term derives from the Greek words *nomicos,* which means legal, according to law, and *plássein,* which means to form, so the concept is adequately characterized."

Many elements of the connective tissue can undergo nomicoplasia, especially mesothelial and endothelial cells, which are normally found lining serous cavities and blood vessels and in this situation they do not form fibrils; however, when they abandon this position such cells can manifest their fibroblastic lineage. These interesting concepts find a definite application in human pathology, especially in the so-called collagen diseases, where increase of intercellular fibers may be a prominent finding, unaccounted for on the basis of the pre-existing population of fibroblasts. Therefore, nomicoplasia is further discussed in Chapter VI.

REFERENCES

1. Weiss, P.: The problem of cellular differentiation, in Proceedings of the First National Cancer Conference, New York, American Cancer Society, 1949.
2. Swann, M. N.: The control of cell division: a review, Cancer Res. *17:*727, 1957; *18:*1118, 1958.
3. Rusch, H. P.: Carcinogenesis: a facet of living processes, Cancer Res. *14:*407, 1954.

4. Harris, H., and Jahnz, M.: The synthesis of protein in the macrophage and the HeLa cell, Brit. J. Exper. Path. *39:*597, 1958.

5. Needham, J.: Biochemistry and Morphogenesis, Cambridge, Cambridge University Press, 1942.

6. Willis, R. A.: The Borderland of Embryology and Pathology, London, Butterworth, 1958.

7. Roessle, R., and Roulet, F.: Mass und Zahl in der Pathologie, Berlin, J. Springer, 1932.

8. Wolbach, S. B., and Coppoletta, J. M.: Body length and normal weights of the more important vital organs between birth and twelve years of age, Am. J. Path. *9:*55, 1933.

9. Saphir, O.: Autopsy Diagnosis and Technique, ed. 4, New York, P. B. Hoeber, 1958.

10. The Autopsy, Washington, D.C., A. F. I. P., 1950.

11. Vogel, F. S., and McClenahan, J. L.: Anomalies of major cerebral arteries associated with congenital malformations of the brain, with special reference to the pathogenesis of anencephaly, Am. J. Path. *28:*701, 1952.

12. Davidson, W. M., and Ross, G. I. M.: Bilateral absence of the kidneys and related congenital anomalies, J. Path. & Bact. *68:*459, 1954.

13. Ashley, D. J. B., and Mostofi, F. K.: Renal agenesis and dysgenesis, J. Urol. *83:*211, 1960.

14. Hilson, D.: Malformation of ears as sign of malformation of genitourinary tract, Brit. M. J. *2:*785, 1957.

15. Liebow, A. A., and Miller, H. C.: Congenital defects in the diaphragm, Am. J. Path. *16:*707, 1940.

16. Silverberg, M., Craig, J., and Gellis, S. S.: Problems in diagnosis of biliary atresia: review and consideration of histological criteria, J. Dis. Child. *99:*574, 1960.

17. Ivemark, B. I.: Implications of agenesis of the Spleen on the pathogenesis of conotruncus anomalies in childhood, Acta paediat. *44:* Suppl. 104. 110, 1955.

18. Brandt, H., and Liebow. A. A.: Right pulmonary isomerism associated with venous, splenic and other anomalies, Lab. Invest. *7:*469, 1958.

19. Emmet, J. L., Alvarez-Ierena, J. J., and McDonald, J. R.: Atrophic pyelonephritis versus congenital renal hypoplasia, J.A.M.A. *148:*1470, 1952.

20. Wilson, J. G.: Factors involved in causing congenital malformations, Bull. New York Acad. Med. *36:*145, 1960.

21. Jackson, C. M.: Recent work on the effects of inanition and of malnutrition on growth and structure, Arch. Path. *7:*1042, 8:81, 273, 1929.

22. Addis, T., Poo, L. J., and Lew, W.: Rate of protein formation in organs and tissues of body after caseous refeeding, J. Biol. Chem. *116:*343, 1936.

23. Berkman, J. M., Weir, J. F., and Kepler, E. J.: Clinical observations on starvation edema, serum protein and effect of forced feeding in anorexia nervosa, Gastroenterology *9:*357, 1947.

24. Terepka, A. R., and Waterhouse, C.: Metabolic observations during the forced feeding of patients with cancer, Am. J. Med. *20:*225, 1956.

25. Hellwegg-Larsen, P., Hoffmeyer, H., Kieler, J., Thaysen, E. H., Thaysen, J. H., Thygesen, P., and Wulff, M. H.: Famine disease in German concentration camps. Complications and sequelae, Acta med. scandinav. *144:* Suppl. 274.93, 1952.

26. Husain, T.: An experimental study of some pressure effects on tissues, with reference to the bedsore problem, J. Path. & Bact. *66:*347, 1953.

27. Adams, R. D., Denny-Brown, D., and Pearson, C. M.: Diseases of Muscle. A Study in Pathology, New York, Paul B. Hoeber, 1953.

28. Whedon, D. G.: Osteoporosis: Atrophy of Disuse, in Rodahl, K., Nicholson, J. T., and Brown, E. M., Jr. (eds.): Bone as a Tissue. New York, McGraw-Hill, 1960.

29. Sokoloff, L., Sharp, J. T., and Kauffman, E. H.: Adrenal cortex in rheumatic disease: pathologic study with special reference to the effect of cortisone and corticotrophin, Arch. Int. Med. *88:* 627, 1951.

30. Sheehan, H. L.: Simmonds' disease due to postpartum necrosis of the anterior pituitary, Quart. J. Med. 8:277, 1939.

31. McKay, D. G., Merrill, S. J., Weiner, A. E., Hertig, A. T., and Reid, D. E.: The pathologic anatomy of eclampsia, bilateral renal cortical necrosis, pituitary necrosis, and other acute fatal complications of pregnancy and its possible relationship to the generalized Shwartzman phenomenon, Am. J. Obst. & Gynec. *66:*507, 1953.

32. Omae, T., and Masson, G. M. C.: Reversibility of renal atrophy caused by unilateral reduction of renal blood supply, J. Clin. Invest. *38:*21, 1960.

33. Bradley, H. C.: Atrophy and autolysis, Physiol. Rev. *18:*173, 1938.

34. Evans, H. M.: The growth hormone of the anterior pituitary, J.A.M.A. *104:*1232, 1935.

35. Landing, B.: Histochemical analysis of anterior pituitary cells of children and the problem of correlation of cytoplasmic proteins with protein hormones, Lab. Invest. *6:*487, 1957.

36. Kellgren, J. H., Ball, J., and Tutton, G. K.: The articular and other limb changes in acromegaly: a clinical and pathological study of 25 cases, Quart. J. Med. *21:*405, 1952.

37. Moore, R. A.: Benign hypertrophy of the prostate. A morphological study, J. Urol. *50:*680, 1943.

38. Moore, R. A.: Number of glomeruli in kidney of adult white rat unilaterally nephrectomized in early life, J. Exper. Med. *50:*709, 1929.

39. Cabrera, E., and Monroy, J. R.: Systolic and diastolic loading of the heart. I. Physiologic and clinical data, Am. Heart J. *43:*661, 1952.

40. Raab, W.: Hormonal factors in heart disease: their role in myocardial hypertrophy, hypoxia and electrolyte imbalance, Ann. Int. Med. *41:*757, 1954.

41. Raab, W.: Hormonal and Neurogenic Cardiovascular Disorders: Endocrine and Neuroendocrine Factors in Pathogenesis and Treatment, Baltimore, William and Wilkins, 1953.

42. Barnard, P. J.: Experimental anoxic cardiac enlargement, Lab. Invest. *7:*81, 1958.

43. Paplanus, S. H., Zbar, M. J., and Hays, J. W.: Cardiac hypertrophy as a manifestation of chronic anemia, Am. J. Path. *34:*149, 1958.

44. Norman, T. D., and McBroom, R. D.: Cardiac hypertrophy in rats with phenylhydrazine anemia, Circulation Res. *6:*765, 1958.

45. Norman, T. D., and Coers, C. R.: Cardiac hypertrophy after coronary artery ligation in rats, Arch. Path. *69:*181, 1960.

46. Connolly, E. P., and Littmann, D.: Coronary arteriosclerosis and myocardial hypertrophy, New Eng. J. Med. *245:*753, 1951.

47. Karsner, H. T., Saphir, O., and Todd, T. W.: The state of the cardiac muscle in hypertrophy and atrophy, Am. J. Path. *1:*351, 1925.

48. Roberts, J. T., and Wearn, J. T.: Quantitative changes in the capillary-muscle relationship in human hearts during normal growth and hypertrophy, Am. Heart J. *21:*617, 1941.

49. Cooley, D. A., Castro Villagrana, B., and Sisteroni, A.: Substitución temporal de la función cardiopulmonar en la cirugía del corazón y aorta, Arch. Inst. cardiol. México *27:*734, 1957.

50. Olson, R. E.: Molecular events in cardiac failure, Am. J. Med. *20:*2, 1956.

51. Willis, R. A.: Metaplasia, in Studies in Pathology presented to Peter MacCallum, New York, Cambridge University Press, 1950.

52. Auerbach, O., Katz, M. L., and Small, M. J.: The effect of streptomycin therapy on the bronchocavitary junction and its relation to cavity healing, Am. Rev. Tuberc. *67:*173, 1953.

53. Auerbach, O.: Pulmonary tuberculosis after the prolonged use of chemotherapy, Am. Rev. Tuberc. *71:*165, 1955.

54. Auerbach, O., Brewster, G. J., Forman, J. B., Petrick, T. J., Smolin, H. J., Muehsman, G. E., Kassouny, D. Y., and Stout, A. P.: Changes in the bronchial epithelium in relation to smoking and cancer of the lung, New Eng. J. Med. *256:*97, 1957.

55. Valentine, E.: Squamous metaplasia of the bronchus, Cancer *10:*272, 1957.

56. Sanderud, K.: Squamous metaplasia of the respiratory tract epithelium, Acta path. et microbiol. scandinav. *43:*47, 1958.

57. Rich, A. R., and Duff, G. L.: Experimental and pathological studies on the pathogenesis of acute hemorrhagic pancreatitis, Bull. Johns Hopkins Hosp. *58:*212, 1936.

58. Gusberg, S. B., and Moore, D. B.: Clinical pattern of intraepithelial carcinoma of the cervix and its pathologic background, Obst. & Gynec. *2:*1, 1953.

59. Fluhmann, C. F.: Squamous metaplasia of the rat uterus, Arch. Path. *59:*238, 1955.

60. Gershoff, S. N., Andrus, S. B., Hegsted, D. M., and Lentini, E. A.: Vitamin A deficiency in cats, Lab. Invest. *6:*227, 1957.

61. Passey, R. D., Leese, A., and Knox, J. C.: Bronchiectasis and metaplasia in the lung of the laboratory rat, J. Path. & Bact. *42:*425, 1936.

62. Ackerman, L. V.: Mucinous adenocarcinoma of the pelvis of the kidney, J. Urol. *55:*36, 1946.

63. Nicholson, G. W.: Studies in Tumor Formation, London, Butterworth, 1950.

64. Sampson, J. A.: The development of the implantation theory for the origin of peritoneal endometriosis, Am. J. Obst. & Gynec. *40:*549, 1940.

65. Huggins, C.: Influence of urinary tract mucosa on the experimental formation of bone, Proc. Soc. Exper. Biol. & Med. *27:*349, 1930.

66. Block, M., and Jacobson, L. O.: Myeloid metaplasia, J.A.M.A. *143:*1390, 1950.

67. Jordan, H. E.: Extramedullary blood production, Physiol. Rev. *22:*75, 1952.

68. Hansemann, D. P.: Ueber azymetrische Zelltheilung in Epithelkrebsen und deren Biologische Bedeutung, Virchows Arch. path. Anat. *119:*299, 1890.

69. Costero, I.: Caracterización del sistema fibroblastico. I. Bases doctrinarias, Arch. Inst. cardiol. México *24:*237, 1954.

70. Costero, I., Barroso-Moguel, R., Pomerat, C. M., and Chévez, A.: Caracterización del sistema fibroblástico. II. Fibrogénesis intracelular en tejido conjuntivo cultivado, Arch. Inst. cardiol. México *24:*337, 1954.

GENERAL PATHOLOGY OF TUMORS

I. INTRODUCTION

An isolated cell performs many finely integrated functions comprised within the general terms of respiration and metabolism, mostly through enzymatic mechanisms. In addition to the continuous maintenance of a dynamic equilibrium between all its constituents, survival of the cellular species demands reduplication of the in-

159

dividual, and mitotic division is the normal mechanism for this important function. Considering respiration, metabolism and mitosis, isolated cells nevertheless develop a very limited number of all their potential abilities, and this is more obvious when the variety of functions of single cells is compared with that of multicellular organisms. Thus, isolated cells have a very limited ability to move; stimuli of many different types awake only a few stereotyped, primitive responses; food is what is found in the immediate environment; survival is possible only under very rigid and narrow conditions, and, as far as is known, amebas have never created a work of art or a philosophic system. In order to gain some independence from the surrounding environment, the single cell must associate with other cells and form organized groups, the functional spectrum of which increases with the number of associated elements. A rapid glance at the zoologic scale should convince us that what the cell loses in individuality is more than compensated by collective freedom and functional differentiation. Even in more complicated animals, different degrees of organization are manifested by greater or lesser ability to perform certain functions such as flying, listening to high frequency sound waves or solving mathematical problems.

The achievement of greater freedom from the surrounding environment by multicellular organisms is possible through specialization of individual or groups of cells; i.e., they have limited the performance of certain functions to a minimum and the remaining potential has been invested in developing (or acquiring) metabolic characteristics contributory to survival of the whole organism. One result of differentiation is the relegation of mitotic division to a second plane by most cells, the remainder keeping this characteristic only at the level of physiologic renewal.[1] It seems that the price paid for developing highly differentiated, specialized functions is the irreversible resignation to mitosis, as is the case with adult nerve cells or the retinal cones and rods. But most cellular members of an organized community preserve, in a more or less recondite fashion, the capacity for multiplication, which is only manifested when the organism

as a whole is in need of it. The general laws of growth are not understood but their results are obvious. Within certain limits, the size and form of individuals and species are constant. Within these limits, too, cellular reduplication contributes to homeostasis, being more active during growth, wound healing or regeneration, and ceasing when the constancy of the internal milieu has been attained again. *When the capacity for reproduction of a cell or a group of cells irreversibly violates homeostasis (the general laws of organization of the individual), the result is a tumor.* This has no pretension of being a definition; at most, it is an attempt at interpreting the nature of neoplastic growth from a general biologic standpoint; at least, it is just a description of the most likely place of tumors in biology. Whatever definition is finally accepted, for the time being, tumors are disturbances of growth. This much seems certain and without exception; probably no other general statement about tumors can be made without specifications, qualifications and exceptions.

Tumors may be contemplated from three different points of view: (a) as a biologic phenomenon, indicating rupture of internal equilibrium in the normal life of a multicellular organism, and offering great opportunities for the study of the intimate mechanisms of cell multiplication and the general laws ruling growth and differentiation, as well as many other phenomena of general interest; (b) as a group of clinicopathologic entities, of specific diseases occurring in man demanding immediate and effective attention, unfortunately not always possible; and (c) in malignant cases, as a human tragedy not only of great significance for the individual but also for society. These three viewpoints are not, and should not, be mutually exclusive; on the contrary, they should constitute the basis of the physician's attitude towards tumors.

It is superfluous to say that cancer as such does not exist, that it is just an abstraction of many diseases differing so much from each other as pneumonia differs from a fracture. There are many different cancers, many more or less well defined diseases, the exact knowledge of which is extremely important for the life and well-being of patients. To abstract is to eliminate, to remove, and in the case of cancer what is done here is to subtract differences and emphasize similarities of all or most neoplastic diseases. When this is done the result is the general pathology of cancer, which is the theme of this chapter; when differences are contemplated and described, the goal is to understand each one of the many varieties of neoplastic entities. It must be emphasized that *a general knowledge of the properties common to all or most tumors is totally insufficient to diagnose and treat an individual case of cancer; a thorough familiarity with each type of tumor, its natural history and best means of diagnosis, as well as the most effective therapeautic methods, is mandatory before undertaking the responsibility involved in this aspect of the practice of medicine.* Of course this is true of any form of disease, but it is even more important in the case of tumors, where only too often the single opportunity of survival open to a patient is in the hands of the first physician consulted.

The literature dealing with different aspects of tumors has attained truly neoplastic proportions, which make it impossible to read more than a fraction of what is published. As in other chapters, in this part of the book care has been exercised to include in the list of references those recent papers with long bibliographic lists. Excellent reviews of the literature from the standpoint of general pathology are available in the books by Payling Wright,[2] Florey,[3] Cowdry,[4] Willis,[5] Mellors[6] and Homburger.[7,8] For more specialized studies the works of Ackerman and del Regato,[9] Willis,[10] Pack and Ariel[11] and the series edited by Raven[12] are especially recommended. The series "Advances in Cancer Research"[13] treats specific subjects with extensive reviews of the literature, and the "Year Book of Cancer,"[14] started in 1957, contains selected abstracts in the English language. Excerpta Medica[15] publishes a monthly fascicle with summaries of the world literature, and the journal "Cancer"[16] contains an extensive section of current cancer abstracts. Other sources may be found in the bibliography at the end of the chapter.

II. DEFINITION, NOMENCLATURE AND CLASSIFICATION

A. DEFINITION

It is not easy to propose a definition of neoplasia which applies to all tumors and at the same time is free of criticism. The reasons for this difficulty appear to be at least two. In the first place, the intimate nature of the biologic disturbances of cells resulting in neoplastic growth is not known. In the second place, tumors follow no inviolable rules; they are bound to no code of behavior, so generalizations are plagued by exceptions. In the present status of knowledge the best definition is merely descriptive, including those general features common to most tumors but leaving room for the many unruly members of the group. It may be comforting to remember that in biology most definitions are of this type and that any attempt to set adequate limits to general concepts is usually defeated by ignorance of intimate mechanisms. Yet, definitions are useful if they present only the central characteristics of phenomena, although the limits with other processes may not be clear. It is with these limitations in mind that the following paragraphs should be examined.

1. Willis' Definition. In his admirable monograph on the pathology of tumors, Willis[10] suggests the following definitions: "A tumor is an abnormal mass of tissue, the growth of which exceeds and is uncoordinated with that of the normal tissues, and persists in the same excessive manner after cessation of the stimuli which evoked the change." This is as good a definition of tumor as is possible today, but the discussion of two aspects of it may clarify certain concepts dealing with the general pathology of cancer. The persistence of neoplastic growth after disappearance of the stimulus (or stimuli) responsible for it has been recognized for some time; indeed, it was included in the joint report on Fundamental Cancer Research, published by a group of experts in 1938, with the following words: "Once malignancy is established in a cell it becomes an automatic process, independent of the presence of a continuously acting agent of outside origin, and the new character of the cell becomes a fixed one which is passed unchanged to the descendants."[17] This implies that the effect of carcinogenic agents is an irreversible and heritable modification of certain metabolic cellular features, especially those related to reduplication, so it would be impossible for the etiologic agent to remain in successive generations of neoplastic cells, and accompany them in metastases, transplantations and tissue culture *in vitro*. There is no doubt that this applies to physical and chemical carcinogens, so in their case it can be accepted that neoplastic growth goes on indefinitely after the action of such agents has been discontinued. In the case of tumors caused by viruses, however, such reasoning loses much weight since it has been shown that the virus persists within cells through many generations and can be found in metastases, transplants and explants; indeed, it is characteristic of tumor viruses that they do so. In view of these facts it may be tentatively postulated that neoplastic growth is an irreversible and heritable cellular modification which continues irrespective of disappearance or persistence of the causal agent.

One other aspect of tumors which has been considered as the most important characteristic by many authors and is apparently not mentioned by Willis is their "autonomy." It has been widely held that neoplastic growth is autonomous in the sense that it fails to obey the "laws governing and restricting the growth of normal tissues." In his authoritative discussion of this issue, Willis points out that tumors often show remarkable organization not only as adult tissues but even as organs, so they cannot be considered as autonomous; furthermore, it is also mentioned that the laws of normal tissue proliferation have not been defined. Similar objections against autonomy as a prominent characteristic of tumors are raised by Berenblum,[18] and Harris.[19] It is not possible, however, to deny that even perfectly organized tumors show no departure from the general pattern of the organism; that a glandular tumor shows exquisitely formed glands is very important, but that they may be present in a metastatic nodule in the brain is even more important, since it reveals the degree to which tumor cells fail to contribute to homeostasis. Furthermore, although the "laws" of cell growth and differentiation have not been defined there can be no doubt that organisms adhere to some sort of general pattern; otherwise variations in weight, height and morphology would be the rule and the limits of species would not exist. This appears to be a purely semantic problem, since such "laws" are implied in Willis' definition when he says that neoplastic growth "is not coordinated with that of normal tissues." This obviously means that normal tissues grow in a coordinated fashion, and what is this coordination if not a "law"? To deny that there are general principles ruling normal cellular multiplication because they have not been clearly enunciated and at the same time accept that normal tissue growth is coordinated is logically inconsistent.

The polemic style of the preceding paragraphs has been adopted only to show that even the best definition of tumor is not without fault. Those are minor criticisms and Willis' definition stands as the most complete characterization of neoplasia. It should be added that the "abnormal mass of tissue" does not necessarily imply an increase in size, since some tumors appear grossly as ulcerations or localized destructions of organs, as may be seen in some carcinomas of the larynx, while in other cases the neoplastic tissue replaces normal structures without any apparent macroscopic change, as observed in carcinoma *in situ* of the cervix or other surface epithelia. The abnormal mass of tissue is always present and when not obvious on gross examination the microscopic study of involved organs will not fail to reveal it.

2. Other Definitions of Tumor. The following is a list of definitions of tumor which appear in some recent and/or widely used textbooks of pathology:

Anderson:[20]   "A neoplasm is an uncontrolled new growth of tissue (Warren)."

Boyd:[21]   "A tumor or neoplasm may be defined as a local growth of new cells which proliferate without control and

Florey:[18] "A tumor is an actively-growing tissue, composed of cells derived from one that has undergone an abnormal type of irreversible differentiation; its growth is progressive, due to a persistent delay in maturation of its stem cells. The essential nature of the irreversible differentiation, whether in biological or chemical terms, is still unknown (Berenblum)."

Robbins:[22] "A tumor represents a pathologic overgrowth of tissue."

Smith, et al.:[23] "Neoplasia is best defined as new growth arising from the individual body cells, (which) is not purposeful and has no expected end point."

B. NOMENCLATURE

Knowledge of the existence of tumors is as old as humanity and many of the names given to different types are inherited from remote times. Several systems of nomenclature have been suggested, but tradition is stronger than logic and time-honored names are usually preferred. Therefore, it is not possible to establish general rules of nomenclature without many exceptions; even the use of the suffix *oma* to indicate the neoplastic nature of some process immediately brings to mind such words as rhinoscleroma, lymphogranuloma venereum and granuloma inguinale, which are chronic inflammations. Perhaps the best thing is to write a list of the names in use and memorize it. Some considerations may be useful, however, before such a list is presented. It is important that the name given to a tumor be as revealing as possible of all those characteristics which are significant in diagnosis, prognosis and treatment, which are (1) histogenesis and behavior, (2) topography and extension and (3) if any, previous treatment and results. A brief comment of each one of these points will clarify their importance.

1. Histogenesis and Behavior. Most of the names in current use for neoplasms imply both the nature of the cell or tissue of origin and the probable behavior of the tumor. Thus, papilloma is a tumor derived from surface epithelium and has a benign evolution, while carcinoma is a tumor arising in epithelium but with a malignant course. However, when the name is only indicative of histogenesis it is imperative to add a term descriptive of the expected behavior of the tumor, as in mesothelioma, a neoplastic growth arising from mesothelial cells which may be benign or malignant. Sometimes the specimen submitted for histologic diagnosis contains only a few cells or the tumor is so anaplastic that a reasonable suggestion as to histogenesis is not possible; in these cases an effort must be made to determine the probabilities of evolution of the disease, which means whether a benign or malignant course should be expected. In practice, the behavior of a tumor is more important than its histogenesis. Some pathologists are inclined to add additional observations, based on microscopic study, such as "grading" or a statement as to the degree of differentiation, an estimate on the speed of growth based on the number of mitosis, etc. These are discussed in some detail in Section V of this chapter.

2. Topography and Extension. Many tumors with identical histogenesis may appear in different organs or tissues. Liposarcomas occur in the retroperitoneal space and in the soft tissues of the thigh; chordomas are seen mainly in the extremes of the vertebral column; lymphomas may appear in lymph nodes or in extraganglionar locations such as stomach or breast. Treatment and prognosis vary a great deal in each one of these instances, so it is convenient always to mention the topographic location of tumors. Similar considerations can be made in relation to extension, which may be conveniently exemplified by carcinoma of the uterine cervix; in this instance there is an international classification in five stages, each one of them defined as follows:

Stage O: Carcinoma *in situ,* preinvasive carcinoma, intraepithelial carcinoma, and similar designations.

Stage I: The carcinoma is strictly confined to the cervix.

Stage II: The carcinoma extends beyond the cervix, but has not reached the pelvic wall, or involves the vagina but not the lower third.

Stage III: The carcinoma has reached the pelvic wall or the lower third of the vagina.

Stage IV: The carcinoma involves the bladder or the rectum (or both) or has extended beyond the limits previously described.

Adequate staging is extremely important for prognosis in carcinoma of the cervix; in addition, the use of such classification is so extended that reports of series of this tumor pretending to demonstrate the results, beneficial or otherwise, of different types of treatments which fail to include staging are almost meaningless. Thus, an adequately labeled tumor of the uterine cervix would read as follows: "epidermoid carcinoma of the uterine cervix, stage III" if that is the particular stage of the case. Although clinical staging has not been developed for all tumors,[23] an idea should always be given of extension, which is the single most important factor in prognosis.

3. Previous Treatments and Results. When a tumor has been treated by whatever means and has failed to be cured, the situation is frequently hopeless. It is therefore imperative to investigate and register all previous treatments and their results; some terms are used with a more or less specific meaning, such as "persistent," when treatment has induced little or no change in tumor growth and extension, "recurrent" when there has been clinical disappearance of tumor activity after treatment but it reappears some time later, and "residual" if the effect of therapy has been a considerable decrease, without disappearance, of tumor growth. When treatment has included radiotherapy the tumor should be classified according to its response and the basis for such classification should be given (*see* Section V). To continue using the example of carcinoma of the uterine cervix, an adequately labeled case of such tumor would be as follows: "epidermoid carcinoma of the

uterine cervix, stage III, radiated, persistent." There is no substitute for the amount of information derived from this label, so every effort should be made to complete it in cases of this or any other type. *To determine the extension, previous treatment and its results is more important for the prognosis and treatment of tumors than the details of their histologic structure.*

C. CLASSIFICATION

Another series of considerations is pertinent before presenting a list of names of tumors, this time dealing with their classification. It has been mentioned that histogenesis and prognosis are the first two requirements of any name, and fortunately this is reflected in most designations of tumors. Some special cases, however, require separate mention, so in the following paragraphs these two aspects of classification are briefly discussed.

1. Histogenetic and Prognostic Classification. From the clinical standpoint, the single most important aspect of the pathology of tumors is their behavior, and they are accordingly separated into two groups: benign and malignant. A benign tumor grows slowly, does not invade neighboring structures and interferes with the patient's well-being mainly because of its position, internal secretions or degenerative phenomena. On the other hand, a malignant tumor grows rapidly, invading and destroying surrounding tissues and organs and producing metastases, and if untreated will finally end the patient's life. The separation between benign and malignant behavior is not distinct, and occasionally a benign tumor undergoes malignant transformation; rare instances of the opposite situation, a malignant tumor becoming a benign growth, have been published.[24, 25] Furthermore, nothing qualitatively different exists in a biologic sense between a benign and a malignant tumor; basically, they both are disturbances of cellular growth and differentiation. The prognostic significance of this difference is so great, however, that in medicine it must be considered before anything else. That in some few cases behavior cannot be predicted at all with any degree of certainty is no reason for declaring that a prognostic classification is artificial or superfluous, as

Table 15. Classification and Nomenclature of Some Tumors

TISSUE OF ORIGIN	BENIGN	MALIGNANT
Epithelium		
covering and lining membranes	Papilloma	Carcinoma
glandular	Adenoma	
trophoblast	Mole	Choriocarcinoma
Connective tissue		
fibrous	Fibroma	Fibrosarcoma
adipose	Lipoma	Liposarcoma
muscular		
smooth	Leiomyoma	Leiomyosarcoma
skeletal	Rhabdomyoma	Rhabdomyosarcoma
cartilage	Chondroma	Chondrosarcoma
bone	Osteoma	Osteosarcoma
notochord		Chordoma
vascular		
blood vessels	Hemangioma	Hemangiosarcoma
lymph vessels	Lymphangioma	Lymphangiosarcoma
glomus	Glomus tumor	Hemangiopericytoma
lymphoid	Benign lymphoma	Malignant lymphoma
mesothelium	Mesothelioma	Malignant mesothelioma
synovium	Synovioma	Synovial sarcoma
Nervous tissue		
peripheral nerves	Neuroma	
nerve sheaths	Neurofibroma, neurilemmoma	Neurogenic sarcoma
glia	Glioma	Glioma
nerve cells	Ganglioneuroma	Neuroblastoma
Other tissues		
pigmented cells	Nevus	Melanoma
adrenal medulla	Pheochromocytoma	Pheochromocytoma
multipotential cells	Teratoma, mixed tumor	Teratoma, mixed tumor

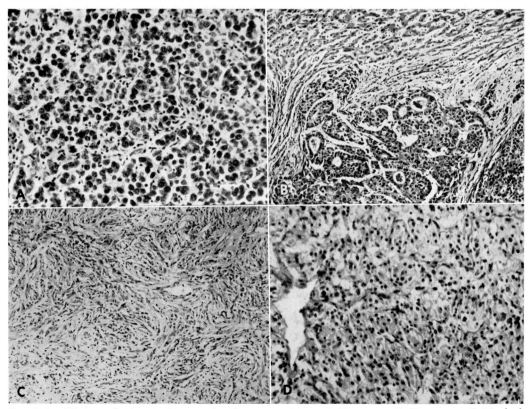

FIG. 5–1. Microscopic aspect of tumors bearing organ names. *A*, Thymoma. *B*, Hepatoma. *C*, Meningioma. *D*, Carotid body tumor.

has been contended by some authors. It is well that the experimentalist and the biologically minded laboratory investigator should consider behavioral differences of tumors as incidental to the intimate nature of neoplastic growth. The practicing physician and the patient are, on the other hand, highly interested in the final outcome of the disease, which among other factors will determine the most adequate form of treatment.

The classification adopted in this book is histogenetic and prognostic (Table 15). Although tumors are cell disturbances, the names used follow the same pattern of division of tissues as in histology. A thorough discussion of other systems of classification can be found in Willis' book.[10]

2. Special Cases. Some special names require separate mention.

a. Names of Organs. Some tumors are known after the organ, and not the tissue, from which they derive. Instances of this practice are meningioma, thymoma, hepatoma, carotid body tumor, etc. This designation indicates not only the seat of the tumor but also that it arises from the parenchymatous cells and reproduces its histologic organization (Fig. 5–1). Some of these terms were introduced at a time when the embryologic derivation of such elements was not known (in some cases it is still not known), and tissues were classified more in accordance with their blastodermic origin than with their morphology and function. The idea that the embryonal layers are specific has lost much ground and today it is not sacrilegious to call renal or adrenal malignancies carcinoma, in spite of their mesodermal origin.

b. Names of Cells. When the tumors arise from cells not organized as tissues, or when only one tissue element is involved in neoplastic growth, the name given is usually that of the cell plus the suffix *oma:* for instance, plasmacytoma, osteoclastoma (a poor designation; giant cell tumor of bone is preferable), interstitial cell tumor of the testis, hilar cell tumor of the ovary, etc. (Fig. 5–2).

c. Eponymic Names. There are many neoplasms known by the name of an author who either described the tumor for the first

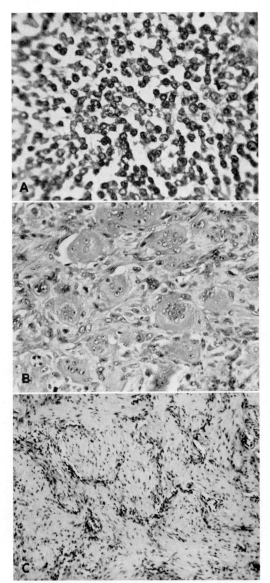

FIG. 5–2. Microscopic aspect of tumors bearing cell names. *A,* Reticulum cell sarcoma. *B,* Giant cell tumor of bone (osteoclastoma). *C,* Hilar cell tumor of ovary. (Tissue courtesy of Dr. Edward S. Murphy.)

time or distinguished himself by the thoroughness of his work, such as Hodgkin's disease, Ewing's tumor or Wilms's tumor (Fig. 5–3). Classic mistakes may also be perpetuated, as in Grawitz's tumor, or awkward designations are replaced by eponyms, as in Brenner's tumor (oöphoroma folliculare) or Krukenberg's tumor (fibrosarcoma ovarii mucocellulare carcinomatodes).

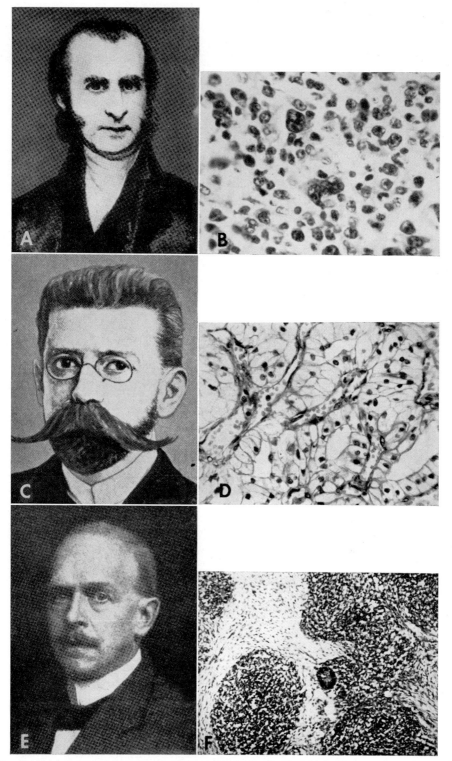

FIG. 5–3.   Some eponyms of tumors. *A*, Thomas Hodgkin. *B*, Hodgkin's disease. *C*, Paul Grawitz. *D*,
Grawitz's tumor. *E*, Max Wilms. *F*, Wilms's tumor.

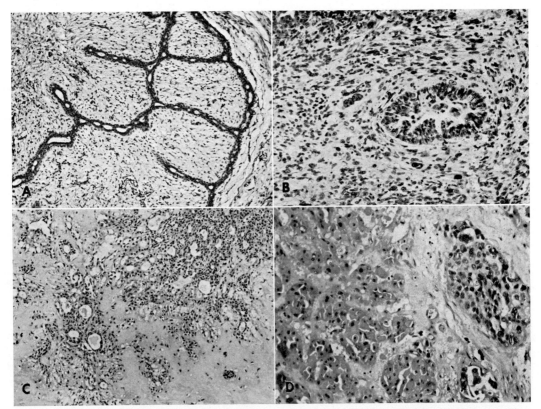

FIG. 5–4. Some tumors with combined names and structures. *A*, Fibroadenoma of breast. *B*, Carcinosarcoma of uterus. *C*, Mixed tumor of salivary gland. *D*, Metastasis of bronchogenic carcinoma in carcinoma of the kidney.

d. Compound Names. There are some tumors where proliferation encompasses two different types of cells and/or tissues, so a double name is used to designate them; for instance, fibroadenoma of the breast, in which both epithelium and stroma are involved in benign multiplication, or carcinosarcoma, a rare tumor in which both epithelial and mesenchymal elements are malignant.[26] These true mixed tumors should not be confused with two other forms of coexistence of two or more tissues in the same tumor. The first form corresponds to metaplasia of neoplastic cells, as in lipomas with myxoid stroma or the so-called "mixed tumor of salivary glands," which is mixed in structure but not in histogenesis. The second form is the "collision" tumor, in which two distinct and separate tumors grow next to each other and may even penetrate into each other, or those rare cases where one malignant tumor metastasizes to another (Fig. 5–4). Gore and Barr[27] have published two such cases and reviewed the literature; curiously enough, more than half of the extant reports show that the recipient tumor was carcinoma of the kidney. To create complicated names for tumors of varied morphology but single histogenesis is a pernicious pastime of ivory-tower histopathologists who in this way pretend to escape the clinical reality.

e. Teratomas. These are tumors formed by elements derived from more than one blastodermic layer, usually showing certain tendency to tissue organization, and which are not normally present in the organ involved. Fibroadenoma is not a teratoma because both epithelial and fibrous tissue are normal components of the breast; on the other hand, ovarian "dermoid cysts" are true teratomas since, in addition to skin with adnexae, other tissues may be found such as teeth, thyroid, nervous tissue, etc. (Fig.

5–5). Both benign and malignant forms of teratoma exist and the final decision should not be reached until completing a detailed study of the specimen.[28]

f. Other Names. Finally, many other names exist of entirely capricious derivation, such as "mesenchymoma," a tumor composed of several mesodermal tissues; "chordoma," a neoplasm presumably aris-

ing from rests of the notochord, etc. In 1904, Albrecht[29] introduced the terms "hamartoma," to characterize congenital, tumor-like malformations composed of tissue elements normally present in organs, but with a bizarre architecture, and "choristoma," to designate congenital neoplasms formed by tissues displaced from their normal position (Fig. 5–6). These are classic

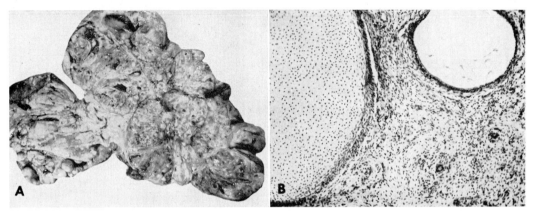

FIG. 5–5. Teratoma. *A*, Gross aspect of solid ovarian teratoma. *B*, Cartilage, epithelium, fibrous tissue and other structures in the same case.

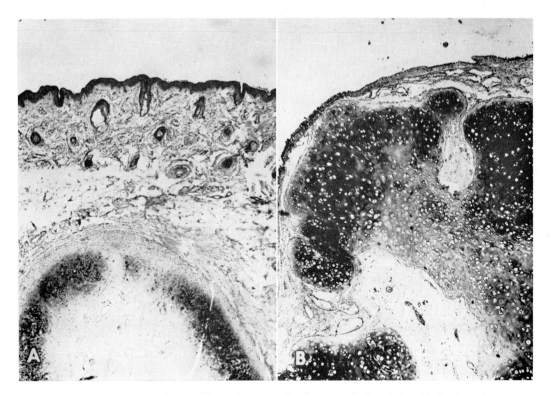

FIG. 5–6. Congenital tumor-like malformations. *A*, Choristoma (displaced tissues) in the subcutaneous tissue of the neck. *B*, Hamartoma of bronchus.

terms serving a well defined purpose and have been widely accepted; would-be innovators suggesting such horrendous terms as "insuloma," for the functional adenoma of islands of Langerhans, or "aldosteroma," for the adrenal cortical adenoma secreting large amounts of aldosterone, should pause to reflect on the already confused status of the nomenclature of tumors before deciding to increase it.

III. THE ETIOLOGY OF TUMORS

Etiology is the study of the cause or causes of disease while pathogenesis refers to the mechanisms by which the causal agent brings about the ailment. Thus, in infectious diseases the etiologic agents are microorganisms while the pathogenesis is a complex interaction known as the host-parasite relation. In neoplastic diseases the etiologic agents seem to be legion; indeed, it is doubtful that in the most frequent forms of human cancers the etiology is ever single. Rather, a constellation of etiologic agents are probably at work for a long period be-

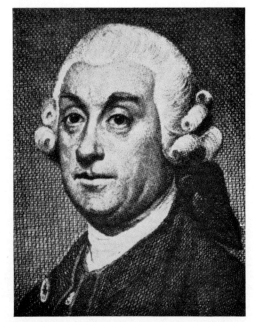

FIG. 5–7.   Sir Percival Pott.

fore normal cells are irreversibly changed into tumor cells. Yet, the effect of carcinogens, or the pathogenesis of neoplasia, is postulated as being always the same: an irreversible, heritable modification in cellu-

ſuch frequent and acute internal pains, as have ſufficiently proved a diſeaſed ſtate of ſome of the viſcera, and which have ſoon been followed by a painful death.

If extirpation ever bids fair for the cure of a cancer, it ſeems to be in this caſe; but then the operation ſhould be immediate, and before the habit is tainted. The diſeaſe, in theſe people, ſeems to derive its origin from a lodgment of ſoot in the rugæ of the ſcrotum, and at firſt not to be a diſeaſe of the habit. In other caſes of a cancerous nature, in which the habit is

FIG. 5–8.   Page in Pott's book where the suggestion occurs that cancer may be due to an exogenous agent.

lar biology leading to unlimited and uncoordinated proliferation.

The study of the etiology of tumors was started in 1775, when Sir Percival Pott, an elegant British surgeon (Fig. 5–7), recognized the association between cancer of the scrotum and the presence of soot in the skin and clothing of chimney sweepers with the following words:[30]

". . . but there is a disease as peculiar to a certain set of people, which has not, at least to my knowledge, been publicly noticed: I mean the chimney sweeper's cancer. It is a disease which always makes its first attack on, and its first appearance in the inferior part of the scrotum; where it produces such frequent and acute internal pains, as have sufficiently proved a diseased state of some of the viscera, and which have soon been followed by a painful death.

"If extirpation ever bids fair for the cure of a cancer, it seems to be in this case; but then the operation should be immediate, and before the habit is tainted. The disease, in these people, seems to derive its origin from a lodgment of soot in the rugae of the scrotum, and at first not to be a disease of the habit . . ." (Fig. 5–8).

With these words was started the search for the etiologic agents of different forms of tumors, which has produced such brilliant results while at the same time showing the extreme complexity of the problem. In the following paragraphs a summary of some of the information available has been attempted, and some remarks have been included on the relation of trauma, heredity and environment to the causation of tumors, the role of endocrine glands and some theories on the intimate nature of neoplastic disease.

A. EXPERIMENTAL STUDIES

Very useful reviews of this subject have been published recently, to which the reader should refer for additional data;[8, 12] in the following paragraphs no attempt has been made to be complete, but only to summarize some of the highlights of this field, a very active one in modern research.

1. Extrinsic Factors. Experimental studies on extrinsic carcinogens may be divided according to the nature of the different agents into: (a) physical, (b) chemical and (c) biologic. This is certainly an artificial separation since in many cases it is not easy to decide if a biologic agent is acting through chemical mechanisms, or if the effect of a chemical substance is due to physical action; nevertheless, the division is adhered to because it serves descriptive purposes.

a. Physical Agents. For a long time it has been suspected that sunlight[31] and ultraviolet radiation[32, 33] can induce neoplastic growth, especially of the skin, because of evidence including the fact that skin cancers are largely limited to uncovered areas— principally the face— of people usually exposed to sunlight for long periods, such as sailors and farmers. Experimentally it has been shown with animals that prolonged exposure to sunlight will end in the production of epithelial tumors, especially in the rat's ear; mice exposed to mercury arc lamp light develop connective tissue tumors, perhaps because the thickness of epithelium in these animals allows passage of ultraviolet light to deeper layers. Carcinogenic wavelength of ultraviolet radiation is from 2600 to 3400 Å.[34]

Ionizing radiations are powerful carcinogens,[35] a fact recognized soon after Roentgen's discovery in 1895; in 1902 the first case of carcinoma of the skin clearly related to the effect of x-radiation was published.[36] With the Curies' discovery of radium came a new impulse to the study of ionizing radiation as a carcinogen, and the atomic bomb and other forms of fission energy have also been able to stimulate neoplastic growth. Experimentally it has been shown that whole-body radiation of some animal species will increase the incidence of leukemia, lymphoma, ovarian and pulmonary tumors, whereas local radiation induces the appearance of skin, colon, lung and other tumors.[37, 38] Absorbed radioactive material such as radium results in osteogenic sarcoma in rats and mice,[39] but it should be remembered that in these species the effective dose is at least 150 times greater than in man. Although not experimental, the appearance of malignant tumors many years after the administration of thorium dioxide, a radiopaque and β-emitter substance with a long half-life, is a sad instance of the carcinogenic effect of ionizing radiation in man.[40] A similar situation followed the use of radium and other radioactive substances in the luminous paint for watch dials, since painters would achieve a fine point on their brushes by compressing them between tongue and lips. The result was the late development of aplastic anemia, aseptic necrosis of bone and bone tumors.[41]

For years, Virchow's theory of "chronic irritation" as a cause of cancer was very popular, but experimental studies have failed to validate it; for instance, Woglom produced chronic irritation in the breasts of virgin rats and compared the incidence of mammary tumors and tumors of other sites with control animals, without finding any difference.[42] Other forms of "chronic irritation" probably have a chemical basis.

b. Chemical Agents. After a few attempts by different experimenters to produce cancer by means of chronic application of chemical agents to the skin of various animal species (and which probably failed because of the short period or the species used), in 1915 two Japanese workers, Yamagiwa and Ichikawa, were able to obtain tumors in the inner surface of the rabbit's ear by chronic painting of this area with tar.[43] This experimental demonstration came 140 years after Pott's clever observation, and served as a starting point for Kennaway's monumental work. Yamagiwa and Ichikawa used the inner surface of the rabbit's ear because no spontaneous tumors are known to occur in this area, and at the end of two or three months observed the appearance of skin papillomas first and carcinomas later, which metastasized to the regional lymph nodes. These studies were confirmed in the same year by Tsutsui, who used tar and mice.[44]

The organized search for the carcinogenic agent in tar and other materials was carried out in the laboratories of the Free Cancer Hospital (today Marsden Hospital) in London, under the direction of the late Sir Ernest Kennaway (Fig. 5–9), who has left an account of it.[45] In collaboration with Goulden, Hieger, Mayneord, Cook and Hewett, who progressively joined the team, Kennaway isolated from tar, crude oil and other materials a series of compounds identified by their fluorescent spectrum and carcinogenic effect in mice; in another line of research, the working team synthesized a series of compounds with the same physical

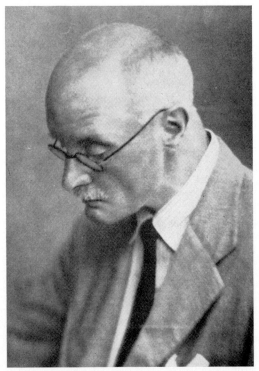

FIG. 5–9.   Sir Ernest Kennaway.

and biologic properties but of known composition. In the beginning this work was carried out with small amounts of material, but when greater concentrations of carcinogenic agents became necessary, two tons of coal tar were processed and after pyrolysis, distillation and repeated extraction with alcohol yielded 7 Gm. of a yellowish crystalline powder with potent carcinogenic action. After 17 years of work, Kennaway and his group were able to announce that synthetic carcinogens were identical with those obtained by pyrolysis and alcoholic extraction from coal tar: they were polycyclic hydrocarbons of the type of perylene, 1,2-benzopyrene and 3,4-benzopyrene.

Much important information continued to come from this group of workers, and the significance of it has been summarized by Haddow[46] as follows: "What undoubtedly emerged from almost thirty years of brilliant work was a satisfying and indeed entrancing correlation between chemical constitution and biological action, whereby the carcinogenic subclasses—benzophenanthrenes, dibenzophenanthrenes, chrysenes, pyrenes and benzanthracenes—could clearly be related to the parent phenanthrene, in a system suggesting dependence upon certain optimal features of molecular size, shape, substitution and chemical reactivity. But we must not minimize another result, namely the profound practical influence which was exerted upon the whole of cancer research, and indeed biology widely, from the mere availability of these potent carcinogens, so rendering possible numberless other investigations and additions to knowledge which could not have been attained without them." Some 1500 compounds have been tested for carcinogenic activity, of which approximately 400 have been positive.[47] It is impossible, however, to generalize on the relation between chemical composition and carcinogenic activity. Within a single group of compounds it is feasible to identify the important foci of activity, but different groups show extraordinary variations in composition, ranging from highly complicated, as in polycyclic hydrocarbons, to very simple, as urethane or chloroform[48] (Fig. 5–10).

Another interesting aspect of chemical carcinogens is the different susceptibility of various animal species; mice are the most susceptible, monkeys are the least. Some substances have not revealed their carcinogenic activity until tested in the susceptible animal, as with β-naphthylamine, a dye capable of producing carcinoma of the bladder in man.[49] Many species were tested until the use of large doses and several years of observation in dogs gave positive results.[50] Another instance is arsenic, which so far has been shown to be carcinogenic only for man.[51]

The mechanism of action of chemical carcinogens is not known, but there are several interesting observations. Cowdry and Paletta[52] found epithelial changes in mice treated with methylcholanthrene for 18 days; these changes were hyperchromatism and loss of regularity of the basal cells, which became more prominent with passage of time. Ultracentrifugation revealed that viscosity of nuclear particles was decreased. This may be in keeping with Haddow's suggestion that the primary step in chemical

carcinogenesis may be the inhibition of certain fundamental processes of genetic or enzyme synthesis, followed by the generation of a new fibre or template, chemically modified and hence genetically also.[53] Nuclear changes are prominent in tumors, and they may be caused by modifications in the heterochromatic regions of the chromosomes, which are probably related to nucleic acid synthesis.[54] The application of a chemical carcinogen to the skin, however, is not followed immediately by the appearance of a tumor; a variable period must elapse which is known as the "latent period."[55] This has also been observed in man, in whom carcinoma of the bladder secondary to β-naphthylamine has a 5 year latent period;[56] benzidine skin cancer takes approximately 8 years to appear;[57] and an extreme case is arsenic cancer.[58] Friedenwald and Rous suggested that carcinogenic action could be separated into two different parts: initiation and promotion.[59] Initiation would be the true carcinogenic effect, produced initially by the agent as an irreversible cell change. The cell is then potentially neoplastic, but latent. An additional factor would then act in this changed cell releasing the capacity for unlimited proliferation. This factor is referred to as promoter or cocarcinogen, and the transformation of a benign into a malignant tumor is known as epicarcinogenesis. Hieger and Pullinger[60] believe that these ideas may find application in cases where chronic irritation seems related to the presence of a malignant tumor, such as a nevus becoming melanoma after multiple trauma; in this instance, nevic cells would represent initiated elements and irritation would act as the promoting agent.

Other interesting concepts which may find practical application are the summation of subminimal doses of two carcinogens applied in successive periods, or their synergistic effect when given at the same time; in some combinations, however, the result is the opposite, since one carcinogen inhibits the other. The latter phenomenon should be distinguished from anticarcinogenesis, in which an active substance is inhibited by a noncarcinogen, as when benzopyrene fails to induce tumor formation because of the influence of bromobenzene. Some experi-

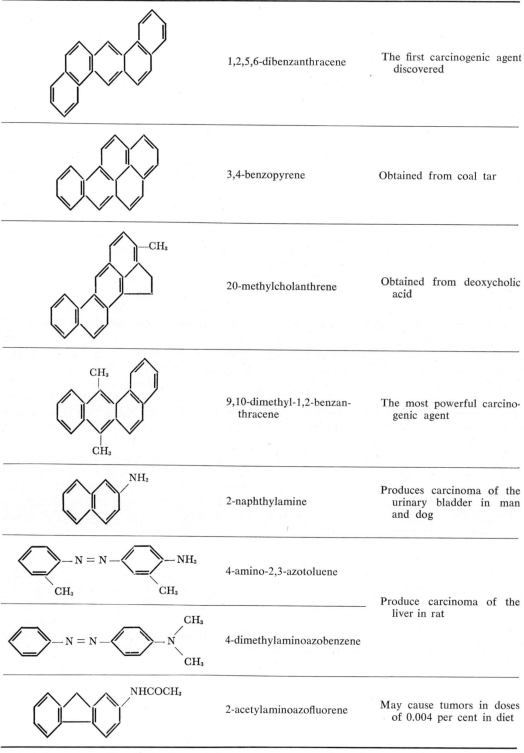

	1,2,5,6-dibenzanthracene	The first carcinogenic agent discovered
	3,4-benzopyrene	Obtained from coal tar
	20-methylcholanthrene	Obtained from deoxycholic acid
	9,10-dimethyl-1,2-benzan-thracene	The most powerful carcinogenic agent
	2-naphthylamine	Produces carcinoma of the urinary bladder in man and dog
	4-amino-2,3-azotoluene	Produce carcinoma of the liver in rat
	4-dimethylaminoazobenzene	
	2-acetylaminoazofluorene	May cause tumors in doses of 0.004 per cent in diet

FIG. 5–10. Some of the most common carcinogenic agents.

mental tumors are conditioned by the presence of a carcinogenic substance, but when the stimulus is discontinued the tumor regresses, as is observed in some tumors produced by coal tar in rabbits. The dose required for induction of neoplastic growth varies according to the agent and the susceptibility of the animal species, but it can be extremely small; in mice, 0.00195 mg. of benzopyrene suffice to produce tumors.[61]

c. Biologic Agents. Bacteria, rickettsiae and fungi are not known or suspected to play any role in the causation of tumors, but it is beyond doubt that viruses and some helminths are capable of inducing neoplastic growth. The first suggestion of the participation of viruses in the etiology of neoplastic growth was made by Borrel,[62] who following his studies on other viruses found that they exerted a proliferative action in tissues. This was followed in 1908 by the classic demonstration of Ellerman and Bang of the viral nature of fowl leukosis[63] and in 1911 by Rous' discovery of the viral origin of spontaneous mesodermal tumors in chicken.[64] The latter is a spindle cell sarcoma (probably a fibrosarcoma) appearing in the breast of the Plymouth Rock chicken. Rous prepared a tumor extract, passed it through a Berkefeld filter and injected the filtrate into the breast of the same type of chicken. The tumor grew again and produced pulmonary metastases. An osteosarcoma and an angiosarcoma were also described in the same epoch, both produced by filtrable viruses. These discoveries were made precisely at the time when Kenna-

way's work was attracting the attention of the scientific world, and their significance was not fully appreciated until in 1932 Shope found a fibromatous tumor in wild cotton-tail rabbits which proved to be transmissible by cell-free extracts.[65] In the following year the same author found another neoplasm with the same transmissibility but of epithelial nature; incidentally, the latter tumor appeared as an epidemic among wild cotton-tail rabbits.[66] These discoveries opened the door to many others and at present a whole series of viral tumors are known to occur in cold-blooded animals, birds and mammals[7] (Table 16).

Many of these filterable agents have been identified as viruses by means of analytic ultracentrifugation, ultrafiltration, electron microscopy and immunology. Some are rather well characterized, such as the virus of Rous carcinoma I, which is not greater than 70 to 100 mμ in diameter and has the composition of a complex nucleoprotein with 40 per cent lipid content and resembling ribonucleic acid;[67] the minimal dose to induce sarcoma in chicken is approximately 2000 particles or 4×10^{-13} Gm. dry weight.[68] Another relatively well known virus is the "milk factor," discovered by Bittner in the milk of mice[69] and which plays an important part in the development of breast cancer in mice, together with a genetic and a hormonal factor.[70] This virus is present in many organs and tissues of high-cancer-strain mice but not in their excreta, although the male transmits the virus by the spermatic fluid;[71] this virus goes

Table 16.   Neoplasms of Viral Etiology

TYPE OF NEOPLASM	ANIMAL SPECIES	REFERENCES
Chicken leukoses	Fowl	Ellerman and Bang (1908)
Chicken sarcomas	Fowl	Rous (1911)
Chicken sarcomas	Fowl	Fujinami and Inamoto (1914
Mill-Hill endothelioma	Fowl	Foulds (1934)
Chicken fibrosarcomas	Fowl	Duran-Reynals (1946)
Mammary cancer (adenocarcinoma)	Mice	Bittner (1936)
Maxillary gland tumors	Mice	Gross (1953)
Leukemia	Mice	Gross (1952)
Papillomatosis	Rabbit, Cattle, Horse	Shope (1933), Olson (1941)
Adenocarcinoma of kidney	Leopard frog	Lucke (1934, 1938)
Papilloma (warts)	Humans	Green, *et al.* (1940)
		Strauss, *et al.* (1950)

through Berkefeld and Seitz filters, is thermolabile, survives freezing for months and multiplies in the chick embryo. Its molecular weight is 3 to 5 million and it is antigenic, stimulating formation of neutralizing antibodies. Attempts at isolation and purification of the virus of mammary cancer have, so far, been disappointing or have yielded results which lack uniformity.[72] Many data on tumor-viruses can be found in the excellent review by Dmochowski.[73]

Many parasites have been held responsible for the production of tumors in animals. In 1931, Strong[74] listed 13, but it is doubtful that all should be accepted. *Taenia multilocularis* and *Spirocerca sanguinolenta* which infest the dog induce fibrous nodules around the parasites which are probably just chronic inflammatory reactions; on the other hand, *Taenia crassicollis* and *Trichosomoides crassicauda* produce malignant tumors in the liver and bladder of the rat. Heading the list was the notorious *Gongylonema neoplasticum,* described by Fibiger as the causal agent of carcinoma of the stomach in the rat; the story of this episode has been well told by Oberling.[75]

2. Intrinsic Factors. Intrinsic factors studied in experimental animals have also been of three general types: (1) hereditary, (2) endocrine and (3) endogenous.

a. Heredity. The fact that tumors occur spontaneously in small laboratory animals, easy to handle and with a relatively short life expectancy, has greatly facilitated studies of heredity as a factor in the production of tumors. To designate a tumor as "spontaneous" is to declare ignorance of its causation. For some time it was thought that breast cancer in mice was spontaneous and genetically determined, but Bittner's studies on "milk factor" have thrown some light on its cause. The establishment of inbred strains has made it possible to study experimentally the influence of genetic constitution (genotype) and environment on the development of cancer; thus, mammary cancer in mice is the result of genetic constitution, estrogenic hormones and the "milk factor."[76] Heston has shown that in lung tumors there are at least four different genes,[77] which are: (1) lethal yellow, a gene related to hair pigmentation, obesity and death of the homozygous embryo, and favoring the appearance of pulmonary tumors, while (2) shaker, (3) hairless and (4) flexed-tail decrease the incidence. Leukemia in mice is extremely important because it resembles that disease in man; McDowell, *et al.* have studied it by means of strain C58 (with a 90 per cent incidence of leukemia), and Storrs-Little strain, which is a highly resistant line. The results indicate that susceptibility to leukemia depends on several genes,[78] and that there is a maternal resistance factor transmitted through milk, egg and placenta.[79] Other factors are also at play, as shown by the fact that the carcinogen-induced leukemia incidence in CBA mice is reduced from 69.7 to 22.0 per cent after thymectomy, but if the operation is followed by autografting of the thymus then the incidence is restored to 69.1 per cent.[80] Other instances might be quoted but the foregoing should suffice to demonstrate that experimental genetic studies are revealing many important aspects of carcinogenesis.

b. Endocrine Glands. The relation of endocrine glands to experimental tumors is of a double nature; hormones may be used as carcinogenic agents, or else once the tumor is established they may influence its course.[81] Studies on the relationship of hormones to the induction of neoplasia have been made almost exclusively in mice, mainly because of the availability of inbred strains with known genetic makeup; other animal species such as rat, rabbit and hamster have also been used. On the other hand, data on the effect of hormones on established tumors are mainly derived from human material, since only few experimental cancers are influenced by endocrine secretions.[82]

Some of the work done inducing tumors with hormones resembles chemical carcinogenesis, since administration is extrinsic and doses are much greater than normal endogenous secretions. Estrogens and gonadotropins are the only hormones implicated so far, and they have produced pituitary, ovarian, renal, testicular, mammary, uterine and other tumors.[83] Many of these neoplastic growths fail to metastasize and require the use of inbred strains to appear.

An interesting experiment was reported by Biskind and Biskind:[84] bilateral ovariectomy in mice, followed by intrasplenic autotransplant of one ovary, results in inactivation of most estrogens secreted before they reach systemic circulation because the first organ they come to is the liver; therefore, there is no normal regulation of secretion of pituitary gonadotropin and this hormone is produced in excess. Gonadotropins stimulate the intrasplenic ovary and granulosa-cell tumors are produced; [85] these tumors will not appear if the animal is treated with either estrogens or androgens. The malignant nature of some of these neoplasms has been manifested by their ability to metastasize.[86] The same effect may be obtained with ionizing radiation, destructive of ovarian germ cells and follicles, which eliminates estrogenic secretion, or with administration of high doses of pituitary gonadotropin.[87]

c. Endogenous Factors. It has been suggested that, other than hormones, the organism can produce carcinogenic substances either under the influence of exogenous factor or "spontaneously." In the first case, exogenous factors would not be considered carcinogenic *per se* but would only serve as a stimulus for the production of endogenous

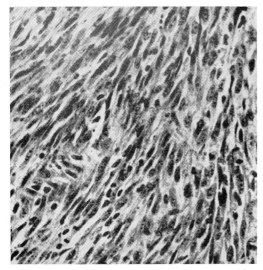

FIG. 5–11. Sarcoma in male stock mouse, which appeared 18 months after commencement of injections of purified cholesterol in olive-oil. (Courtesy of Dr. I. Hieger and the Editor, British Medical Bulletin.)

carcinogens; in the second case, such agents could be the result of a metabolic aberration. These ideas are purely theoretical and the majority are based on the similarity between some potent carcinogens and normally existing substances in the organism, such as methylcholanthrene and estrogens or deoxycholic acid. Even though methylcholanthrene has been prepared from deoxycholic acid,[88] the latter has never been shown to be carcinogenic; with cholesterol, on the other hand, spindle-cell sarcomas have been induced in the subcutaneous tissue of mice (Fig. 5–11).[89, 90] Many natural products have been examined in search of carcinogenic activity, such as urine, bile, extracts of different organs, etc., and although a few tumors have been observed, especially with liver extracts, results are interpreted as negative. Hieger believes that even if carcinogenic substances were normally present in tissues, their concentration would be too low to be of any significance.[91]

B. THE SIGNIFICANCE OF EXPERIMENTAL STUDIES IN HUMAN CARCINOGENESIS

The following paragraphs are a condensation of Steiner's excellent review on the meaning of experimental studies in human tumors.[92] Animal work can be considered in three different groups: (a) those with immediate application to man because identical conditions are present, (b) those with a possible practical usefulness but in need of further investigations and (c) experiments with no human analogy because conditions are too artificial. Instances of the third group of experimental studies would be those carried out with highly inbred strains of mice, with massive doses of carcinogenic agents, or with elaborate modifications of the endocrine equilibrium.

Foremost among experimental observations with application to man is the finding of chemical carcinogens, which have been demonstrated in many materials with which man is in daily contact, such as 3,4-benzopyrene, arsenic, beryllium, urethane, etc. Animal studies have also served to build the viral theory of cancer, which is discussed below. Latency or induction periods are observed in man and contribute to the difficutlies encountered in etiologic studies, since they average 5 to 15 years; of some significance has been the experimental demonstration of the effectiveness of very small doses. The combination of prolonged induction periods and minute concentrations of carcinogens, together with synergistic action and anticarcinogenesis, have probably been responsible for the delay in recognizing etiologic agents in human tumors. In addition, it has been shown experimentally that the same polycyclic hydrocarbons can induce formation of different tumors, such as osteosarcoma, fibrosarcoma, lyphosarcoma, lymphoma, intracranial neoplasms and carcinomas in various organs, including stomach, intestine, lung, skin, prostate, etc. The latter is especially important since it supports Willis' contention that an etiologic classification of tumors, even if possible, would be useless.[10]

C. CLINICAL STUDIES

1. Some Instances of Carcinogenic Action in Man. It has been mentioned that there are few, if any, simple or single causes in biology; instead, there are complex situations and environments in which the probability of certain events is increased. This is certainly true of human cancer, where the irreversible transformation of normal cells results from the combined effect of many factors, such as genetic constitution, susceptibility, endocrine equilibrium, environmental conditions favoring contact with carcinogens, the actual presence of the agent, dosage, time, etc. Nevertheless, there are cases where in the middle of such a constellation of etiologic agents, one or a few stand out as of greater significance than the others and seem to throw light on causation and bring hope for prevention. Some instances are briefly described in the following paragraphs.

a. Carcinoma of the Skin. Reasons to consider ultraviolet radiation as the predominant factor in causation of carcinoma of the skin have been mentioned[33] and may be summarized as follows: (1) carcinoma of the skin is more frequent in people with prolonged exposure to sunlight, such as sailors and farmers; (2) tumors appear in uncovered areas, as the face and dorsum of the hands; (3) the frequency of carcinoma of the skin is higher in light- than in dark-

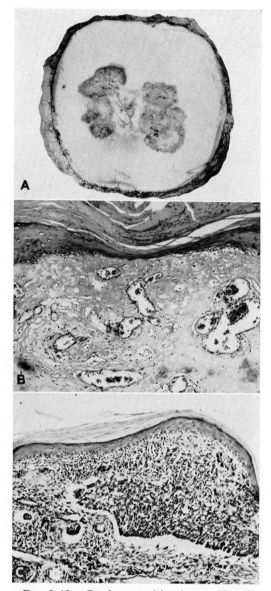

FIG. 5–12. Carcinoma arising in an old radiodermatitis. *A,* Gross aspect of the lesion. *B,* Radiodermatitis. *C,* Carcinoma in the same case.

skinned subjects, probably because the former absorb less ultraviolet radiations and also because the epithelium is thinner; (4) among colored people, skin carcinoma is more frequent in albinos.

In spite of these facts, sunlight is not the only factor responsible for skin carcinoma; malignant epithelial tumors appear frequently in the margins of chronic, usually varicose, leg ulcers (Marjolin's ulcer).[93] Partisans of the "chronic irritation" theory of cancer cite this evolution of leg ulcers, submitted for years to chronic inflammation plus the pseudotherapeutic use of many and varied substances.[94] Another important etiologic agent is ionizing radiation ("malignant irradiation for benign conditions")[95] which is only too often found in the history of patients with carcinoma of the skin; Totten, et al. recorded it in 20 of 105 cases of carcinoma of the upper lip[96] (Fig. 5–12). Finally, arsenic is also carcinogenic for the skin, as reported by Arheleger and Kremen,[97] especially after being used as treatment for different dermatoses. It goes without saying that many other cases of carcinoma of the skin have no apparent etiologic agent.

b. *Carcinoma of the Uterine Cervix.* Many factors have been suggested as important in the etiology of carcinoma of the cervix, such as chronic cervicitis, multiple deliveries, syphilis, cervical lacerations, diet, estrogenic hormones, racial factors, etc.

In an impressive paper, Kennaway collected data on the incidence of carcinoma of the uterine cervix from all over the world, and after an exhaustive analysis concluded that two factors seem to be significant: "1. A factor which is opposed by the Jewish practice of abstention from intercourse during most of the first half of the ovulatory cycle; and 2. A factor which is intensified in both married and single women by descent in the economic scale."[98]

An extensive analysis was carried out by Wynder, et al.[99] including several environmental features plus all the local and general conditions mentioned above and many others; different racial and religious groups were interviewed in the United States and India represented by Jews, non-Jews, Negroes, Hindus, Moslems, Christians and Parsis. The salient conclusions of this survey were that women with carcinoma of the cervix are significantly younger at the time of first sexual contact and marriage than controls, that multiple marriages were much more common among patients with carcinoma and that the latter were exposed more often to uncircumcised partners. Wynder, et al. conclude that, "The present results are compatible with the concept that those population groups having a late age at first coitus and first marriage and a low

re-marriage rate, whose men are circumcised, have a low rate of carcinoma of the cervix."

This brief resume does no justice to the careful study of Wynder, et al., who have succeeded in demonstrating the great significance of environmental factors in this type of tumor; some authors have failed to confirm this report[100] but others are in full agreement.[101] There can be no doubt that other circumstances are also present since carcinoma of the cervix has been observed in virgins and in women with circumcised sexual partners.[102] It is of interest to point out that smegma contains carcinogenic substances which are capable of producing experimental tumors, and that the aforementioned data refer only to epidermoid carcinoma; adenocarcinoma of the cervix has not been found to follow racial or socioeconomic influences.

c. *Carcinoma of the Penis.* In close association with the preceding carcinoma of the cervix is carcinoma of the penis, which is much more frequent in subjects with phimosis or uncircumcised than in otherwise normal men[103] (Fig. 5–13). This fact suggests again that smegma may be important in causation and if this is true, then it would represent an endogenous carcinogen for men and exogenous for women. It may be of interest in this respect that Heins, et al. have been able to produce carcinoma of the cervix in d b a-1 strain mice by repeated local application of human smegma.[104]

d. *Carcinoma of the Mouth and Esophagus.* Ahlbom observed that more than 70 per cent of women with cancer of the oral mucosa or upper esophagus in Sweden had a chronic history of Plummer-Vinson syndrome,[105] which is characterized by sideropenic anemia, cheilitis, leukoplakia of the oral mucosa and fingernail changes. This syndrome probably results from a complex vitamin and iron dietetic deficiency which improves with addition of iron to the diet. The association of carcinoma of the oral mucosa and esophagus with the Plummer-Vinson syndrome is statistically highly significant and it is considered that lesions in the oral and upper esophageal mucosa are the antecedent of cancer.[106] Should this prove to be true it would represent a very interesting type of causation, where an ex-

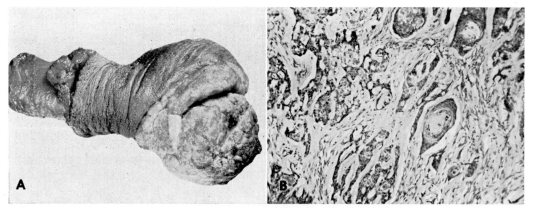

Fig. 5–13. Carcinoma of penis. *A*, Gross aspect of the lesion. This is the most frequent type of tumor, without extensive invasion of surrounding tissues. *B*, Well differentiated epidermoid carcinoma of penis.

ogenous, dietetic deficiency induces tissue changes which then become the seat of neoplastic growth; another possibility is that the susceptibility of oral and esophageal epithelium to carcinogenic agents is increased by the deficiency in food.[107]

e. Carcinoma of the Lung. In recent years there has been a growing interest in bronchogenic carcinoma, mainly because of the phenomenal rise in frequency, although the not-too-scientific publicity given to the relation between smoking and this form of cancer has also been at play. There can be no doubt that the frequency of bronchogenic carcinoma has increased in the last 20 or 30 years, and although there is a widespread belief that this rise in frequency is partially apparent and due to better diagnostic means, some well documented studies have shown that this factor accounts for only a minimal fraction of the increase.[108] Since cellular protoplasm is not known to change in such a short period, the increase suggests a modification in extrinsic, possibly environmental, factors. The problem of the etiology of carcinoma of the lung is, therefore, of a double nature. It is necessary to determine both the cause of bronchogenic carcinoma as well as the cause of the recent rise in frequency.

Bronchogenic carcinoma has been known for a long time, especially in the mining areas of Bohemia and Saxony, where 44 to 75 per cent of the miners died as a consequence of "Bergkrankheit" or "mountain disease."[109] In Joachimsthal (Bohemia) and Schneeberg (Saxony) the mines have been worked for nickel, silver, cobalt, bismuth, radium and finally for uranium, and each one of these metals has been considered the cause of "Bergfertig." The disease was recognized as cancer in 1879, and it has been calculated that miners in Joachimsthal were nearly 30 times more liable to develop it than adult men of Vienna; the average induction time was found to be 17 years and no cases appeared with less than 13 years of exposure.[110] Histologically almost all tumors were epidermoid, oat-cell or undifferentiated carcinomas (Fig. 5–14). Radioactive ores have been considered directly responsible for this form of carcinoma of the lung, and calculations of the amount of radiation present in the air of the mine are consistent with doses with definitive carcinogenic effect.[111] It should be remembered that it was precisely from Joachimsthal that the Austrian government obtained the ton of mineral ore used by the Curies for their transcendental discovery in 1898. Other industrial factors considered as possible etiologic agents of bronchogenic cancer are nickel refining, chromates, asbestos, the combustion and distillation products of coal, arsenic, etc. In general, the risk of developing carcinoma of the lung for workers of these industries is 5 to 15 times greater than for the unexposed population.[112]

The reason for considering atmospheric pollution responsible for some cases of pulmonary cancer is that higher mortality has consistently been reported in urban than in rural areas; it is also significant that substances known to be carcinogenic for animals have been isolated from the urban atmosphere. But the evidence is far from being conclusive, since occupational studies of men heavily exposed to pollution have so far failed to provide evidence of a direct relation between cancer and air contamination with urban products. Furthermore, the carcinogenic substances obtained from the atmosphere are arsenic, radioactive elements, 3,4-benzopyrene, other polycyclic hydrocarbons and, possibly, the oxidation products of aliphatic hydrocarbons. Arsenic can be discarded on a quantitative basis, since Doll has calculated that the amount inspired by an average man in London in 10 years would be of the order of 5 mg., which is little more than would be volatilized in smoking one cigarette a week

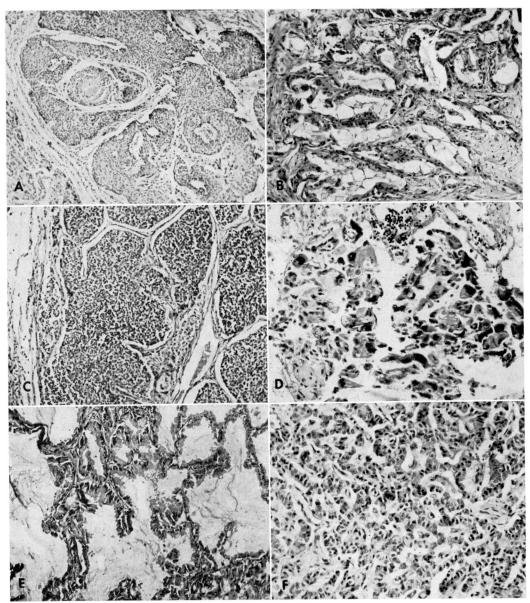

FIG. 5–14. Histologic types of bronchogenic carcinoma. *A,* Epidermoid carcinoma. *B,* Adenocarcinoma. *C,* Undifferentiated, "oat-cell" carcinoma. *D,* Undifferentiated, giant cell carcinoma. *E,* Bronchiolar (alveolar) carcinoma. *F,* So-called bronchial adenoma.

Table 17. Principal Characteristics of the Smoking Histories of Men with and without Lung Cancer, Reported by Various Authors

AUTHOR	DATE	COUNTRY	NUMBER OF MEN		PERCENTAGE OF "NONSMOKERS" AMONG MEN		PERCENTAGE OF "HEAVY SMOKERS" AMONG MEN	
			with lung cancer	without lung cancer	with lung cancer	without lung cancer	with lung cancer	without lung cancer
Müller	1939	Germany	86	86	3.5	16.3	65	36
Schairer and Schöniger	1943	Germany	93	270	3.2	15.9	52	27
Wassink	1948	Holland	134	100	4.5	19.0	55	19
Shrek, et al.	1950	U.S.A.	82	522	14.6	23.9	18	9
Mills and Porter	1950	U.S.A.	444	430	7.0	31.0	..	..
Levin, et al.	1950	U.S.A.	236	481	15.3	21.7	..	..
Wynder and Graham	1950	U.S.A.	605	780	1.3	14.6	51	19
Doll and Hill	1950	Britain	649	649	0.3	4.2	26	13
McConnell, et al.	1952	Britain	93	186	5.4	6.5	35	22
Doll and Hill	1952	Britain	708	708	0.7	4.8	24	14
Sadowsky, et al.	1953	U.S.A.	477	615	3.8	13.2	..	..
Wynder and Cornfield	1953	U.S.A.	63	133	4.1	20.6	68	29
Koulumies	1953	Finland	812	300	0.6	18.0	66	31
Lickint	1953	Germany	224	1000	1.8	16.0	74	29
Breslow, et al.	1954	U.S.A.	518	518	3.7	10.8	74	42
Watson and Conte	1954	U.S.A.	265	277	1.9	9.7	73	57
Randig	1954	Germany	415	381	1.2	5.8	34	18
Gsell	1956	Switzerland	150	150	1.3	19.3	67	15
Kreyberg	1956	Norway	213	4158	1.4	13.2	18	7
Schwartz and Denoix	1957	France	602	1204	3.1	15.8	13	7

(From Doll[115])

over the same period.[113] On the other hand, 3,4-benzopyrene does occur in adequate concentrations, but Steiner has found that cancer of the skin appears in mice treated with extracts of smoke particles, but not by the application of smoke itself, which is against the hypothesis that atmospheric benzopyrene is a cause of the disease.[114] In general, the evidence favoring air pollution is difficult to interpret because there are differences which characterize urban and rural life other than atmospheric contamination, the most important being cigarette smoking.

Finally, data incriminating cigarette smoking as a cause of lung cancer have been obtained by three different methods: first, the retrospective study of patients with bronchogenic carcinoma and the comparison of their smoking habits with the habits of patients with other diseases or with the habits of healthy subjects; second, the prospective analysis of the causes of death of groups of people whose smoking habits had previously been defined; and third, the investigation of the experimental carcinogenic

effect of different types of cigarette smoke preparations.

Over twenty retrospective studies from eight different countries are available, comparing the proportion of lung cancer between smokers and nonsmokers[115] (Table 17). Although not all of them include the same data, it is possible to summarize their main results as follows: (a) there are more heavy smokers and fewer nonsmokers among patients with lung cancer than among patients with other diseases, and this difference is of a high order of significance; (b) there is a steady increase in the relative proportion of lung cancer to control patients as the amount smoked daily increases; (c) the difference in smoking habits holds for both sexes, but is more marked in men than in women; (d) the proportion of inhalers is greater among the cancer patients; (e) persons with bronchogenic carcinoma started smoking earlier and kept the habit longer than controls without pulmonary tumors; (f) the relation between smoking and cancer of the lung is confined to patients with epidermoid, oat-cell and undifferentiated carcinoma; other forms, such as adenocarcinoma, bronchiolar carcinoma and bronchial adenoma fail to show any statistical association. The results of retrospective studies, therefore, strongly support the suggestion that smoking is a cause of carcinoma of the lung.

Prospective studies have not been so numerous but have thrown additional light on the problem. Doll and Hill,[116] in England, and Hammond and Horn,[117, 118] and Dorn[119] in the U.S.A., examined the smoking habits of large numbers of subjects and then recorded the frequency of later occurrence of lung cancer, other respiratory diseases, other cancers, and other causes of death, with the type and intensity of smoking. A positive correlation was found only with pulmonary tumors, which increased with the amount smoked; this result is in entire agreement with that obtained by retrospective work (Fig. 5–15).

Laboratory studies have been directed to examine the effect of smoking in the respiratory tract of men and experimental animals, and to detect the presence of carcinogenic agents in tobacco smoke. Auerbach, et al.[120] studied the entire tracheobronchial tree of 117 subjects aged 50 to 70 by means of serial sections (a total of 28,638 slides). In this group, 34 patients had died of carcinoma of the lung and of the remainder, 16 had never smoked cigarettes, 20 smoked less than one pack a day and 47 smoked one pack or more daily. Epithelial changes were tabulated according to 4 different lesions, and their results are shown in Table 18. It is clear that the proportion showing each of the changes increased steadily from nonsmokers to heavy smokers and was highest in men dying of lung cancer. Similar studies were published by Sanderud[121] and Knudtson[122] with comparable results.

Search for carcinogenic agents in tobacco

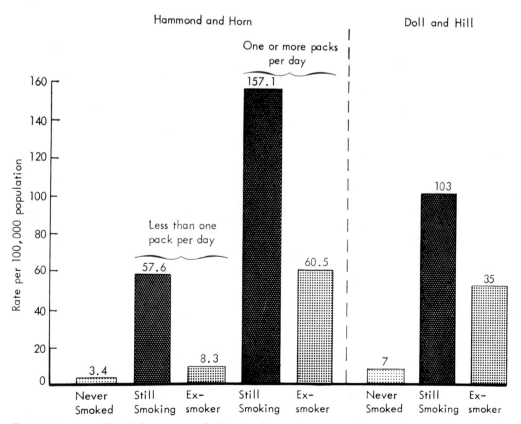

FIG. 5–15. Age-adjusted lung cancer death rates for smokers, ex-smokers, and nonsmokers, based on prospective studies of Hammond and Horn (187,783 subjects) and Doll and Hill (40,701 subjects). (Courtesy of Dr. L. E. Burney and the Editor, Journal of the American Medical Association.)

Table 18. Histologic Changes in the Respiratory Tract of Persons of Different Smoking Habits

HISTOLOGICAL CHANGE	PER CENT OF SLIDES SHOWING CHANGE AMONG:			
	MEN DYING OF DISEASES OTHER THAN LUNG CANCER			MEN DYING OF LUNG CANCER
	Never smoked regularly	Cigarette smokers		
		Less than 20 a day	20 or more a day	
Basal cell hyperplasia	18.6	22.0	36.1	43.5
3 or more cell rows	2.9	5.6	10.8	15.0
5 or more cell rows				
Stratification	4.2	7.1	10.4	13.4
Squamous metaplasia	1.9	6.3	9.5	11.7
Carcinoma in situ	1.0	4.1	6.0	6.3
Number of men	16	20	47	34

(Data from Auerbach et al.[120])

has revealed that there are substances capable, under suitable conditions, of causing cancer in animals. In this respect, Wynder, et al.[123] were the first to produce skin tumors in mice with chronic applications of tar extracted from the smoke of cigarettes. The first papilloma appeared in 8 weeks, the first carcinoma in one year, and at the end of two years 58 per cent of the surviving animals had malignant tumors, 44 per cent with metastases; similar results were obtained in other strains tested and in rabbits. Other workers have confirmed these findings.[124] Carcinogenic substances in tobacco smoke have been identified, such as arsenic, 3,4-benzopyrene, 1,2-benzopyrene, 1,2-benzanthracene, 1,12-benzoperylene, etc.,[125] but the amounts are minute and, according to Wynder and Wright,[126] are quite insufficient to account for the known activity of tar on the skin of mice; these authors believe that the actual carcinogen responsible for tobacco tar activity is yet to be identified.

The evidence summarized in the preceding paragraphs has not gone without criticism. It has been said that statistical analyses are biased and selected,[127] that no true lung cancer has been produced experimentally with tobacco derivatives,[128] that genotypic influences determine both the amount of smoking and the frequency of cancer,[129] that decrease in mortality due to tuberculosis has brought to the fore a disease which is primarily genetic in nature,[130] etc. Many of these criticisms are answered on

statistical grounds by Bross,[131] who points out that they not only fail to prove the association between smoking and lung cancer wrong, but are also unable to offer a tenable counterhypothesis.

The Medical Research Council in Britain advised the Minister of Health in 1957[133] that:

"In scientific work, as in the practical affairs of everyday life, conclusions have often to be founded on the most reasonable and probable explanation of the observed facts and, so far, no adequate explanation for the large increase in the incidence of lung cancer has been advanced save that cigarette smoking is indeed the principal factor in the causation of the disease. The epidemiological evidence is now extensive and very detailed, and it follows a classical pattern upon which many advances in preventive medicine have been made in the past. It is clearly impossible to add to the evidence by means of an experiment in man. . . . Evidence from many investigations in different countries indicates that a major part of the increase is associated with tobacco smoking, particularly in the form of cigarettes. In the opinion of the Council, the most reasonable interpretation of this evidence is that the relationship is one of direct cause and effect."

Summarizing the results of the International Cancer Congress held in London in 1958, Reif stated:[134]

"The conclusion drawn here is that all investigators reporting epidemiological studies of the effect of cigarette smoking on lung-cancer incidence agreed unanimously that cigarette smoking is the main cause for the present increase in this disease. Also, all investigators reporting experimental studies in which cigarette smoke was specifically studied for carcinogenic effects agreed unanimously that cigarette smoke is a carcinogen for man. From these two sets of agreements it follows that the papers presented establish decisively that cigarette smoking is *a* cause of human lung cancer, and, beyond reasonable doubt, that cigarette smoking is the *main* cause of the present increase in lung-cancer incidence."

In 1959, the Surgeon General of the United States Public Health Service issued the following statements:[135]

"1. The weight of evidence at present implicates smoking as the principal etiological factor in the increased incidence of lung cancer. 2. Cigarette smoking particularly is associated with an increased chance of developing lung cancer. 3. Stopping cigarette smoking even after long exposure is beneficial. 4. No method of treating tobacco or filtering the smoke has been demonstrated to be effective in materially reducing or eliminating the hazard of lung cancer. 5. The nonsmoker has a lower incidence of lung cancer than the smoker in all-controlled studies, whether analyzed in terms of rural areas, urban regions, industrial occupations, or sex. 6. Persons who have never smoked at all (cigarettes, cigars, or pipe) have the best chance

of escaping lung cancer. 7. Unless the use of tobacco can be made safe, the individual person's risk of lung cancer can best be reduced by the elimination of smoking."

A comprehensive review of the entire controversy has been published by Davis,[136] which should be consulted for further information; after a thoughtful discussion, this author sums up his views on tobacco smoke and lung cancer as follows: "The evidence in favor of such a relationship is extraordinarily abundant and consistent. The several alternative suggestions are largely speculative and consistency among their proponents is lacking."

f. Leukemia. Although most cases of leukemia appear "spontaneously," a suggestive statistical correlation has been established with one particular group of the population, namely physicians.[137] The incidence of leukemia is 3.5 per cent of all malignant tumors in the general population and 8.5 per cent among physicians; analysis of doctors

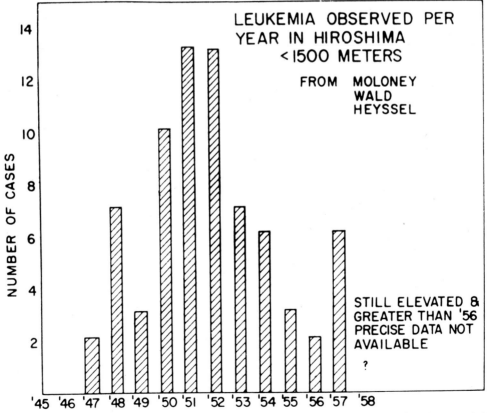

FIG. 5–16.   Histogram of cases of leukemia found per year at Hiroshima between 1945 and 1958. (Courtesy of Dr. E. P. Cronkite and the Editor, American Journal of Medicine.)

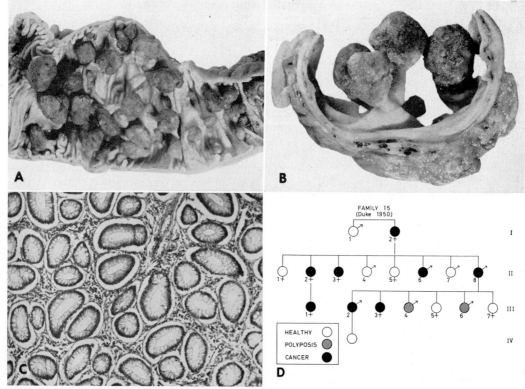

Fig. 5–17. Multiple intestinal polyposis. *A*, Numerous polyps in the colon of an 18 year old patient. *B*, Cut surface of large intestine in the same case. *C*, Microscopic aspect of polyps. *D*, Genealogy of a family with multiple intestinal polyposis.

in different specialties shows that leukemia is at least 9 times more frequent in radiologists than in any other specialists. Mortality due to leukemia per 100,000 is as follows:

General population (male)	9.5
Physicians in general	12.5
Dermatologists	45.0
Radiologists	69.0

These figures indicate that leukemia should be considered as a professional risk for people handling ionizing radiation with medical uses. In their recent review of this problem, Cronkite, *et al.*[138] suggest that for a high level, single dose exposure of man, the incidence of leukemia is approximately linear with dose, but that below dose levels of approximately 100 r equivalent the available data are inadequate for prediction. The same uncertainty applies to the effect of small and repeated doses, which were held responsible for some cases of myeloid and acute leukemia by Lewis.[139] A famous case

was that of Walter B. Cannon, late Professor of Physiology at Harvard. Early in his career, Cannon was quite interested in the movements of the digestive tract, which he studied by means of radiopaque meals and x-rays. At that time no full awareness of the dangers involved in overexposure had developed and the result was a chronic, life-long dermatitis, complicated by an episode of lymphoid leukemia and ending in mycosis fungoides. The entire process took 35 years from the first exposure, and the diagnosis of mycosis fungoides was made by Wolbach 14 years before Cannon's death.[140]

It has been established that among survivors of atomic explosions in Hiroshima and Nagasaki leukemia is at least 10 times more frequent than in the general population.[141] The incidence is even higher in the group which had been within a radius of 2000 meters from the epicenter of explosion. It is not known whether the incidence will continue rising with time,[142] but on the basis of more recent data, showing a decrease in incidence of cases of leukemia during the past 7 years[143] (Fig. 5–16) and the suggestion that probably 90 per cent of the cases occur within 10 years after exposure,[144] it does not appear that the incidence of leukemia will continue increasing at a constant rate throughout the duration of these people's lives. On the other hand, Murphy and Yasuda[145] have called attention to the fact that carcinoma of the stomach, the most frequent malignant tumor in Japan, has not increased in frequency since the atomic explosion in Hiroshima.

g. Genetically Determined Tumors. There are at least four types of genetically determined tumors: familial intestinal polyposis, retinoblastoma, multiple neurofibromatosis or von Recklinghausen's disease and multiple osteocartilaginous exostoses or Ollier's disease. Another disease which will be mentioned, xeroderma pigmentosum, is not a tumor but a precancerous lesion.

Multiple intestinal polyposis is characterized by the presence of numerous adenomatous polyps in the colon (Fig. 5–17, *A, B, C*) becoming clinically manifest at a very early age;[146] one or several polyps undergo malignant transformation, usually in youth. The disease is inherited as a dominant character, one of every two children of affected individuals presenting the lesions regardless of sex[147] (Fig. 5–17, *D*).

Retinoblastoma is a malignant tumor of the retina with a tendency to be multiple and bilateral (Fig. 5–18). Genetic determination is demonstrated in the series of 190 cases studied by Reese, of which only 6 survivors had children; the total number of children was 10, of which 9 developed bilateral retinoblastomas.[148]

Multiple neurofibromatosis or von Recklinghausen's disease is characterized by the presence of various cutaneous marks such as nevi, hirsutism, "café au lait" spots and

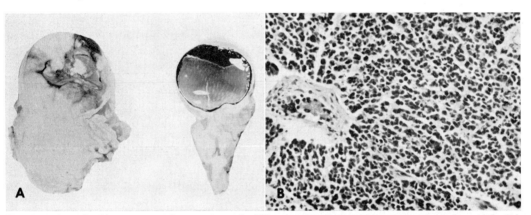

FIG. 5–18.   Retinoblastoma. *A,* Gross aspect. *B,* Microscopic picture. No rosettes were formed in this case.

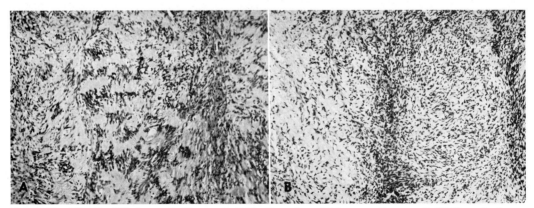

FIG. 5–19.   Von Recklinghausen's disease. *A,* Palisading of nuclei in neurofibroma. *B,* Malignant schwannoma in the same case.

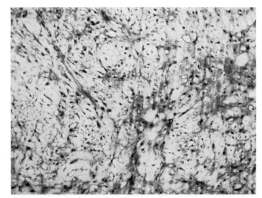

FIG. 5–20.   Ollier's disease. Chondrosarcoma developing in one exostosis.

subcutaneous tumors of different types as lipoma, neurofibroma, hemangioma, etc.[149] It is inherited as a dominant character, but occasionally patients are seen with no apparent family history; approximately 5 to 10 per cent of patients develop malignant tumors, usually by epicarcinogenesis, which may be fibrosarcomas, malignant schwannomas (Fig. 5–19), liposarcomas or malignant melanomas.[150]

Multiple osteocartilaginous exostoses or Ollier's disease appears as multiple, more or less symmetrical, osteocartilaginous growths of the skeleton with a predominance for long bones and pelvis; it is transmitted by a dominant gene and in approximately 10 to 15 per cent of the cases chondrosarcomas develop which may be multiple[151] (Fig. 5–20).

Xeroderma pigmentosum is transmitted by heterozygous parents by a recessive gene, since only one fourth of the descendants are affected; consanguinity in parents has been demonstrated in 30 per cent of a series of 43 families.[152] It is characterized by light, dry skin with many areas of pigmentation and hypersensitivity to sunlight; after exposure the skin shows hyperkeratosis, atrophy and ulceration (Fig. 5–21). Multiple malignant tumors develop usually in childhood and these are mostly epidermoid carcinomas, although sarcomas and malignant melanomas may also be present (Fig. 5–22). Koller studied three families, in one of which several members were affected and showed some unusual features, such as the

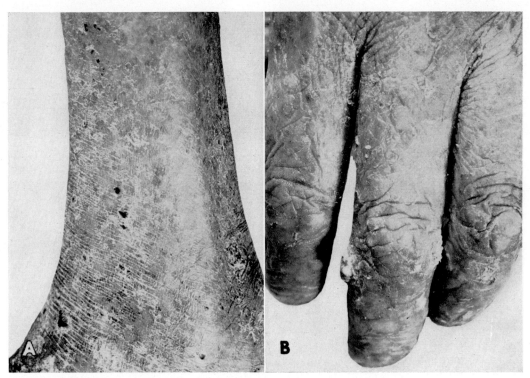

FIG. 5–21.   Xeroderma pigmentosum. Skin lesions in a 17-year-old girl with extensive cutaneous involvement. The small excrescence in the middle finger proved to be epidermoid carcinoma.

late development of complications and a predominance for females.[153]

Although in the five conditions mentioned inheritance plays a dominant role, other instances exist in which such a factor seems to be important. One of the most striking instances is the pedigree of family "G," studied by Warthin,[154] where the incidence of cancer in members who reached the "cancer age" was 31.8 per cent; the predominant tumor in males was in the gastro-intestinal tract, and in females in the uterus (Fig. 5–23). Lentz[155] and others[156] have made collections of such pedigrees, showing among other things that close relatives are more frequently affected and that this is true for malignant epithelial tumors only; the incidence in relatives of patients with sar-comas was lower than in the general population. Pedigree studies of patients with carcinoma of the stomach and large intestine,[157] breast, uterus, leukemia and other malignant tumors suggest the existence of genetic factors,[158] but the conclusions are difficult to establish because of the absence of adequate controls.[159]

2. Trauma and Cancer. Chronic and repeated trauma in the same area for a prolonged period is an instance of "chronic irritation" and its role in the causation of tumors has been mentioned. Of interest here is the relation between single trauma and cancer. The problem is important from many viewpoints, including medicolegal complications, and for this reason some authors have established a group of criteria

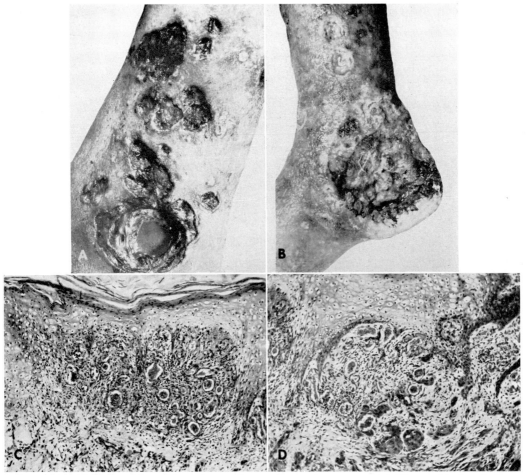

FIG. 5–22. Multiple epidermoid carcinomas in xeroderma pigmentosum. *A,* Ulcerated lesions in lower leg. *B,* Large, fungating epidermoid carcinoma in foot; other lesions may be seen in the leg. *C,* Microscopic aspect of skin lesion with many dilated blood vessels. *D,* A similar field with infiltrating carcinoma in the dermis.

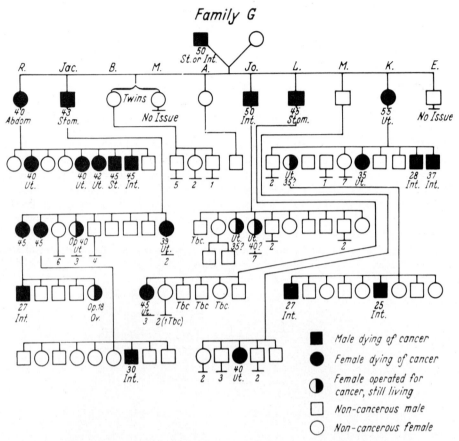

FIG. 5–23. Incidence of cancer in family G, studied by Warthin.

that should be fulfilled before accepting single trauma as the cause of a tumor; the following list was proposed by Ewing:[160]

1. Trauma must be authentic and adequate.

2. The injured part should have been normal before trauma.

3. The tumor should arise in the exact site of trauma.

4. The diagnosis of the presence and nature of the tumor must be objective.

It is obvious that these criteria can be met only rarely, and it is even legitimate to question if they can ever be met, since absolute proof of integrity and normality of the injured area before trauma can only be obtained by histologic study, which requires surgical removal; the not-too-infrequent finding of microscopic tumors in many organs supports this contention.

The relation between trauma and cancer has been suggested in tumors of bone, breast and testes, but in none of these areas are there sufficient data to prove it. Orthopedic surgeons traumatize bones with great energy by means of saws, nails, prostheses, etc., but no sarcomas result from it; fractures are very frequent but malignant tumors arising in them must be extremely rare, if they exist at all. The breast is exposed to many traumas throughout life, but cancer develops mainly in certain age groups. Testicular tumors have a varied morphology, but so far no one has suggested that dysgerminoma, which is an ovarian tumor identical with seminoma, is caused by trauma. Furthermore, 11 per cent of all tumors of the testes occur in ectopic (usually abdominal) organs, where they are better protected against trauma, and in 97.5 per cent of cases of malignant testicular tumors occurring in subjects with unilateral ectopia of the testes, the tumor develops in the ectopic organ.

Trauma is the rule in everyday life and the majority of instances are rapidly forgotten unless something happens to fix the subject's attention; thus, the most prevalent general idea is that the role of single trauma is to call attention to a preexisting tumor. It is also possible that the neoplasm may interfere with adequate functioning of the involved area, increasing its susceptibility to trauma. In a masterful paper, Stewart[161] invites all partisans of the traumatic etiology of cancer to, ". . . concentrate upon observing a group of children at play. They will, I can assure them, in the course of an afternoon witness all the types of injury supposed to cause cancer and unless hard-hearted will return home greatly depressed at the sad outlook for the future these children possess."

3. Hormone Dependent Tumors. Huggins and Scott[162] were the first to employ the terms "hormone dependent" and "hormone independent" to describe tumors which depend upon hormones for their maintenance or those which grow independently of them. Hormone dependent tumors can be temporarily controlled by an alteration of the hormonal environment in which they develop. Furthermore, dependent growths are frequently composed of cells which have been experimentally stimulated to proliferate because of a hormonal imbalance, but in some instances they can be induced by other means such as irradiations or chemical carcinogens. The difference between hormone dependent and hormone independent tumors may not be very basic; it is possible that some malignant growths are composed of both dependent and autonomous cells,[163] and this would explain why some cases which have been held in check by endocrine therapy for some time suddenly lose their responsiveness to a particular hormone or combination of hormones. Of course, the possibility of a change in the intimate nature of cells is also a valid hypothesis.

Hormone dependent human tumors are prostatic and mammary carcinomas. The partial control of advanced prostatic carcinoma by castration and estrogens is the most important advance in the treatment of disseminated cancer since the discovery of roentgen rays.[82] It has been established that from 50 to 75 per cent of patients with carcinoma of the prostate are benefited by castration or physiologic neutralization of androgens by estrogenic administration;[164] of the original 20 patients with metastasizing prostatic carcinoma treated by castration by Huggins in 1946, 4 were free of evidence of tumor 5 years later.[165] Since many cases show a reactivation of the tumor after being asymptomatic for variable periods, it has been postulated that some extragenital source of androgen is present and Huggins and Bergenstal carried out bilateral adrenalectomy in seven patients in 1951.[166] Results are not as beneficial as in breast carcinoma, and this procedure[167] and hypophysectomy require a more extensive trial before interpretations are possible.

Carcinoma of the breast is another form of human hormone dependent tumor. Treatment aimed at changing the hormonal environment in which the cells grow is indicated in patients with inoperable, generalized disease, and is therefore palliative in nature.[168] Ovariectomy and androgens, primarily testosterone propionate, have been tried in women in the premenopausal and menopausal age, sometimes combined with radiotherapy. Beneficial effects appear in only 10 to 15 per cent of the cases, usually as disappearance of bone pain due to metastasis, but subjective improvement occurs in 50 per cent of the patients.[169] Estrogens are also used, especially in older, postmenopausal women in whom the lesions are not amenable to radiotherapy;[170] orchiectomy and estrogens also alleviate many male patients with disseminated mammary cancer.[171] Bilateral adrenalectomy is performed in some women whose cancer escapes partial hormonal control, and approximately 50 per cent of such patients show beneficial effects, while in 20 per cent the relief is gratifying and may be maintained for more than 3 years.[172] Hypophysectomy is also indicated in selected patients with metastatic carcinoma of the breast; one of the largest series is that of Pearson and Ray,[173] who operated on 343 patients and obtained remissions of more than 6 months in 33 per cent. A previous favorable response to oophorectomy in the premenopausal patient is the most reliable index for predicting satisfactory results of hypophysectomy.

4. Environmental Factors in Human Tumors. Table 19 modified from Hueper's

Table 19. Environmental Carcinogenic Agents and Sites of Cancer

CLASSIFICATION	CARCINOGENIC AGENT	TYPE OF CONTACT	SITE OF CANCER
Organic chemicals, aromatic	Benzol	Cutaneous, respiratory	Leukemia, lymphosarcoma, myeloma (?)
	Aromatic amines, beta-naphthylamine, benzidine, 4-aminodiphenyl	Cutaneous, respiratory	Carcinoma of bladder, ureter, renal pelvis
	Coal tar, pitch, asphalt, soot, bitumen, creosote oil, anthracene oil (3,4-benzyprene)	Cutaneous Respiratory (fumes)	Carcinoma of skin Carcinoma of lung
	Shale oil, lubricating oils, crude paraffin oils	Cutaneous	Carcinoma of skin
	Lignite oils, lubricating oils, crude paraffin oils, tar oils	Cutaneous	Carcinoma of skin
	Petroleums and petroleum products, lubricating oils, crude paraffin oils, fuel oils, commercial soots	Cutaneous Respiratory (mist-dust)	Carcinoma of skin Carcinoma of lung
Organic chemicals, aliphatic	Isopropyl oil Mustard gas	Respiratory Respiratory	Carcinoma of nasal sinuses and lung Carcinoma of lung and larynx (?)
Inorganic chemicals	Arsenicals, inorganic and organic	Cutaneous Alimentary	Carcinoma of skin Cancer of liver
	(?)	Respiratory	Carcinoma of lung, alimentary tract (?), bladder (?)
	Chromates	Respiratory	Carcinoma of lung
	Nickel	Respiratory	Carcinoma of nasal sinuses and lung
	Asbestos	Respiratory	Carcinoma of lung
Physical agents	Ionizing radiation of electromagnetic (gamma) and corpuscular types (alpha, beta) from radioactive chemicals	Cutaneous Respiratory Alimentary general body, parental	Carcinoma and sarcoma of skin Carcinoma of lung, nasal sinuses Sarcoma of bones, leukemia, lymphosarcoma, sarcoma of liver (?)
	Ionizing radiation from x-ray tubes	Cutaneous General body, cutaneous	Carcinoma of skin, sarcoma of connective tissues and bones, leukemia, lymphosarcoma
	Ultraviolet radiation, solar radiation	Cutaneous	Carcinoma of skin
		PRECANCEROUS AND PERICANCEROUS CONDITIONS	
Dietary imbalances	Iodine deficiency	Adenomatous goiter	Carcinoma of thyroid
	Vitamin B complex deficiency (?)	Plummer-Vinson syndrome	Carcinoma of nasopharynx
	Vitamin B complex-protein deficiency (?)	Cirrhosis of liver	Carcinoma of liver

CLASSIFICATION	CARCINOGENIC AGENT	PRECANCEROUS CONDITIONS	SITE OF CANCER
Parasitic infections	Schistosoma haematobium	Chronic cystitis	Carcinoma of bladder
	Schistosoma mansoni (?)	Chronic colitis and proctitis	Carcinoma of colon and rectum (?)
	Clonorchis sinensis (?)	Cirrhosis of liver	Carcinoma of liver (?)
Indeterminate	Kangri, kairo, kang (Thermic carbonization of tissue and soot) (?)	Burn ulcers, scars, thermic dermatitis	Carcinoma of skin
	Khaini quid (tobacco-lime)	Chronic gingivitis	Carcinoma of mucosa of lower lip and gum
	Betel quid (areca nut, tobacco, lime, buyo leaf)	Chronic inflammation of oral mucosa	Carcinoma of oral mucosa, gum, cheek, tongue
	Dhoti (loin cloth) (soot ?)	Chronic dermatitis	Carcinoma of skin
	Tobacco extractives ?	Chronic inflammation of oral and/or bronchial mucosa	Carcinoma of oral cavity (?) Carcinoma of lung (?)
	Tobacco combustion products (tar) and thermic burns (chutta)		

(From Hueper[175])

work[174, 175] summarizes the environmental factors definitively established as responsible for some forms of tumor in man. The mechanism of action of these different carcinogens suggests that tumors develop in areas where exposure to the agent is more intense and/or more prolonged. On this basis it is possible to consider the resulting tumors in the five following groups: (1) Tumors developing in sites of primary contact, as skin cancers due to ionizing radiation or sunlight, arsenic, etc.; also, pulmonary tumors caused by asbestosis and other forms of inhalations. (2) Tumors appearing in sites of selective deposition, such as osteogenic sarcomas resulting from the ingestion of radioactive material or thyroid carcinomas produced by radioactive iodine. (3) Tumors in organs with special (functional or toxic) affinity for the carcinogen, as carcinoma of the liver appearing after ingestion of aminofluorene compounds, "butter yellow," thiourea or selenium, and uterine carcinoma caused by prolonged administration of estrogens. (4) Tumors in organs excreting the carcinogen, as carcinoma of the bladder induced by β-naphthylamine. (5) Tumors resulting from dietetic deficiencies, for example carcinoma of the oral mucosa and upper esophagus in Plummer-Vinson's syndrome.

D. THEORIES ON THE "CAUSE" OF CANCER

"Not long ago, in the dark ages of medicine, one could think nearly anything about disease because one knew almost nothing. Theoretical system succeeded system, from humours to homeopathy. Opinions strongly held appeared like realities and were acted upon as such. Now all this is at an end: for most diseases fact has killed fancy. Not as concerns tumors though. Knowledge of these is still so fragmentary that the mind can play at will, devising explanations as in the bad old days: the tumor problem is the last stronghold of metaphysics in medicine."[176] Volumes could be written on the different theories postulated to explain the "cause" of cancer but few occupations would be more useless since the vast majority are based on hypotheses and not on facts. Furthermore, cause and pathogenesis should not be confused as it often has been; for instance, Cohnheim's theory of "embryonal rests," small hypothetical groups of undifferentiated cells persisting in the organism and awaiting the stimulus to grow. In this theory the stimulus is missing, and even if objective demonstration of sufficient "embryonal rests" were available (which it is not) the problem of causation would still be the same, since Cohnheim's hypothesis refers to pathogenesis. Similar remarks are valid for Virchow's chronic irritation theory and for many others. In recent years, however, evidence has accumulated behind two general theories of the "cause" of cancer, and the nature of the intimate change in the biology of the normal cell that makes it neoplastic has been the subject of refreshing speculations.

1. Virus Theory of Cancer. That *some* forms of tumors are caused by viruses is no longer a theory, but an established scientific fact.[177] The virus *theory* of cancer may be considered, therefore, as aspiring to explain most or all types of tumors as induced by viruses. The suggestion, first made by Borrel in 1907, was strongly backed by Ellerman and Bang's demonstration of a filterable agent in avian leukosis, Rous' discovery of the sarcoma bearing his name in chickens and Shope's discovery of viruses as causal agents of tumors in mammals. One of the most decided and imaginative partisans of this theory, Duran-Reynals,[178] has reasoned that the causal agent of cancer should show the following properties: (1) since cancer is characterized by the indefinite growth of cells, the cause must need these cells for survival and must be able to multiply within them; (2) in view of the fact that cancer develops after varied stimuli to appropriate areas, the cause should have some degree of specificity; (3) since cancer frequently appears in selected tissues, but may involve many others, the cause should be highly tissue specific, but should also have an almost infinite capacity for variation; (4) since cancer is more frequent in middle-aged and old people, the cause should remain latent in tissue throughout almost all the life of the subject and find adequate living conditions in cells modified by age. All these features are present in viruses. Furthermore, although in many tumors intentional search for viruses has given negative results, it is not valid to conclude that they are absent; the alternative hypothesis is known as "masking," where viruses assume a state in which they cannot be revealed as free infectious entities, although they can be shown in some cases by indirect serologic methods and other means.[179] In spite of some objections, Bryan, *et al.*[180] concluded that, "The general assumption by investigators in the field of cancer research that the absence of demonstrable virus in tumor-tissue extracts is justification for considering the tumors of 'nonviral' origin, is shown to be invalid." Demonstration of such viruses is hampered, however, because even if they existed as "masked" particles in human tumors, and antibodies were present in sera, detection of such antibodies would not be possible because the nature of the free virus is not known.[181]

Tumor viruses do not differ essentially from ordinary viruses in most of their properties;[182] they, however, induce indefinite multiplication in cells, while ordinary viruses destroy cells. The reasons for this difference are not known, but Rubin has shown that the Rous virus multiplies very slowly in the chick embryo, when compared with other ordinary, necrotizing viruses;[183] Duran-Reynals suggests that slow virus reduplication fails to kill the cell and only liberates it from its normal controlling mechanisms.[181] Another problem is the relation of viruses to known causal agents of tumors, such as chemical carcinogens or ionizing radiation. It has been shown that such agents are capable of inducing the appearance of phages when applied to certain lysogenic bacteria,[184] and the same mechanism could operate in cells, although this extrapolation is very distant in the zoologic scale. Extensive work by Peacock failed to transmit chemically induced tumors by means of cell-free ultrafiltrates, which would be in support of such an idea,[185] but positive results have been reported by McIntosh and Selbie.[186] Another line of evidence, however, has been published by Andrewes,[187] and Foulds and Dmochowski,[188] who found that neutralizing antibodies against sarcoma or leukoses virus develop in pheasants and chickens bearing transplants of chemically induced tumors, and in rabbits immunized against extracts of such tumors. X-irradiation of mice with a low incidence of leukemia has induced leukemia, which could then be transmitted by cell-free extracts to other animals of the same strain. In his discussion of viruses versus mutation as the cause of cancer, Duran-Reynals points out that, ". . . there is no evidence whatsoever that carcinogenesis has ever been observed in the proved absence of viruses."[181] It can be concluded, then, that the virus theory of cancer is the only one with objective facts in its favor, namely, the demonstration that *some* tumors are caused by viruses; how many, is the present and most important problem.

As propounded by Duran-Reynals, Oberling and Guérin[189] and others,[190] the viral theory of cancer places the virus in a continuing and permanent role, inducing a cellular change that might be characterized as extreme hyperplasia. Another view would be that viruses are only biologic carcinogens, capable of activating neoplastic potentialities already existing in cells, in much the same way as other types of carcinogenic agents such as ultraviolet and ionizing radiation, and chemical carcinogens.[191] In this case, the virus would initiate tumor growth and its continuous presence would not be necessary. A third view of the role of viruses in neoplasia would envisage integration of viral nucleic acid with the nucleic acids of the cellular chromosomes and simultaneous replication thereafter, along with the normal genes during subsequent cell divisions.[192] This hypothesis would account for the inherited factor associated with the development of spontaneous tumors in certain inbred laboratory animals such as pulmonary adenoma in mice, but not for extrachromosomal factors as the one responsible for mammary carcinoma in inbred strains of mice (Bittner's "milk factor").

2. Somatic Mutation Theory of Cancer. In 1912, Boveri[193] published the first suggestion of the somatic mutation theory of cancer in his book entitled "The Origin of Malignant Tumors"; according to this author, different types of stimuli can induce abnormal distribution of chromatin material in daughter cells, some of which could continue to show excessive cell proliferation of the type encountered in tumors. It was suggested that the essence of the neoplastic state was a certain abnormal chromatin complex, irrespective of its origin; among the possible etiologic agents mentioned were intracellular parasites, external influences and diseased chromosomes. Such diseased chromosomes would arise from mutation of genes, either spontaneous or due to the influence of mutagenic agents. This theory

was supported by Boycott,[194] Lockhart-Mummery[195] and others, on the basis of the following observations: (a) Single gene mutation is an established fact in both plants and animals, as is also gene-block mutation. Since genes control enzymatic reactions and, through them, normal development and cellular function, mutations might occur in a gene or gene-block controlling the level of mitotic activity, the result being neoplastic growth. (b) Carcinogens often are mutagens in moulds and bacteria, and there are data favoring the same role in mice. Ionizing and ultraviolet radiations are both carcinogens and mutagens,[196] and Muller has attributed the carcinogenic effect of radiation to its property of producing gene mutations.[197] (c) Tumors in *Drosophila* depend on one or several specific genes; a malignant neoplasm reported by Shatoury[198] is determined by a lethal gene located in the sex chromosome. This tumor kills the larvae before pupation.

The long latent period between carcinogenic stimulus and the appearance of cancer is a serious objection to the somatic mutation theory, since it would be expected that neoplastic growth should appear immediately after mutation. In addition, Blum[199] has shown that the rate of proliferation of tumor cells is progressively accelerated by successive doses of ultraviolet radiation. These objections have been met with the alternate hypothesis of multiple mutations, based on the age incidence of cancer; Nordling,[200] and others, have suggested that six to seven mutations are necessary before cancer appears as a clinical entity. A variation of the somatic mutation theory was presented by Darlington in 1944, called the plasmagene theory of cancer.[201] Plasmagenes are assumed cytoplasmic particles composed of ribonucleic acid and playing an important role in protoplasmic heredity, demonstrable only through mutations; some examples are known in yeast, *Drosophila* and other organisms. Darlington suggested that a plasmagene can mutate into a "cancer agent" which may or may not have complete autonomy like a true virus; the main difference between plasmagenes and viruses is their mode of transmission, since plasmagenes are transmitted by cytoplasmic heredity while the virus is transmitted by infection.[202] It should be clear by now that the somatic mutation theory of cancer is not referring to the cause of the change but to the mechanism by which cells become neoplastic; if mutations are "spontaneous," then the cause remains unknown, and if mutations are caused by chemical carcinogens, ionizing radiation, viruses, and all the other factors mentioned, then these are the "causes" of cancer.

Warburg's important finding that cancer cells have a decreased oxidative and an increased anaerobic metabolism when compared to normal cells[203] has been construed by this author as the underlying cause of cancer, while others consider it simply as an accompaniment of neoplastic transformation. Warburg believes that mitochondria, the seat of oxidative metabolism, are self-replicating elements which carry on an extranuclear hereditary transmission of the respiratory enzymes; therefore, mitochondria may also undergo mutation or irreversible damage, which would be perpetuated in descendant cells. The stimulus for anaerobic metabolism is considered to be "the energy deficiency under which the cells operate after destruction of their respiration, which forces the cells to replace the irretrievably lost respiration energy in some way."[204] This is similar to the plasmagene theory of Darlington mentioned above, with the addition that altered mitochondria are considered the continuing causative agents of cancer. Another speculation of the biochemical mechanism by which normal cells become neoplastic postulates that a deletion of certain protein constituents deprives cells of their capacity to obey restraining and controlling influences of the organism as a whole. Some support to this idea has been lent by Miller and Miller's observation that carcinogenic aminoazo dyes form firm complexes with normally occurring proteins of the liver, but that no similar binding takes place in the hepatic neoplasms produced by these dyes.[205] Other carcinogens acting on different tissues have been shown to behave in a similar way. Potter[206] suggests that loss of cellular enzymatic proteins is due to deletion of nucleic acid templates. Once phrased like this, the deletion hypothesis is compatible with the somatic mutation theory and even with the viral theory, since the same metabolic end-result could be achieved through the competitive superiority of viruses in supplying their own "templates" for enzyme synthesis, to the exclusion of normal, but nonparticipating cellular templates.[207]

Finally, Greene's immunologic theory of carcinogenesis[208] should be mentioned briefly. After observing that polycyclic hydrocarbons inhibited transplantable tumors and that this effect was abolished by cortisone, Greene postulated that normal cells are endowed with certain specific antigens known as "self-markers" and that these antigens are recognized by the normal growth-regulating mechanism. The effect of carcinogens would be to combine with the self-marker, the resulting complex being self-replicating.[209] The new complex would then excite the formation of antibody, which upon combining with the carcinogen self-marker antigen would eliminate it, producing a new race of cells lacking in some degree their tissue-specific pattern; these cells would not be recognized by the growth-regulating mechanisms and, therefore, would be free to proliferate indefinitely, giving rise to a tumor. Within the general context of his clonal selection theory of acquired immunity Burnet[210] is in favor of a somatic mutation as the first event in the production of cancer; according to this author: "Somatic mutation results in a change by which a cell and its descendants are released from one or more of the controls that maintained its type in normal spatial and numerical relation with the rest of the body."

Many other theories on the cause of cancer could be mentioned. There is no doubt that time and knowledge have changed the rather simple outlook on the etiology of cancer that characterized the first experimentalists; they were primarily interested in finding a specific chemical substance as the cause of neoplastic growth. "Instead of asking what chemical turns a normal cell into a cancer cell, much better questions are being formulated. What are the factors which in complex organisms transcend the cell, to unify and control a mass of protoplasm into orderly development and maintenance of a whole? What intracellular mechanisms of synthesis are chiefly concerned with growth and differentiation? In what ways do the interplay between these two, without which there is no life, become disturbed, so that tissue malformation occurs? What inherent mechanisms allow tissues once involved in this process to progress further and further away from dependence on normal organismic controls towards independent expression of their modified potentialities to form a new whole? To such questions as these we have a right to expect complicated but detailed answers in terms of organization and its disturbance; to the question 'What is the cause of cancer?' we have no right to expect any civil answer at all."[211]

IV. ANATOMY, PHYSIOLOGY AND BIOCHEMISTRY OF TUMORS

The search for differences between normal and neoplastic cells has been conducted at three different levels of organization: anatomic, physiologic and biochemical. There is a massive amount of data accumulated on each of these aspects, and extensive reviews can be found in the volumes by Cowdry[4] and Mellors.[6] Some of the differences between healthy and tumor cells are summarized in this section, but it is convenient to emphasize at the outset that none of the features studied, be they morphologic,

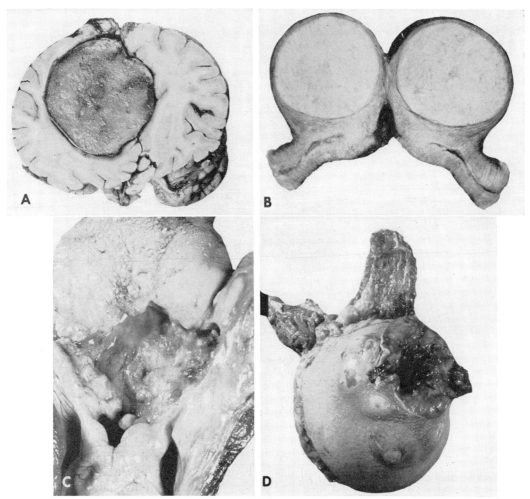

Fig. 5–24. The three main gross aspects of tumors. *A* and *B,* A tumor mass, represented by meningioma and uterine fibroleiomyoma. *C,* Ulcerating carcinoma of the base of the tongue. *D,* Ulcerated mass, a fungating carcinoma of the breast.

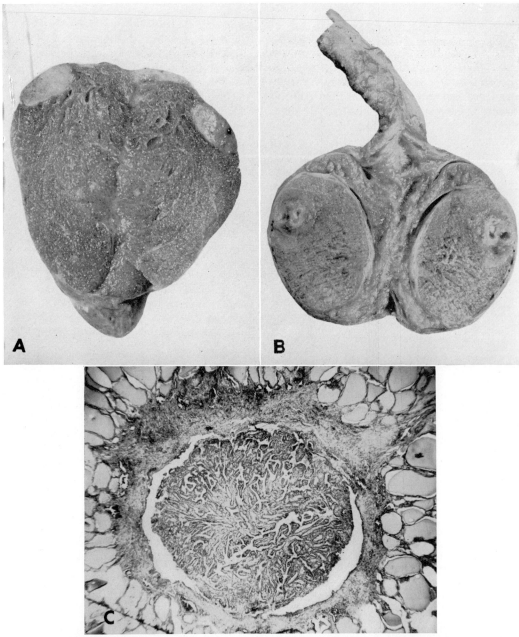

FIG. 5–25. Occult carcinomas. *A,* Small carcinoma of the thyroid, which became manifest by diffuse, bilateral pulmonary metastases. *B,* Seminoma of the testis, which was unsuspected until autopsy. *C,* Papillary carcinoma of the thyroid.

functional or chemical, establish a qualitative separation between normal and neoplastic elements. The only fundamental difference lies in the irreversible and unlimited capacity of tumor cells to proliferate, and even this is more conceptual than factual, since explanted normal cells preserved in tissue culture can multiply for long or indefinite periods. Dedifferentiation, if it truly exists as such, is the normal status of embryonal cells; invasiveness is depicted by the trophoblast in normal pregnancy; homologous and heterologous transplantation can be accomplished with embryonal tissues, etc. No single, isolated property distinguishes normal from neoplastic cells, but

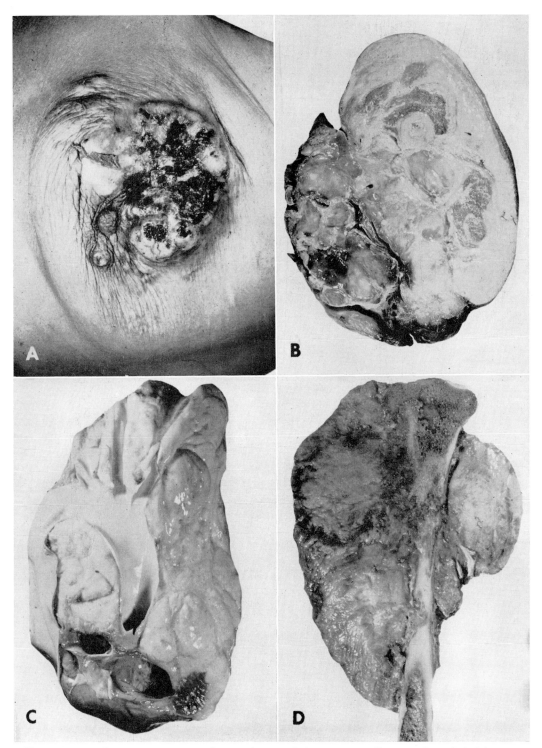

FIG. 5–26.   Large tumors. *A*, Fungating carcinoma of the breast. *B*, Cross section of rhabdomyosarcoma of thigh. *C*, Malignant thymoma with extensive involvement of the heart and great vessels. *D*, Osteogenic sarcoma of tibia.

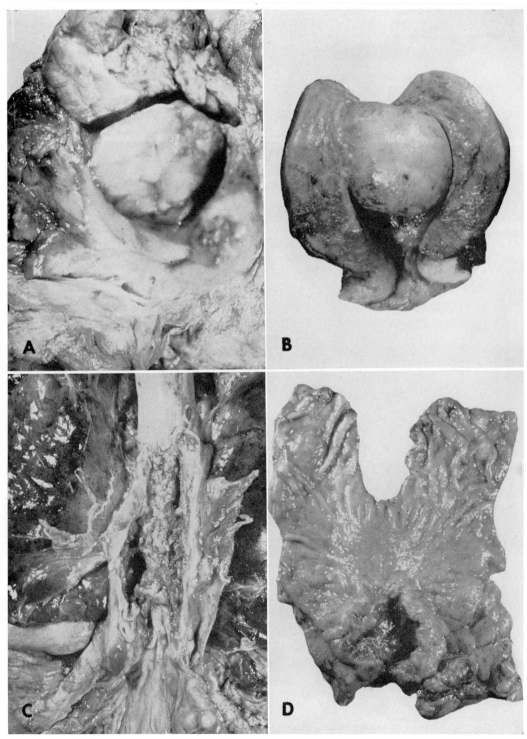

FIG. 5–27. The shape of tumors. *A*, Fibroadenoma of breast. *B*, Fibroleiomyoma of uterus. *C*, Ulcerated carcinoma of esophagus. *D*, Ulcerated leiomyoma of stomach.

rather the high frequency with which the latter exhibit a group of features. In other words, *neoplasia is a form of abnormal cellular behavior,* the result of many properties manifested by anatomic, functional and biochemical changes in tissues.

A. ANATOMY OF TUMORS

The morphology of tumors may be studied with the unaided eye or by microscopic and ultramicroscopic techniques. A thorough familiarity with the gross aspect of neoplasms is extremely important for clinical diagnosis, since in many cases the tumor mass is the reason for consultation and in many others physical examination, endoscopic procedures, radiologic studies and/or surgical explorations will reveal different aspects of the pathologic anatomy of cancer. The single, most representative gross feature of tumors is their variability; yet, within their protean morphology certain patterns are discernible, often for specific neoplasms, and they must be learned for each tumor. The microscopic structure of tumors is the basis of the best diagnostic method available, and the details belong to more specialized works; some generalizations, however, may serve to round off the biologic concept of cancer, which is the aim of this presentation.

1. Macroscopic Anatomy of Tumors. Grossly, tumors may appear in three general forms: (a) a mass, which corresponds to the usual connotation of the word "tumor," (b) an ulcer or loss of tissue and (c) a combination of the preceding two forms, or an ulcerated mass (Fig. 5–24). Benign tumors usually manifest themselves in the first form, i.e., as tissue masses, while malignant tumors may show destruction and ulceration. Exceptions to this statement are legion, but it can be said that a tumor showing loss of tissue is malignant (or should be considered as such) until proved otherwise; on the other hand, absence of necrosis is no guarantee of benign behavior.

The size of tumors varies from microscopic to very large, sometimes monstrous masses; in general, size is no indication of prognosis since very small carcinomas may metastasize widely, as observed in carcinomas of the thyroid, breast, lung, prostate and many others ("occult" carcinomas)

which become clinically manifest by their metastases (Fig. 5–25). Tumors may be so small that a biopsy can include the entire lesion, as has occurred in some carcinomas *in situ* of the uterine cervix.[212] On the other hand, some tumors may reach enormous dimensions, as the fibroleiomyoma reported by Novak and Novak[213] which weighed 360 pounds. Sarcomas, especially retroperitoneal or of the extremities, may reach large sizes in terminal states[214] (Fig. 5–26). Loss of tissue may also be extensive, and this is seen more often in basal cell carcinomas of the skin, usually the face.

The shapes of tumors vary according to the type of growth. If it is eccentric and there is compression of surrounding tissues, the neoplastic mass tends to be spherical, as uterine fibroleiomyoma or fibroadenoma of the breast. When growth is infiltrative the tumor appears as an irregular, indurated area without definite margins, as carcinoma of the stomach or rhabdomyosarcoma. With rapid growth there is necrosis and ulceration, so the tumor appears as an irregular loss of tissue with indurated margins, as in epidermoid carcinoma of the lower lip. Necrosis, however, is not exclusive of malignant tumors; some neoplasms, considered benign on all other counts, may undergo ischemic or hemorrhagic necrosis, as leiomyoma of the stomach or chromophobe adenoma of the pituitary (Fig. 5–27).

Great variations are also observed on the surfaces of tumors, which may be smooth, uniform or nodular in encapsulated neoplasms, as uterine fibroleiomyoma; finely granular in papillary tumors, as carcinoma of the ovary or of the thyroid; umbilicated in rapidly growing metastatic tumors; fungating in ulcerated, infected and necrotic neoplasms as carcinoma of the breast or of the uterus (Fig. 5–28). Color may sometimes serve to suggest the diagnosis and it was part of the reason for the establishment of classic names such as cancer and sarcoma: cancer was the term used for tumors resembling the whitish color of crab meat, while sarcomas were red and fleshy, simulating striated muscle.[215] Some tumors have characteristic color, such as bile-producing liver carcinomas, which are green; melanomas and some deeply pigmented basal cell carcinomas, which are dark brown or black;

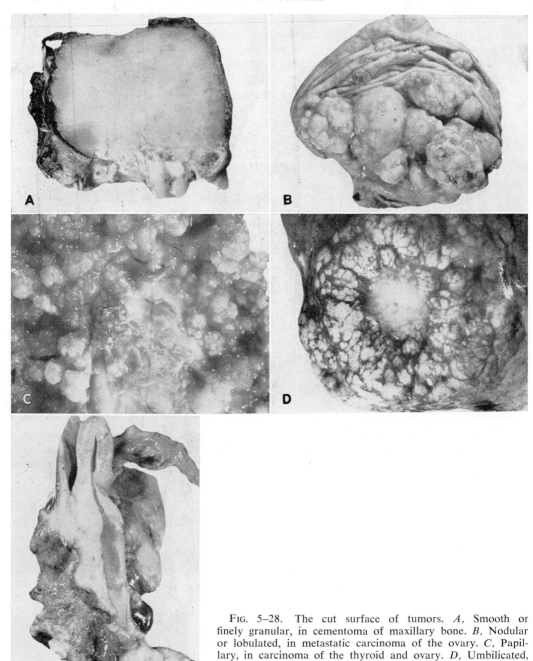

FIG. 5–28. The cut surface of tumors. *A,* Smooth or finely granular, in cementoma of maxillary bone. *B,* Nodular or lobulated, in metastatic carcinoma of the ovary. *C,* Papillary, in carcinoma of the thyroid and ovary. *D,* Umbilicated, in metastatic bronchogenic carcinoma in liver. *E,* Fungating and ulcerated, in carcinoma of the uterine cervix.

or carcinomas of the kidney, whose intense yellow color is caused by fatty infiltration, etc. Hemorrhage, necrosis and fibrosis may give the cut surface of tumors a variegated appearance, to which cyst formation, calcification and infection also contribute (Fig. 5–29). Pulsation, although rarely observed, is sufficiently characteristic of some tumors

such as metastatic carcinoma of thyroid, kidney or liver, as to be suggestive of the diagnosis; murmurs may be perceived on auscultation.

Complete encapsulation is very important as revealing failure to infiltrate, but it should not be confused with clear limitation without true deposit of connective tissue, which is frequently seen in metastatic tumors of the lung or liver, nor with the apparently good macroscopic limitation of some sarcomas, especially fibrosarcoma, which dissolves under the microscope.

2. Microscopic Anatomy of Tumors. In the same manner as the gross aspect, the microscopic structure of tumors is characterized by variability; with all due exceptions, however, tumors are tissues and show a similar pattern of organization in parenchyma and stroma, the latter containing blood and lymph vessels, nerves and all the other components of connective tissue. It is customary to consider the tumor cells as parenchymatous, regardless of their epithelial or mesenchymatous origin; thus, in carcinoma of the liver the parenchyma is formed by hepatic cells or intrahepatic biliary duct cells, which proliferate indefinitely, while in liposarcoma undifferentiated lipoblastic cells are viewed as parenchymatous. On the other hand, the stroma is always composed of connective tissue, which may be very abundant, as in scirrhous carcinoma

of the breast or stomach, or extremely scarce, as in Ewing's tumor or medulloblastoma. It is usually accepted that metastatic nodules arise by distant seeding of parenchymatous tumor cells which induce formation of stroma in their new habitat. Reactive proliferation of connective tissue is known as "desmoplastic."

Tumor cells may be morphologically indistinguishable from their normal counterparts; furthermore, they may reproduce the structure of the parent tissue so faithfully as to defy anatomic differentiation, which is then based exclusively on behavior. It has been remarked before that in most cases the potentialities of cells can be predicted from their morphology, but that some exceptions exist in this correlation. In the presence of "benign" structure with "malignant" behavior or vice versa, it is nonsense to grant superiority to the microscopic picture by means of semantic chimeras as "metastasizing adenoma." Tumors are inclined to ignore verbalistic controversies and, clad in their "benign" disguise, will relent-

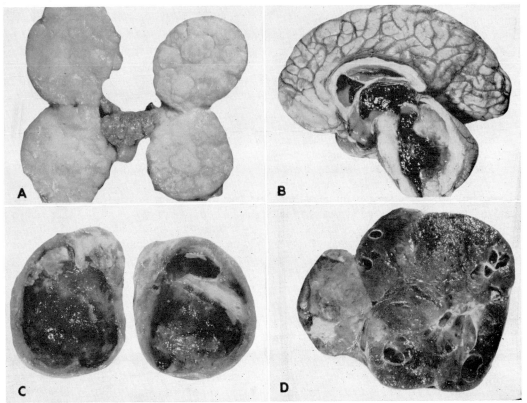

FIG. 5–29. Degenerative phenomena in tumors. *A,* Extensive necrosis in malignant lymphoma. *B,* Hemorrhage in cerebellar glioma. *C,* Hemorrhage and cyst formation in parathyroid adenoma. *D,* Cyst formation in struma ovarii.

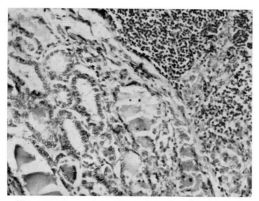

FIG. 5–30. Well differentiated, metastatic follicular carcinoma of the thyroid in cervical lymph node. (Courtesy of Dr. Edmundo Rojas.)

lessly continue to grow and metastasize until the end of the patient's (and their own) life. "Intrinsic," "histologic," and "cytologic" malignancy have meaning only as far as they correspond to the actual behavior of tumors and are not, as such designations imply, separate and unrelated concepts. An instance of this confusion is the so-called "lateral aberrant thyroid" or "metastasizing adenoma of the thyroid," which is nothing but a well differentiated, follicular carcinoma of this organ;[216] in this case one or more lymph nodes of the jugular group are found partially or totally replaced by what appears to be normal thyroid tissue (Fig. 5–30). Ignorance of embryology lies behind the designation of "lateral aberrant thyroid," since it is well known that the thyroid develops in the midline and always within the confines of the deep cervical fascia, while the lymph nodes lie outside this structure.[217] Unrealistic veneration of morphology leads to violation of the term "adenoma" in the second designation mentioned, when by definition it indicates a benign (and therefore a nonmetastasizing) growth.

On the other hand, tumor cells may partially or completely depart from the normal structure of cells or tissues and become organized as more or less uniform masses which make it very difficult to recognize their origin. When a tumor reproduces the histologic structure of the parent tissue it is known as "well differentiated," while progressive degrees of departure from this structure are referred to as "poor differentiation" or "undifferentiation." A change in

histologic pattern has also been mentioned as metaplasia, as in adenoacanthoma of the endometrium or mucoepidermoid carcinoma in salivary glands; similar metaplastic transformations occur in sarcomas, as in liposarcoma with spindle-celled, fibrosarcomatous elements. Variability in histologic structure is important because it points out the need of examining different areas of the same tumor before rendering a diagnosis as to site of origin, and also because it represents one of the main objections to histologic grading as a method for determining prognosis (see below) (Fig. 5–31). As a rule, metastatic nodules preserve the same degree of differentiation as the primary tumor, so when the latter is well differentiated it is possible to establish the site of origin from the microscopic study of the metastasis; this, however, is not always so. Instances are occasionally observed where the structure is better preserved in the metastatic nodule or vice versa.

In considering the structure of the isolated malignant cell it must be emphasized again that no qualitative differences exist with the normal o rnonneoplastic cell and that no morphologic change, regardless of how bizarre or extreme it may be, that is found in tumor cells may not be encountered also in nonneoplastic elements. It is the combination of several structural features that permits one to distinguish between them, and this distinction has increased in significance since the advent of exfoliative cytology in the diagnosis of tumors.

In general, a tumor cell has irregular shape and abnormal size; the shape may sometimes be characteristic, as tadpole cells in rhabdomyosarcoma, and the size may be enormous, as with giant cells in glioblastoma multiforme. The amount of cytoplasm is variable but the significant change seems to be a loss of the cytoplasmic/nuclear ratio, which may be caused by decrease in size of cytoplasm, increase of nucleus or a combination of both factors. The cytoplasm may contain fat, glycogen, pigment granules and many other inclusions, which are sometimes characteristic, as with the physaliphorous cell of chordoma or with melanoma. At other times functional differentiation may be structurally apparent, as with crossed striations in rhabdomyosarcoma or fibrog-

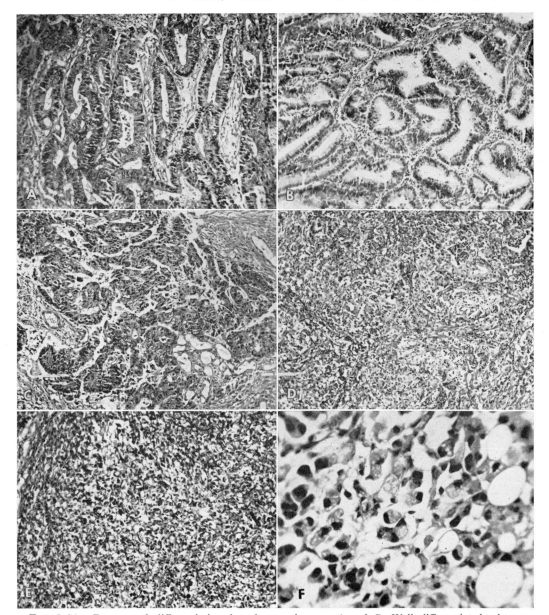

FIG. 5–31. Degrees of differentiation in adenocarcinoma. *A* and *B,* Well differentiated adenocarcinoma. *C* and *D,* Poorly differentiated adenocarcinoma. *E* and *F,* Undifferentiated or anaplastic adenocarcinoma, showing small cells with vacuolated, foamy cytoplasm.

lia fibrils in fibrosarcoma. But the most suggestive changes in morphology reside in the nucleus, where modifications of size, shape, density and distribution of chromatin are the rule in malignant neoplasms; the nucleolus is frequently prominent and shows atypical staining. Mitotic figures may be numerous, and this is so constantly seen in malignant tumors that it serves as a rough appreciation of the speed of growth; they

may also be abnormal, sometimes giving rise to almost incredible figures with several spindles or many more chromosomes than normal (Fig. 5–32). A description of all or the most frequent variations in cytologic structure of tumors is out of place here; the preceding brief and incomplete enumeration should suffice to emphasize two major points: (a) the more malignant the tumor, the less "differentiated" will be its structure,

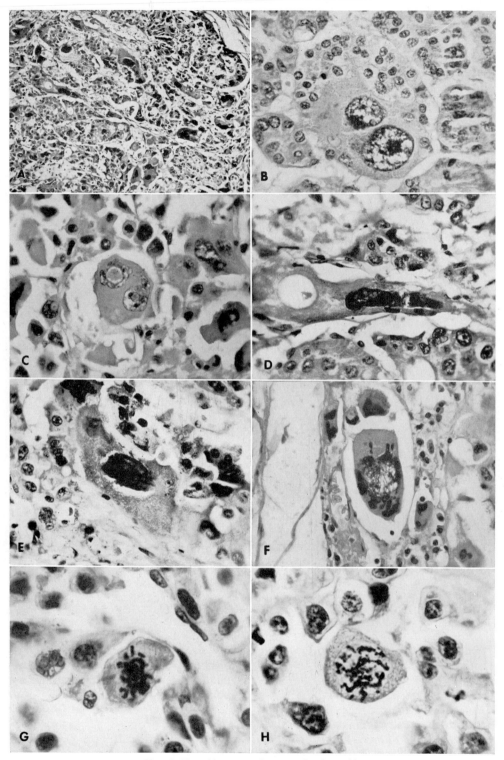

FIG. 5–32. (*See opposite page for legend.*)

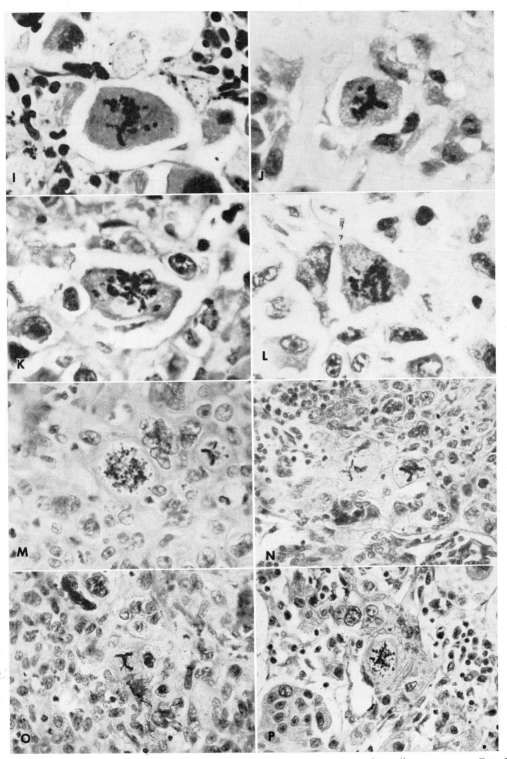

Fig. 5–32. Atypical cells in malignant tumors, *A* to *F*. Abnormal mitoses in malignant tumors, *G* to *P*.

Table 20.   Some Functional Tumors of Endocrine Glands

ORGAN	TUMOR	SECRETION	EFFECT
Pituitary gland	Acidophilic adenoma	Growth hormone	Acromegaly
Parathyroid	Adenoma or carcinoma	Parathormone	Hyperparathyroidism
Thyroid	Adenoma or carcinoma	Thyroid hormone	Hyperthyroidism
Islands of Langerhans	Adenoma or carcinoma	Insulin	Hyperinsulinism
Adrenal medulla	Pheochromocytoma	Adrenalin	Hypertension
Adrenal cortex	Adenoma or carcinoma	Corticosteroids	Cushing's syndrome
		Aldosterone	Hyperaldosteronism
Ovary	Arrhenoblastoma		
	Adrenocortical rest	Androgens	Masculinization
	Hilar cell tumor		
	Brenner tumor		
	Thecoma or luteoma	Estrogens	Feminization
	Granulosa cell tumor		
Testes	Interstitial cell tumor	Androgens	Masculinization (precocious puberty)

but there are prominent exceptions to this generalization underlining that behavior may sometimes be unpredictable from morphology; (b) no single structural feature is specific for tumor cells; recognition depends on a group of morphologic changes, more apparent in tissues than in isolated elements.

The stroma or supporting tissue of tumors may be formed by fibrous, osseous, lymphoid, adipose, glial and other structures, depending on the site of neoplastic growth. Fibroblastic stroma is, however, more frequently seen than any other, probably because of nomicoplasia of connective tissue cells. The blood vessels of many tumors have been studied by special techniques, revealing that tumors are often more vascularized than normal tissues, and that their blood is derived mainly from arterial circulation. For instance, primary carcinomas of the lung and liver, as well as metastatic tumors in the latter organ, show abundant proliferation of blood vessels arising from the bronchial arteries and the hepatic artery, respectively.[218, 219]

B. PHYSIOLOGY OF TUMORS

Two different aspects are of interest in the study of tumors from a functional point of view: the physiology of neoplastic cells, and the functional effects of a tumor on the host.

1. Physiology of Neoplastic Cells. Many tumors preserve the function of the parent tissue, sometimes exaggerated, often diminished, rarely distorted and modified in quality, and this is taken as proof of the fact that the neoplastic change is not incompatible with maintenance of highly specialized mechanisms. Indeed, only very anaplastic tumors fail to show any sign of functional activity, which makes the con-

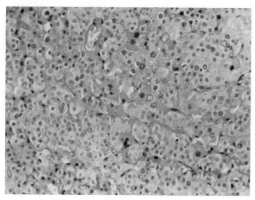

FIG. 5–33.   Microscopic aspect of a parathyroid adenoma.

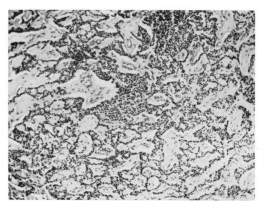

FIG. 5–34.   Adenoma of islands of Langerhans. (Courtesy of Dr. Edmundo Rojas.)

cept of undifferentiation or reversion to embryonic state difficult to accept as such. The best instances of functioning tumors are found in the endocrine glands, and Table 20 presents a list of some of them.

Acidophilic adenoma of the pituitary gland is usually associated with acromegaly, a disease characterized by increase in size of all organs except the brain, persistence of the thymus, gonadal hypofunction, overgrowth of bones and soft tissues of head, hands and feet, fatigue and muscular pains.[220] Furthermore, in half of the cases there are pressure symptoms caused by the adenoma, with visual disturbances and headache. Hyperthyroidism and diabetes mellitus may also be present, the latter being typically resistant to insulin. Acidophilic cells in the pituitary gland secrete growth hormone but the disease is very complex and probably there is participation of other pituitary hormones as well.[221] Some adenomas and carcinomas of the thyroid may be associated with an exaggerated secretion of thyroid hormone and the clinical picture of hyperthyroidism; this is rare, however, with malignant tumors, where it has been estimated to occur in no more than 2 to 4 per cent of them.[222] Of special interest are those rare cases in which the tumor cells preserve their ability to incorporate iodine,[223] a radioactive isotope of which (I^{131}) may be used to diagnose their presence. Parathyroid adenomas give rise to the well known picture of hyperparathyroidism (von Recklinghausen's disease) (Fig. 5–33). Pancreatic island tissue may give rise to adenomas responsible for the clinical picture of hypoglycemic crises associated with hyperinsulinism;[224, 225] most of these tumors are found in the body and tail of the pancreas, measure from 2.0 to 5.5 cm. in diameter, are rarely well encapsulated, but frequently "shell out" and have a reddish, dark color. In 10 to 20 per cent of the cases the tumors are carcinomas, with liver metastasis[226] (Fig. 5–34). Of special interest are some rare, fibroblastic or mesothelial neoplasms associated with hypoglycemia which have been described in recent years.[227] No adequate explanation exists for their hypoglycemic effect although the secretion of an insulin-like substance has been postulated[228] and denied.[229] There are tumors of the adrenal gland with secretions which give rise to clinical symptoms of hyperfunction, such as pheochromocytoma,[230] with paroxysmal or permanent arterial hypertension, and cortical adenomas which produce Cushing's syndrome.[231] Some localized, tumor-like hyperplasias have been described which secrete aldosterone and produce the syndrome of primary hyperaldosteronism characterized by hypertension, hypernatremia, renal loss of potassium and absence of edema,[232] although the latter has been present in some cases.[233]

But perhaps the area where functioning tumors are more characteristic is the gonads, ovaries and testes. In the ovary, tumors with a functional effect on the organism are classified as masculinizing and feminizing.[234] The former are arrhenoblastoma,[235] adrenocortical cell tumor, hilar cell tumor[236] and some rare cases of Brenner tumor;[237] feminizing are the granulosa cell tumor and the thecoma, with or without luteinization.[238, 239] In the testes the interstitial cell tumor will produce hypergonadism or precocious puberty.[240] Furthermore, teratomas are frequent in the ovary and occasionally they may contain functioning tissues such as thyroid or chorionic villi; the latter, whether they are in a teratoma or as part of a molar or normal pregnancy, constitute the parent tissue of one of the most malignant tumors, choriocarcinoma, which is feminizing and is characterized, among other things, by the presence of high titres of chorionic gonadotropin in the urine[241] (Fig. 5–35).

Carcinoid tumors of the intestine or other locations may give rise to a peculiar syndrome, recently described under the name of "carcinoid syndrome," characterized by cyanosis rubra of the face, polycythemia, gastrointestinal disturbances and malformations of the right side of the heart, with elimination of large amounts of 5-hydroxyindolacetic acid and other metabolites of tryptophan in the urine.[242] Carcinoid tumors are derived from enterochromaffin cells and secrete large amounts of serotonin or 5-hydroxytryptamine, the substance which is held responsible for most of the lesions, although experimentally they have not been reproduced either by administration of large amounts of exogenous serotonin[243] or by

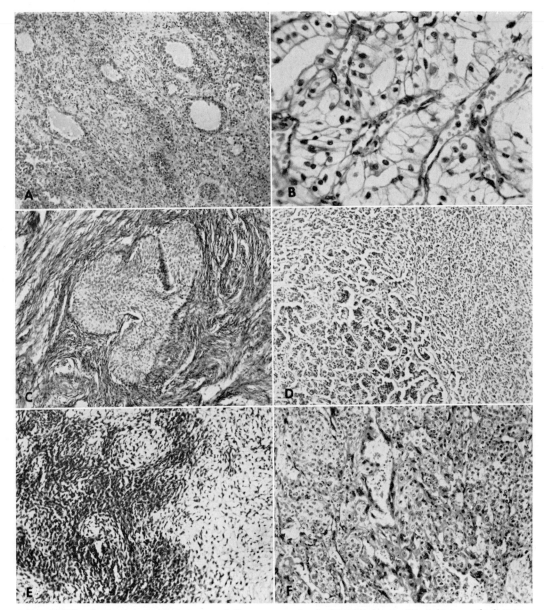

FIG. 5–35. Some functional tumors of the ovary. *A,* Arrhenoblastoma. *B,* Adrenocortical tumor (masculinovoblastoma). *C,* Brenner tumor. *D,* Granulosa cell carcinoma. *E,* Thecoma. *F,* Choriocarcinoma.

transplantation to mice of a mastocytoma which produced large amounts of serotonin.[244]

Endocrine functions are not the only ones preserved by tumor cells. Other specialized activities may still be present in tumors, and may be extremely useful for microscopic diagnosis; indeed, tumor cells are recognized mainly by searching for evidence of what they are doing or trying to do. For instance, fibrosarcomatous cells are usually engaged in laying down reticulum and collagen, and the more differentiated they are the more abundant the intercellular substances will be.[245] In osteogenic sarcoma, malignant osteoblasts are forming bone or osteoid tissue, and in this particular case the definitive microscopic diagnosis depends precisely on this feature since the cells tend to be extremely pleomorphic.[246] In adenocarcinomas arising in mucus-producing glandular epithelium the presence of basophilic and amorphous material within the glandular lumen is a sign of functional activity of the cells, which may be better characterized by certain histologic techniques. But, even in more anaplastic tumors the formation of mucus is preserved and isolated cells may appear as bloated, spheric elements with the nucleus displaced to the periphery and compressed against the cytoplasmic membrane, giving the appearance of a "signet ring." Adenocarcinomas of this type are encountered in almost any organ with mucus-secreting glands but are more frequent in breast, lung, gallbladder, gastrointestinal tract and urinary bladder.[247] Well differentiated epidermoid carcinomas show epithelial whorls with keratin formation; malignant melanomas synthesize melanin; some liver cell carcinomas produce bile, etc. (Fig. 5–36). The instances can be multiplied but they only emphasize the concept that neoplastic cells preserve specialized functions and that the microscopic recognition of this activity is one of the bases for histologic diagnosis; in other cases, however, no signs of functional differentiation are manifested in structure and the diagnosis rests on recognition of morphologic patterns of unknown meaning, as in medulloblastoma of the cerebellum and oatcell carcinoma of the lung.

2. Functional Effects of Tumors on the Host. Many of the symptoms produced by tumors result from three main properties: their location in the organism, their endocrine function and the degenerative phenomena which they undergo.[10] In the vast majority of benign tumors these three features suffice to explain the entire clinical picture. For instance, craniopharyngioma is a developmental neoplasm devoid of endocrine secretion arising in the area of the sella turcica, which produces compression of the pituitary gland, the optic chiasm, the hypothalamus and other neighboring structures. The results are intracranial hypertension, visual disturbances, delayed somatic development, diabetes insipidus and somnolence.[248] A fibroleiomyoma of the uterus will produce menstrual disturbances caused by compression and distortion of the uterine cavity, atrophy and ulceration of the over-lying endometrium, etc. The endocrine function of many neoplasms has been mentioned in the preceding paragraphs and degenerative phenomena are rare in benign, but frequent in malignant, tumors.

Some patients, however, present symptoms and signs that are not so easily explained by the three factors mentioned, so other mechanisms must be at play. Meigs' syndrome is characterized by ascites, right hydrothorax and ovarian tumor; when first described the syndrome was thought to occur only with ovarian fibromas, but ever since it has been observed with many other solid and even cystic tumors of the ovary.[249] All explanations offered so far to account for this peculiar combination of findings are unsatisfactory. Another instance of a benign tumor with unexpected manifestations is hemangioblastoma of the cerebellum, which is sometimes associated with polycythemia; again there is no adequate explanation.[250]

A similar situation exists with regard to malignant tumors, since mechanical, endocrine and degenerative factors account for many, but not all, the clinical manifestations. Weight loss, unexplained fever, localized pain, etc., are frequently the only complaints of patients with deep-seated malignant neoplasms. Willis[10] makes a vigorous defense of the idea that the cachexia of advanced cancer patients is only the result of unspecific factors such as, ". . . starvation, haemorrhage, ulceration, bacterial infection, destruction of functionally vital tissues, pain, sleeplessness and anxiety." It is of interest, however, that patients in which none of these factors have been at play *die* in an almost perfect state of health. Not only death, but also other findings cannot easily be explained as results of unspecific factors. Which one of them would account for the precocious appearance of hypertrophic osteoarthropathy in cases of pleural mesothelioma and some bronchogenic carcinomas?[251] It is also difficult to account for the rapid disappearance of such a complication after removal of the tumor. The suggestion that tumor cells produce large amounts of hyaluronic acid and that this substance is deposited in the neighborhood of bone inducing it and the soft tissues to proliferate, is purely speculative.[252] Another

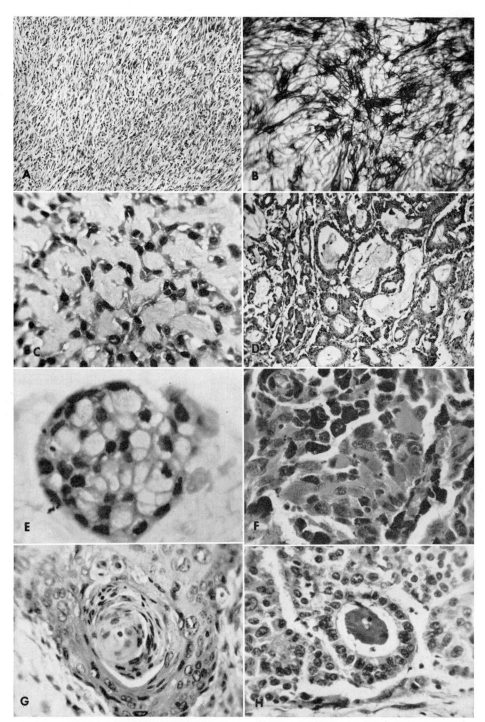

Fig. 5–36. Histophysiology of some malignant tumors. *A*, Fibrosarcoma. *B*, Reticulum-producing cells in fibrosarcoma. *C*, Osteogenic sarcoma, with osteoblasts laying down osteoid tissue. *D*, Mucus-producing adenocarcinoma. *E*, Another adenocarcinoma showing mucus secretion by single cells ("signet-ring" cell carcinoma). *F*, Malignant melanoma with abundant melanin formation. *G*, Keratinization in epidermoid carcinoma. *H*, Bile formation in cholangiocarcinoma.

important problem in cancer patients is anemia, which is present even in hospitalized cases without hemorrhage, ulcerations, infections, etc., and who take all their food. It has been shown that in many of these cases the anemia is hemolytic and that there is a circulating autoantibody which destroys red blood cells.[253] This is not a specific mechanism, but it is present in cancer patients and cannot be ascribed to insomnia and anxiety. Approximately from 1 to 4 per cent of renal carcinomas are associated with polycythemia, which has been shown to disappear with surgical cure of the tumor.[254] Rare cases of Wilms's tumor have been accompanied by arterial hypertension, returning to normal after radiotherapy and recurring with development of pulmonary metastasis.[255] Finally, many patients with malignant tumors are in negative nitrogen balance and in spite of force feeding continue to eliminate more nitrogen than the amount ingested. This is seen in cases without extensive destruction of tissue or disseminated metastatic disease; intermediary metabolism is fundamentally disturbed and the cause is unknown.[256]

This should not be taken as support of the naïve ideas which picture tumors as devouring the food ingested by the patient and the patient itself, or as producing "toxic" substances which mysteriously damage the organism but spare the tumor cells; Willis has discussed these and other mistaken conceptions with forceful arguments. But to deny that neoplasms influence the organism through unknown mechanisms is to negate the existence of the problem; this probably results in peace of mind, but it is doubtful that knowledge about tumors is advanced.

C. BIOCHEMISTRY OF TUMORS

The study of tumors at a biochemical level of organization has been conducted in two general ways. In the first place, pieces of neoplasm have been analyzed to determine their composition and to compare it with normal tissues; in the second place, the metabolism of living neoplastic cells has been compared with that of normal cells. Both types of studies are extremely complicated and the results are difficult to interpret with reference to a general concept of

the nature of neoplasia, not only because of conflicting data but also because no such concept is available. The best introduction to the extensive literature on this subject is Greenstein's "Biochemistry of Cancer," a veritable storehouse of information.[257]

The chemical analysis of a fragment of tissue provides data related to the large mass of examined protoplasm, which includes not only tumor cells, but also stroma, inflammatory elements, etc.; furthermore, tumor cells are not all identical but some may be intermitotic, others are degenerated, dying or dead, near or far from blood vessels, etc., and all these factors are not discriminated in this type of study. In addition, unless the different cellular components are separated, the results of chemical determinations in tumor tissue reveal the presence of a series of substances but provide no information as to their precise location within the cell.[258] Finally, as with the histologic study with which it must always be compared, the biochemical analysis of neoplasms refers to an instant in the life of tumors but tells nothing of the entire process, as dynamic and changing as life itself. To overcome this last difficulty it is convenient to examine the chemical composition of "precancerous" tissue, meaning areas undergoing the neoplastic change but not quite tumoral as yet, spontaneous and induced tumors, metastasis, transplanted and explanted neoplasms. In fact, the introduction of transplanted tumors in the experimental study of neoplasms has provided a precious tool, since in each transplant a purer cellular strain is obtained and the tumor shows a greater degree of autonomy; many of the data summarized below have been obtained from transplanted tumors.

The quantitative analysis of tumor tissue fragments has revealed the following facts: (a) The amino acid composition,[259] the nature of the soluble protein fraction[260] and the enzymatic potentialities[261] are variable in different types of normal tissues; however, when different tumors are compared to each other they are found to be quite similar or, at least, they resemble each other more than their respective tissues of origin. (b) No differences are apparent between the amounts and characteristics of nucleic acids.[262] (c) The calcium, zinc and copper content of the epidermis is considerably decreased after neoplastic transformation.[263] (d) There is a slight fall in the lipid concentration.[264] (e) The water content of neoplastic cells is higher than normal.[265]

The enzymatic pattern of each normal tissue is a distinguishing characteristic which permits their separation as with their histologic structure; both the quality and quantity of enzymes are specific for liver, pancreas, brain, lymphoid tissue, etc. Tumors have not been found to differ qualitatively from normal tissues in their enzymatic pattern; i.e., there is no "cancer enzyme" which appears only in neoplastic cells, nor the systematic deletion of an enzyme or a group of enzymes drawing a line between tumor and normal tissue.[266] Another interesting characteristic is that the enzymatic pattern of tumors bears no relation to age, speed of growth or the animal species in which it is transplanted. This is indicative of the high degree of autonomy of neoplastic cells, which are totally independent of the surrounding environment. The actual variation in the enzymatic pattern of tumor cells when compared to normal elements may be summarized as follows.[267] (a) The range of enzymatic activity and of concentration of different compounds such as vitamins is much narrower in tumors than in normal tissues; i.e., when normal lung is compared with bronchogenic carcinoma the enzymatic activity of the latter is seen to correspond to the average activity of the former while the extremes are never reached, and the same is true for the concentration of vitamins A and B_{12}. (b) The pattern of enzymatic activity of normal tissues is different, but in their tumors the differences tend to disappear; i.e., when normal lung is compared with normal lymph node from a chemical standpoint they show important differences, but between carcinoma of the lung and lymphosarcoma there are almost no variations (the difficulties in establishing the microscopic differentiation between oat-cell carcinoma of the lung and lymphosarcoma are brought to mind). From an enzymatic standpoint, tumors converge to a common type of tissue. (c) As a corollary of the preceding characteristic of tumors, when normal tissues undergo neoplastic transformation many of their specific functions

decrease or are completely lost; i.e., normal liver has a high concentration of arginase, catalase and flavin, but in transplanted hepatoma these enzymes are either decreased or absent. The result of all these changes in the enzymatic pattern of tumors is that the "enzymatic reserve" decreases or is entirely lost, so neoplastic cells seem to be using their catalytic proteins at a maximum.

The conclusion is that, whatever their origin, tumors resemble each other biochemically more than they resemble their tissues of origin and more than these tissues in between, and that neoplastic transformation is accompanied by a metabolic simplification of cells. It is interesting that the greater the autonomy of tumors the lesser their biochemical resemblance to their tissues of origin, and the greater their simplification and their similarity to other tumors. For instance, regenerating liver is very similar to normal liver, hepatic cells under the influence of carcinogenic agents already show some differences; hepatoma is quite different from normal liver, and transplanted hepatoma bears no resemblance to normal liver while it is indistinguishable from transplanted lymphosarcoma. From these and other results Greenstein[257] concludes that, apparently, tumors show ". . . a remarkable chemical uniformity . . . as a class of tissue, and suggests that mechanisms involved in malignant uncontrolled growth are common to all tumors regardless of etiology, histogenesis, or animal species in which they are found." The parallelism between biochemical and histologic observations is apparent and, after all, only to be expected, since for years histologists have believed that tumor cells are simplified and tend to a common type: "Biochemistry is anatomy at the molecular level."

V. THE DISSEMINATION OF TUMORS

The capacities to invade surrounding structures and to metastasize are characteristic properties of malignant tumors; they reveal a fundamental modification in the biology of neoplastic cells, the achievement of a maximum degree of autonomy. Benign tumors are no less neoplasms because they lack these properties; indeed, it has been mentioned that the acquisition of the ability to invade and to metastasize seems incidental to the basic process of neoplastic transformation, although it is extremely important from a practical standpoint, and it is for this reason that invasion and metastasis are treated separately. In addition, a brief review of some of the findings obtained by transplantation of tumors is included in this discussion.

The spread of tumors is the result of two different mechanisms: invasion and metastasis. Invasion is the presence of neoplastic cells away from their site of origin without loss of continuity between the primary tumor and the secondary tissue mass. For instance, bronchogenic carcinoma may invade the parietal pleura and grow into the thoracic wall, destroying soft tissues and ribs; a carcinoma of the stomach may penetrate all the walls of this organ, become adherent to the liver and grow within the hepatic parenchyma, etc. On the other hand, metastasis is the presence of tumor cells away from the primary neoplasm and without anatomic continuity with it; bronchogenic carcinoma will present metastatic nodules in the brain, adrenals and bones; carcinoma of the stomach may have secondary growths in the perigastric lymph nodes, liver and pelvic peritoneum, etc. In none of these instances is there continuity between the primary tumors and the secondary growths. Invasion and metastasis are separately discussed in the following paragraphs.

A. INVASION

Invasiveness is the capacity of cells to penetrate the surrounding tissues. This definition includes tumors and normal elements which share the ability to travel in the intimacy of the organism, such as leukocytes, macrophages and trophoblast. Therefore, any hypothesis explaining invasiveness of tumor cells should also account for the same property exhibited by nonneoplastic elements. Indeed, some of the most strongly held views on invasiveness have been derived from observations made with freely moving, normal cells. Perhaps the idea of tissue damage should be added to the concept of neoplastic invasion, but it is not easy to decide if this property of tumor cells is due solely to their ability to grow indefinitely; neoplastic cells not only invade tissues but do it aggressively, producing lesions in normal cells. In this respect it is interesting to note that a pure culture of fibroblasts is invaded and destroyed by a pure culture of mammary carcinoma of Walker 256 strain.[268]

Many factors have been considered responsible for the invasiveness of neoplastic cells, such as their speed of multiplication, loss of growth inhibition, the production of cytolytic and/or histolytic substances (which is a rebirth of the "universal solvent") or spreading factors, their ameboid movements or phagocytic properties, etc.[269] Coman, one of the few investigators who has studied the problem experimentally, reasons that leukocytes and macrophages owe their invasive properties to the fact that they are isolated, freely moving elements; therefore, it would be of interest to see if tumor cells are endowed with the same properties.[270] Ameboid movements of neoplastic cells were observed by Virchow a little less than 100 years ago in small fragments of freshly removed human tumors, and ever since they have been studied by many techniques, including tissue culture. It has been shown that, whatever their origin, tumor cells present ameboid movements, as the cells of carcinoma of the breast, which move at an average speed of 0.7 μ/min., but may reach a maximum speed of 2.4 μ/min., and small groups of 3 to 5 cells of a skin carcinoma of the rabbit can displace as a unit.[271] Of special interest is the fact that benign tumor cells (which show no tendency to invade surrounding tissues) will show ameboid movements as long as they become detached, isolated elements. The problem can be reduced, therefore, to a study of the factors that keep normal cells adherent to each other and the examination of the same factors in invasive tumor cells. By means of the micromanipulator, Coman found that the force required to separate normal epithelial cells is greater than that necessary to isolate tumor cells of an epidermoid carcinoma of

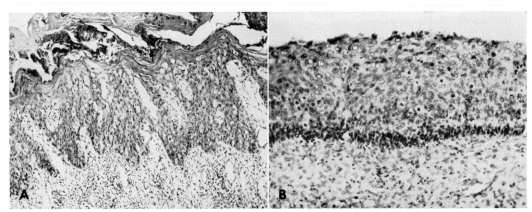

FIG. 5–37. *A,* Epithelial invasion by malignant cells in Paget's disease of the nipple. *B,* Neoplastic transformation of epithelial cells in carcinoma *in situ* of uterine cervix.

the same organ.[272] Furthermore, mechanical agitation of several human adenocarcinomas revealed that tumor cells are more easily separated than homologous glandular epithelium submitted to the same procedure.[273] These studies show that neoplastic elements are less strongly adherent to each other than normal cells and, therefore, it is easier for them to become detached and invasive.

The next step in this interesting work was to determine which are the factors responsible for adherence of normal cells, and the results seem to indicate that calcium plays a very important role in it. It has been mentioned (p. 63) that calcium deficiency will induce increased capillary permeability, possibly because of changes in the intercellular cement. Many authors have shown that cancerous tissues have a lower calcium concentration than normal, and the application of methylcholanthrene to the skin epithelium is followed by a rapid fall in calcium,[263]

simultaneous with an increase in the facility of cells to become detached. Since calcium is bound to the cell surface, electron microscope studies were carried out of the surface of invasive tumor cells and irregularities in the macromolecular structures were found. It was postulated that such irregularities were the basis of decreased adhesiveness and, therefore, of the ability of tumor cells to invade.[274] Quantitative studies of calcium content, correlated with the invasiveness of tumors, would be of great interest. The problem presents many other facets when human material is studied since variables are enormously multiplied, but within the simplified system of experimental tumors, it may be tentatively concluded that invasiveness depends on the ameboid movements of neoplastic cells, released from their attachment to each other by a decrease in the concentration of calcium ions on their surface.

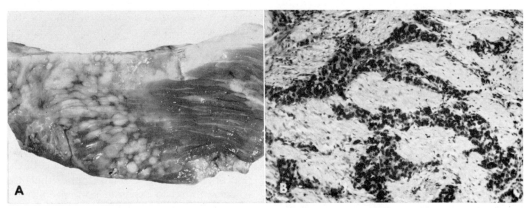

FIG. 5–38. Invasion of muscle by malignant cells. *A,* Interfascicular invasion of skeletal muscle in carcinoma of the breast. *B,* Invasion of smooth muscle by carcinoma in the wall of the stomach.

The routes of invasion of surrounding tissues are those offering the least resistance to penetration by tumor cells; i.e., interstitial spaces and preformed cavities or ducts. The last structures to be invaded are those physically more resistant, as cartilage and bone; even epithelium is invaded, although often it is difficult to distinguish between penetration by a malignant tumor and neoplastic transformation of neighboring cells. Probably, both processes occur. Epithelial invasion is seen in Paget's disease of the nipple, which is intraepithelial growth of carcinoma cells of an underlying ductal tumor in the breast, while neoplastic transformation of epithelial cells is apparent in carcinoma *in situ* of the uterine cervix or bronchus (Fig. 5–37). Of course, the most frequent invasion occurs along interstitial spaces where cells can move more freely and are seen forming groups or even as isolated elements; this is clearly seen in epithelial tumors invading hollow organs

with muscular layers such as the stomach, where smooth muscle bundles are separated by lines of glandular or undifferentiated elements (Fig. 5–38). Preformed ducts are represented by lymph and blood vessels, usually of small caliber (Fig. 5–39); larger blood vessels, especially veins, may become permeated by tumor cells in rare cases. Invasion of lymphatic and blood capillaries is very frequent and has great prognostic significance, since tumor cells may escape through them from the primary site and establish a metastasis (Fig. 5–40); any tumor invading interstitial spaces will find lymphatic and blood capillaries in its way, but the number of cases with distant metastases is lower than could be expected from this situation. Reasons for this disparity are mentioned below. Once within the lumen of a vessel, neoplastic cells may follow one of three possible fates or a combination of them. In the first, the vessel is obliterated by continuous growth and be-

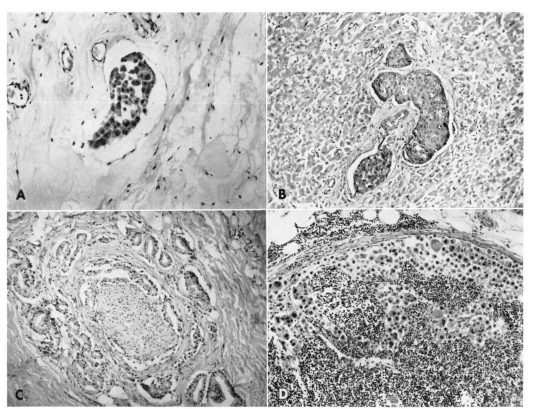

FIG. 5–39.   Lymphatic invasion by malignant tumors. *A*, Carcinoma of the breast invading lymphatics in subcutaneous soft tissues. *B*, Bronchogenic carcinoma within myocardial lymph vessels. *C*, Perineural lymphatic invasion in carcinoma of the prostate. *D*, Invasion of peripheral sinus in lymph node by malignant melanoma.

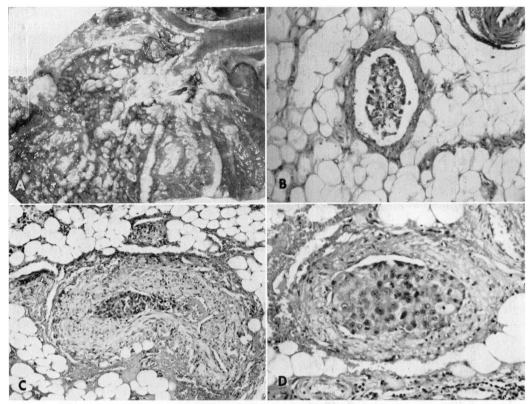

FIG. 5–40. Invasion of lymph and blood vessels by tumor cells. *A,* Peribronchial and perivascular lymphatic invasion in carcinoma of the breast. *B,* Small vein with tumor thrombus. *C* and *D,* Two arterioles containing malignant epithelial cells.

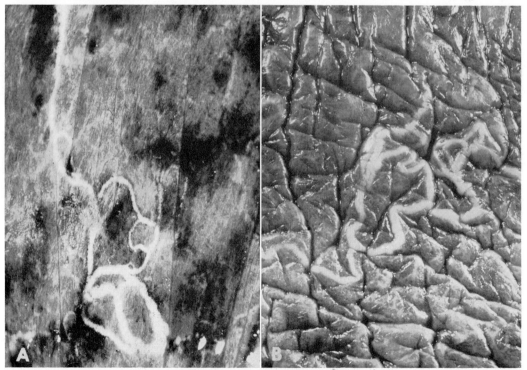

FIG. 5–41. Two instances of lymphatic permeation in the pleura.

comes one more of the interstitial elements destroyed by the tumor; in the second, a continuous mass grows for variable distances within the lumen of the vessel without losing continuity with the primary tumor, a process known as permeation, which is more frequent in lymphatics; in the third, a group of neoplastic cells becomes detached from the rest of the tumor and travels for some distance until it becomes established in a new position, where it may continue to grow. This is known as metastasis.

Lymphatic permeation is the rule in carcinoma of the prostate, and is frequently encountered in carcinoma of the breast, stomach and colon; some times it may be observed grossly in subserous lymphatic networks (Fig. 5–41), as in the pleura or diaphragm in cases of carcinoma of the thyroid, pancreas and breast; when it is very extensive, lymphatic permeation is referred to as "carcinomatous lymphangitis," an inadequate term since the process is neoplastic and not inflammatory. Tumor cell cords grow both in the direction of lymph flow as well as in the opposite direction, a form of retrograde permeation. This type of growth may reach the thoracic duct and continue for variable distances within this structure without actually giving rise to metastases. Willis[275] found this phenomenon in 3 per cent of 500 autopsy cases of malignant tumors and in 6 per cent of malignant abdominal neoplasms, while Young[276] found it in 40 per cent of his 100 autopsies. The significance of these findings is discussed in the next section.

Venules are also frequently invaded by tumors, especially in carcinomas of the thyroid, stomach and intestine; careful examination may show this change grossly. Special stains for elastic fibers obtained routinely in all cases of gastrointestinal malignant tumors reveal an unsuspected high frequency of venular invasion. In well differentiated carcinoma of the thyroid vein invasion may be the only sign of malignancy, but once established there should be no doubt about the nature of the tumor. It was mentioned before that not only venules but also large veins may be invaded in some cases; carcinoma of the kidney has a notorious tendency to grow within the renal vein, continue into the inferior vena cava

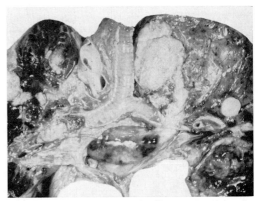

Fig. 5–42. A metastatic fibrosarcoma in the lung, growing into a pulmonary vein which drains in the left atrium; a huge tumor mass fills this cardiac cavity and probably contributed to death. (Courtesy of Dr. Raul Cicero and the Editor, Revista Mexicana de Tuberculosis.)

and may even reach the heart and fill the right atrium, a situation also observed with neuroblastoma and occasionally with chondrosarcoma. Bronchogenic carcinoma may invade the superior vena cava, especially when it arises in the right upper lobe; Cicero, et al.[277] found this complication in 6 out of 20 autopsy cases, and in 3 of the 6 patients the tumor was located in the upper right lobe of the lung. An extraordinary case, published by Amador and Cicero,[278] was that of a metastatic fibrosarcoma in the lung. One of the pulmonary nodules broke into a pulmonary vein in the left upper lobe and grew into the left atrium where a huge tumor mass was formed which probably contributed to death by obstruction of the mitral orifice (Fig. 5–42). The microscopic study of invaded veins shows fibrous thickening of the intima with thrombosis; often, tumor cells invade the thrombus and use it as a basis for continued growth within the lumen. Arteries are more resistant than veins, perhaps because of their greater concentration of elastic fibers. Although this is purely conjectural, the fact is that they are less frequently invaded than veins. Perhaps the tumor penetrating more often within arteries is bronchogenic carcinoma, which may invade a branch of a pulmonary artery or a bronchial artery.[279] The frequency of this phenomenon has been correlated with prognosis and it has been shown to be a more faithful sign than lymph node metastases and other forms of invasion of surrounding structures.[280] Carcinoma of the tonsil may erode the carotid artery and produce death by massive hemorrhage.

B. METASTASIS

Neoplastic cells capable of leaving the primary tumor and continuing to grow away from it in a different organ may do so through a series of steps which may be summarized as follows: (a) invasion, when they reach and penetrate lymphatic or blood vessels, a serous cavity or a preformed organic duct; (b) embolism or transportation, whence tumor cells are carried away by lymph, blood, serous fluid or epithelial secretions, until they reach the end of their journey in a distant organ or a serous or epithelial surface; (c) cellular multiplication with formation of a nodule, which invades surrounding structures and stimulates stromal reaction. In some part of this odyssey the cell becomes fundamentally different from others unable to imitate it, and this difference represents a high degree of autonomy from the conditions of the new environment.

There are many problems related to this mechanism of dissemination of malignant tumors, some of which have been studied both experimentally and in autopsy material. The experimental literature is summarized by Coman,[281] and Zeidman,[282] while Willis[275] and Walther[283] have published valuable monographs with ample information based on human material and with long bibliographic lists. The significance of metastasis is double. On one hand, it reveals the degree to which tumor cells have become autonomous and, therefore, it is a measure of their biologic transformation; on the other hand, it clearly represents the difference between curability and incurability of malignant tumors. Few neoplasms with distant metastases are curable, although in rare cases promising results have been obtained.

1. Routes of Metastatic Dissemination. Tumor cells may follow five different routes for metastatic spread, which are: (a) lymphatic, (b) hematogenous, (c) mixed or lymphohematogenous, (d) transcelomic, (e) preformed epithelial-lined ducts.

a. Lymphatic Route. This type of metastasis is more often seen in carcinomas, but it cannot be considered exclusively associated with them, nor is it true that malignant epithelial tumors do not disseminate through other routes. A lymphatic metastasis consists of the penetration of tumor cells within a lymphatic vessel where they travel up to the corresponding lymph node; this structure is invaded and the neoplastic elements may then continue their way within the lumen of the efferent lymphatic channel until a new lymph node is reached and the process is repeated. The first lymph nodes involved by tumor are those corresponding to the normal lymphatic drainage of the site of origin of neoplastic growth, and this is why a thorough knowledge of the distribution of lymph nodes in the organism is necessary for the proper diagnosis and treatment of tumors. Bronchogenic carcinoma, for instance, will metastasize first to lymph nodes in the pulmonary hilus; carcinoma of the breast goes to the axillary and/or to the internal mammary lymph node groups; carcinoma of the thyroid involves first the lower jugular chain, etc. Rarely, a tumor may jump the first "relay" of lymph nodes and appear at another, more distant group, as in carcinoma of the lower lip, which instead of appearing first in the submental group may show metastases in the cervical lymph nodes, or carcinoma of the breast with lymphatic metastasis in the opposite axilla. When some of these cases are carefully studied, however, the lymph nodes of the first relay may also be found to be involved, although not sufficiently to have been palpated or shown to be affected in a routine microscopic examination.

The ability of tumor cells to jump a lymph node has been experimentally studied by Zeidman,[284] who injected cells of a transplantable tumor in the afferent lymph vessel of the popliteal lymph node of rabbits. He observed that tumor emboli stopped in the peripheral sinus, without continuing into the efferent vessel until several weeks after the injection. It was concluded that lymph nodes were an adequate barrier against that particular tumor. Once the lymph node is occupied by cancer it "closes" to other elements, a fact shown both experimentally and in human patients with injections of dyes or radioactive material into the draining areas of lymph nodes occupied by neoplastic cells. Neither dye nor radioactive material would penetrate into the tumor nodule in the lymph node, and if the entire lymph node was replaced by tumor then the injected elements would not reach it.[285] It has been said that lymph nodes draining certain malignant tumors show peculiar changes before the arrival of neoplastic cells.[286, 287] Nadel and Ackerman have reported a histologic picture identical to Boeck's sarcoid which has been interpreted as a reaction to products of necrosis of the tumor mass,[288] an observation confirmed by others.[289]

The "closure" of lymph nodes occupied by malignant cells provides a possible explanation for anomalous or retrograde lymphatic disseminations, of which Willis[275] gives numerous examples and Zeidman[290] has made an experimental analysis. It is not always possible to be certain that tumor cells have traveled against the normal lymphatic flow, but the beautiful experiments of Celis described below have clearly shown that the occlusion of lymphatic circulation modifies the direction of flow and facilitates the appearance of collaterals which may carry neoplastic elements.

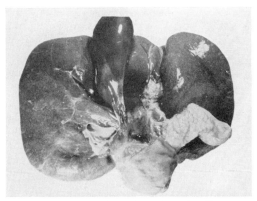

FIG. 5–43. Obstruction of extrahepatic biliary tract by metastatic carcinoma of the lung.

Lymphatic metastasis may give rise to three different complications: (a) compression of neighboring structures with the corresponding clinical manifestations, such as jaundice resulting from pressure caused by enlarged hilar lymph nodes (Fig. 5–43) or hydronephrosis and uremia secondary to ureteral compression by metastatic hypogastric lymph nodes in carcinoma of the uterine cervix[291] (Fig. 5–44); (b) invasion and rupture of veins, occasionally seen in

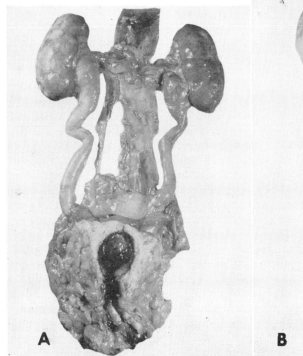

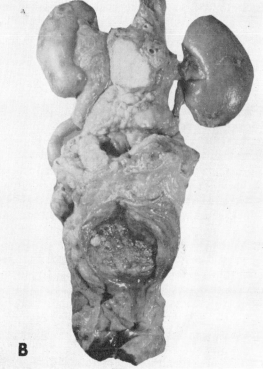

FIG. 5–44. Two instances of extensive involvement of pelvic lymphatic structures by carcinoma of the uterine cervix, with partial occlusion of ureters, hydroureter and hydronephrosis.

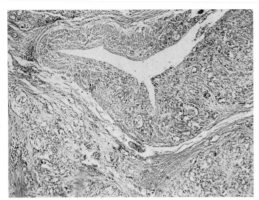

FIG. 5–45.   Invasion of the wall of a vein by adenocarcinoma of parotid gland.

cervical metastasis of carcinoma of the
larynx[292] (Fig. 5–45); (c) lymphedema of
an extremity, as is sometimes observed in
unoperated patients with carcinoma of the
breast and extensive occlusion of axillary
lymph nodes.[293]

An important type of lymphatic metastasis arises from another secondary deposit;
for instance, hematogenous or blood-borne
lung metastases may be accompanied by
tumor in the pulmonary hilar lymph nodes.
Unfortunately, however, these cases are difficult to interpret, since such tumors can
also give direct metastasis to the lymph
nodes.

b. Hematogenous Route. The penetration
of a blood vessel by a group of neoplastic
cells and their transportation by the blood
to a distant organ, where they become established and form another tumor mass, is
known as hematogenous or blood-borne metastasis. It is especially frequent in sarcomas, but as was remarked for lymphatic
dissemination in carcinomas, it is neither
exclusive of them nor is it acceptable that
carcinomas do not use the blood to disseminate. In discussing invasion it was mentioned that malignant cells often penetrate
within the lumen of venules, but that the
frequency of hematogenous metastasis is
lower than could be expected. Engel showed
that 50 per cent of 107 carcinomas of the
stomach, colon and breast had tumor cells
in the blood of the veins draining the tumor,
but no correlation could be established between this fact and the presence of metastasis or prognosis,[294] and other similar
studies have been published.[295, 296] This

may be due to a series of factors determining
the fate of tumor cells reaching a blood
vessel, some of which are as follows:

(1) THE TUMOR EMBOLUS. It is apparent
from a pathologic standpoint that in order
to have a hematogenous metastasis it is
necessary that the tumor embolus be formed
by a minimum number of cells and that if
this minimum is not reached then neoplastic
embolism is possible, but the cells will not
survive in their new environment.[297]
Willis[275] calls attention to the fact that it is
not rare to see small groups of neoplastic
cells in the pulmonary veins, surrounded by
a blood clot and in all stages of degeneration. It is believed that such cell groups are
unable to proliferate and establish a metastasis, but experimental data seem to be
against this idea. By means of transplantable tumors in rabbits and rats, Zeidman
and Buss[298] showed that tumor cells can
pass through the lungs and produce systemic metastases, and that this passage was
not determined by the size of the cells, since
those that were larger passed the lungs more
easily. There can be no doubt that in order
to traverse the lung capillaries tumor cells
must be associated in very small groups or
even travel alone, and yet they are capable
of producing metastases in other organs;
furthermore, the explanation cannot be
based on arteriovenous anastomosis allow-
ing the passage of larger cells since under
identical experimental conditions both tumors behave in a different manner. Other
than the passage through the lung of small
groups of cells, the size of the tumor embolus requires additional conditions in order
to become established as a metastasis. When
Krebs-2 tumor cells, for example, are injected intravenously in mice only pulmonary
metastases appear, but when cortisone is
administered at the same time there are
metastases in many other organs.[299]

(2) THE SIZE OF THE INVOLVED VESSEL.
In close association with the preceding facts
is that the frequency of blood-borne metastases bears no relation to the invasion of
venules, but is well correlated with the involvement of large veins. This assertion is
based on autopsy observations, after the
tumor has had all opportunities to develop
metastases even before invasion of large
veins, which would be secondary. Further-

more, the end of all lymphatic circulation is the blood and it is not known how frequently tumor cells reach blood vessels through the lymph. Nevertheless, it is a fact that patients with extensive metastatic disease usually have involvement of larger veins.

(3) THE THREE GREAT ROUTES OF VENOUS CIRCULATION. Hematogenous metastases are more frequently seen in lungs, liver and bones. Part of the explanation of this phenomenon is based on the anatomic distribution of the venous system in man, since the liver receives all the splanchnic circulation and the lungs are the final station of all venous circulation (and directly of all blood from the upper half of the body and the lower extremities). Therefore, it could be expected that these two organs, lung and liver, would be the most frequently involved by blood-borne metastases. Batson gave the accepted explanation for the high frequency of metastases in bones, based on his study of carcinoma of the prostate;[300] he observed that tumor emboli could penetrate into the vertebral veins and through them reach the bones of the pelvis, the vertebral column and the cranium. This was especially frequent with an increase in intra-abdominal pressure, as obtained with cough and strain, since the change in pressure would send the blood from the vena cava into the vertebral veins.[301] Coman and de Long injected suspensions of tumor cells into the femoral veins of rabbits and rats while the intra-abdominal pressure was slightly elevated and found numerous neoplastic emboli obstructing the ramifications of vertebral veins.[302] Since the vena cava is anastomosed with the vertebral veins along the entire spinal column from the pelvis to the cranium, it may be conceived as a third venous system, comparable to the portal or caval systems, which accounts for the frequency of metastasis in bone. For instance, internal mammary veins are anastomosed with the vertebral system through intercostal and subclavian veins, and this would explain why carcinoma of the breast frequently shows bone metastasis. It must be emphasized that the vertebral venous system accounts for only part of the skeletal metastases, namely those occurring in the central part, and the shoulder and pelvic

girdles; metastases in distal bones must be explained by other mechanisms.

(4) THE PARADOXICAL DISTRIBUTION OF METASTASIS. For a long time it has been observed that some tumors rarely metastasize to certain organs; for example, metastatic tumors of the bronchi are extremely rare regardless of the origin of the primary neoplasms. These cases, together with the high frequency of secondary tumors in lungs, liver and bones, have been explained according to two different theories: (a) The "soil" theory, proposed by Stephen Paget in 1889, compares tumor cells to seeds thrown into fields of different fertility which grow only where they find adequate environment for survival. According to this theory, lung carcinoma cells would find in the adrenal an environment conducive to their metabolism and growth while in the spleen or striated muscle they succumb because there are none of the substances necessary for survival.[303] (b) The "mechanical" theory, attributed to Ewing by Coman,[281] explains the differences in the distribution of metastases as due to the anatomic distribution of the blood vessels in various organs and tissues "because there are no data supporting the idea that any organ is better adapted than others to the growth of tumor cells."

The "soil" theory is favored by most pathologists, and Willis gives many reasons in its support. Indeed, the problem is not so much the distribution of venous metastases, which may be explained anatomically by the three main venous systems (vena cava, portal vein and vertebral veins), but the distribution of systemic, arterial metastases. Experimentally, the injection of V_2 tumor cells into the left ventricle of rabbits will result in metastatic nodules in almost all organs, but when this tumor is allowed to run its natural course there will be metastases only in the regional lymph nodes and in the lungs.[304] In this case, the tumor follows the "soil" theory in spontaneous behavior and the "mechanical" theory when the cells are placed in the systemic circulation.

The question still remains, however, of why spontaneous metastases of many tumors show preference for certain organs while ignoring others. Coman, et al.[305] have made some experimental studies by means of Brown-Pearce tumor and rabbits. Tumor cells were fixed, stained in order to facilitate recognition and injected into the left ventricle of rabbits; the animals were sacrificed immediately, sections were prepared of all organs and the number of emboli in arterioles and capillaries were counted and expressed as the number of emboli per square centimeter in eight different organs. The same experiment was carried out again, this time with living tumor cells and waiting until metastases had developed. No correlation was found between the total number of emboli and the number of metastatic nodules, but an excellent correlation was possible when capillary emboli alone were compared with metastatic tumors. Furthermore, the number of emboli produced by stained tumor cells was greater in organs with a higher incidence of spontaneous metastases. With these data, Coman, et al. concluded that, at least for Brown-Pearce tumor in rabbits, the distribution of metastases is due to the manner of arrival of neoplastic cell emboli at different organs and not to metabolic peculiarities of tissues. It is also suggested that metastases arise primarily from small, capillary emboli and not from larger groups of cells lodged in arterioles; apparently, tumors find it as difficult to leave arterial vessels as to penetrate them.

On the other hand, Lucké, et al.[306] injected V_2 tumor cells into the portal and caval circulations, observing that in both cases metastases were more numerous in the liver than in the lungs, and their results were interpreted as favoring the "soil" theory of metastatic distribution. It is difficult to escape the impression that both theories are true and that bizarre patterns of metastasis will eventually be explained by different combinations of both mechanisms.

(5) DURATION AND SIZE OF PRIMARY NEOPLASM. It has been suggested that the longer the duration of a malignant tumor the greater the opportunity it has to metastasize and, if so, the more numerous the metastatic nodules. With all exceptions considered this is most probably true for a certain group of neoplasms; certainly, autopsy experience supports such an idea. But the corollary of this assertion, that larger tumor masses are more likely to metastasize than small neoplasms, is not only untrue, but dangerous. The presence or absence of metastasis is not a function of the size of the primary tumor, and this is confirmed by both experimental and clinical material; the concept of "occult carcinoma" has been mentioned and instances of grossly unapparent tumors with widespread metastases could be multiplied *ad nauseam*. Willis[10] devotes an entire chapter to "latent" neoplasms and mentions cases from the oral cavity, pharynx, esophagus, stomach, intestine, pancreas, liver, gallbladder, lungs, thyroid, kidney, urinary bladder, breast, testes, melanomas, etc. Indeed, there seems to be no organ, where malignant, usually metastasizing tumors occur, that will not occasionally lodge a very small primary growth, becoming clinically manifest through dissemination. To ignore this relatively frequent combination will result in two unfortunate situations. First, patients will be mistakenly treated for the metastatic tumor by means that should be used only for primary growths, as is sometimes seen in intracranial metastases of bronchogenic carcinoma;[307] second, inadmissible temporization with malignant tumors "because they are small and the probability of metastasis is low" may well destroy the only opportunity for cure of many patients.

Perhaps this is the best place to mention MacDonald's "biologic predeterminism," a synoptic expression of the balance between host and neoplasm.[308, 309] According to this author, the ultimate outcome of a malignant tumor is determined before the neoplastic process becomes clinically detectable, and is the result of the struggle for power between the developing tumor and the enigmatic defensive reactions of the host. Thus, each cancer would have certain biologic characteristics which tend to remain more or less constant throughout its life, so the time factor would be of secondary importance, especially in determining the presence or absence of metastases. This concept was offered as an alternative to the more widely supported idea of cancer starting as a localized disease and spreading as time passes to the regional lymph nodes, and with further passage of time to other parts of the body. When the latter idea of cancer is accepted, there is full justification for hoping that the earlier the diagnosis the more likely the cure, but data published from several sources seem to oppose this simple cause-and-effect relation for all tumors. Biologic predeterminism in cancer is the recognition of an obvious fact, namely that with the same type of tumor some patients will show a rapid evolution, with early and widely disseminated metastases, while others will run a more chronic course and, even though lymphatic or blood-borne metastases may be present, live for many years. Furthermore, it leaves ample room for those types of cancer that do have a natural history conforming to the traditional doctrine that curability is directly related to the earliness of diagnosis and the immediacy of treatment; for instance, epidermoid carcinomas of the lip, uterine cervix and skin. But to generalize from these cases to all tumors is to invite failure in many cases; speaking of public education in cancer, Kreyberg remarks that: "It is not correct and not fair to publish such statistics in a manner that makes the public believe that if the women examine themselves regularly and carefully, and pay a visit to a competent doctor at the first suspicion of a symptom from the breast, their chance of a complete cure is in the vicinity of 90 per cent."[310] After all, deep within the rationale of malignant tumor metastasis there is one factor more important than time and/or size (and which in fact also determines the influence of these two features): the biologic nature of the tumor.[311]

(6) INFLUENCE OF PHYSICAL EXAMINATION AND SURGERY. Palpation of a tumor is a theoretical cause of detachment of neoplastic cells and metastasis, and there is some experimental evidence showing that tumor "massage" will increase the number of secondary deposits.[312, 313] This danger is certainly overrated, since "massage" bears little relation to careful clinical palpation.

A different problem is the demonstration by Fisher and Turnbull[314] that manipulation of a rectal cancer at the time of operation may shower the blood stream with cancer cells. The influence of surgery on the frequency of metastases has been the subject of some experimental work. (1) Paschkis, et al.[315] observed that the growth of subcutaneous tumors was accelerated when partial hepatectomy was performed at the time that tumor cell suspensions were injected. (2) Buinauskas, et al.[316] reported that celiotomy just prior to subcutaneous tumor cell inoculation resulted in increased take and growth of such tumors when compared with unoperated controls. (3) Fisher and Fisher, in a very interesting study,[317] have narrowed down the influence of surgery to liver damage, since laparotomy and liver manipulation increased fourfold the number of hepatic metastases after intraportal injection of Walker carcinosarcoma cells. Furthermore, other operative procedures such as dorsal incision or laparotomy without liver manipulation failed to elicit a similar response; partial hepatectomy produced a threefold increase in liver metastases when compared with controls, the same as when the liver was damaged with chloroform. "Stressful" situations such as anesthesia, removal of other organs such as a kidney, intraperitoneal air injection, etc., did not increase the number of liver metastases which were present in adrenalectomized animals treated with supportive doses of steroids. A very interesting finding is that after 8 weeks of the intraportal administration of tumor cells the incidence of liver metastasis is no greater than after two weeks, but successive weekly laparotomies will increase this frequency to 100 per cent. The authors suggest that: "These findings would lend credence to the possibility that circulating cancer cells, if they are alive to begin with, might forever remain capable of growth should conditions be favorable." Judiciously, they add that whatever clinical significance their studies may have must await further investigation.

A different type of surgical influence on metastasis is that directly caused by the surgeon's scalpel, which may be apparent in the operative scars[318] at the lines of suture after resection of the large intestine for carcinoma. This has been observed by Goligher, et al.[319] after operations on the rectosigmoid or sigmoid in which an attempt was made to save the anal sphincter, and by Beahrs, et al.[320] in cases where exfoliated cells from cancers high in the colon implanted themselves in the incisions of hem-

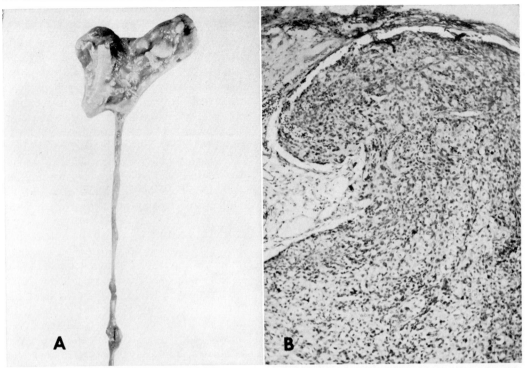

FIG. 5–46. Thoracic duct involvement in anaplastic carcinoma of the stomach. *A,* Thoracic duct showing a low enlarged lymph node and a large tumor mass located in the supraclavicular region, *B,* Complete filling of the lumen by tumor cells.

orrhoidectomy. Special precautions in handling the intestine have been devised to avoid this form of surgical implantation of tumor,[321, 322] but perhaps the most important rule is to be fully aware of the possibility. The possible role of biopsy in the dissemination of tumors is discussed in the next section of this chapter.

Several authors have described the principal cellular events associated with the development of intravascular cancer cells by means of histologic examination of both human and experimental material.[323, 324] Of special interest are the observations by Wood,[325] who visualized the fate of blood-borne cancer cells *in vivo* by means of the rabbit ear chamber technique and V_2 carcinoma, derived from the Shope virus papilloma. It was shown that metastasis formation occurs only from capillaries and that the site where cancer cells will become adherent to the capillary wall cannot be predicted, since sometimes tumor cells adhered in vessels whose diameters were three times larger than the cancer cell and without cessation of blood flow. Endothelial adherence of tumor cells was apparently independent of leukocytic sticking, vasomotor activity or capillary flow rate. A few minutes later a thrombus was formed. Since it had been shown previously that the administration of heparin or bishydroxycoumarin (Dicumarol) reduces the resulting number of pulmonary metastases after the intravenous inoculation of tumor cells (and likewise the incidence of visceral metastases in animals bearing transplanted neoplasms), such intravascular thrombi were considered as an essential process in the development of secondary blood-borne tumor deposits. The endothelium is damaged some time later and leukocytes are seen to migrate through the capillary wall leaving an endothelial defect through which cancer cells emigrate from the blood vessel into the connective tissue. The earliest that tumor cells were observed to reach the perivascular area was within 3 hours and neoplastic growth was progressive in the extravascular tissues in 6 hours. An interesting observation was the proliferation of capillaries arising from preexisting vessels and entering the tumor within 24 hours.

c. Lymphohematogenous Route. The

lymphohematogenous path of metastasis is followed when tumor cells reach the blood from a lymphatic channel such as the thoracic duct or the great lymphatic vein. Another possibility may be observed rarely, namely the perforation of a venous channel by a lymph node containing tumor cells. There are many communications between the lymphatic and venous systems other than the thoracic duct and the lymphatic vein, which become apparent especially after obstruction of large lymphatic vessels. (One was described by Celis, et al.[326] in the dog between an abdominal lymph vessel and the inferior vena cava.) The true frequency with which abdominal tumors use this route for dissemination is not known, but it is probably greater than usually considered, since careful examination of the thoracic duct in cases with abdominal cancers shows it to be involved in 6 to 25 per cent. In 129 cases of carcinoma, Young found involvement of the thoracic duct in 37 per cent, while in 21 cases of sarcoma it was involved in 53 per cent;[276] Kansel, et al. found metastatic involvement of the thoracic duct in 30 per cent of 13 autopsies of malignant disease.[327] Watne, et al. cannulated the thoracic duct in 30 patients with far advanced carcinomas and sarcomas, and found tumor cells in 7; in addition, tumor cells were also found in 15 of 91 autopsy cases of advanced malignancies.[328] It is interesting that no correlation was established between the presence of pulmonary metastasis and tumor emboli in the lymph. For many years it has been known that carcinoma of the stomach is sometimes associated with enlargement of the left supraclavicular lymph nodes, and Troisier noted in 1889 that this is also observed with other abdominal cancers (Fig. 5–46). It was believed that the Virchow-Troisier node was the result of invasion of the thoracic duct, and this belief has been confirmed experimentally by Zeidman[329] by means of injection of dyes within the duct, which resulted in staining of the supraclavicular lymph nodes. Incidentally, in this work Zeidman also showed the presence of collaterals of the thoracic duct draining into the intercostal and mediastinal lymph nodes. A very complete study of the lymphatics of the thorax has been published by Kuthy and Celis,[330] and the significance of the thoracic duct in the spread of malignant tumors is analyzed by Celis, et al.[331]

d. Transcelomic Route. This form of metastatic dissemination occurs in serous cavities and consists of the passage of neoplastic cells from one area of the cavity to a distant place within the same cavity, where they proliferate and form secondary deposits. This type of seeding is also known as implantation metastases. It is especially frequent in the pleura with carcinomas of the lung and in the peritoneum with carcinomas of the gastrointestinal tract and the ovary (Fig. 5–47). It may be observed in the meninges almost exclusively with ependymomas and malignant meningiomas, but this is rare.[332] Transcelomic metastases appear usually when the primary tumor is within the same serous cavity or in its immediate neighborhood. Only rarely do they represent the extension of another metastatic

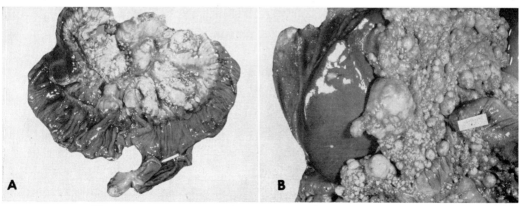

Fɪɢ. 5–47.   Transcelomic dissemination of carcinoma of the ovary.

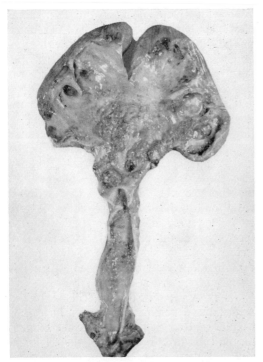

FIG. 5–48. Ureteral seeding of papillary carcinoma of renal pelvis, a form of metastases through previously formed, epithelium-lined ducts.

nodule, and when this occurs it is usually a metastatic lymph node that ruptures into the serous cavity. The presence of cancer cells is usually followed by a transudation of fluid, frequently (although not necessarily) hemorrhagic; it is important that tumor cells be well preserved in serous effusions since this facilitates recognition in cytologic studies.[333] Occasionally serous metastases stimulate the formation of fibrous adhesions and, through this mechanism, cause intestinal subocclusive or occlusive accidents. Rapid formation of serous transudate may be a disturbing complication of some cancers, especially of the ovary, but it may be avoided by the use of radioactive gold deposited in the involved cavity.[334] Sometimes the omentum becomes thickened and rolls up in the abdomen; in this situation it may be palpated as a firm, horizontal mass in the epigastrium and both upper quadrants, but this condition may also be present in peritoneal tuberculosis. Grossly, some forms of diffuse peritoneal carcinomatosis may be difficult to distinguish from primary mesothelioma, but careful search for the primary tumor and microscopic examination are usually sufficient to establish the correct diagnosis in most cases.

e. Metastasis through Preformed, Epithelial-Lined Ducts. The respiratory, digestive and urinary tracts are the paths followed by neoplastic cells in this type of dissemination. Furth has shown that the experimental inoculation of leukemic or cancer cells into the trachea will result in pulmonary tumors;[335] a suggestion is obtained of this process in humans when bronchiolar, multicentric tumors are examined, but no proof exists that it occurs.[336] It has been mentioned before that in tumors of the lower digestive tract there is frequent desquamation of cancer cells into the lumen and that the surgeon may implant them in the wall during resections. Finally, in the urinary tract transitional cell tumors tend to be multiple; therefore, when several growths appear at different levels between renal pelves and urinary bladder, the decision between metastases and multicentric origin may be well nigh impossible (Fig. 5–48). Sargent reviewed the literature in reference to carcinoma of the kidney and found that intraluminal metastases in the ureter are extremely rare.[337]

Another possibility is transtubal dissemination of adenocarcinoma of the uterus, which has been considered alternatively as real or illusory. In a recent study, Dahle[338] made smears of the Douglas' cul de sac and of both tubes in 21 patients with adenocarcinoma of the uterus treated by radical hysterectomy and found tumor cells in the cul de sac in 7 cases and in one or both tubes in 11 cases. Since it cannot be predicted whether these cells are capable of producing peritoneal metastases, Dahle suggested the deposition of Au^{198} in the pelvic peritoneum at the end of the operation.

C. DIFFICULTIES IN DETERMINING ROUTE OF NEOPLASTIC DISSEMINATION

Once the possible paths of metastases are known it is of interest to inquire how often and how accurately they may be determined in individual cancer cases. Clinically, this problem emerges in cases of "occult" tumors which are manifested by their metastases. When recognized, the routes of dissemination may suggest the possible site of the primary tumor, as axillary deposits in homolateral carcinoma of the breast, jugular lymphatic chain metastases in carcinoma of the thyroid, etc. Distant metastases, be they lymphatic or hematogenous, complicate the issue almost beyond possibility of a reasonable suggestion as to the site of origin before a biopsy is examined. For instance, Virchow-Troisier's node is usually associated with an abdominal malignancy, frequently (but not always) of the stomach, although it may also appear in intrathoracic tumors such as carcinoma of the lung. "Occult" carcinomas metastasizing mainly by the hematogenous route may sometimes be suspected from the pattern of distribution of secondary nodules, as in bronchogenic carcinoma, which usually shows involvement of brain, bones, adrenals and liver. Many other cases, however, constitute a real challenge to the clinician's sagacity and knowledge, and very often the final opinion must rest on histologic examination.

The clinical difficulties just mentioned are shared by the pathologist at autopsy, although there is no doubt that direct examination of organs will help to solve some otherwise puzzling cases. Death, however, usually occurs at the end of a more or less prolonged course during which the tumor has had ample time and opportunity to use many or all the metastatic paths, thus creating a most complex anatomic picture. Experience with a reasonably large series of autopsies of cancer patients should show that in discussing the frequency of the different routes used by various tumors to metastasize, the data are only suggestive of general trends and should not be taken as absolute figures.

A special problem is presented by the so-called systemic or generalized tumors, such as lymphomas or leukemias; it is a matter of controversy if these neoplasms arise simultaneously in many sites of the organism or if they have a unicentric origin with precocious metastases. There seem to be clear examples of both possibilities occurring in different cases. Extraganglionar lymphomas are usually localized and may even be cured with treatment aimed exclusively at the primary site of origin before they have a chance to metastasize, as with lymphoma of the stomach or reticulosarcoma of bone; on the other hand, Hodg-

kin's disease, lymphatic lymphosarcoma and all varieties of leukemia tend to appear simultaneously or in rapid succession in many separate lymph node groups.

D. THE SINGLE, ISOLATED METASTASIS

One of the most important principles of cancer surgery is that tumors should be removed *en bloc* with the draining lymph nodes of the first, and sometimes second, relay, which naturally includes all lymphatic channels joining the site of origin of the tumor with lymph nodes. This is only possible, however, when the route of dissemination is lymphogenous; surgical treatment is not curative in the presence of blood-borne metastases. The exception to this rule is the rare patient with a single, isolated metastasis, usually in the lungs, when the metastatic nodule may be removed surgically if: (a) The primary tumor is under control, which may be achieved by surgery or other means. (b) Extensive clinical and laboratory examinations have convinced the surgeon that there is only one metastasis. Encouraging results have been published in a group of 43 cases by Hood, et al.[339] and in 20 cases by Strieder.[340] Habein, et al.[341] reported what is the largest group of patients who had pulmonary resections for metastatic malignant lesions; of their 93 patients, 16 were living without evidence of recurrence three or more years after the pulmonary operation.

E. FREQUENCY AND DISTRIBUTION OF METASTASES

Willis' excellent monograph "The Spread of Tumors in the Human Body"[275] is based on 500 autopsy cases of malignant tumors, and Abrams, et al. have published an extensive analysis of metastases in 1000 cases of carcinomas.[342] Obviously, the most frequently involved organs will vary according to the different concentrations of various types of tumors; nevertheless, in both Willis' and Abrams' series, metastases are more often present in abdominal lymph nodes, liver and lungs. Brandt, et al.[343] analyzed a series of 500 autopsies of malignant tumors performed at the Pathology Unit of the National University of Mexico Medical School. His results are presented in Tables 21, 22 and 23. In large series the true

Table 21. General Distribution of Metastases in 420 Cases of Carcinoma

PRIMARY TUMOR	NUMBER OF CASES	REGIONAL LYMPH NODES	DISTANT LYMPH NODES	LUNG	LIVER	PERITONEUM	PLEURA	KIDNEY	ADRENALS	BONE	DIGESTIVE TRACT	DIAPHRAGM	SPLEEN	THYROID	BRAIN	MENINGES	PERICARDIUM	HEART	PANCREAS	GENITAL ORGANS
Uterine cervix	135	85	50	23	23	11	6	5	2	2	2	6	1	—	—	—	1	2	2	2
Lung	42	37	22	15	14	5	6	8	12	9	7	4	2	5	8	4	4	3	2	1
Breast	31	28	27	20	18	3	12	5	7	6	4	5	3	6	4	4	6	3	4	1
Stomach	22	14	11	4	8	8	2	2	2	—	1	2	3	—	—	2	1	1	2	1
Skin	20	8	4	1	2	1	—	—	—	1	—	—	—	—	—	—	—	—	—	—
Thyroid	17	8	5	7	—	—	1	3	1	2	—	1	—	—	2	1	1	—	—	—
Biliary tract	15	11	6	7	11	5	2	2	2	—	1	3	—	1	—	—	—	1	—	3
Pancreas	13	8	5	5	9	3	3	1	2	—	2	2	1	—	—	—	1	—	—	1
Liver	13	1	3	4	—	—	1	1	—	—	—	—	—	1	—	1	—	1	—	—
Pharynx and tongue	13	11	—	1	—	—	1	—	—	—	—	—	—	1	—	—	—	—	—	—
Ovary	11	5	7	1	5	9	3	—	—	—	—	—	3	—	—	—	—	—	—	1
Urinary bladder	10	1	1	—	—	—	—	1	—	—	1	—	1	—	—	—	—	—	1	—
Larynx	10	9	2	1	1	—	—	—	1	—	—	—	2	1	—	—	—	—	—	—
Intestine	9	2	1	1	3	—	—	1	—	—	2	1	—	—	—	—	—	—	—	1
Prostate	8	3	2	2	—	1	—	—	—	2	—	—	—	—	—	—	—	—	—	—
Melanoma	7	5	4	5	3	1	—	—	2	1	2	—	1	1	—	1	1	1	2	1
Others	51	28	21	16	10	—	4	4	—	6	3	1	6	3	3	4	2	4	3	1
Total	427	264	171	113	107	47	41	33	31	29	25	24	23	19	17	17	17	16	16	13

(Brandt et al.[343])

Table 22. General Distribution of Metastases in 32 Cases of Sarcoma

TUMOR	NUMBER OF CASES	LUNG	REGIONAL LYMPH NODES	LIVER	BONE	DISTANT LYMPH NODES	PLEURA	PERITONEUM	KIDNEY	HEART	DIAPHRAGM	DIGESTIVE TRACT	ADRENALS	BRAIN	MENINGES	THYROID	PERICARDIUM
Fibrosarcoma	4	4	2	2	3	1	1	2	—	2	1	1	1	1	—	—	1
Osteosarcoma	4	4	1	—	1	—	—	—	—	—	—	1	—	—	—	—	—
Rhabdomyosarcoma	4	2	1	1	—	1	—	—	—	—	—	—	—	—	—	—	—
Mesothelioma	4	1	1	—	—	—	1	—	—	—	—	—	—	—	—	—	—
Lymphoma of digestive tract	4	—	3	1	—	1	—	—	2	—	—	—	—	—	—	1	—
Liposarcoma	3	—	—	—	—	—	—	—	—	—	—	—	—	—	—	—	—
Sarcoma of the breast	3	1	1	—	—	—	—	—	—	—	—	—	—	—	—	—	—
Ewing's tumor	2	2	1	—	1	2	2	1	2	—	1	—	—	—	1	—	—
Mesenchymoma	1	—	—	1	—	—	—	—	—	—	—	—	1	—	—	—	—
Leiomyosarcoma	1	—	—	1	—	—	—	—	—	—	—	—	—	—	—	—	—
Synovial sarcoma	1	—	—	—	—	—	—	—	—	—	—	—	—	—	—	—	—
Malignant schwannoma	1	—	—	—	—	—	—	—	—	—	—	—	—	—	—	—	—
Total	32	14	10	6	5	5	4	3	4	3	2	2	2	1	1	1	1

(Brandt et al.[343])

V. THE DISSEMINATION OF TUMORS / **231**

Table 23. Frequency of Organ Involvement in 41 Systemic Tumors

TUMOR	NUMBER OF CASES	LIVER	KIDNEY	LUNG	DIGESTIVE TRACT	BONE	PLEURA	HEART	DIAPHRAGM	ADRENALS	PANCREAS	GENITAL ORGANS	PERICARDIUM	PERITONEUM	BRAIN	MENINGES	THYROID
Lymphoma	28	14	11	12	9	7	4	4	6	3	3	2	4	4	3	2	2
Leukemia	11	10	7	5	2	2	2	2	—	3	2	3	—	—	—	1	1
Multiple myeloma	2	—	—	—	—	—	—	—	—	—	—	—	—	—	—	—	—
Total	41	24	18	17	11	9	6	6	6	6	5	5	4	4	3	3	3

(Brandt et al.[343])

frequency of metastases in organs usually considered as rarely involved becomes apparent. In 241 consecutive autopsies of malignant tumors excluding brain neoplasms, González, *et al.* found 17.9 per cent of involvement of heart and/or pericardium,[344] and Arenas, in an analysis of 625 autopsies of cancer cases, found 4.1 per cent with metastatic involvement of the spleen.[345]

F. TRANSPLANTATION OF TUMORS

Tissue transplantation was discussed in Chapter III, where reference was made to a series of principles and facts that hold for both nonneoplastic and tumor tissues. In the case of tumor transplantation, however, results are especially interesting because they reveal a series of facts related to their metastasizing ability and to their prognosis. According to Shimkin,[346] the first description of a heterologous tumor transplant (man to dog) was made by Novinsky in 1887. Isolated reports continued to appear sporadically, but not until 1938, when Greene published his first results with a case of carcinoma of the breast,[347] did research in tumor transplantation begin to gain in importance. At present it is one of the most intensely studied fields in experimental oncology. Almost all types of human tumors have been transplanted to animals varying from mice to monkey, and the characteristics of failures are as important as those of successes. Not only do human tumors grow in animals, but also spontaneous or carcinogen-induced tumors may be homo- or heterotransplanted, which is an excellent research tool. Some of the most important data taken from the excellent paper by Greene[348] are as follows:

(1) No morphologic differences have been observed between transplantable and nontransplantable human tumors; both may have the same degree of differentiation, the same number of mitoses, etc. The only important difference is not related to the tumor itself, but to the amount of accompanying stroma, which when very abundant or very scarce may make transplantation difficult or impossible. There seems to be an optimal amount of stroma for transplantation, which may be responsible for failure either by excess (as in scirrhous carcinomas) or by defect.

(2) Once the tumor has "taken" the speed of growth is more or less uniform, but pregnancy, starvation and other conditions may stop it; the time elapsing between inoculation and onset of growth is variable and cannot be predicted from morphology.

(3) After transplantation, tumors usually tend to preserve their morphology, and when they change it is to become better differentiated, which phenomenon has been used for diagnosing otherwise highly undifferentiated neoplasms.[349]

(4) Transplantability is closely related to prognosis; 93.8 per cent of the patients from whom it was possible to transplant tumors died, whereas 79.3 per cent of those from whom transplantation was not possible survived.

(5) Transplantability is related to average survival; in the same series, patients with tumors "taking" in heterotransplantation survived an average of 6.4 months, while average survival of patients with nontransplantable tumors was 39.2 months.

(6) In some cases it was shown that, although on first inoculation the tumor

failed to "take," ulterior experiments were successful and these patients eventually succumbed to their disease.

(7) In relation to metastasis, patients without clinical and/or laboratory evidence of secondary growths had positive transplants in only 28.8 per cent; those with regional lymphatic involvement were transplanted successfully in 39.0 per cent; the group with distant lymphatic metastasis gave 88.8 per cent of positive "takes," and the tumors of patients with hematogenous dissemination were transplantable in 100 per cent of the cases.

Greene's results have been extensively quoted because they clearly show the relation between the biology of the tumor and its capacity to grow in a heterologous host and the interaction existing between host and tumor. Indeed, they are reminiscent of the separation mentioned in Section II of this chapter, where tumors were considered as either dependent or autonomous. A dependent tumor is susceptible to the defenses of the host, which may be artificially decreased by means of ionizing radiation, cortisone, blocking of the properdin system, etc.;[350] the result of conditioning the host is that dependent tumors will gain the ability to grow in it. On the other hand, autonomous neoplasms require no conditioning to "take" in homo- or heterotransplantation, and this capacity has been shown to parallel their ability to metastasize. That a positive or negative "take" in tumor transplantation depends both on the tumor and the host is a most important theoretical finding which may throw much light on the biology of neoplasms and may even prove of significance in a more rational treatment, since increasing the resistance of the host is one way to limit tumor growth.

Some preliminary work published by Southam, et al.[351, 352] may have some bearing on the problem of host resistance in cancer. These authors transplanted human tumors to volunteers, both normal and cancerous, and observed that in normal subjects tumor cells grew for several days but disappeared at the end of 4 weeks, while of 14 cancer patients with tumor homotransplants 4 showed local recurrence after biopsy and progressive growth of tumor nodules. The possible relation of these results to the existence of general constitutional factors must await further studies.

VI. DIAGNOSIS

In this section no attempt is made to present a comprehensive discussion of the different methods available for the diagnosis of tumors; such presentation is outside the scope of this book and can be found in specialized works.[9, 11, 12] Some remarks on various selected aspects of the microscopic diagnosis of tumors by biopsy and by exfoliative cytology, as well as on the pathologic study of resected tumor specimens, may well serve to round off the general biologic concept of neoplasms, the presentation of which is the aim of this chapter.

A. BIOPSY

Biopsy means literally "study *in vivo*," but common usage has identified this word with the surgical operation required to obtain the tissue, or with the tissue fragment itself. The purpose of a biopsy, whether it is used in a patient with a tumor or with any other form of disease, is to provide histopathologic evidence of the nature of the patient's illness. In a thoughtful paper, Wartman[353] has pointed out that when biopsy was first proposed in the middle of the nineteenth century it was hailed as a great medical discovery; with accumulating experience the limitations of the procedure became apparent and for some time it fell into disrepute. Even Virchow[354] opposed the use of biopsies for the diagnosis of tumors "and his opposition naturally became harder after his misdiagnosis of the Kaiser's laryngeal cancer." But this reaction was soon overcome and early in this century the biopsy was established as a useful diagnostic procedure. Today the accuracy and reliability of diagnoses established by this means are widely accepted and there is even some unconscious tendency to end all discussions on difficult cases after they have been "proved by biopsy."

Objective analysis of the validity of biopsy diagnosis in different fields is badly needed, as revealed by the disturbing results of Siegler's study.[355] He submitted 20 slides of cervical biopsies to 25 different pathologists without their having any knowledge of the patient or of the nature of the biopsy. In this study there was no slide about which there was complete agreement by all pathologists; of course, the study was set up in such a way as to almost assure the result, since this is one of the most subjective areas of today's pathology and no information was given to the participants. In other fields where objective criteria of diagnosis are better defined and more widely accepted, and with all clinical information available, the result would be obviously quite different. Indeed, Shea's rigorous analysis of the consistency of microscopic diagnosis of liver hyalin shows that when criteria are objectively defined several observers can agree both with themselves in several tests, as well as with each other.[356]

There are several procedures used to obtain tissue for the microscopic study of tumors, and the selection of each one will depend on the conditions of the tumor, the experience of surgeon and pathologist with each one of the procedures and the time available for study.[357]

1. Types of Biopsies. The different methods for obtaining tissue for microscopic study can be summarized as follows: (1) incisional biopsy, (2) excisional biopsy, (3) aspiration biopsy and (4) quick or "frozen" section.

a. Incisional Biopsy. This method consists of the removal of a portion of the lesion, usually with a margin of healthy tissue. It should not be performed with the electric knife, especially when the fragment to be obtained is very small, because heat distorts cells beyond any possibility of recognition; if bleeding is expected it should be stopped after the biopsy has been obtained. Besides esthetic considerations, there is no reason to use this technique in small lesions which should be removed entirely. Although complications of biopsies are discussed below, it must be emphasized that the only possible contraindication of incisional biopsy seems to be large, non-ulcerated malignant melanomas because of the possibility of causing dissemination. Care should be exercised to obtain the fragment away from necrotic and/or infected areas of the tumor, where the structure is distorted and the diagnosis is more difficult to establish.

b. Aspiration Biopsy. This type of biopsy is very popular with experienced practitioners in some centers;[358] it consists of the removal of a cylinder of tumor tissue by means of a needle introduced within the tumor mass.[359] The needle may be very fine, or else a thick trocar can be used (punch biopsy); the main indications for this procedure seem to be those cases where no other type of biopsy is possible because of the condition of the patient, the number of patients examined or the location of the tumor. In some cases no formed tissue is obtained but only serosanguineous fluid, which is also useful for diagnosis since a smear may be prepared with it. Since it is less elaborate than incisional or excisional methods, it has the added advantage that it can be performed in the office and repeated more easily and with less discomfort for the patient in case of failure. The main disadvantages are that it is a blind technique, and that microscopic interpretation requires extensive experience. But the latter, which can be said of any other method, should not be construed as a criticism but only as a warning against overconfidence in diagnosis.

c. Excisional Biopsy. This is the procedure of choice in small lesions and consists in complete removal of the entire lesion with an adequate margin of healthy tissues; the latter is very important, since it is preferable to give a wide margin than to leave tumor cells in the margins of the excision.

d. Quick or "Frozen" Section. Introduced by William H. Welch, the rapid examination of the histologic characteristics of a tumor during surgical intervention is a widely used technique. The one and only indication for this procedure is to aid in the decision as to the type of surgery that will be carried out in a given patient, whether it be by diagnosing an obscure lesion or by determining the presence or absence of malignant cells in the margins of an excision. It should not be requested by the surgeon, nor carried out by the pathologist to satisfy the curiosity of any member of the team in charge of the patient, since it involves a risk of mistake and no harm is done by waiting a few more hours until definitive sections are obtained. In experienced hands, sectioning and staining of tissue fragments should take no more than a few minutes and the interpretation, since it should be based on the recognition of definite structures, is also very rapid; as many sections should be prepared as necessary to remove any possible vestige of doubt in the histologic diagnosis. Uncertainty as to the nature of the lesion, of whatever remote nature, should preclude the establishment of a diagnosis since it carries definite therapeutic implications which no amount of repentance can undo.

Success in any of the different types of biopsy described depends mainly on three fundamental factors, namely the selection of an adequate fragment, the histologic interpretation by an experienced and responsible pathologist and the closest collaboration between clinician and pathologist. Not very often is the pathologist called upon to decide the particular site from which the specimen should be obtained for microscopic study, so the responsibility rests with the clinician to remove tissue with changes representative of the lesion; frequently, the entire procedure fails simply because the tissue obtained did not include the lesion or shows too much necrosis and/or inflammation. On the other hand, when the specimen is large as many blocks should be obtained for microscopic study as may be necessary to render a satisfactory diagnosis; it is not enough to take a biopsy of the biopsy, which may not show important features of the lesion and may even fail to include it.

It has been mentioned that the pathologist should be experienced and responsible. Experience is necessary in order to recognize the many different microscopic aspects of tumors in small fragments of tissue, to request and actually perform when necessary as many special stains as the case may demand to clarify the diagnosis, etc. Responsibility is measured by the number of times and the assuredness with which the pathologist will say, "I don't know" instead of hiding his ignorance in obscure verbalisms or ambiguous statements. It is easier to be dogmatic than to be right, but cancers are not easy to fool and will usually refuse to cooperate with clumsy or dishonest diagnosis. There is almost no need to emphasize that the closer the collaboration between the clinician and the pathologist the more accurate the diagnosis and, therefore, the more benefit accrued to the patient, which is precisely the goal of the entire procedure.

B. HISTOLOGIC DIAGNOSIS OF CANCER

The histologic diagnosis of cancer is more than just a name indicating histogenesis and probable behavior; it suggests treatment and implies prognosis of the individual case and will influence the treatment of many more future patients since such diagnoses will become one of the "facts" deciding the frequency and curability of different types of tumors.[360] The histologic diagnosis of neoplasms is the best of all available diagnoses, but by no means is an absolute truth, since personal factors are involved which qualify all procedures requiring human experience and which, therefore, are subject to error. To minimize this error it is necessary to interpret the histologic features together with the entire clinical picture of the patient. The time when this correlation is carried out varies according to different practices, since some pathologists prefer to have the clinical information available before the slides are examined, while others believe that microscopic analysis should be entirely objective and once a conclusion has been reached the clinical information should then be brought to bear on it. In either case, the final idea should be the result of a combined and objective weighing of all factors and not a brilliant (but often wrong) microscopic guess; according to Ackerman, "The pathologist can make enough errors with all available information without trying to be dramatic."[361]

In addition to diagnosing the tumor, the pathologist is frequently requested to provide additional information on several features of the neoplasm, namely a semiquantitative estimate of the degree of differentiation which is supposedly correlated with prognosis, a definite statement as to radiosensitivity and, in case of a nonneoplastic or benign condition, the likelihood of its developing into a malignant tumor. A brief discussion of each one of these three points may help to dispel some widely held but mistaken ideas.

1. Grading of Tumors. Using the concept of anaplasia proclaimed by von Hansemann in 1890 (p. 155), Broders suggested a method of establishing the histologic grade of malignancy of tumors and, through it, of gaining a more or less exact idea of the prognosis.[362] This method consists of grading tumors ". . . according to differentiation and mitoses, with special emphasis on differentiation." Four grades were defined. The first or grade I included those tumors showing poor differentiation in 25 per cent of the cells and the remaining 75 per cent well differentiated; grade II had equal numbers of well differentiated and undifferentiated cells; grade III showed 75 per cent of the cells in a state of poor differentiation; grade IV had more than 75 per cent of the cells in the same condition. In his study of 537 epidermoid carcinomas of the lower lip, Broders[362] found that no grade I tumor caused the death of the patient, that 54.9 per cent with grade II carcinomas died as a consequence of this disease, that 84.21 per cent of the patients with grade III neoplasms were killed by their tumor, and that 100 per cent of the patients with grade IV carcinomas died as a consequence of the malignant tumor. In addition, while no patient with grade I carcinoma showed metastases, 91.66 per cent of those with grade IV tumors had disseminated disease. In many additional papers Broders extended his method to tumors of the skin, genitourinary tract, head and neck, rectum, esophagus, etc.[11]

The main tenets of histologic grading were summarized by Goyanna, et al.[363] as follows: (1) the degree of anaplasia may be determined by histologic study; (2) with variable and practically insignificant exceptions, the grade of malignancy is the same throughout the tumor; (3) as a general rule, a tumor preserves the same grade of malignancy throughout all phases of its evolution, its metastases and recurrences; (4) prognosis is directly related to the histologic grade of malignancy. This last tenet was so certain for Broders that in 1925 he wrote, "The day is not far when not only the physician but also the patient and his family, as well as insurance companies, will be interested in the grade of malignancy of cancer."[364]

Broders' ideas gained rapid popularity and even today there are clinicians requesting (and pathologists providing) histologic grading as a means of learning the prognosis of tumors; criticisms were not wanting, which would be unnecessary to repeat here.[365, 366] Suffice it to say that the four basic tenets or postulates of this method are either inexact or simply wrong, but very especially the last one, which holds that prognosis is closely correlated with the degree of anaplasia of the tumor. Similar methods were also proclaimed, with groups and with various pseudo-objective criteria. An extreme example was Hueper's "histologic malignogram,"[367] based on 20 well defined histologic characteristics such as the special type of cancer, the nucleo-cytoplasmic ratio, the irregularity in the size of cells, etc. It may be mentioned in passing that once this "malignogram" was determined, it was to be compared with a "clinical index of malignancy" of equally complex elaboration.

What can be said now, 40 years after histologic grading was proclaimed? Indeed, it was a brave attempt to give semiquantitative expression to a series of histologic observations made by all pathologists. It may be dangerous to replace an estimate of anaplasia by an integer which says little or nothing of the individual case, and what is even worse, the grade of malignancy of the sample may be taken for that of the whole tumor. Furthermore, anaplasia or undifferentiation has no well defined criteria and to replace it by a figure may give the false impression of uniformity and objectivity, when actually subjective and highly personal intuitions are involved. The immediate success of Broders' method was due to the fact that it was believed to be an easy and simple way to determine the prognosis of tumors. At that time it was an important contribution to pathology, but greater experience and better knowledge have revealed that there is no easy and simple way to establish the prognosis in tumors. Indeed, there is not even a single difficult and complicated way to do it with reasonable success in all cases. Prognosis is the result of *all* factors present in a given cancer patient: age, sex, nutritional status, nature, size and location of tumor, presence

Table 24. Radiosensitivity of Normal Tissues

Bone marrow	More sensitive
Reproductive tissue	
Alimentary tract	
Skin	
Connective tissue	
Bone	
Glandular tissue	
Kidney	
Muscle	
Nervous tissue	Least sensitive

or absence of metastasis, number of lymph nodes involved, form of treatment, result, etc. In each type of tumor factors important in prognosis are legion and should be learned for each clinicopathologic entity; instances involving almost any tumor might be quoted, but the following example should suffice to illustrate the complexity of the problem. Two women have epidermoid carcinoma of the uterine cervix with the same histologic grade of malignancy. The first patient shows a tumor limited to the uterus, without any invasion or infection, has a good nutritional status, accepts and follows treatment regularly and returns to periodic consultation. The second patient has a lesion with ureteral compression, bilateral hydroureter and hydronephrosis, anemia and poor nutritional status, extensive necrosis and infection of the tumor mass, lymphatic and distant metastases, refuses treatment or is following it in a very irregular manner. Obviously the prognosis of these two patients will be different, in spite of having identical histologic grades of malignancy. When grading is practiced *en lieu* of a thorough clinical and laboratory examination, and prognosis is established in ignorance of all the other factors mentioned, it becomes a pernicious and dangerous habit; if, on the other hand, histologic grading is simply one more of the complex of phenomena which are weighed together to reach an idea of prognosis, it becomes a minor item of secondary, if any, significance.

2. Radiosensitivity. It should be mentioned at the outset of this discussion that the histologic features are no indication of the type of response to radiotherapy that can be expected from a given tumor. The pathologist can say when a tumor is or is not radiosensitive for the same reasons as the clinician and the radiotherapist: because

similar tumors have been radiated and their responses have been observed. It is the experience accumulated after radiating many cases of the same histologic type of tumor that reveals whether a similar neoplasm will respond or not to radiotherapy; a tumor with a new or infrequent histologic aspect must be treated before anything can be said about the results of radiation.

That the radiosensitivity of cells varies in inverse relation to their degree of differentiation was established in 1908 by Bergonie and Tribondeau;[369] i.e., the more undifferentiated the cell the more radiosensitive. Table 24 shows the radiosensitivity of normal tissues,[370] which follows Bergonie and Tribondeau's rule; a classification of tumors according to radiosensitivity given by Warren,[371] however, reveals that their distribution follows no rule and is rather capricious (Table 25). In an extensive and valuable review of the radiosensitivity of tumors, Stewart[372] points out, among others, the following significant facts: "Certain tumors seem to exhibit inherent qualities of radioresistance, . . . as, for example, in the neurosarcoma, glioma and melanoma groups." He also shows that radiosensitivity increases with the embryonal quality of tumors and higher degrees of anaplasia; infection interferes with the normal response to radiation; desmoplastic tumors are frequently radioresistant; the tumor bed is of great significance; metastatic tumors in lymph nodes may be more or less radiosensitive than primary neoplasms, and tumors of large size may become radioresistant after infarction and liquefaction, though belonging to usually radiosensitive types. Stewart's statements serve to emphasize that there are many factors participating in the response of a tumor to radiation, and that some of them are not apparent on histologic examination.

There are several types of well defined responses to radiation in tumors. *Radiocurability* is the property of some tumors to be destroyed or controlled by radiation, and this characteristic bears no relation to *radiosensitivity,* which is the susceptibility of a given tumor to radiation when compared to another. Radioresistance is the reverse of any of the two concepts previously mentioned, so that when reference is made

Table 25.   Radiosensitivity of Human Tumors

GROUP I	GROUP II	GROUP III
(Sensitive tumors: disappearance of tumors with doses lesser than 2500 r; normal tissues unaffected)	(Intermediate tumors: regression with doses of 2500 to 5000 r.)	(Resistant tumors: more than 5000 r with irreversible changes in normal tissues)
Lymphosarcoma	Basal cell carcinoma	Carcinoma of the breast
Lymphoepithelioma	Some epidermoid carcinomas	Carcinoma of the stomach
Ewing's sarcoma	of the skin and uterine	Osteogenic sarcoma
Chronic leukemia	cervix	Chondrosarcoma
Some parotid tumors	Carcinoma of the thyroid	Malignant melanoma

(From Warren[271])

to radioresistance it is necessary to specify if it is in relation to curability and/or sensitivity. These three types of response to radiation are relative and require further study.

3. Precancerous Lesions. According to Ewing,[373] precancerous lesions are those preceding and favoring the development of cancer, but without possessing the essential elements of the cancerous process. Again it must be pointed out that there is nothing in the histologic picture of these lesions that will permit predicting which one is "preceding and favoring the development of cancer"; it is the ulterior development of similar lesions that is brought to mind when such a prediction is made. Precancerous lesions have very little in common; Table 26 gives a list of diseases considered as precancerous, together with another list of conditions wrongly presumed at one time or another to precede the formation of tumors. The concept of precancerous lesion is purely statistical; it is true that most precancerous lesions are proliferative in nature,

but there are many other lesions, even more proliferative, which are not precancerous.[374] Once the statistical relation has been established by observing the behavior of different lesions, the microscopic diagnosis will serve to decide whether they are or are not precancerous, but not because of any peculiar histologic markings.

C. COMPLICATIONS OF BIOPSY

There are two theoretical complications of biopsy: the seeding of tumor cells in normal tissues along the path of incision or along a needle tract, and metastatic dissemination aided by the opening of lymphatic and blood vessels within the tumor mass at the time of obtaining the fragment. Both complications have been shown to occur and should be taken into account when deciding what procedure is to be followed in a given patient, but it should be emphasized that much more damage is done by avoiding the biopsy and treating patients on the basis of clinical impressions than by performing it carefully and guiding therapy

Table 26.

PRECANCEROUS LESIONS	NONPRECANCEROUS LESIONS
Arsenic dermatitis	Fibroadenoma of the breast
Xeroderma pigmentosum	Chronic cystic disease of the breast
Senile keratosis	Intraductal papilloma of the breast
Radiodermatitis	Paget's disease of the nipple
Chronic ulcers (varicose, Marjolin's)	Gastric or duodenal peptic ulcer
Plummer-Vinson syndrome	Queyrat's erythroplasia
Leukoplakia	Carcinoma *in situ*
Gastric and colonic polyposis	Benign tumors in general
Cholelithiasis	Jadassohn-Tieche nevus
Cirrhosis of the liver (postnecrotic, hemochromatosis)	Bowen's disease
Multiple cartilaginous exostoses	
Dermoepidermal nevi	
Paget's disease of bone	

by its result. Ackerman and Myron[375] observed the presence of tumor nodules in the needle tract of aspiration biopsies but other authors with a great deal of experience in this type of procedure have not encountered this complication.[376] Incisional biopsy has been cited as a cause of metastatic dissemination, but this has been more on the basis of arm-chair theorizing than on objective evidence; the latter is very difficult to obtain since blood-borne metastases cannot be ruled out with clinical and radiologic examinations. Some time ago Wood[377] submitted the suggestion that incisional biopsy increases the risk of metastasis to experimental examination by transplanting a tumor to a group of animals and performing biopsies in one half of them; when the entire group was sacrificed no differences were found in the incidence of metastases. In a series of 300 cases of carcinoma of the breast examined by Lockhart and Ackerman incisional biopsy was not correlated with a larger number of metastases.[378] Instances of this type of work cannot be multiplied because the logical possibility has been confused with reality, and also because nobody would like to do the experiment with patients. The absence of evidence, however, is no proof that biopsy increases the danger of metastases. Probably the best attitude is to perform a biopsy and proceed with treatment as soon as possible, as suggested by Greenough for tumors of the breast.[379]

D. EXFOLIATIVE CYTOLOGY

The presence of desquamated malignant cells in the different secretions of the body has been known and used for diagnosis for many years. According to Bamforth and Osborn,[380] clear descriptions and illustrations of cancer cells in the urine of women with advanced carcinoma of the uterine cervix were published by Beale in 1854, although he was still opposed to Virchow's cell theory. Other isolated efforts were made in different parts of the world, but the definite introduction of exfoliative cytology as a useful diagnostic tool in oncology is the contribution of George Papanicolaou, whose interest in cytology arose from a study of the cyclic changes in endometrium of guinea pigs. In 1923 Papanicolaou extended his animal studies to women and before long

realized that he could recognize cancer cells; this "new cancer diagnosis" technique appeared in print in 1928,[381] but was unfortunately ignored or considered superfluous. More intense work of Papanicolaou with Traut ended in the publication in 1943 of their monograph "Diagnosis of Uterine Cancer by the Vaginal Smear,"[382] which marks the true beginning of world-wide acceptance of the method, despite some bitter but brief opposition by many pathologists. Cytologic diagnosis of cancer is no doubt the greatest advance in oncology in the last decade, and this form of study has been finding new fields of use other than diagnosis, such as follow-up of treated patients, determination of radiosensitivity and/or radiation response, etc.

It should be remembered that biopsy diagnosis remains the ultimate criterion for establishing the diagnosis of cancer. Any technique suggested as alternative for biopsy must be at least as accurate, reproducible and simple in execution, and have some additional and definite advantages over the biopsy; exfoliative cytology meets all these requirements.[383] Accuracy and reproducibility have been shown in many studies, but the one reported by Graham, et al.[384] may be cited; in 181 cases of carcinoma of the uterine cervix the biopsy was positive in 90 per cent, cytology in 91 per cent and both methods combined in 99 per cent of the cases. Accuracy is not so high in other areas of the organism, but for sputum it has been reported to be 80 per cent,[385] for stomach 50 per cent,[386] for urine 61 per cent,[387] etc. The advantages of exfoliative cytology are as follows: (1) it is a simple and painless office procedure; (2) it is relatively rapid and results may be obtained in the same day; (3) it is inexpensive; (4) it can be repeated as often as necessary without harm to the patient; (5) it permits diagnosis in very early stages of neoplastic growth, including carcinoma *in situ*; (6) it is useful for screening large groups of patients; (7) it does not conflict with other established diagnostic procedures. Perhaps the main disadvantage of this technique is that it requires specialized training, but since this is true of any other human activity it can be discarded as the last of the ill-aimed criticisms made by those pathologists who found it hard to learn a new method. In relation to its role in cancer diagnosis, Bamforth and Osborn[380] remark that, "It is only one way of looking at a diagnostic problem, but when correlated with other diagnostic methods it is always interesting and often of the greatest value, and may lead to the correct diagnosis of cancer when inspection and biopsy fail. . . . If cytology reveals some of the limitations of inspection and biopsy,

these in their turn reveal some of the limitations of cytology, and most diagnoses are made when all methods are used."

Cytologic smears are reported according to different usages and nomenclatures; Papanicolaou[388] devised one in five groups which is quite elaborate, whereas in many other laboratories they are simply classified as "positive," "negative" and "suspicious," the last category indicating that more smears

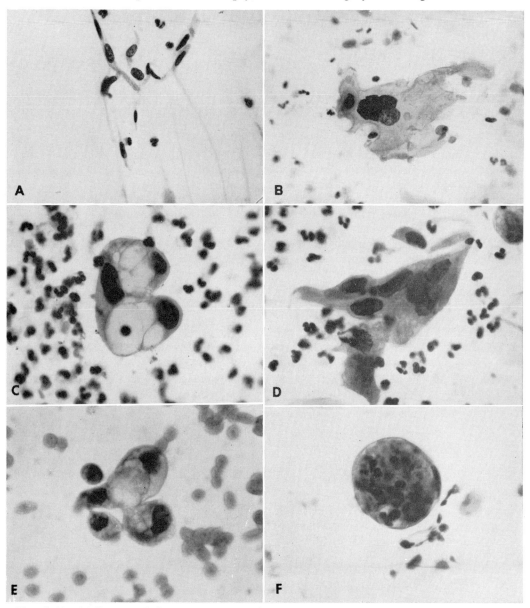

FIG. 5–49.   Malignant cells in smears. *A*, "Fibroid" cells in epidermoid carcinoma of the uterine cervix. *B*, Large epithelial cell with irregular, lobulated and hyperchromatic nucleus in epidermoid carcinoma of uterine cervix. *C*, Adenocarcinoma of the lung. *D*, Epidermoid carcinoma of the lung. *E*, Adenocarcinoma of the endometrium. *F*, A clump of malignant cells in undifferentiated carcinoma of the lung.

would be desirable before rendering a definite opinion. A negative report is no proof that the patient has no cancer; it simply means that no cells with the characteristics usually identified with malignancy have been observed. Of course, the cells may be there and be missed or confused by the observer, or else no desquamation occurred at the time the specimen was obtained; in both cases the result is falsely negative and is an important index of accuracy. On the other hand, abnormal but benign cells may be mistaken for malignant elements and this is a "false positive" report. These two types of errors make up no more than 5 to 10 per cent of all reports in many series of vaginal or sputum smears, but are larger with other fluids such as urine, gastric washings, mammary secretion, etc.

Recognition of tumor cells is entirely based on morphology, since mitoses are only rarely observed in smears. Structural changes identified with malignancy are mainly nuclear and may appear as irregularities in size and shape, hyperchromatism and loss of nucleo-cytoplasmic ratio; some special cells have been described as being suggestive of different histologic types of tumors, such as carcinoma in situ,[389] epidermoid carcinoma, adenocarcinoma, etc. (Fig. 5–49). Cytologic "typing" is being practiced in some centers with surprising accuracy[390] and its usefulness is based on the belief that different histologic types are indicative of differences in prognosis; if this is true it only applies to very large series of cases and has little or no significance for the individual patient.

E. THE STUDY OF THE SURGICAL SPECIMEN

Once a tumor has been removed the specimen should be examined by a pathologist in such a way that at the end of his study all data of any significance for prognosis are available. They include the histology, extension of the tumor, presence or absence of neoplastic cells in the margins of excision and/or within lymphatics and blood vessels, metastases in lymph nodes with careful description of number and location, etc. This requires a detailed dissection according to preestablished methods which should be modified following the needs of individual cases. It is convenient to use diagrams of the surgical specimens and mark with conventional signs all positive and negative findings. Anatomic features of prognostic significance vary in different tumors. For instance, the level of invasion of axillary lymph nodes in radical mastectomy specimens has been shown by Berg[391] to be important in statistical analysis of large series, since the lowest level has approximately the same five year survival as the complete absence of metastatic nodes. Histologic grading bears relation to prognosis in giant cell tumors of bone.[392] The depth of invasion of the wall of the urinary bladder in carcinomas of this organ appears as the single most important factor in determining length of survival.[393] Duke has shown that the same holds true for carcinoma of the colon.[394] Capsular invasion and vascular penetration are significant in carcinoma of the kidney, etc. Although some techniques have been devised to increase the yield of lymph nodes dissected in surgical specimens, nothing is more valuable than the care and interest of the pathologist who knows the significance of his work. A rapid and superficial dissection with only a few blocks taken for microscopic study may create in the surgeon a false impression of complete removal and may destroy the opportunity for adequate, additional treatment for the patient. The pathologist's responsibility in diagnosing cancer and in studying the surgical specimen goes beyond the labeling of small bits of tissue; he should be conscious that his is an aspect of the practice of medicine that may be more important for the welfare of the patient than the surgeon's scalpel or the radiotherapist's x-ray tube.

REFERENCES

1. Rusch, H. P.: Carcinogenesis: a facet of living processes. Cancer Res. *14:*407, 1954.
2. Payling Wright, G.: Introduction to Pathology, ed. 2, London, Longmans and Greene, 1956.
3. Florey, H. W. (ed.): General Pathology (Chapters 21 to 26), ed. 2, Philadelphia, W. B. Saunders, 1958.
4. Cowdry, E. V.: Cancer Cells, Philadelphia, W. B. Saunders, 1955.
5. Willis, R. A.: Principles of Pathology, London, Butterworth, 1950.
6. Mellors, R. C.: Cancer, in Mellors, R. C. (ed.): Analytical Pathology, New York, Blakiston, 1957.

7. Homburger, F.: The Biologic Basis of Cancer Management, New York, Hoeber and Harper, 1957.
8. Homburger, F. (ed.): The Physiopathology of Cancer, New York, Hoeber and Harper, 1959.
9. Ackerman, L. V., and del Regato, J. A.: Cancer. Diagnosis, Treatment and Prognosis, ed. 2, St. Louis, C. V. Mosby, 1954.
10. Willis, R. A.: Pathology of Tumors, ed. 2, London, Butterworth, 1953.
11. Pack, G. T., and Ariel, I. M.: The Treatment of Cancer and Allied Disease, ed. 2, New York, Hoeber, 1958.
12. Raven, R. W. (ed.): Cancer, London, Butterworth, 1957.
13. Greenstein, J. P., and Haddow, A.: Advances in Cancer Research, New York, Academic Press, 1953–56.
14. Clark, R. L., Jr., and Cumley, R. W. (eds.): Year Book of Cancer, Chicago, Year Book Publishers, 1956–59.
15. Excerpta Medica. Section on Oncology (IX), Excerpta Med., Holland.
16. Cancer, A Journal of the American Cancer Society, Stewart, F. (ed.): Philadelphia, J. B. Lippincott.
17. Bayne-Jones, S., Harrison, R. G., Little, C. C., Northrop, J., and Murphy, J. B.: Fundamental cancer research, Publ. Health Rep. 53:2121, 1930.
18. Berenblum, I.: The Nature of Tumor Growth, in Florey, H. W. (ed.): General Pathology, ed. 2, Philadelphia, W. B. Saunders, 1958.
19. Harris, H.: Cell Growth and Multiplication, in Florey, H. W. (ed.): General Pathology, ed. 2, Philadelphia, W. B. Saunders, 1958.
20. Anderson, W. A. D. (ed.): Pathology, ed. 3, St. Louis, C. V. Mosby, 1956.
21. Boyd, W.: Textbook of Pathology, ed. 5, Philadelphia, Lea and Febiger, 1948.
22. Robbins, S. L.: Textbook of Pathology, Philadelphia, W. B. Saunders, 1957.
23. Smith, E. B., Beamer, P. R., Vellios, F., and Schulz, D. M.: Principles of Human Pathology, New York, Oxford University Press, 1959.
24. Cushing, H., and Wolbach, S. B.: Transformation of malignant paravertebral sympathicoblastoma into benign ganglioneuroma, Am. J. Path. 3:203, 1927.
25. Fox, F., Davidson, J., and Thomas, L. B.: Maturation of sympathicoblastoma into ganglioneuroma, Cancer 12:108, 1959.
26. Bergman, M., Ackerman, L. V., and Kemler, R. L.: Carcinosarcoma of the lung, Cancer 4:919, 1951.
27. Gore, I., and Barr, R.: Metastasis of cancer to cancer, Arch. Path. 66:293, 1958.
28. Willis, R. A.: Teratomas, Washington, D.C., A. F. I. P., 1954.
29. Albrecht, E.: Ueber Hamartome, Verhandl. deutsch. path. Gesellsch. 7:153, 1904.
30. Pott, P.: The Chirurgical Works of Percival Pott, London, J. Williams, 1788.
31. Blum, H. F.: Sunlight as a causal factor in cancer of the skin in man, J. Nat. Cancer Inst. 9:247, 1948.
32. Blum, H. G.: On the mechanism of cancer induction by ultraviolet radiation, J. Nat. Cancer Inst. 11:463, 1950.
33. Blum, H. F.: Carcinogenesis by Ultraviolet Light, Princeton, Princeton University Press, 1959.
34. Kline, B. E., and Baumann, C. A.: Carcinogenesis by ultraviolet rays with reference to wavelength and energy, Arch. Path. 31:135, 1941.
35. Tullis, J. L.: Delayed effects of ionizing radiation in man, Arch. Path. 66:403, 1958.
36. Frieben: Abstract in "Vereine und Kongresse," Fortschr. Roentgen, 6:106, 1902.
37. Furth, J., and Lorenz, E.: Carcinogenesis by ionizing radiations, in Hollaender, A. (ed.): Radiation Biology, New York, McGraw-Hill, 1954.
38. Brues, A. M.: Radiation as a carcinogenic agent, Radiation Res. 3:272, 1955.
39. Dunlap, C. E., Aub., J. C., Evans, R. D., and Harris, R. S.: Transplantable osteogenic sarcomas induced in rats by feeding radium, Am. J. Path. 20:1, 1944.
40. Morgan, A. D., Jayne, W. H. W., and Marrack, D.: Primary liver cell carcinoma 24 years after intravenous injection of thorotrast, J. Clin. Path. 11:7, 1958.
41. Martland, H. S.: The occurrence of malignancy in radioactive persons, Am. J. Cancer 15:2435, 1931.
42. Woglom, W. H.: Chronic inflammation and carcinogenesis, Cancer Res. 5:576, 1945.
43. Yamagiwa, K., and Ichikawa, K.: Experimental study of the pathogenesis of carcinoma, J. Cancer Res. 3:1, 1918.
44. Tsutsui, H.: Artificially-induced cancroids in mouse, Gann 12:17, 1918.
45. Kennaway, E.: The identification of a carcinogenic compound in coal-tar, Brit. M. J. 2:749, 1955.
46. Haddow, A.: Causation of cancer: Introduction, Brit. Med. Bull. 14:73, 1958.
47. Hartwell, J. L.: Survey of Compounds Which Have Been Tested for Carcinogenic Activity, ed. 2, U. S. Public Health Service No. 149: 1951.
48. Haddow, A.: The Chemical and Genetic Mechanisms of Carcinogenesis. I. Nature and mode of action, in Homburger, F. (ed.): Physiopathology of Cancer, ed. 2, New York, Hoeber and Harper, 1959.
49. Price, J. M., Wear, J. V., Brown, R. R., Satter, E. J., and Olson, C.: Studies on etiology of carcinoma of urinary bladder, J. Urol. 83:376, 1960.
50. Bonser, G. M.: Epithelial tumors of the bladder in dogs induced by pure β-naphthylamine, J. Path. & Bact. 55:1, 1943.
51. Neubauer, O.: Arsenical cancer: a review, Brit. J. Cancer 1:193, 1947.
52. Cowdry, E. V., and Paletta, F. X.: Changes in cellular, nuclear and nucleolar sizes during methylcholanthrene epidermal carcinogenesis, J. Nat. Cancer Inst. 1:745, 1941.
53. Haddow, A.: Chemical carcinogens and their modes of action. Brit. M. Bull. 14:79, 1958.
54. Koller, P. C.: Origin of malignant tumor cells, Nature 151:244, 1943.
55. Orr, J. W.: The mechanism of chemical carcinogenesis, Brit. M. Bull. 14:99, 1958.
56. Hueper, W. C.: Occupational bladder cancer, Proceedings of the Second National Cancer Conference 1:361, 1952.
57. Hueper, W. C.: Carcinogens and carcinogenesis, Am. J. Med. 8:355, 1950.
58. Anderson, N. P.: Arsenic as the cause of cancer of mucous membranes, Arch. Dermat. & Syph. 42:647, 1940.
59. Friedenwald, W. F., and Rous, P.: The initiating and promoting elements in tumor production, J. Exper. Med. 80:101, 1954.
60. Hieger, I., and Pullinger, B. D.: Chemical Carcinogenesis, in Hadfield, G. (ed.): Recent Advances in Pathology, London, J. & A. Churchill, 1953.

61. Bryan, W. R., and Shimkin, M. D.: Quantitative analysis of dose-response data obtained with three carcinogenic hydrocarbons in strain C3H male mice, J. Nat. Cancer Inst. *3:*503, 1943.

62. Borrel, A.: Epithélioses infectieuses et épiteliomas, Ann. Inst. Pasteur *17:*81, 1903.

63. Ellerman, V., and Bang, O.: Experimentelle Leukämie bei Huebnern, Zentralbl. Bakt. *46:* 595, 1908.

64. Rous, P.: Transmission of a malignant new growth by means of a cell free filtrate, J.A.M.A. *56:* 198, 1911.

65. Shope, R. E.: A transmissible tumor-like condition in rabbits, J. Exper. Med. *56:*793, 1932.

66. Shope, R. E.: Infectious papillomatosis of rabbits, with a note on histopathology by E. W. Hurst, J. Exper. Med. *58:*607, 1933.

67. Claude, A.: Chemical composition of the tumor-producing fraction of the chicken tumor I., Science *90:*213, 1939.

68. Claude, A., and Rothen, A.: Properties of the causative agent of a chicken tumor. XIV. Relation between a tumor nucleoprotein and the active principle, J. Exper. Med. *71:*619, 1940.

69. Bittner, J. J.: Some possible effects of nursing on the mammary gland tumor incidence in mice, Science *84:*162, 1936.

70. Bittner, J. J.: The genesis of breast cancer in mice, Texas Rep. Biol. & Med. *10:*160, 1952.

71. Müllbock, O.: Mammary tumor agent in the sperm of high-cancer-strain male mice, J. Nat. Cancer Inst. *10:*861, 1950.

72. Dmochowski, L.: The milk agent in the origin of mammary tumors in mice, in Greenstein, J. P., and Haddow, A. (eds.): Advances in Cancer Research *1:*103, 1953.

73. Dmochowski, L.: The part played by viruses in the origin of tumors, in Raven, R. W. (ed.): Cancer, Vol. 1, London, Butterworth, 1957.

74. Strong, R. P.: The role played by helminths in the production of tumors in man and animals, Internat. Clin. *4:*68, 1931.

75. Oberling, C. H.: The Riddle of Cancer, New Haven, Yale University Press, 1952.

76. Koller, P. C.: The genetic component of cancer, in Raven, R. W. (ed.): Cancer, Vol. 1, London, Butterworth, 1957.

77. Heston, W. E.: Localization of gene action in the causation of lung and mammary gland tumors in mice, J. Nat. Cancer Inst. *15:*775, 1954.

78. MacDowell, E. C., Potter, J. S., and Taylor, M. J.: Mouse leukemia. XII. The role of genes in spontaneous cases, Cancer Res. *5:*65, 1945.

79. MacDowell, E. C., and Taylor, M. J.: Mouse leukemia. XIII. A maternal influence that lowers the incidence of spontaneous cases, Proc. Soc. Exper. Biol. & Med. *68:*571, 1948.

80. Law, L. W., and Miller, J. H.: The effect of thymectomy on the incidence, latent period and type of leukemia in the high leukemia strains of mice, Cancer Res. *10:*230, 1950.

81. Kirschbaum, A.: The role of hormones in cancer: laboratory animals, Cancer Res. *17:*432, 1957.

82. Shimkim, M. B.: Hormones and neoplasia, in Raven, R. W. (ed.): Cancer, Vol. 1, London, Butterworth, 1957.

83. Bielschowsky, F., and Horning, E. S.: Aspects of endocrine carcinogenesis, Brit. M. Bull. *14:*106, 1958.

84. Biskind, M. S., and Biskind, G. S.: Development of tumors in the rat ovary after transplantation into the spleen, Proc. Soc. Exper. Biol. & Med. *55:*176, 1944.

85. Biskind, G. R., and Biskind, M. S.: Experimental ovarian tumors in rats, Am. J. Clin. Path. *19:* 501, 1949.

86. Gardner, W. U.: Development and growth of tumors in ovaries transplanted into the spleen, Cancer Res. *15:*109, 1955.

87. Biskind, G. R., Bernstein, D. E., and Gospe, S. M.: The effect of exogenous gonadotrophins on the development of experimental ovarian tumors in rats, Cancer Res. *13:*216, 1953.

88. Cook, J. E., and Haslewood, G. A. D.: The conversion of a bile acid into a hydrocarbon derived from 1:2-benzanthracene, J. Chem. Soc. Ind. *52:*758, 1933.

89. Kennaway, E. L.: The carcinogenic effect of cholesterol, in Raven, R. W. (ed.): Cancer, Vol. 1, London, Butterworth, 1957.

90. Hieger, I.: Carcinogenesis by cholesterol, Brit. J. Cancer *13:*439, 1960.

91. Hieger, I.: Carcinogenic substances in human tissue, Cancer Res. *6:*657, 1946.

92. Steiner, P.: Human significance of experimental carcinogenesis, Arch. Path. *55:*227, 1953.

93. Treves, N., and Pack, G. T.: Development of cancer in burn scars; analysis and report of 34 cases, Surg. Gynec. & Obst. *51:*749, 1930.

94. Bowers, R. F., and Young, J. M.: Carcinoma arising in scars, osteomyelitis, and fistulae, Arch. Surg. *80:*564, 1960.

95. Cannon, B., Randolph, J. G., and Murray, J. E.: Malignant irradiation for benign conditions, New Eng. J. Med. *260:*197, 1959.

96. Totten, R. S., Atypas, P. G., Dupertuis, S. M., Gaisford, J. C., and White, W. L.: Preexisting roentgen-ray dermatitis in patients with skin cancer, Cancer *10:*1024, 1957.

97. Arhelger, S. W., and Kremen, A.: Arsenical epitheliomas of medical origin, Surgery *30:*977, 1951.

98. Kennaway, E. L.: Racial and social incidence of cancer of uterus, Brit. J. Cancer *8:*177, 1948.

99. Wynder, E. L., Cornfield, J., Schroff, P. D., and Doraiswami, K. R.: A study of environmental factors in carcinoma of the cervix, Am. J. Obst. & Gynec. *68:*1016, 1954.

100. Jones, E. G., MacDonald, I., and Breslow, L.: Study of epidemiologic factors in carcinoma of uterine cervix, Am. J. Obst. & Gynec. *76:*1, 1958.

101. Dunn, J. E., Jr., and Buell, P.: Association of cervical cancer with circumcision of sexual partner, J. Nat. Cancer Inst. *22:*749, 1959.

102. Wynder, E. L., Mautel, N., and Licklider, S. D.: Statistical considerations on circumcision and cervical cancer, Am. J. Obst. & Gynec. *79:* 1026, 1960.

103. Furlong, J. H., Jr., and Uhle, C. A. W.: Cancer of penis; report of eighty-eight cases, J. Urol. *69:*550, 1953.

104. Heins, H. C., Jr., Dennis, E. J., and Pratt-Thomas, H. R.: The possible role of smegma in carcinoma of the cervix, Am. J. Obst. & Gynec. *76:*726, 1958.

105. Ahlbom, H. E.: Simple achlorhydric anemia, Plummer-Vinson syndrome, and carcinoma of the mouth, pharynx and esophagus in women, Brit. Med. J. *2:*331, 1936.

106. Wynder, E. L., and Fryer, J. H.: Etiologic considerations of Plummer-Vinson (Patterson-Kelly) syndrome, Ann. Int. Med. *49:*1106, 1958

107. Linvall, N.: Hypopharyngeal carcinoma in sideropenic dysphagia, Acta radiol. *39:*17, 1953.

108. O'Neal, R. M., Taik-Lee, K., and Edwards, D. L.: Bronchogenic carcinoma. An evaluation from autopsy data, with special reference to incidence,

sex ratio, histological type, and accuracy of clinical diagnosis, Cancer *10:*1031, 1957.

109. Weller, C. V.: Causal Factors in Cancer of the Lung, Springfield, Charles C Thomas, 1953.

110. Sikl, H.: The plesent status of knowledge about the Jachmymov disease, Acta Unio internat. contra cancrum *6:*1366, 1960.

111. Evans, R. D.: Quantitative aspects of radiation carcinogenesis in humans, Acta Unio internat. contra Cancrum *6:*1229, 1950.

112. Doll, R.: Etiology of lung cancer, in Greenstein, J. P., and Haddow, A. (eds.): Advances in Cancer Research *3:*1, 1955.

113. Doll, R.: Present Knowledge of the Causation of Carcinoma of the Lung. Atmospheric Pollution, in Bignall, J. R. (ed.): Carcinoma of the Lung, London, E. & S. Livingstone, 1958.

114. Steiner, P. E.: The conditional biological activity of the carcinogens in carbon blacks, and its elimination, Cancer Res. *14:*103, 1954.

115. Doll, R.: Present Knowledge of the Causation of Carcinoma of the Lung. The Smoking of Tobacco, in Bignall, J. R. (ed.): Carcinoma of the Lung, London, E. & S. Livingstone, 1958.

116. Doll, R., and Hill, B.: Lung cancer and other causes of death in relation to smoking: second report on mortality of British doctors, Brit. M. J. *2:*1071, 1956.

117. Hammond, E. C., and Horn, D.: Smoking and death rates. Report on 44 months of follow up of 187,783 men: total mortality, J.A.M.A. *166:*1159, 1958.

118. Hammond, E. C., and Horn, D.: Smoking and death rates. Report on 44 months of follow up of 187,783 men: death rates by cause, J.A.M.A. *166:*1294, 1958.

119. Dorn, H. F.: Tobacco consumption and mortality from cancer and other diseases, Pub. Health Rep. *74:*581, 1959.

120. Auerbach, O., Gere, J. B., Forman, J. B., Petrick, T. G., Smolin, H. J., Muehsam, G. E., Kassouny, D. Y., and Stout, A. P.: Changes in the bronchial epithelium in relation to smoking and cancer of the lung: a report of progress, New Eng. J. Med. *256:*97, 1957.

121. Sanderud, K.: Squamous metaplasia of the respiratory tract epithelium. An autopsy study of 214 cases. 2. Relation to tobacco smoking, occupation and residence. Acta path. et microbiol. Scandinav. *43:*47, 1958.

122. Knudtson, K. R.: The pathologic effects of smoking tobacco on the trachea and bronchial mucosa, Am. J. Clin. Path. *33:*310, 1960.

123. Wynder, E. L., Graham, E. A., and Croninger, A. B.: Experimental production of carcinoma with cigarette tar, Cancer Res. *13:*47, 1958.

124. Engelbreth-Holm, J., and Ahlmann, J.: Production of carcinoma in St/Eh mice with cigarette tar, Acta path. et microbiol. Scandinav. *41:*267, 1957.

125. Gellhorn, A.: Carcinogenic activity of cigarette tobacco tar, Cancer Res. *18:*510, 1958.

126. Wynder, E. L., and Wright, G.: Study of tobacco carcinogenesis: the primary fractions, Cancer *10:*255, 1957.

127. Berkson, J.: Smoking and lung cancer; some observations on two recent reports, J. Am. Stat. Assn. *53:*28, 1958.

128. Little, C. C.: Statement. Ca, Bull. Cancer Progr. *8:*2, 1958.

129. Fisher, R. A.: Lung cancer and cigarettes? Nature *182:*108, 1958.

130. Herdan, G.: Increase in mortality due to cancer of lung in light of distribution of disease among different social classes and occupations, Brit. J. Cancer *12:*492, 1958

131. Bross, I. D. J.: Statistical criticism, Cancer *13:*394, 1960.

132. Joint Report of Study Group on Smoking and Health, Science *125:*1129, 1957.

133. Tobacco smoking and cancer of lung. Statement of British Medical Research Council, Brit. M. J. *1:*1523, 1957.

134. Reif, A. R.: International Cancer Congress, Science *128:*1512, 1958.

135. Burney, L. E.: Smoking and lung cancer. A statement of the Public Health Service, J.A.M.A. *171:*1829, 1959.

136. Davis, D. F.: A review of the evidence on the relationship between smoking and lung cancer, J. Chron. Dis. *11:*579, 1960.

137. Peller, S., and Pick, P.: Leukemia and other malignancies in physicians. Am. J. Med. Sc. *224:*154, 1952.

138. Cronkite, E. P., Moloney, W., and Bond, V. P.: Radiation leukemogenesis. An analysis of the problem, Am. J. Med. *28:*673, 1960.

139. Lewis, E. B.: Leukemia and ionizing radiation, Science *125:*965, 1957.

140. Aub, J. C., Wolbach, S. B., Kennedy, B. J., and Bailey, O. T.: Mycosis fungoides followed for fourteen years, Arch. Path. *60:*535, 1955.

141. Lange, R. D., Moloney, W. C., and Yamawaki, T.: Leukemia in atomic bomb survivors. I. General considerations, Blood *9:*574, 1954.

142. Moloney, W. C., and Kastenbaum, M. A.: Leukemogenic effects of ionizing radiation on atomic bomb survivors in Hiroshima City, Science *121:*308, 1955.

143. Heyssel, R., Brill, B. A., Woodbury, L. A., Nishimura, E. T., Ghose, T., Hoshino, T. and Yamasaki, M.: Leukemia in Hiroshima atomic bomb survivors, Blood *15:*313, 1960.

144. Cobb, S., Miller, M., and Wald, N.: On the estimation of the incubation period in malignant disease, J. Chron. Dis. *9:*385, 1959.

145. Murphy, E. S., and Yasuda, A.: Carcinoma of the stomach in Hiroshima, Japan, Am. J. Path. *34:*531, 1958.

146. Coleman, S. T., and Eckert, C.: Preservation of the rectum in familial polyposis of the colon and rectum, Arch. Surg. *73:*635, 1956.

147. Dukes, C.: Familial intestinal polyposis, Ann. Eugenics *17:*1, 1952.

148. Reese, A. B.: Tumors of the Eye, New York, P. B. Hoeber, 1951.

149. Stout, A. P.: Tumors of the Peripheral Nervous System, Washington, A.F.I.P., 1953.

150. Hosoi, K.: Multiple neurofibromatosis (von Recklinghausen's disease), Arch. Surg. *22:*258, 1931.

151. Jaffe, H. L.: Tumors and Tumorous Conditions of the Bones and Joints, Philadelphia, Lea and Febiger, 1958.

152. Cockayne, E. A.: Inherited Abnormalities of the Skin and its Appendages, London, Oxford University Press, 1933.

153. Koller, P. C.: Inheritance of xeroderma and its chromosome mechanism, Brit. J. Cancer *2:*149, 1948.

154. Warthin, A. S.: The further study of a cancer family, J. Cancer Res. *9:*279, 1925.

155. Lentz, O.: Krebs und Vererbung, Arb. Stat. Inst. exp. Ther., Frankfr. 45, 1947.

156. Schintz, H. R., Cocchi, U., and Neuhaus, J.: Die Vererbung des Krebses bei Menschen, Arch. Klaus. Stift. VererbForsch. *23:*1, 1948.

157. Macklin, M. T.: Inheritance of cancer of the stomach and large intestine in man, J. Nat. Cancer Inst. *24:*551, 1960.

158. Gorer, A.: Cancer, in Clinical Genetics, London, Butterworth, 1953.

159. Macklin, M. T.: Inheritance of cancer in man, Eugenics News *38:*112, 1953.

160. Ewing, J.: Modern attitude toward traumatic cancer, Arch. Path. *19:*690, 1935.

161. Stewart, F. W.: Occupational and post-traumatic cancer, Bull. New York Acad. Med. *23:*145, 1947.

162. Huggins, C., and Scott, W. W.: Bilateral adrenalectomy in prostatic cancer, Am. Surgeon *122:* 1031, 1945.

163. Franks, L. M.: Estrogen treated prostatic cancer. The variation responsiveness of tumor cells, Cancer *13:*490, 1960.

164. Huggins, C.: Control of cancers of man by endocrinologic methods, Cancer Res. *16:*825, 1956.

165. Huggins, C.: Prostatic cancer treated by castration: the five-year results, J.A.M.A. *131:*576, 1946.

166. Huggins, C., and Bergenstal, D. M.: Inhibition of human mammary and prostatic cancers by adrenalectomy, Cancer Res. *12:*134, 1952.

167. MacFarlane, D. A., Thomas, L. P., and Harrison, J. H.: A survey of total adrenalectomy in cancer of the prostate, Am. J. Surg. *99:*562, 1960.

168. Current status of hormone therapy of advanced mammary cancer, Council on Pharmacy and Chemistry, A.M.A., J.A.M.A. *146:*471, 1951.

169. Baker, W. H., Kelley, R. M., and Sohier, W. D.: Hormonal treatment of metastatic carcinoma of the breast, Am. J. Surg. *99:*538, 1960.

170. Nathanson, I. T., and Kelley, R. M.: Hormonal treatment of cancer, New Eng. J. Med. *246:* 135, 1952.

171. Treves, N.: The treatment of cancer, especially inoperable cancer, of the male breast by ablative surgery (orchiectomy, adrenalectomy and hypophysectomy) and hormone therapy (estrogens and corticosteroids): an analysis of 42 patients, Cancer *12:*820, 1959.

172. Frachia, A. A., Holleb, A. I., Farrow, J. H., Treves, N. E., Randall, H. T., Finkbeiner, J. A. and Whitmore, W. F., Jr.: Results of bilateral adrenalectomy in the management of incurable breast cancer, Cancer *12:*58, 1959.

173. Pearson, O. H., and Ray, B. S.: Hypophysectomy in the treatment of metastatic mammary cancer, Am. J. Surg. *99:*544, 1960.

174. Hueper, W. C.: Newer developments in occupational and environmental cancer, Arch. Int. Med. *100:*487, 1957.

175. Hueper, W. C.: Environmental Cancer, in Homburger, F. (ed.): Physiopathology of Cancer, ed. 2, New York, Hoeber-Harper, 1958.

176. Rous, P.: The virus tumors and the tumor problem, Harvey Lect. *74:*1935–36.

177. Furth, J., and Metcalf, D.: An appraisal of the tumor-virus problem, J. Chron. Dis. *8:*88, 1958.

178. Duran-Reynals, F.: Neoplastic infection and cancer, Am. J. Med. *8:*490, 1950.

179. Shrigley, E. W.: Virus-induced tumors of animals, Ann. Rev. Microbiol. *5:*241, 1951.

180. Bryan, W. R., Calnan, D., and Moloney, J. B.: Biological studies on the Rous sarcoma virus. III. The recovery of virus from experimental tumors in relation to the initiating dose, J. Nat. Cancer Inst. *16:*317, 1955.

181. Duran-Reynals, F.: Virus-Induced Tumors and the Virus Theory of Cancer, in Homburger, F. (ed.): Physiopathology of Cancer, ed. 2, New York, Hoeber-Harper, 1958.

182. Dmochowski, L.: Viruses and tumors. An old problem in the light of recent advances, Bacteriol. Rev. *23:*18, 1959.

183. Rubin, H.: Quantitative relations between causative virus and cell in the Rous No. 1 chicken sarcoma, Virology *1:*445, 1955.

184. Lwoff, A.: Lysogeny, Bact. Rev. *17:*269, 1953.

185. Peacock, P. R.: Studies of fowl tumors induced by carcinogenic agents. I. Attempted transmission by cell-free material, Am. J. Cancer *25:*49, 1935.

186. McIntosh, J., and Selbie, F. R.: Further observations of filterable tumors induced in fowls by injection of tar, Brit. J. Exper. Path. *20:*49, 1939.

187. Andrewes, C. H.: Evidence for the presence of a virus in a nonfilterable tar sarcoma of the fowl, J. Path. & Bact. *43:*23, 1936.

188. Foulds, L., and Dmochowski, L.: Neutralizing and complement-fixing properties of antisera produced by fractionated extracts of a nonfilterable dibenzathracene fowl sarcoma, Brit. J. Exper. Path. *20:*458, 1939.

189. Oberling, C., and Guérin, M.: The Role of Viruses in the Production of Cancer, in Greenstein, J. P., and Haddow, A. (eds.): Advances in Cancer Research *2:*353, 1954.

190. Andrewes, C. H.: The bearing of recent work on the virus theory of cancer, Brit. M. J. *1:*81, 1950.

191. Syverton, J. T.: The pathogenesis of the rabbit papilloma-to-carcinoma sequence, Ann. New York Acad. Sc. *54:*1126, 1952.

192. Luria, S. E.: General Virology, New York, John Wiley and Sons, 1953.

193. Boveri, T.: The Origin of Malignant Tumors, Baltimore, Williams and Wilkins, 1929.

194. Boycott, A. E.: Discussion on experimental production of malignant tumors, Proc. Roy. Soc. Med. *113:*291, 1933.

195. Lockhart-Mummery, J. P.: The Origin of Cancer, London, J. & A. Churchill, 1934.

196. Burdette, W. J.: The significance of mutation in relation to the origin of tumors, Cancer Res. *15:*201, 1955.

197. Muller, H. J.: The nature of the genetics effects produced by radiation, Radiat. Biol. *1:*351, 1954.

198. Shatoury, El. H. H.: A genetically controlled malignant tumor in *Drosphila,* Arch. Entw. Mech. Org. *147:*496, 1955.

199. Blum, H. F.: Ultraviolet radiation and cancer, Radiat. Biol. *2:*529, 1955.

200. Nordling, C. O.: A new theory on the cancer-inducing mechanism, Brit. J. Cancer *7:*68, 1953.

201. Darlington, C. D.: The plasmagene theory of the origin of cancer, Brit. J. Cancer *2:*118, 1948.

202. Darlington, C. D.: Plasmagene Theory and Cancer Genesis, in Cancer and Genetics, Austin, University of Texas Press, 1959.

203. Warburg, O.: On respiratory impairment in cancer cells, Science *124:*269, 1956.

204. Warburg, O.: On the origin of cancer cells, Science *123:*309, 1956.

205. Miller, J. A., and Miller, E. C.: The Carcinogenic Aminoazo Dyes, in Greenstein, J. P., and Haddow, A. (eds.): Advances in Cancer Research *1:*339 1954.

206. Potter, V. R.: The biochemical approach to the cancer problem, Fed. Proc. *17:*691, 1958.

207. Bryan, W. R.: A reconsideration of the nature of the neoplastic reaction in the light of recent advances in cancer research, J. Nat. Cancer Inst. *24:*221, 1960.

208. Greene, H. N.: Immunological basis of carcinogenesis, Brit. M. Bull. *14:*101, 1958.

209. Westrop, J. W., and Greene, H. N.: Binding of a hepato carcinogen to the structural lipoprotein of rat liver: its bearing on the immunological theory of cancer, Nature *186:*350, 1960.

210. Burnet, M.: The Clonal Selection Theory of Acquired Immunity, London, Cambridge University Press, 1959.

211. Smithers, D. W.: On the pathogenesis of cancer. Lancet *1:*589, 1959.

212. Stoddard, L.: The Problem of Carcinoma *in situ* with Reference to the Human Cervix, in McManus, J. F. A. (ed.): Progress in Fundamental Medicine, Philadelphia, Lea and Febiger, 1952.

213. Novak, E., and Novak, E. R.: Gynecologic and Obstetric Pathology, ed. 4, Philadelphia, W. B. Saunders, 1958.

214. DeWeerd, J. H., and Dockerty, M. B.: Lipomatous retroperitoneal tumors, Am. J. Surg. *84:* 397, 1952.

215. Bett, W. R.: Historical Aspects of Cancer, in Raven, R. W. (ed.): Cancer, Vol. 1, London, Butterworth, 1957.

216. Warren, S., and Feldman, J. D.: The nature of lateral "aberrant" thyroid tumors, Surg. Gynec. & Obst. *88:*31, 1949.

217. Kind, W. L., and Pemberton, J.: So-called lateral aberrant thyroid tumors, Tr. Am. Goiter A., 1941.

218. Liebow, A. A., Hales, M. R., Harrison, W., Bloomer, W., and Lindskog, G. E.: The genesis and functional implications of collateral circulation of the lungs, Yale J. Biol. & Med. *22:*637, 1950.

219. Balfour, D. C., Jr., Reynolds, T. B., Mikkelsen, W. P., Patterson, A. C., and Hales, M. R.: Portal hypertension, Arch. Int. Med. *9 :*853, 1954.

220. Kellgren, J. H., Ball, J., and Tutton, G. K.: The articular and other limb changes in acromegaly: a clinical and pathological study of 25 cases, Quart. J. Med. *21:*405, 1952.

221. Russfield, A. B., Reiner, L., and Klaus, H.: The endocrine significance of hypophyseal tumors in man, Am. J. Path. *32:*1055, 1956.

222. Cole, W. H., Slaughter, D. P., and Majarakis, J. D.: Carcinoma of the thyroid gland, Surg. Gynec. & Obst. *89:*349, 1949.

223. Fitzgerald, P. J., Foote, F. W., Jr., and Hill, R. F.: Concentration of I[131] in thyroid cancer, shown by radioautography: a study of 100 consecutive cases showing the relation of histological structure to the function of thyroid carcinoma, Cancer *3:*86, 1950.

224. Howard, J. M., Moss, N. H., and Rhoads, J. E.: Hyperinsulinism and islet cell tumors of the pancreas, with 398 recorded tumors, Surg. Gynec. & Obst. *90:*417, 1950.

225. ReMine, W. H., Scholz, D. A., and Priestley, J. T.: Hyperinsulinism. Clinical and surgical aspects, Am. J. Surg. *99:*413, 1960.

226. Sieracki, J., Marshall, R. B., and Horn, R. C., Jr.: Tumors of the pancreatic islets, Cancer *13:*347, 1960.

227. Miller, D. R., Bolinger, R. E., and Friesen, S. T.: Hypoglycemia due to nonpancreatic mesodermal tumors: report of two cases, Ann. Surg. *150:*684, 1959.

228. August, J. T., and Hiatt, H. H.: Severe hypoglycemia secondary to nonpancreatic fibrosarcoma with insulin activity, New Eng. J. Med. *258:* 17, 1958.

229. Sellman, J. C., Perkoff, G. T., Null, F. C., Kimmel, J. R., and Tyler, F. H.: Hypoglycemia associated with massive intra-abdominal mesothelial-cell sarcoma, New Eng. J. Med. *260:*847, 1959.

230. Hume, D. M.: Pheochromocytoma in the adult and in the child, Am. J. Surg. *99:*458, 1960.

231. Cope, O., and Raker, J. W.: Cushing's disease.

The surgical experience in the light of 26 cases, New Eng. J. Med. *253:*119, 1955.

232. Hewlett, J. S., McCullagh, E. P., Farrell, G. L., Dustan, H. P., Poutasse, E. P., and Prondfit, W. L.: Aldosterone-producing tumors of the adrenal gland; report of three cases, J.A.M.A. *164:*719, 1957.

233. Ross, E. J., Crabbé, J., Renold, A. E., Emerson, J., Jr., and Thorn, G. W.: A case of massive edema in association with an aldosterone-secreting adrenocortical adenoma, Am. J. Med. *25:* 278, 1958.

234. Morris, J. M., and Scully, R. E.: Endocrine Pathology of the Ovary, St. Louis, C. V. Mosby, 1958.

235. Iverson, L.: Masculinizing tumors of the ovary, Surg. Gynec. & Obst. *84:*213, 1947.

236. Sternberg, W. H.: The morphology, androgenic function, hyperplasia, and tumors of the human ovarian hilus cells, Am. J. Path. *25:*493, 1949.

237. Biggart, J. H., and MacAffee, C. H. G.: Tumors of the ovarian mesenchyme. A clinicopathological survey, J. Obst. Gynaec. Brit. Emp. *62:* 829, 1955.

238. Busby, T., and Anderson, G. W.: Feminizing mesenchymomas of the ovary. Includes 107 cases of granulosa, granulosa-theca cell and theca cell tumors, Am. J. Obst. & Gynec. *68:*1391, 1954.

239. Mansell, H., and Hertig, A. T.: Granulosa-theca cell tumors and endometrial carcinoma. A study of their relationship and a survey of 80 cases, Am. J. Obst. & Gynec. *6:*385, 1955.

240. Jungck, E. C., Trash, A. M., Ohlmacher, A. P., Knight, A. M., Jr., and Dyrenforth, L. Y.: Sexual precocity due to interstitial-cell tumor of the testes: report of two cases, J. Clin. Endocrinol. *17:*291, 1957.

241. Smalbraak, J.: Trophoblastic Growths, Amsterdam, Elsevier Publishing, 1957.

242. Schneckloth, R. E., Page, I. H., and Corcoran, A. C.: The malignant carcinoid syndrome, Circulation *19:*766, 1959.

243. MacDonald, R. A., Robbins, S. L., and Mallory, G. K.: Morphologic effects of serotonin (5-hydroxytryptamine), Arch. Path. *65:*369, 1958.

244. Gottlieb, L. S., Broitman, S. A., Vitale, J. J., and Zamcheck, N.: Failure of endogenous serotonin to produce lesions of the carcinoid syndrome, Arch. Path. *69:*77, 1960.

245. Stout, A. P.: Fibrosarcoma: the malignant tumor of fibroblasts, Cancer *1:*30, 1948.

246. Lichtenstein, L.: Bone Tumors, ed. 2, St. Louis, C. V. Mosby, 1957.

247. Saphir, O.: Signet-ring cell carcinoma, Mil. Surgeon *109:*360, 1951.

248. Tytus, J. S., and Pennybaker, J.: Pearly tumors in relation to the central nervous system, J. Neurol. Neurosurg. *19:*241, 1956.

249. Meigs, J. V.: Fibroma of the ovary with ascites and hydrothorax: Meigs' syndrome, Am. J. Obst. & Gynec. *67:*962, 1954.

250. Starr, G. F., Stroebel, C. F., Jr., and Kearns, T. P.: Polycythemia with papilledema and infratentorial vascular tumors, Ann. Int. Med. *48:*978, 1958.

251. Benoit, H. W., Jr., and Ackerman, L. V.: Solitary pleural mesotheliomas, J. Thoracic Surg. *25:*246, 1953.

252. Clagett, O. T., McDonald, J. R., and Schmidt, H. W.: Localized fibrous mesothelioma of the pleura, J. Thoracic Surg. *24:*3, 1952.

253. Hyman, G., and Harvey, J. E.: The pathogenesis of anemia in patients with carcinoma, Am. J. Med. *19:*350, 1955.

254. Damon, A., Holub, D. A., Melicow, M. M., and Uson, A. C.: Polycythemia and renal carcinoma. Report of 10 new cases, two with long hematologic remission following nephrectomy, Am. J. Med. 25:182, 1958.

255. Bradley, J. E., and Drake, M. E.: Effect of preoperative roentgentherapy on arterial hypertension in embryoma (kidney), J. Pediat. 35:710, 1949.

256. Terepka, A. R., and Waterhouse, C.: Metabolic observations during the forced feeding of patients with cancer, Am. J. Med. 20:225, 1956.

257. Greenstein, J. P.: Biochemistry of Cancer, ed. 2, New York, Academic Press, 1954.

258. Winzler, R. J.: The Chemistry of Cancer Tissue, in Homburger, F. (ed.): Physiopathology of Cancer, ed. 2, New York, Hoeber-Harper, 1957.

259. Toennies, G.: Protein-chemical aspects of cancer, Cancer Res. 7:193, 1947.

260. Roberts, E., and Frankel, S.: Free amino acids in normal and neoplastic tissues of mice as studied by paper chromatography, Cancer Res. 9:645, 1949.

261. Weinhouse, S.: Oxidative Metabolism of Neoplastic Tissues, in Greenstein, J. P., and Haddow, A. (eds.): Advances in Cancer Research 3:269, 1955.

262. Kit, S.: The Deoxyribonucleic Acids of Normal and Malignant Tissues, in Genetics and Cancer, Austin, University of Texas Press, 1959.

263. Carruthers, C.: Chemical studies on the transformation of mouse epidermis to squamous cell carcinoma, Cancer. Res. 10:255, 1950.

264. Wicks, L. F., and Suntzeff, V.: Changes in epidermal cholesterol during methylcholantrene carcinogenesis in mice, Cancer Res. 5:464, 1945.

265. Suntzeff, V., and Carruthers, C.: The water content in the epidermis of mice undergoing carcinogenesis by methylcholanthrene, Cancer Res. 6:574, 1946.

266. Fishman, W. H.: Enzymes and Cancer, in Homburger, F. (ed.): Physiopathology of Cancer, ed. 2, New York, Hoeber-Harper, 1957.

267. Griffin, A. C.: The Metabolism of the Cancer Cell, in Nowinski, W. W. (ed.): Fundamental Aspects of Normal and Malignant Growth, New York, Elsevier Publishing, 1960.

268. Earle, W. R.: Further study of Walker rat mammary carcinoma No. 256 in vitro, Arch. exper. Zellforsch. 20:140, 1937.

269. Willis, R. A.: The Dissemination of Tumors, in Raven, R. W. (ed.): Cancer, Vol. 2, London, Butterworth, 1957.

270. Coman, D. R.: Mechanism of invasiveness of cancer, Science 105:347, 1947.

271. Enterline, H. T., and Coman, D. R.: The ameboid motility of human and animal neoplastic cells, Cancer 3:1033, 1950.

272. Coman, D. R.: Decreased mutual adhesiveness, a property of cells from human squamous carcinomas, Cancer Res. 4:625, 1944.

273. McCutcheon, M., Coman, D. R., and Moore, F. B.: Studies on the invasiveness of cancer. Adhesiveness of malignant cells of various human adenocarcinomas, Cancer 1:460, 1948.

274. Coman, D. R., and Anderson, T. F.: A structural difference between the surfaces of normal and of carcinomatous epidermal cells, Cancer Res. 15:541, 1955.

275. Willis, R. A.: The Spread of Tumors in the Human Body, ed. 2, London, Butterworth, 1952.

276. Young, J. M.: The thoracic duct in malignant disease. Am. J. Path. 32:253, 1956.

277. Cicero, R. S., Pérez-Tamayo, R., and Pacheco, C. R.: La flebografía mediastinal en el carcinoma broncogénico, Rev. méx. tuberc. 17:460, 1956.

278. Cicero, R. S., and Amador, E. W.: Alteraciones pulmonares en un caso de sarcoma metastásico. Rev. méx. tuberc. 16:389, 1955.

279. Collier, F. C., Enterline, H. T., Kyle, R. H., Tristan, T. T., and Greening, R.: The prognostic implications of vascular invasion in primary carcinoma of the lung. A clinicopathologic correlation of 225 cases with 100 per cent follow up, Arch. Path. 66:594, 1958.

280. Salas, J.: Cancer del pulmón. Invasión vascular y otros caracteres patológicos en relación con el pronóstico, Acta Médica Cost. 2:173, 1960.

281. Coman, D. R.: Mechanisms responsible for the origin and distribution of blood-borne tumor metastases, Cancer Res. 13:397, 1953.

282. Zeidman, I.: Metastasis: a review of recent advances, Cancer Res. 17:157, 1957.

283. Walther, H. E.: Krebsmetastasen, Basel, Benno Schwabe, 1948.

284. Zeidman, I.: Experimental studies in the spread of cancer in the lymphatic system. I. Effectiveness of the lymph nodes as a barrier to the passage of embolic tumor cell, Cancer Res. 14:403, 1954.

285. Seaman, W. B., and Powers, W. E.: Studies on the distribution of radioactive colloidal gold in regional lymph nodes containing cancer, Cancer 8:1044, 1955.

286. Black, M. M., and Speer, F. D.: Lymph node reactivity in cancer patients, Surg. Gynec. & Obst. 110:477, 1960.

287. Wartman, W. B.: Sinus cell hyperplasia of lymph nodes regional to adenocarcinoma of the breast and colon, Brit. J. Cancer 13:389, 1960.

288. Nadel, E., and Ackerman, L. V.: Lesions resembling Boeck's sarcoid, Am. J. Clin. Path. 20:952, 1950.

289. Gresham, G. A., and Ackerley, A. G.: Giant cell granulomata in regional lymph nodes of carcinoma, J. Clin. Path. 11:244, 1958.

290. Zeidman, I.: Experimental studies on the spread of cancer in the lymphatic system. IV. Retrograde spread, Cancer Res. 19:1114, 1959.

291. Marcial-Rojas, R. A., and Meigs, J. V.: Cancer of the cervix uteri. A review of 169 necropsied cases, Am. J. Path. 31:1077, 1955.

292. Martin, H. E., Del Valle, B., Ehrlich, H., and Cahan, W. G.: Neck dissection, Cancer 4:441, 1951.

293. West, J. P., and Ellison, J. B.: A study of the causes and prevention of edema of the arm following radical mastectomy, Surg. Gynec. & Obst. 109:359, 1959.

294. Engell, H. C.: Cancer cells in the circulating blood, Acta chir. scandinav. Suppl. 201:1, 1955.

295. Sandberg, A. A., and Moore, G. E.: Examination of blood for tumor cells, J. Nat. Cancer Inst. 19:1, 1957.

296. Pruitt, J. C., Hilberg, A. W., and Kaiser, R. F.: Malignant cells in peripheral blood, New Eng. J. Med. 259:1161, 1958.

297. Watanabe, S.: The metastasizability of tumor cells, Cancer 7:215, 1954.

298. Zeidman, I., and Buss, J. M.: Transpulmonary passage of tumor cell emboli, Cancer Res. 12:731, 1952.

299. Pomeroy, T. C.: Studies on the mechanism of cortisone-induced metastasis of transplantable mouse tumors, Cancer Res. 14:201, 1954.

300. Batson, O. V.: The role of the vertebral veins in

metastatic processes, Ann. Int. Med. *16:*38, 1942.

301. Wack, J. P., Dubuque, T., and Wyatt, J. P.: The role of the vertebral venous plexus in the dissemination of labeled emboli, Arch. Path. *65:* 675, 1958.

302. Coman, D. R., and deLong, R. P.: The role of the vertebral venous system in the metastasis of cancer to the spinal column, Cancer *4:*610, 1951.

303. Paget, S.: The distribution of secondary growths in carcinoma of the breast, Lancet *1:*571, 1889.

304. Coman, D. R., Eisenberg, R. B., and McCutcheon, M.: Studies on the mechanisms of metastasis. Experiments with V2 carcinomas of rabbits, Cancer Res. *9:*649, 1949.

305. Coman, D. R., deLong, R. P., and McCutcheon, M.: Studies on the mechanisms of metastasis. The distribution of tumors in various organs in relation to the distribution of arterial emboli, Cancer Res. *11:*648, 1951.

306. Lucké, B., Breedis, C., Woo, Z. P., Berwick, L., and Nowell, P.: Differential growth of metastatic tumors in liver and lung. Experiments with rabbit V2 carcinoma, Cancer Res. *12:*734, 1952.

307. Halpert, B., Erickson, E. E., and Fields, W. S.: Intracranial involvement from carcinoma of the lung, Arch. Path. *69:*93, 1960.

308. MacDonald, I.: Biological predeterminism in human cancer, Surg. Gyn. & Obst. *92:*443, 1951.

309. MacDonald, I.: The individual basis of biologic variability in cancer, Surg. Gynec. & Obst. *106:* 227, 1958.

310. Kreyberg, L.: Significance of "early diagnosis" in breast cancer: study of some common usages of the term, Brit. J. Cancer *7:*157, 1953.

311. Crile, G., Jr.: Factors influencing the spread of cancer, Surg. Gynec. & Obst. *103:*342, 1956.

312. Marsh, M. C.: Tumor massage and metastasis in mice, J. Cancer Res. *11:*101, 1927.

313. Know, L. C.: The relationship of massage to metastases in malignant tumors, Ann. Surg. *75:* 129, 1922.

314. Fisher, E. R., and Turnbull, R. B., Jr.: The cytologic demonstration and significance of tumor cells in the mesenteric venous blood in patients with colorectal carcinoma, Surg. Gynec. & Obst. *100:*102, 1955.

315. Paschkis, K. E., Cantarow, A., Stasney, J., and Hobbs, J. H.: Tumor growth in partially hepatectomized rats, Cancer Res. *15:*579, 1955.

316. Buinauskas, P., McDonald, G. O., and Cole, W. H.: Role of operative stress on the resistance of the experimental animal to inoculated cancer cells, Ann. Surg. *148:*642, 1958.

317. Fisher, B., and Fisher, E. R.: Experimental studies of factors influencing hepatic metastases. III. Effect of surgical trauma with special reference to liver injury, Ann. Surg. *150:*731, 1959.

318. Smith, R. R., Thomas, L. B., and Hilberg, A. W.: Cancer cell contamination of operative wounds, Cancer *11:*53, 1958.

319. Goligher, J. C., Dukes, G. E., and Bussey, H. J. R.: Local recurrences after sphincter-saving excisions for carcinoma of the rectum and rectosigmoid, Brit. J. Surg. *39:*199, 1951.

320. Beahrs, O. H., Phillips, J. W., and Dockerty, M. B.: Implantation of tumor cells as a factor in recurrence of carcinoma of the rectosigmoid, Cancer *8:*831, 1955.

321. Precautions in the spread of carcinoma of the colon and rectum, Editorial, Ann. Surg. *140:* 135, 1954.

322. Cole, W. H., Roberts, S., Watne, A., McDonald, G., and McGrew, E.: The dissemination of cancer cells, Bull. New York Acad. Med. *34:* 163, 1958.

323. Saphir, O.: The fate of carcinoma emboli in the lung, Am. J. Path. *23:*345, 1947.

324. Baserga, R., and Saffioti, U.: Experimental studies on histogenesis of blood-borne metastasis, Arch. Path. *59:*26, 1955.

325. Wood, S., Jr.: Pathogenesis of metastasis formation observed in vivo in the rabbit ear chamber, Arch. Path. *66:*550, 1958.

326. Celis, A., Kuthy, J. P., and del Castillo, H.: The importance of thoracic duct in the spread of malignant disease, Acta radiol. scandinav. *45:* 169, 1956.

327. Kansel, H. W., Reeve, T. S., Stein, A. A., Alley, R. D., and Shanahan, A.: Anatomic and pathologic studies of the thoracic duct, J. Thor. Surg. *34:*631, 1957.

328. Watne, A. L., Hatibogen, I., and Moore, G. E.: A clinical and autopsy study of tumor cells in the thoracic duct lymph, Surg. Gynec. & Obst. *110:*339, 1960.

329. Zeidman, I.: Experimental studies on the spread of cancer in the lymphatic system. III. Tumor emboli in the thoracic duct. The pathogenesis of Virchow's node, Cancer Res. *15:*719, 1955.

330. Celis, A., and Kuthy, J. P.: Lymphatics of the thorax: an anatomical and radiologic study, Acta radiol. scandinav. *38:*461, 1952.

331. Celis, A., Kuthy, J. P., del Castillo, H., Hidalgo, F., and Cosio, M. P.: La via linfohematógena en las diseminaciones neoplásicas intrapulmonares, Rev. méd. Hosp. Gen. *21:*81, 1958.

332. McMenemey, W. H., and Cumings, J. N.: The value of the examination of the cerebrospinal fluid in the diagnosis of intracranial tumors, J. Clin. Path. *12:*400, 1959.

333. Foot, N. C.: Identification of types and primary sites of metastatic tumor from exfoliated cells in serous fluids, Am. J. Path. *30:*661, 1954.

334. Osborne, M. P., and Copeland, B. E.: Intracavitary administration of radioactive colloidal gold (Au198) for the treatment of malignant effusions: a report of thirty-nine cases and an appraisal of results, New Eng. J. Med. *255:* 1122, 1956.

335. Furth, J.: Experiments on the spread of neoplastic cells through the respiratory passages, Am. J. Path. *22:*1101, 1946.

336. Liebow, A. A.: Tumors of the Lower Respiratory Tract, Washington, A.F.I.P., 1955.

337. Sargent, J. W.: Ureteral metastasis from renal adenocarcinoma, J. Urol. *83:*97, 1960.

338. Dahle, T.: Transtubal spread of tumor cells in carcinoma of the body of the uterus, Surg. Gynec. & Obst. *103:*332, 1956.

339. Hood, R. T., Jr., McBurnery, R. P., and Clagett, O. T.: Metastatic malignant lesions of lungs treated by pulmonary resection: report of 43 cases, J. Thoracic Surg. *30:*81, 1955.

340. Strieder, J. W.: Surgical management of neoplastic pulmonary metastasis, New Eng. J. Med. *254:* 1059, 1956.

341. Habein, H. C., Clagett, O. T., and McDonald, J. R.: Pulmonary resection for metastatic tumors, Arch. Surg. *78:*716, 1959.

342. Abrams, H. L., Spiro, R., and Goldstein, N.: Metastasis in carcinoma. Analysis of 1000 autopsied cases, Cancer *3:*74, 1950.

343. Brandt, H., Flores Barroeta, F., and Villa Treviño, S.: Algunos datos sobre 680 autopsias de tumores malignos, Prensa méd. México *24:*119, 1959.

344. González, A. A., Villa Treviño, S., and Pérez Tamayo, R.: Tumores secundarios del corazón y pericardio, Arch. Inst. cardiol. México 26: 672, 1956.

345. Arenas, W. R.: Tumors Metastáticos del Bazo. Tésis Profesional, Escuela Nacional de Medicina, U.N.A.M., 1958.

346. Shimkin, M. B.: M. A. Novinsky: a note on the history of transplantation of tumors, Cancer 8: 653, 1955.

347. Greene, H. S. N.: Heterologous transplantation of human and other mammalian tumors, Science 88:357, 1938.

348. Greene, H. S. N.: The significance of heterologous transplantability of human cancer, Cancer 5: 24, 1951.

349. Greene, H. S. N.: The microscope or the guinea pig? Yale J. Biol. & Med. 18:239, 1946.

350. Towbin, A.: Heterologous transplantation of malignant tumors to the anterior chamber of the eye in guinea pigs treated with cortisone, Am. J. Path. 3:483, 1957.

351. Southam, C. M., More, A. E., and Rhoads, C. P.: Homotransplantation of human cell lines, Science 125:158, 1957.

352. Southam, C. M., and Moore, A. E.: Induced immunity to cancer cell homografts in man, Ann. New York Acad. Sc. 78:635, 1958.

353. Wartman, W. B.: Evaluation of biopsy diagnosis, Am. J. Clin. Path. 32:468, 1959.

354. Virchow, R.: Zur Diagnose und Prognose des Carzinoms, Arch. path. Anat. 111:1, 1888.

355. Siegler, E. E.: Microdiagnosis of carcinoma in situ of the uterine cervix, Cancer 9:463, 1956.

356. Shea, S. M.: The method of paired comparisons in histopathological ranking, Arch. Path. 65:77, 1958.

357. Hardy, J. D., Griffin, J. C., Jr., and Rodriguez, J. A.: Biopsy Manual, Philadelphia, W. B. Saunders, 1959.

358. Robbins, G. F., Brothers, J. H., III, Eberhart, W. F., and Quan, S.: Is aspiration biopsy of breast cancer dangerous to the patient? Cancer 7:774, 1954.

359. Smetana, H. F.: The needle biopsy in diagnosis, Am. J. Clin. Path. 24:395, 1954.

360. Park, W. W.: On diagnosing cancer histologically, Lancet 1:701, 1956.

361. Ackerman, L. V.: Surgical Pathology, ed. 2, St. Louis, C. V. Mosby, 1958.

362. Broders, A. C.: Squamous cell epithelioma of the lip, J.A.M.A. 92:817, 1920.

363. Goyanna, R., Torres, E. T., and Broders, A. C.: Graduacao histologica dos tumores malignos, O Hosp. 39:791, 1951.

364. Broders, A. C.: The grading of carcinoma, Minnesota Med. 8:726, 1925.

365. Plaut, A.: The relation between the histologic picture and prognosis in tumors, Arch. Path. 3: 340, 1927.

366. Reinman, S. P.: The issues at stake in the grading of tumors, Arch. Path. 8:803, 1929.

367. Hellwig, C. A.: The scientific basis of biopsy in tumors, Arch. Path. 14:517, 1932.

368. Hueper, W. C.: Carcinomas of the uterine cervix: their histologic structure, malignancy, and prognosis, Arch. Path. 6:1064, 1928.

369. Bergonie, J., and Tribondeau, L.: Interpretation des quelques resultats de la radiotherapie et essai de fixation d'une technique rationnelle, Compt. rend. Acad. sc. 143:983, 1906.

370. Scarff, R. W., and Andrews, P. S.: The histological

aspects of tumor radiosensitivity, Brit. J. Radiol. 29:478, 1956.

371. Warren, S.: The radiosensitivity of tumors, Am. J. Roentgenol. 45:641, 1941.

372. Stewart, F. W.: Radiosensitivity of tumors, Arch. Surg. 27:979, 1933.

373. Ewing, J.: Neoplastic Diseases, 4th ed., Philadelphia, W. B. Saunders Co., 1940.

374. Stewart, F. W.: The problem of the precancerous lesion, Postgrad. Med. 27:317, 1960.

375. Ackerman, L. V., and Myron, W. W., Jr.: The implantation of cancer. An avoidable surgical risk? Surgery 37:341, 1955.

376. Fernández, E. M.: Valoración de la biopsia por aspiración basada en 731 casos. Tésis Recepcional, Escuela Nacional de Medicina, U.N.A.M., 1958.

377. Wood, F. C.: Diagnostic incision of tumors, J.A.M.A. 73:704, 1919.

378. Lockhart, C., and Ackerman, L. V.: The implications of local excision or simple mastectomy prior to radical mastectomy for carcinoma of the breast, Surgery 26:577, 1949.

379. Greenough, R. B.: Early diagnosis of cancer of the breast, Ann. Surg. 102:233, 1935.

380. Bamforth, J., and Osborn, G. R.: Diagnosis from cells, J. Clin. Path. 11:473, 1958.

381. Papanicolaou, G. N.: New cancer diagnosis, Proc. Race Betterment Conf., pp. 528, 1928.

382. Papanicolaou, G. N., and Traut, H.: Diagnosis of Uterine Cancer by the Vaginal Smear, New York, The Commonwealth Fund, 1943.

383. Kasdon, S. C.: Applied Exfoliative Cytology, in Homburger, F. (ed.): Physiopathology of Cancer, ed. 2, New York, Hoeber-Harper, 1957.

384. Graham, R. M., Sturgis, S. H., and McGraw, J.: A comparison of the accuracy in diagnosis of the vaginal smear and the biopsy in carcinoma of the cervix, Am. J. Obst. & Gynec. 55:303, 1948.

385. Jackson, E., Bertoli, F., and Ackerman, L. V.: Exfoliative cytology: adjunct in diagnosis of bronchogenic carcinoma, J. Thoracic Surg. 21: 7, 1951.

386. Pollard, H. M., Bryant, H. C., Block, M., and Hall, W. C.: Diagnosis of gastric neoplasms by cytologic examination of gastric secretions, J.A.M.A. 139:71, 1949.

387. Foot, N. C., Papanicolaou, G. N., Holmquist, N. D., and Seybolt, J. F.: Exfoliative cytology of urinary sediments, Cancer 11:127, 1958.

388. Papanicolaou, G. N.: Atlas of Exfoliative Cytology, Cambridge, Harvard University Press, 1954.

389. Pund, E. R., and Auerbach, S. H.: Preinvasive carcinoma of the cervix uteri, J.A.M.A. 131: 960, 1946.

390. Supjut, H. J., Fier, D. J., and Ackerman, L. V.: Exfoliative cytology and pulmonary cancer: histopathologic and cytologic correlation, J. Thoracic Surg. 30:90, 1955.

391. Berg, J. W.: The significance of axillary node levels in the study of breast carcinoma, Cancer 8:776, 1955.

392. Jaffe, H. L., Lichtenstein, L., and Portis, R. B.: Giant cell tumor of bone, Arch. Path. 30:993, 1940.

393. Jewett, H. J.: Carcinoma of the bladder: influence of depth of infiltration on the five-year results following complete extirpation of the primary growth, J. Urol. 67:672, 1953.

394. Dukes, C. E.: The surgical pathology of rectal cancer, J. Clin. Path. 2:95, 1949.

PART II

CHAPTER VI

GENERAL PATHOLOGY

OF CONNECTIVE TISSUES

I. INTRODUCTION

A special chapter on the general pathology of connective tissues in this book is justified only if enough data are at hand to consider these different areas of the body as parts of a well defined anatomicophysiologic unit, closely integrated with the rest of the organism through homeostatic mechanisms. It is the purpose of the following pages to show that the available information is compatible with this concept, although there are still many gaps in knowledge. Since standard textbooks of physiology are uniformly silent on the intercellular substances, a review of pertinent information on the anatomy, physiology and biochemistry of connective tissues precedes the section on general pathology, which is then followed by an analysis of the so-called collagen diseases and some congenital disorders of the mesenchyme. In keeping with the rest of the book, no attempt is made to treat diseases as isolated entities but rather they are viewed as instances of the general mechanisms by which homeostasis is disturbed at the level of connective tissues.

The concept of connective tissue as an integrated system is of recent acceptance. Delay in its development was probably due to two different causes. In the first place, connective tissues are widely disseminated throughout the organism, without obvious anatomic continuity or limits, intimately interwoven with other organs and tissues and showing local variations in morphology, as in cartilage, tendon and fatty tissue. It was not until certain diseases were shown to involve apparently unre-

251

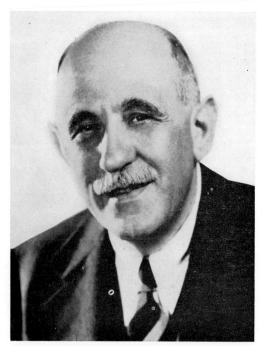

FIG. 6–1. Paul Klemperer.

lated areas of the organism that the idea of a system was grasped. The other cause of the late development of such an idea was the monumental work of Virchow in favor of the cellular concept of disease; in the words of Schade, "Since connective tissues as a part of the organism are characterized by the large mass of extracellular elements in comparison with cells, no attention has been paid to them in the era of cellular pathology."[1] Although medical historians are sure to find previous contributions of significance to the concept of connective tissues as a system, in 1913 Schade[2] referred to the "organ functions of connective tissue" and described colloidomechanic, diffusion, water and food storage and other physiologic mechanisms in the mesenchyme. In his classic book "Physical Chemistry in Internal Medicine," published in 1923, Chapter 9 is entitled "On the Field of Connective Tissue Diseases" and deals with changes in elasticity such as aneurysms, hemorrhoids and varices, etc., as well as with myxedema, edema, wound healing, immune reactions, etc. The list is quite different from that accepted today under the general term of collagen diseases, but the concept is the same: connective tissues are an integrated organic system and as such share in anatomy, physiology and pathology. A few years later Jäger,[3] Rössle,[4] and Klinge[5] postulated that certain diseases due to hypersensitivity show changes in different areas of connective tissue (die Rheumatische Formenkreiss) and although their work provided a great impulse to the idea of connective tissue as an organ, it was contaminated with the concept of a specific pathogenesis, which is still lingering in many publications today.

In 1942, Paul Klemperer (Fig. 6–1) and his associates at the Mount Sinai Hospital in New York published their classic paper on "Diffuse Collagen Disease"[6] and definitely opened the field of connective tissue pathology; in this paper they say, "The justification for the concept of a systemic disease of the connective tissues depends on the actual existence of a connective tissue system." They then go on to give anatomic and physiologic data supporting the reality of such a system. These data have been multiplied in recent years by means of biophysical, biochemical and histochemical techniques, and constitute the content of the first section of this chapter. Good introductions to the literature can be found in papers by Klemperer,[7, 8, 9] Costero, et al., [10–15] the Josiah Macy Jr. Foundation series,[16] the volumes edited by Randall,[17] Asboe-Hansen,[18] and Tunbridge, et al.,[19] as well as in reviews published by Ragan,[20] Baker and Abrahms,[21] and Bunim and Black.[22]

II. ORGANIZATION OF CONNECTIVE TISSUES

There are two general types of mesenchymal tissues in the organism, namely loose or undifferentiated, and differentiated connective tissues; the latter show extraordinary variations in morphology and function, as in muscle, bone and blood, so here reference will be made only to the loose variety. Other than striated and smooth muscle, loose connective tissue is the most abundant form of mesenchyme in the organism and its structure is the least special-

Table 27. Some Cells of Connective Tissues†

CELL	MORPHOLOGY	FUNCTION
Histiocyte	Pale, ovoid cytoplasm; round and small, hyperchromatic nucleus	Multipotent cell, with capacity to differentiate in other connective tissue elements
Fibroblast	Bipolar and sometimes fibrillary, elongated cytoplasm; spindle-shaped nucleus with pointed ends and visible nucleolus	"Chief" cell in connective tissues; producer of acid mucopolysaccharides and intercellular fibers
Mast cell	Ovoid cytoplasm with abundant metachromatic granulations; round and small, hyperchromatic nucleus	Numerous around capillaries; contain heparin, histamine and 5-hydroxytryptamine
Macrophage	Round or ovoid cytoplasm, dark and small nucleus	Part of the reticuloendothelial tissue
Lymphocyte	Scarce cytoplasm, round and hyperchromatic nucleus	Unknown function; "trephocyte" (?) participates in antibody synthesis

† There are also adipose cells, plasma cells, polymorphonuclear leukocytes, nerves, etc., which seem to play a secondary role in the production and maintenance of connective tissues.

ized. It is formed by three basic elements which are cells, intercellular fibers and ground substance; these three components are intimately related not only structurally, but also in physiology and metabolism, but for descriptive purposes it is convenient to separate them for discussing their anatomy and biochemistry, and consider them together again when reviewing their functions.

A. MORPHOLOGY AND BIOCHEMISTRY

1. Cells. Many of the recent contributions on connective tissues deal with intercellular substances, apparently a reaction of investigators in favor of long forgotten elements; in comparison, cells have been relegated to a secondary plane although there is unanimous agreement that they are the source and masters of extracellular components. Connective tissues contain many cells, some of them native and permanent residents while others are only transitory visitors, passing through interstitial spaces at one moment or another. Connective tissue cells proper may be listed as in Table 27, where some of their morphologic and functional characteristics are given. The most important elements are histiocytes, fibroblasts and mast cells; macrophages have been discussed in Chapter II and lymphocytes are dealt with mainly in Chapter VIII, in relation to their role in the synthesis of antibodies.

Histiocytes are undifferentiated connective tissue cells from which all others are supposedly derived; there is so much variation of opinion as to their morphology that

the term is rather more conceptual than specific. Maximow and Bloom's description of histiocytes follows:

"In form the outstretched macrophages vary from flat, rounded or oval cells to elongated, spindle-shaped elements which sometimes have branched processes. . . . The nucleus is smaller than that of the fibroblast, has a heavy, slightly folded membrane, and is irregular, oval or kidney-shaped. It contains no large nucleoli; the chromatin particles are coarser and stain darker than in the fibroblasts. The cytoplasm has distinct, ragged outlines and stains darkly. Near the nucleus there is a distinct diplosome and a Golgi net; the mitochondria are short rods or granules and are assembled mainly around the cytocentrum. The cytoplasm usually contains a number of small vacuoles which stain supravitally with neutral red."[23]

There can be no doubt that such cells exist in loose connective tissue. Their multipotentiality has been inferred from *in vitro* studies, but it is extremely difficult to demonstrate *in vivo,* especially when different elements are given the same name, or various designations are used for the same cell. Transitions between one and another cellular type are difficult to observe in fixed and stained slides; some good luck and more imagination are required, and doubt is always left as to the direction in which the change was being effected. Anyway, and although the study of single cells in histologic preparations may not provide certainty as to the identity of transitional elements, from a theoretical point of view it is convenient to admit the existence of histiocytes with ample capacity to differentiate into several connective tissue elements.

Fibroblasts are the central and most important cells of connective tissues; they play an important role in the deposition of intercellular substances and probably also in their maintenance, metabolism and turn over. The term fibroblast is somewhat loosely used for different elements, some of which are unable to form fibers; the reason is that the name is descriptive of a certain morphology, usually (but not always) associated with fibroblastic activity. Fibroblasts are spindle-shaped elements with undulating and ribbon-like cytoplasm which shows fine intracytoplasmic fibrils; when these fibrils emerge on the sides of the cellular membrane they are known as "fibroglia" or Mallory fibrils. The nucleus is dark and elongated with pointed ends, which serve to distinguish it from smooth muscle cells, where nuclei are also elongated, but paler and with rounded ends (cigar-shaped). It was mentioned in Chapter III that the morphology of fibroblasts changes with different functional activities. The one described above corresponds to the most typical stage of fiber-forming cells, while rounded elements are migrating and polysaccharide-producing cells, and smaller and darker fibroblasts are seen at the end of healing and in loose connective tissue (fibrocytes); their function is not known.[24]

Fibroblastic cytoplasm contains alkaline phosphatase[25] and small amounts of glycogen,[26] especially during active proliferation, when the nucleic acid content is increased;[27] *in vitro,* fibroblasts can carry out transaminations since the addition of C^{14}-labeled glucose will result in radioactive amino acids.[28] Bouceck and Noble believe that fibroblasts can synthesize cholesterol.[29]

"Mast cells are large connective tissue cells with an approximately central nucleus and ample cytoplasm with more or less densely arranged granules. Their shape and size show considerable variation. The granules are evenly distributed over the cytoplasm and stain metachromatically with certain dyes."[30] Mast cells were described by Ehrlich in 1879[31] and for many years were almost forgotten by most investigators until in 1937 Holmgren and Wilander[32] suggested that they form and contain heparin, and ever since mast cells have continued to receive growing attention. Their origin is assumed from perivascular histiocytes, partly because mast cells are very numerous around capillaries,[33] although Asboe-Hansen has suggested that they may derive from the basophil leukocyte of the blood[30]; mitoses are extremely rare and the time they survive in tissues is unknown. The problem that has attracted more attention, however, is the nature of their cytoplasmic granulations. In addition to heparin,[34] it has been shown by Riley and West,[35] and others[36] that mast cells contain histamine, and Benditt, *et al.* demonstrated the presence of 5-hydroxytryptamine or serotonin.[37] Asboe-Hansen has suggested that mast cells secrete hyaluronic acid and possibly other polysaccharides,[38] but this has not been confirmed by several authors.[39,40] Sylvén believes that heparin is found in the intergranular cytoplasm and that granulations contain no anticoagulant[41]; mast cells are not the only sources of heparin, histamine and serotonin in the body. The mechanisms by which all these substances are released from the cytoplasm of mast cells has been examined by many authors,[42] and it is agreed that rupture of the cell with scattering of granules results from the use of most agents that produce an increase in local and/or systemic heparin, histamine and serotonin.[43] The existence of such important and active substances in mast cells should not cloud the fact that there are also lipid constituents[44] and enzymes[45, 46] in the cytoplasm. The important role ascribed to mast cells in inflammation has been mentioned in Chapter II; some remarks on their function in connective tissue homeostasis are presented below.

2. Fibers. It is impossible (and undesirable) to present here a summary of the tremendous amount of data accumulated in recent years on the intercellular, fibrillary components of connective tissue; rather, a brief review of some significant observations made by histologic, histochemical, biochemical, biophysical and immunologic techniques is attempted, with emphasis on those aspects related to fibrogenesis, metabolism and pathology. Those interested in amplifying their information in this fascinating field are referred to the works of Jackson,[47] Gross[48] and Gustavson.[49]

Before entering such description, however, it may be of interest to comment briefly on a simple principle, which tends to

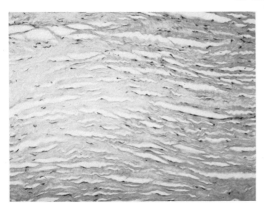

FIG. 6–2. Collagen fibers in rat tail tendon, stained with hematoxylin and eosin.

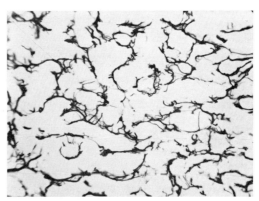

FIG. 6–3. Reticulum fibers in the liver, stained with silver.

be swamped under the baconian deluge of data. Each one of the methods mentioned for obtaining information has given results on a specific and well delimited area of the structure and composition of intercellular fibers, and these results cannot replace those obtained by any of the other methods. Histologic morphology shows at least three general types of fibers with well defined differential characteristics, but many of the differences decrease or vanish when chemical composition or ultrastructure are analyzed. The erroneous conclusion, revealing a certain degree of technique-worship, is that the different types of fibers are identical; histologic differences will not disappear because they are ignored, and even though electron microscopy is a very elegant and relatively new research tool, it has its own field of application, as the ordinary microscope has its own. It cannot be accepted that "collagen and reticulum fibers are identical" because it is not true; rather, it should be suggested that "under the electron microscope there are few or no differences between collagen and reticulum," which violates no facts observed under the ordinary microscope and adds a very interesting and puzzling feature of intercellular fibers. The meaning of these remarks will become clearer in the following paragraphs.

a. Histologic Observations. In ordinary histologic sections and with the aid of some special stains it is possible to distinguish three general types of fibers in the intercellular spaces, namely collagen, reticulum and elastic fibers. Collagen fibers are relatively wide, undulating, acidophilic struc-

tures with fine longitudinal fibrillation and weakly birefringent; seldom, if ever, these fibers anastomose or fuse with each other under normal circumstances (Fig. 6–2). The name collagen has been applied to them because on boiling they are transformed into a gelatinous substance (in Greek "kolla"). With silver stains, collagen fibers take a reddish brown color which changes into dark purple after toning with gold. The general aspect of these fibers varies in different areas of the organism; for instance, in the subcutaneous tissues they are loosely arranged, undulating and with blood vessels, skin adnexae and clear spaces between them, while in tendons collagen fibers are straight, closely attached to each other and arranged along the traction axis.

Reticulum fibers are much finer, of irregular course and widely anastomosed with each other, show no birefringence and are not demonstrated by routine stains such as hematoxylin-eosin. Special stains, of which silver impregnations give the clearer picture, show reticulum fibers in uniform black color (Fig. 6–3); the name "reticulum" derives from the peculiar networks formed by these fibers in many organs, especially parenchymatous. With additional techniques at least three varieties of reticulum have been distinguished;[50] (a) precollagenic fibers, which eventually become collagen, are seen mainly in embryonal tissue and during wound healing;[51] (b) reticular fibers, which are present in the spleen and lymphoid organs and apparently are cytoplasmic prolongations of reticulum cells;[52] (c) argyrophilic fibrils, which are neither dependent on reticulum

Table 28. Some Characteristics of Four Different Types of Reticulum Fibers

PRECOLLAGEN	"RETICULUM"	ADULT STROMA	OVARIAN STROMA
Appear in embryonal tissues and during wound healing	Occur in spleen and lymphoid tissues	The classic reticulum of Kupffer and Mall; kidney, liver, muscle, etc.	Resistant to *Cl. welchii* collagenase
Become (or are replaced by) collagen	They depend on (and probably are) cytoplasm of reticulum cells	Not a precursor of collagen	Are hydrolyzed by trypsin
Formed by fibroblasts in tissue culture where transformation in collagen is evident	They are not collagen precursors	Unaltered by phosphate buffers and acetic acid	Have been identified only in the ovary
Lose their argyrophilia when exposed to phosphate buffer followed by acetic acid.	Are differentially stained by Lillie's allochroic procedure (resembling basement membranes) Bind insulin		

(Based on Robb-Smith's data)

cells, nor do they mature into collagen fibers, such as are present in the stroma of the kidney or liver.[53] These three types are usually referred to under the designation of reticulum, but it would perhaps be convenient to separate them since not only their morphology and fate are different but also their behavior in disease.[54] Furthermore, histochemical techniques have revealed other varieties of "reticulum"[55] and there are probably some more;[56] some features of four different types appear in Table 28.

Elastic fibers are the third general form of intercellular fibers of connective tissue; in some places they become organized as membranes or sheets, as in the aorta or the ligamentum nuchae, while in other areas they appear as fibrils. Elastic material is birefringent and requires special stains for its demonstration.[57]

b. Histochemical Analysis. Many histochemical tests have been applied to the intercellular fibers of connective tissues and some conspicuous differences have become apparent; unfortunately, most of these techniques are yet to be defined specifically in biochemical terms and are difficult to interpret. Lillie[58] and McManus[59] have summarized most of the literature and from their data Table 29 has been prepared. Probably the most discussed point is whether or not collagen stains with the periodic acid-leukofuchsin technique (PAS). This is of special interest since the PAS method re-

Table 29. Some Histochemical Data of Connective Tissue Fibers

METHODS	PURPOSE	COLLAGEN	RETICULUM	ELASTIC FIBERS
Silver impregnation	Not exactly "histochemical"; perhaps depends on carbohydrates	+ Reddish brown without gold; purple violet with gold	+ Jet black	0 or +
Sakaguchi	Presence of arginine	+	+	?
Tetrazolium	Reducing groups	+	+	?
Metachromasia	Sulphate groups? Polymerization of carbohydrates? Acid mucopolysaccharides	0 Positive after trypsin	−	−
PAS	Glycoproteins (aldehyde groups)	0 or + Weak, according to technique	+ Intense	0 or + Weak
Orcein	Hydrogen bonds	−	−	+
Allochroic procedure (PAS + methyl blue)	?	Change from red to blue	Variable according to type	?

Table 30. Chemical Compositions of Collagen Fibers

	% OF DRY WEIGHT		% OF DRY WEIGHT
Total nitrogen	18.60	Threonine	2.4
Amino nitrogen	0.46	Methionine	0.8
Glycine	26.2	Phenylalanine	2.5
Proline	15.1	Arginine	8.8
Hydroxyproline	12.83	Histidine	0.8
Lysine	4.5	Hydroxylysine	1.3
Tyrosine	1.4	Aspartic acid	6.3
Tryptophan	0.0	Glutamic acid	11.3
Cystine	0.0	Amido nitrogen	0.66
Alanine	9.5	Hexosamine	0.33
Leucine ⎱ Isoleucine ⎰	5.6		
Valine	3.4		
Serine	3.4		

(Includes reticulum fibers.) (Bowes, Elliot and Moss)

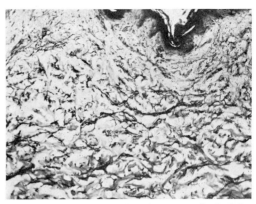

FIG. 6–4. Elastic fibers in skin (Gomori's fuchsin-paraldehyde technique).

veals aldehydes (acyclic or aromatic) and carbohydrates; since chemical analysis of collagen, reticulum and elastic fibers has shown them to have glycoproteins, the problem is really why in some cases carbohydrates are visible and in other cases they are not. Histochemical methods have a better localizing value than chemical analysis of fragments of tissue, but on the other hand specificity of techniques is often decreased and negative results can be interpreted only as unavailability of reactive groups, either because of combination or because of absence from tissues.

c. Biochemistry. Collagen, reticulum and elastic fibers are scleroproteins characterized by insolubility in water, aqueous solutions of neutral salts and organic solvents; digestible by trypsin and pepsin; and when boiled they dissolve and become water-soluble gelatin, an irreversible transformation the product of which is more rapidly digested by proteolytic enzymes.[47] The amino acid composition of collagen and reticulum is shown in Table 30 where it is apparent that some of them occur in high concentrations, such as glycine, lysine, proline and hydroxyproline; that others are missing, such as tryptophan and cystine; that the concentration of methionine and tyrosine is very low as compared with other proteins, and that collagen is the only protein with hydroxylysine, which makes up 1.3 per cent of the molecule.[60, 61] All these data

represent a "fingerprint" for collagen, which may be extracted and determined quantitatively with relative ease in many tissues; the most frequently used technique is that of Neuman and Logan[62] with some modifications, where the amount of collagen is derived from the hydroxyproline content.

Values in Table 30 refer to hide collagen after tanning and, most probably, are those of insoluble collagen. For many years it has been known, however, that dilute organic acids can extract protein from rat-tail tendon;[63] and in 1927 Nageotte showed that such protein could be precipitated in fibrous form having all the tinctorial properties of native collagen fibers.[64] This soluble fraction has been shown to be identical with insoluble collagen in amino acid composition,[65] x-ray diffraction pattern,[66] and ultramicroscopic structure.[67] With some minor technical modifications, Orekhovitch, et al.[68] also extracted some crystalline soluble proteins from collagen and named them "procollagen." Furthermore, Gross, et al[69] isolated other fractions by means of neutral or slightly alkaline salt solutions and labeled them "tropocollagen." It appears that some of these different soluble collagens are precursors of the insoluble form (*vide infra*); some of their chemical properties appear in Table 31. In a thorough study of these extractable collagens, Jackson and Bentley[70] have concluded that at any given time in developing connective tissue there is a continuous spectrum of collagen aggregates of varying degrees of strength of cross linkage, and that the various extraction media used remove a particular cross section of these

Table 31. Some Varieties of Collagen

Tropocollagen (Gross, et al.)	Extractable with dilute alkaline or neutral solutions; shows fibers with periodicity of 2000 Å; solutions are stable at 4 and 37° C. Metabolically very active. Present in the ground substance of growing or healing connective tissues.
Procollagen (Orekhovitch, et al.)	Extractable with dilute acid solutions; precipitates with neutral or alkaline solutions; shows fibers with periodicity of 650 Å; dissolves when heated at 37° C in acid solutions. Metabolically less active. Present in newly formed collagen-fibers.
Collagen	"Condensed" fibers, insoluble in neutral or weak alkaline solutions; show fibers with periodicity of 650 Å. Metabolically inert. It makes up the main bulk of connective tissue.

(Modified from Orekhovitch and Shpikiter)

aggregates. Additional types of collagen have been postulated, such as collastromin and metacollagen, but they result from a combination of acid pH and heat which will lead to an irreversible partial degradation of the constituent collagen molecules with drastic changes in their structural integrity; for these reasons, they are dismissed by Jackson[71] as having no biologic significance.

Reticulum in healing wounds is soluble in acid citrate buffer and its positive silver staining is abolished by extraction with neutral salt solutions,[72] whereas reticulum from parenchymatous organs such as the kidney seems to be a complex of collagen, lipid and a polysaccharide, which can be dissociated only by complete acid hydrolysis giving rise to myristic acid, at least two hexoses and amino acids with the characteristic pattern of collagen.[73]

Amino acid analyses of highly purified elastin from ligamentum nuchae have been performed by Partridge and Davis,[74] and Lansing,[75] whose results appear in Table 32. There is a very high concentration of nonpolar amino acids which compares well with the nonpolar nature of rubber and gives elastin similar properties of reversible extensibility; further data on the results of hydrolysis have been presented by Partridge, et al.[76]

It has been suggested by Burton, et al.,[77] and Keech[78] that there exists a range of proteins intermediate in composition between collagen and elastin and that collagen can be converted *in vitro* into elastin by many chemical and enzymatic reactions, but Partridge,[79] and Jackson[71] have criticized this view on several grounds, one of which is that in order to obtain the correct amino acid pattern for elastin it would be necessary to break the collagen molecule into very small peptides to retain the proline while removing the hydroxyproline, since the sequence gly-pro-hypro-gly is an essential structural element of crystalline collagen.[80] There is some evidence favoring the presence of cellulose in normal human dermis[81] and if it is confirmed it will be necessary to consider it as another fibrous protein component of connective tissues.

d. Biophysical Properties. The biophysical properties of collagen, reticulum and elastic proteins have been the subject of intense study; results will surely find application in pathology, but so far their meaning in disease is not clear. Those of more immediate interest are results obtained with x-ray diffraction techniques and the electron microscope.

Information obtained with x-ray diffraction analysis refers to protein configuration, both in relation to peptide linkages as well as to spatial structure. The collagenous proteins are considered as macromolecules containing three chains more or less elongated of peptides wound in helical fashion about

Table 32. Amino Acids of Elastic Fibers

	AMINO ACID RESIDUE g/100 g
Alanine	25.1
Glycine	22.5
Proline	13.4
Valine	12.5
Leucine, isoleucine	10.1
Phenylalanine	4.4
Glutamic acid	2.4
Hydroxyproline	1.7
Tyrosine	1.4
Threonine	0.9
Arginine	0.9
Serine	0.7
Aspartic acid	0.4
Lysine	0.4
Cystine	0.3
Methionine	0.2
Tryptophan	0.0
Histidine	Traces

one another to form a coil.[82] The proposed triple-stranded structure would complete a turn each 2.86 Å (Fig. 6–5). Gustavson[83] has suggested that forces maintaining those three chains firmly bound together are peptide linkages between hydroxyproline molecules. The most widely accepted model of collagen macromolecules, that of a three-stranded helical structure, need not be the only configuration present over its entire extent. Other arrangements are possible, and even two types of helical models have been suggested, based on variations in the position of hydroxyproline bonding.[84] In small angle x-ray diffraction collagen manifests a well defined pattern consisting of many orders of a large axial repeat; Bear showed this repeat to be 640 Å in air dried fibers and close to 700 Å in moist fibers.[85] In the beginning it was thought that this axial repeat represented the molecular length of the collagen molecules, and some support for this view was provided by the similar periodicity observed under the electron microscope, but at present it is believed that the collagen macromolecule has a length of four times the 700 Å period, i.e., about 2800 Å. Kellgren, et al.[86] have attempted an analysis of fibrinoid necrosis by means of x-ray diffraction and found little evidence of the presence of macromolecules of the collagen type; more studies of this sort are needed.

Electron microscopy provides an almost direct photograph of the protein molecule; when teased collagen fibrils are stained with phosphotungstic acid and studied under the electron microscope[87, 88] a characteristic banding is observed formed by dark lines which appear depressed and are separated by periods falling into two groups: 210 Å and 650 Å (Fig. 6–6). Fibers with the 210 Å periodicity are thinner and more abundant in younger animals, and for this reason Porter has suggested that they may transform into fibers of the other group.[89] Dark bands represent the regular repeat of some structure in the molecule where a greater amount of nonvolatile material is concentrated. Bear[90] believes that these bands represent regions of relative disorder due to the interaction of side chains of relatively large size, while the interbands represent regions of relative order due to interaction of the smaller side chains, which

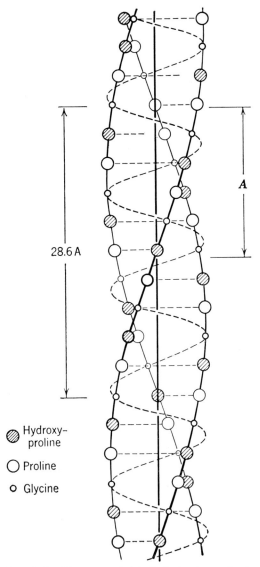

FIG. 6–5. Three-stranded helical structure of collagen macromolecules, according to A. Rich.

are found in considerable abundance in collagen. Periodicity is identical in collagen and reticulum fibers, but they may be distinguished under the electron microscope by silver staining; according to Schwartz, silver granules appear only on the surface of reticulum fibers, along the dark bands, while they penetrate into collagen fibers always in relation to the dark periods.[91] Therefore, under the electron microscope reticulum fibers are argyrophobic and collagen fibers are argyrophilic, and this difference has been attributed to carbohydrates, which are present within collagen fibers and absent inside,

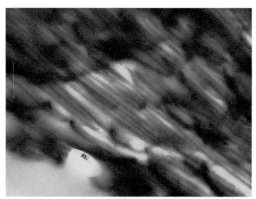

Fig. 6–6.   Electron microscope picture of collagen fibers. (Courtesy of Dr. G. C. Godman.)

but not on the surface, of reticulum fibers.

Of great interest has been the finding that soluble collagen can be reversibly precipitated in fibrous form by appropriate adjustment of pH and ionic strength of the acid solution. Electron microscopy showed that the reprecipitated fibrils, after staining with phosphotungstic acid, possess structures depending on the conditions of precipitation; with increasing ionic strength, typical 650 Å periodicity is obtained[92] while, with the addition of α-1 acid glycoprotein to an acetic acid solution of collagen followed by dialysis against water, the axial repeat obtained is about four times that of normal collagen ("long-spacing" types).[93] These observations are of interest in relation to the nature of the precursor of insoluble collagen as observed in connective tissues, and are further discussed below.

Some studies have failed to reveal changes in the ultramicroscopic structure of collagen fibers in pathologic tissues,[94, 95] and Schmitt[84] has remarked, "What is pathological collagen? How would one even know what collagen is unless one purified it and determined its structural and chemical properties as a molecule or macromolecule? Can we say that a collagen fibril that looks a little different or stains differently is 'pathological'? Certainly not until we have explored the full range of states possible for normal, purified collagen." On the other hand, Wolpers[96] has described the absence of axial periodicity in collagen fibers from necrotic areas of old rheumatic nodules, and Rich, *et al.*[97] found other changes in collagen at the seat of reaction in the Arthus phenomenon. Certainly this is a most in-

teresting field of pathology, which goes beyond the cellular level of organization familiar to all students of disease.

e. Immunologic Studies. It has been shown that collagen is antigenic and species specific.[98] An especially interesting finding is the preparation of an antigenic substance from reticulum of renal cortex, which reacts with reticulum fibers but not with collagen,[99, 100] thus providing an indication of a basic difference between reticulum and collagen, probably on the basis of carbohydrates.[101]

A summary of some of the data presented in the previous paragraphs, comparing collagen and reticulum fibers, appears in Table 33; elastic fibers are not included because data on these structures are still quite incomplete.

3. Ground Substance. "Recognized and labeled for many decades, coincident in most cases with Claude Bérnard's *milieu interne,* made to fit the current knowledge on metabolic functions, accused of having spaces and holding, physiologically, free water, identified by some rudimentary reactions of the so-called mucins, in brief, supposed rather than studied, the ground substance has been denied a personality of its own."[102] It is not difficult to explain the situation presented above by Duran-Reynals since one of the best ways to characterize ground substance is negative, i.e., ground substance is what is left of the connective tissue after cells and fibers have been removed. Dorfman suggested that the term ground substance be reserved for "the amorphous continuum separating cells, fibers and vessels in connective tissues."[103] This amorphous continuum is formed by two general types of substances: those belonging to the connective tissue proper, and those which are in transit and make up what is known as "interstitial circulation." Therefore, ground substance consists of acid mucopolysaccharides, proteins, water, salts, amino acids and ions such as Na^+, Cl^-, K^+, etc. Whatever final definition of ground substance is accepted, it must be emphasized that it is a continuously changing, dynamic structure, the composition of which will partly depend at a given moment on the metabolism of the parenchymatous organ where it is found. The structure, chemical

Table 33.   Comparison between Reticulum and Collagen Fibers

METHOD	COLLAGEN	RETICULUM
Histology		
Hematoxylin-eosin	Undulating and acidophilic, fibrillary, single	Almost invisible, eosinophilic, thin, branching
Silver impregnation (without toning)	Reddish brown	Jet black
Acid fuchsin	Intense red	Pale red
Histochemistry		
Metachromasia (after trypsin)	Positive	Negative
Metachromasia (after SO$_4$)	Negative	Positive
PAS (aldehydes)	Weakly positive	Intensely positive
Ultrastructure		
Periodicity at 640 Å	Present	Present
Thickness	750 Å	280 Å
Localization of silver	Within the fibers	Outside of the fiber
Biochemistry		
Protein with abundant lysine, glycine, hydroxylysine, hydroxyproline	Present (80 %)	Present (80%)
Carbohydrate	1.3%	4.2%
Lipids	?	Myristic acid (10.9%)
Immunology		
Antigenicity	+	+
Crossed reaction	0	0

composition and histochemistry of the ground substance are briefly discussed in the following paragraphs.

Ground substance is rarely visible in normal tissues under the light microscope, with the one exception of the umbilical cord, where most of the viscous, jelly-like interstitial material is formed by hyaluronic acid;[104] this material is basophilic and, therefore, stains blue with hematoxylin eosin (Fig. 6–7). Histochemical techniques are necessary to reveal ground substance, which in no case shows any recognizable structure. With the electron microscope, however, some details have been observed. In the developing rat-tail tendon fixed by freezing and drying and with postfixation by alcoholic phosphotungstic acid or platinum tetrabromide, which made the colloidal structure of ground substance sufficiently insoluble to preserve the submicroscopic structure, Bondareff[105] found that the intercellular regions were filled in by tightly packed vacuoles (about 500 to 2000 Å) of low density, enclosed by denser walls (about 150 Å or more thick). The vacuoles were considered to have more water than the denser walls. Similar results have been obtained by Chase,[106] and Dennis,[107] using the mouse diaphragm muscle injected previously with ferrocyanide. In these studies, Prussian blue was seen to be distributed extracellularly, as discrete droplets of about 0.25 μ, which were aggregated as clusters about 1 to 2 μ in diameter. With the electron microscope each droplet of 0.25 μ was seen to be further divided into submicroscopic droplets of 600 to 1200 Å in diameter. These studies sug-

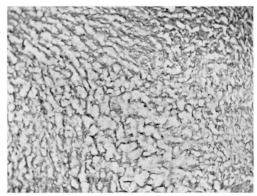

FIG. 6–7.   Photomicrograph of umbilical cord, showing the abundant interstitial mucoid material, known to be hyaluronic acid.

Table 34. Acid Mucopolysaccharides

1. Nonsulphated mucopolysaccharides
   A. Hyaluronic acid
   B. Chondroitin

2. Sulphated mucopolysaccharides
   A. Chondroitin sulphate A
   B. Chondroitin sulphate B
   C. Chondroitin sulphate C
   D. Heparitin sulphate
   E. Keratosulphate

gest that ground substance is organized as a two-phase system, the vacuoles and their walls, and this system is assumed to be in equilibrium. The high potential for rapid and reversible change in the minute relations of the two phases lies in part in their small dimensions and may be inferred from the rapidity with which ground substance is shown to react to hormones and other stimuli. The concept of ground substance organized at the submicroscopic level as a two phase colloidal system was assumed by Joseph, et al.[108] and permitted a thermodynamic treatment of the ground substance by means of electrometric measurements. According to Gersh and Catchpole,[109] the two-phase system should replace their earlier suggestion that ground substance was organized as a polymer.[110] Participation of connective tissues in fluid and electrolyte homeostasis of the organism can be explained by this hypothesis, which is further discussed in the following section of this chapter.

The identification of organic compounds forming part of the ground substance has not been completed as yet; it is known that there is a group of complex substances formed by acid mucopolysaccharides and proteins (mucoproteins) as well as neutral sugars, non-protein nitrogenated substances, etc.[111] Acid mucopolysaccharides have been extensively studied by Meyer and his group,[112] while the other components have received less attention although it is certain that they are of great significance, both in metabolism and in pathology of connective tissue. Technical difficulties, however, are numerous and formidable, and require the perfecting of methods that at present are crude and unspecific. From the analysis of many different connective tissues, Meyer, et al.[113] have isolated at least 7 different types of acid mucopolysaccharides (Table 34); those of more significance are hyaluronic acid and the different types of chondroitin sulphates.

Hyaluronic acid is a nonramified polymer built from the repetition of a disaccharide formed by N-acetyl-hyalobiuronic acid (D-glucuronic acid and N-acetyl-D-glucosamine) (Fig. 6–8); it is found mainly in the umbilical cord, in synovial fluid, in vitreous humor and in some mesotheliomas. In some areas there are variations in molecular weight or polydispersion, but not in chemical composition.[114] Chondroitin, the other nonsulphated acid mucopolysaccharide, resembles hyaluronic acid but instead of D-glucosamine there is D-galactosamine in the molecule; it has been found only in the cornea.[115]

Chondroitin sulphates have been separated into three different types A, B and C, on the basis of differences in solubility, optic rotation and enzymatic hydrolysis; in addition, they have peculiar distributions in the organism[116] (Table 35). Chondroitin sulphates are polymers formed by equimolec-

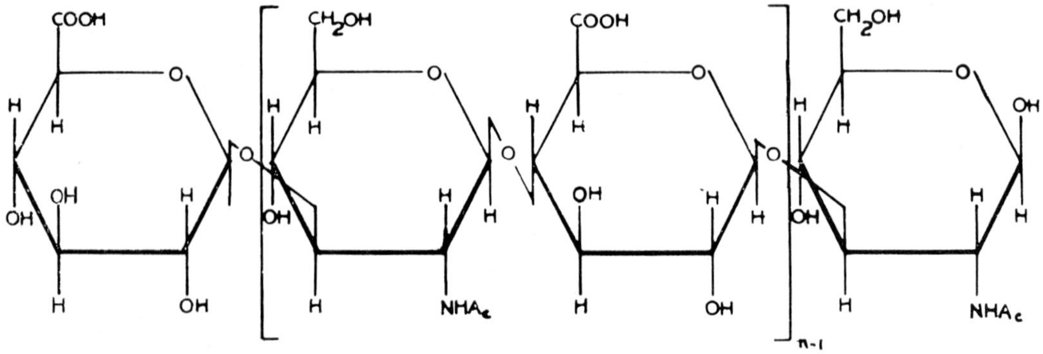

FIG. 6–8. Chemical structure of hyaluronic acid.

Table 35. **Distribution of Acid Mucopolysaccharides in Connective Tissue**

	TISSUE	HYALURONIC ACID	CS A	CS B	CS C	CHONDROITIN	KERATOSULPHATE
Group I	Vitreous humor	+	−	−	−	−	−
	Synovial fluid	+	−	−	−	−	−
	Mesothelioma	+	−	−	−	−	−
Group II	Hyaline cartilage	−	+	+	+	?	
Group III	Heart valves	−	−	+	+	?	
	Tendon	±	−	+	+	?	
	Aorta	−	−	+	+	?	
Group IV	Skin	+	−	+	−	?	−
	Umbilical cord	+	−	−	+	?	
Group V	Cornea	−	+	−	−	+	+

(Meyer and Rapport[116])

ular amounts of N-acetylgalactose, glucuronic acid and sulphate (Fig. 6–9); keratosulphate is the only sulphated acid mucopolysaccharide without uronic acid and is formed by equimolecular amounts of N-acetylglucosamine, galactose and sulphate. It is found in large amounts in the cornea and in lesser concentration it is present in growing bone.[117] The structure of heparin, the anticoagulant mucopolysaccharide, is not known; it has been shown that it contains glucosamine, glucuronic acid and sulphuric acid, the latter as a sulphate ester in amidic linkage with the amino group of glucosamine.[118]

One of the most important characteristics of these compounds is their polymerization, which has led some authors to consider them as linear polyelectrolytes (*vide infra*) playing an important role in the intermediary metabolism of water and electrolytes. Hyaluronic acid obtained from the umbilical cord has a molecular weight of 8 millions and the shape of dissolved particles seems to be a coil formed by chains of hydrated molecules of approximately 10 Å in diameter.[119] Other polysaccharides have even greater molecular weights.

The histochemical determination of acid mucopolysaccharides is carried out by four general types of procedures, all related to the polysaccharide in the molecule, which

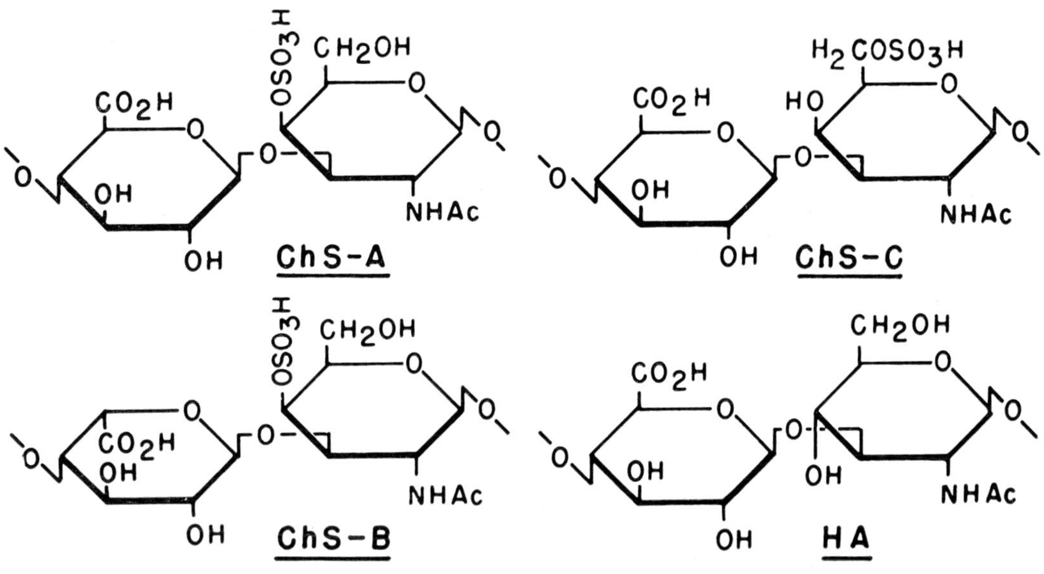

FIG. 6–9. Comparison of structure of chondroitin sulphates (ChS) with hyaluronic acid (HA).

Table 36. **Some Histochemical Properties of Ground Substance**

PROPERTY	TECHNIQUE	MEANING
1. Metachromasia	Toluidine blue Thionine blue Azur dyes Methyl violet	Change of color (blue to pink) indicates presence of acid muco-polysaccharides, SO_4 groups or other compounds. Highly specific when used after treatment with enzymes (hyaluronidase); in general it is very variable and difficult to standardize.
2. Iron Adsorption	Hale's method Rinehart-Abul-Haj Ritter-Oleson	Iron adsorption by acid mucopolysaccharides, which are then stained for iron. High specificity.
3. Glycol groups in 1–2 position	PAS stain (Lillie, McManus)	Suggests presence of glyco- or lipoproteins; it is specific only for glycol groups revealed as aldehydes.
4. Enzymes	Hyaluronidase Proteinase	Increase the specificity of other methods, especially metachromasia.

are: (a) metachromasia, (b) iron absorption, (c) staining of 1-2 glycols or other reactive groups in the same position and (d) utilization of the previous techniques after the effect of certain enzymes. Each one of these methods has different meaning and limitations, which appear in Table 36.

Metachromasia is produced by basic dyes such as toluidine blue, thionine, methyl violet and some azure derivatives. Michaelis and Granick[120] believed that metachromasia, as a deviation of Beer's law, was due to the presence of highly polymerized compounds which would accumulate dye particles changing their light absorption, but this suggestion found no support in the careful studies of Levine and Schubert.[121] Lison,[122] and Sylvén,[123] proposed that metachromasia was due to the presence of high molecular weight sulphuric esters, but other compounds may be positive and yet have no SO_4, as nucleoproteins.[124] In spite of ignorance regarding the true mechanism of metachromasia, when the reaction is carried out with adequate controls and under rigorous conditions of pH, ionic strength and time, its value as a histochemical technique is very great, especially with complementary enzymatic studies.[125]

Acid mucopolysaccharides have the property of adsorbing iron,[126] and this has been used to develop a series of histochemical tests which, according to Immers, are not quite specific since phospholipids, polynucleotides and phosphoproteins are stained in the same fashion;[127] nevertheless, the use of enzymes and blocking agents increases their usefulness and may even be used in a quantitative fashion, at least for chondroitin sulphate.[128]

The use of different oxidating agents such as chromic or periodic acid has shown that in ground substance there are compounds with neighboring hydroxyl groups which are transformed into aldehydes and may be demonstrated histochemically by means of Schiff's leukofuchsin.[129] This technique is known as PAS and is widely used in any of several variants. In general, metachromatic areas are also PAS-positive although important differences have been noted, especially after the use of enzymes. On the other hand, the majority of aldehyde groups demonstrated by this technique are in glycoproteins (when care has been taken to eliminate glycogen by means of amylase), so a positive reaction strongly indicates, although does not prove, the presence of those compounds.[130]

The most widely used enzymes in the histochemical study of connective tissues are hyaluronidases and proteolytic enzymes, especially trypsin.[131] Hyaluronidase was described by Duran-Reynals in 1928, as a result of a study on the effect of testicular extracts on experimental infections with vaccinia virus, and it has been isolated from certain snake poisons and leech; it is also produced by bacteria such as micrococcus, pneumococcus, streptococcus and *Clostridia,* and by some insects.[132] Hyaluronidase will depolymerize or hydrolyze hyaluronic acid until a disaccharide is produced, and the same effect is observed with chondroitin sulphate, which is broken down in small fragments preserving sulphate. When ground substances is treated with hyaluronidase metachromasia will fail to appear and this result is highly suggestive of the presence of acid mucopolysaccharides.[133] Another enzymatic procedure is proteolytic digestion with trypsin before the application of metachromatic dyes, which has been used by Follis in the skin,[134] and Wagner in other tissues,[135] to unmask the presence of acid mucopolysaccharides; once metachromasia has been demonstrated its sensibility to hyaluronidase may be tested. A summary of histochemical methods used for identification of acid mucopolysaccharides in tissues appears in Table 36.

There are two general types of proteins in the ground substance, namely those belonging to connective tissue proper and those which are transiently present, as a part of interstitial circulation.[136] During the process of collagen deposition soluble protein precursors such as procollagen and tropocollagen are found in the ground substance; in addition, Jackson[137] has described another soluble hydroxyproline compound which is probably also a precursor of low molecular weight. According to Humphrey, et al.,[138] plasma proteins circulate freely in the interstitial fluids, which at any given moment contain half or more of the total plasma proteins of the body; nevertheless, albumin and globulin are found in different concentrations.[139] The existence of other proteins in connective tissue has been suspected for years but only recently one has been isolated from cartilage by Shatton and Schubert.[140] Detailed analysis of the protein of this chondromucoprotein shows that it contains no hydroxyproline and that the entire amino acid pattern is quite different from collagen; in addition, there is 4.5 per cent tyrosine, and glucosamine.[141] Most of the mucopolysaccharide has been shown to be chondroitin sulphate.[142] Very little is known of other proteins in ground substance, however, other than that they have more tyrosine than collagen and that their composition probably varies in different tissues; Slack[111] believes that these mucoproteins are important in the maintenance of the final structures of living connective tissue.

In summary, this brief review of the organization of connective tissue shows it to be a complex formed by cells of various types, intercellular fibers of different aspects and ground substance of diverse composition. It is difficult to escape the idea that variations observed are related to the metabolic and functional peculiarities of the organ or tissue where it is studied, and that in addition to serving as ground for the passage of material between blood vessels and parenchyma, connective tissues carry out two other general types of functions, one group related to the homeostasis of the organism as a whole, and the other imposed by its topographic location. The interrelation of the various components of connective tissues, their functions and metabolism are discussed in the next paragraphs.

B. PHYSIOLOGY AND FUNCTIONS

As with any other organ or system in the organism, in the connective tissue it is convenient to distinguish between physiology and functions. Physiology is represented by all processes occurring in the intimacy of connective tissues, determined by their cellular population, structural organization and chemical composition, while the functions of connective tissue are the consequences of its physiology on general homeostasis, determined by the integration of physiologic mechanisms of connective tissues with the rest of the organism. This is the most fascinating field in the study of connective tissues, but unfortunately is also the one in which there is less factual information. Nevertheless, a brief review of what is known, together with some remarks on the vast areas of ignorance, may be of some use in establishing the validity of the concept of the connective tissue as a system, as well as in facilitating understanding of the general pathology of this section of the organism.

1. Physiology. *a. Morphogenesis.* The mechanisms of morphogenesis and integration of the three elements of connective tissue have received considerable attention. It is accepted that the fibroblast takes its origin from other fibroblasts or from undifferentiated connective tissue elements; certainly, it is frequent to observe mitoses in fibroblasts during wound healing, and nomicoplasia has been described in Chapter III. The interrelation of different connective tissue cells depends a great deal on the definition of each element and on the data accepted as proof of their transformation into each other, but in general there can be no doubt that there is a certain amount of functional and morphologic interchange. Histiocytes, macrophages and fibroblasts are all capable of phagocytosis, fiber formation and, most probably, deposition of some components of ground substance.

Fiber formation has been much discussed, and especially the role of cells in the process, perhaps because from the first studies there was a tendency to adopt dogmatic attitudes, which are so characteristic of the early stages of knowledge, when information is very limited. Schwann, who first described the connective tissue cell,[143] believed that the collagen fiber developed directly from the cell, while Virchow suggested that the cell secreted a soluble substance that became fibrillated outside the cell.[144] These two positions have been maintained on the basis of different observations up to the present time, when the evidence seems to indicate that both mechanisms may be at play. In 1896, von Ebner[145] observed the appearance of fibers in the complete absence of cells in the dorsal cord of certain amphibia and reptiles, and suggested that cells were not necessary for fibrillogenesis; von Ebner identified those fibers as collagen. Studying the clotting of frog's blood, Baitsell showed in 1917 that fibers appeared without participation of cells, and suggested that in the embryo connective tissue fibers are derived from a substance similar to fibrin.[146]

These two observations were the starting point for the widely held opinion that fibroblasts play a secondary, if any, role in fibrogenesis. In addition, it is not easy to establish in fixed and sectioned tissues that extracellular fibers are formed by fibroblasts, since it can be objected that when they appear within the cytoplasm it is only through phagocytosis of fibers formed in the extracellular fluids. It is not clear how far this argument can be carried, since collagen formation is just another instance of protein synthesis, which requires cellular activity; indeed, protein synthesis is one of the basic characteristics of living matter and up to this date it has not been possible to form proteins by means of cell-free systems. Collagen deposition involves many different steps, such as synthesis of amino acids from two-carbon, and probably other, fragments,

the sequential and spatial arrangement of amino acids in peptides and polypeptides, the structural arrangement of polypeptides as various soluble collagen precursors, and finally the precipitation of insoluble collagen.[147] All of these steps require different forms of enzymatic activity, adequate environment, inducing stimuli, etc., and it is simply inconceivable that all of them can be carried out without participation of cells. That collagen fibers can dissolve in acetic acid solutions and reconstitute by the addition of alkali or acid mucopolysaccharides only shows that a small part of the entire cycle of protein synthesis and precipitation can occur by physicochemical changes in the absence of cells, but all the other steps require cellular activity. Therefore, it seems that the problem is not to determine whether collagen deposition occurs in the absence of cells, but to establish which of the many phases of the formation of insoluble collagen can be carried out in the extracellular space under normal and abnormal conditions.

These ideas find support in Robertson and Schwartz'[148] observations with the experimental induction of connective tissue by means of carrageenin, a sulphated polysaccharide derived from sea weeds. When this toxic substance was injected into the subcutaneous tissue of scorbutic animals, the amount of collagen fibers formed at the end of 14 days was very small in comparison to normal controls, but the addition of vitamin C to the experimental group induced deposition of comparable amounts of collagen in only 3 days. These results suggest that fibroblastic activity is blocked in a certain stage of protein synthesis by the absence of ascorbic acid, but that the cell is accumulating precursors; with the addition of vitamin C to the diet the transformation of such precursors into insoluble, extracellular collagen is faster than in controls. Further work by Gould and Woesner[149] has shown that in this experimental situation there is a blockage in the passage of proline to hydroxyproline, since in scorbutic animals there is accumulation of proline and almost no hydroxyproline, but upon addition of vitamin C to the diet the proline concentration decreases, there is a simultaneous increase in hydroxyproline, and extracellular collagen fibers appear. Another line of evidence has been provided by Robbins, et al.,[150] who found that fibrils failed to form in tissue cultures of fibroblasts grown in the presence of an anticollagen serum. Instead, amorphous masses developed extracellularly, having the tinctorial properties of collagen and devoid of a characteristic collagen structure under the electron microscope. These masses were interpreted as antigen-antibody complexes formed in the extracellular space before the soluble collagen precursor had had time to aggregate to form the normal collagen fibril.

The nature of the soluble precursor secreted by the fibroblast has been debated, but it appears that most of the evidence favors a fraction extracted with 0.2 M NaCl; Harkness, et al.[151] found that alkaline buffer-extracted collagen incorporates C^{14}-labeled glycine at a higher rate than any other fraction, and this study was confirmed by Jackson.[152] Citrate-extracted collagen, which was claimed by Orekhovitch and his group to be the earliest precursor of insoluble collagen,[153] is believed to represent recently laid down collagen, probably from the surface of large fibers. In actively growing 8-day-old guinea pigs the neutral salt-extractable collagen (obtained with cold 0.45 M NaCl) accounted for about 10 per cent of the total dermal collagen, which is about equal to the daily increment in total collagen incident to growth.[154] It has been mentioned that many different soluble collagen aggregates of varying degrees of strength of cross linkage are present in developing connective tissue,[70] which probably represent various stages in collagen "maturation." This idea has been represented by Gross[155] as in Fig. 6–10; the elementary particle is known as tropocollagen, a macromolecular monomer of collagen with periodicity of approximately 2800 Å.

Studies in the rabbit ear chamber by Stearns,[156] electron microscopic observations by Porter,[89, 157] and Wasserman,[158] and tissue culture experiments with special techniques by Costero, et al.,[159] have conclusively shown that connective tissue fibers appear both within and without the cytoplasm of fibroblasts as a very fine reticulum. When intracellular, such fine fibrils become thicker as they approach the cellular membrane and acquire the staining characteristics and the 650 Å axial periodicity, which is fully developed when they leave the cell. Costero[159] has illustrated the presence of collagen fibers within the cytoplasm of tissue culture fibroblasts. On the other hand, Fitton Jackson[160] has shown that in the growing chick embryo collagen fibers appear first in the intercellular space and has suggested that the cell secretes a globular, soluble protein which becomes insoluble through the effect of acid mucopolysaccharides. In view of these and other data it can be concluded that in the majority of cases, and especially during embryonic development, fibroblasts participate in the formation of collagen up to the stage of soluble precursor, which under special circumstances may continue to insoluble collagen within the cytoplasm. It will be of great interest to find out what are the relations between these two different forms of collagen maturation.

The formation of elastic fibers is not well understood. Fibroblasts in tissue cultures have not been observed to produce them; they are not found in relation to any type of cell in tissue sections; they regenerate very slowly in wound healing, and their chemical structure is somewhat different from collagen. An elastoblast has been postulated, but more on theoretical grounds than on the basis of objective data.

The formation of ground substance presents even greater problems than collagen fibers, partly because it varies in composition from one tissue to another and partly because so little is known about many of its components; again, most of the information available is on acid mucopolysaccharides, while little or nothing can be said about the deposition of the protein fraction. Grossfeld, et al.[161, 162] have definitively established that fibroblasts are capable of producing acid mucopolysaccharides in tissue cultures. This observation has been placed on firmer basis by Gaines,[163] who performed simultaneous analysis of acid mucopolysaccharides and collagen in the same tissue culture of human synovium and subcutaneous tissues, guinea pig subcutaneous tissue, and chick embryo heart and skin. This author found that the cells derived from the latter source were capable of synthesizing both collagen and acid mucopolysaccharides in the same culture, and the predominant cell type in these

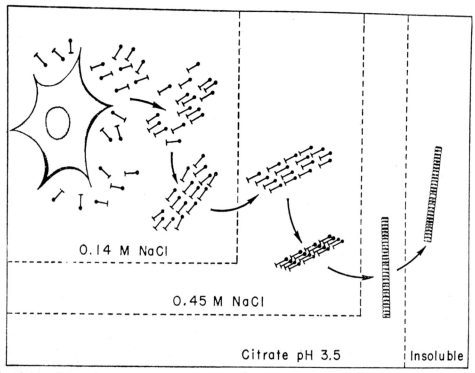

0.14 M NaCl

0.45 M NaCl

Citrate pH 3.5 | Insoluble

FIG. 6–10. Schematic representation of a hypothesis formulated to help explain the occurrence of the different extractable collagen fractions. The rodlike units represent tropocollagen particles. Cold physiologic saline (0.14 M NaCl) extracts the more recently formed collagen molecules (and perhaps also that resulting from physiologic degradation) which are completely dissociated or in the most loose association; hypertonic salt solutions extract the same material plus older collagen in a more ordered state of aggregation; acid citrate buffer extracts all of the above plus some of the older collagen in the typical fibrillar form. The insoluble fibers were of a sufficient age so that the degree of crosslinking has prevented solubilization. (From Gross, J., in Page, I. H., Ed., Connective Tissue, Thrombosis, and Atherosclerosis, The Academic Press, Inc.)

cultures appeared to be the fibroblast. Such function had been suggested by Gersh and Catchpole,[164] who observed PAS positive granulations in the cytoplasm of fibroblasts, and by Mancini and Boccarini,[165] who were able to show that cytoplasmic granulations were metachromatic; it has been mentioned that Asboe-Hansen[38] believed mast cells secrete hyaluronic acid. Grossfeld's demonstration in no way eliminates other possible origins of acid mucopolysaccharides (inferred from metachromatic staining) which have been seen to predominate around the blood vessels in early stages of wound healing and, therefore, could also derive from the circulation.[166]

An extraordinarily interesting aspect is the relation of acid mucopolysaccharides to formation of insoluble, extracellular collagen fibers. Meyer[167] suggested that mucopolysaccharides may serve as templates for the transformation of globular into fibrous protein, because of acidic groups distributed regularly within the molecule, and a similar but more elaborate hypothesis has been presented by Kirby.[168] It has been mentioned (Chapter III) that in wound healing the appearance of collagen fibers coincides with a drop in the amount of tissue hexosamines, which suggests that acid mucopolysaccharides are "used" during collagen formation. Furthermore, it has been shown that collagen fibers contain carbohydrates, although in low concentrations[169] (about 1 per cent) and some of them are glucose, galactose, mannose, glucosamine, fucose, etc. In addition, soluble or dissolved collagen may be precipitated as "long-spacing" fibers by the addition of mucopolysaccharides.[93] Finally, silver stains (Gomori) and PAS are positive in collagen, which has been taken to indicate the presence of carbohydrates (glycoproteins) or, even better, of aldehyde groups.[170] On the other hand, wound healing is interrupted before collagen is deposited during the skin homograft rejection, but the fall in hexosamines is not modified. This suggests that the disappearance of acid mucopolysaccharides (as hexosamines) coincides with, but plays no role in, the deposition of collagen.[171] The use of tissue hexosamine determinations in wound healing as an index of acid mucopolysaccharide concentration has been criticized because most of the hexosamine present seems to derive from the plasma;[172] furthermore, Jackson mentions that chondroitin sulphate and hyaluronic acid account for no more than 5 per cent of the hexosamine, 80 per cent being in the plasma proteins.[173] Nevertheless, histochemical studies have shown that there is a correlation between the rise and fall of tissue hexosamines and the appearance and disappearance of metachromasia, so the problem deserves reexamination with direct measurements of acid mucopolysaccharides as such and not as hexosamines.

Fitton Jackson's[174, 175, 176] studies may be summarized as an instance of the possible interaction between fibroblastic activity and acid mucopolysaccharides in the formation of collagen. Working with chick embryos and by means of cytochemical, x-ray diffraction and electron microscopic techniques, this author has shown that early in the development of bones and tendons fibroblasts contain cytoplasmic granules formed by protein and polysaccharides and, in addition, they show alkaline phosphatase and cytochrome-oxidase activity, which suggests active protein synthesis. In this stage there is no interstitial space and no fibrils are observed; soon thereafter, however, fibrils appear as filaments 80 Å thick without axial periodicity and within the cytoplasm or closely associated with it. At the same time, fibrils become apparent in the interstitial space and increase in number as this space grows until axial repeat of 210 Å appears. X-ray diffraction is typical of collagen and fibrils are present both within and outside the cytoplasm, although they are more numerous in the latter position. Both diameter and axial periodicity of fibers increase until adult collagen is formed, with

a diameter of 750 Å and an axial periodicity of 650 Å. When such fibers become visible with the ordinary microscope the extracellular space is PAS positive and metachromatic, but such reactions disappear progressively and in adult chickens they are no longer present. The sequence suggested by Fitton Jackson[177] is as follows: (1) cellular synthesis of collagen precursors and acid mucopolysaccharides, which are deposited in the intercellular space; (2) transformation of globular, soluble protein into fibrous, insoluble protein through the influence of mucopolysaccharides, within and without the cytoplasm, with extrusion of fibers formed inside the cell; (3) growth and "maturation" of extracellular fibers by the addition of precursors synthesized by the cell; (4) by pinocytosis, the complex formed by fibrils, soluble precursors and acid mucopolysaccharides may pass into the cytoplasm and there continue developing, or else fibrils are phagocytized by the fibroblast and give the appearance of having formed completely within the cell. Such a sequence is schematized in Fig. 6–11.

b. Metabolism. The various collagen fractions (acid-soluble, neutral salt-soluble and insoluble) have been shown to have extremely different rates of turnover. This has been studied with C^{14}-labeled glycine and the rate of incorporation of this amino acid to collagen. The extent to which different components of connective tissue participate in the dynamic status of the rest of the organism is variable. Results of studies performed by means of radioactive isotopes seem to indicate that "mature" or insoluble collagen fibers have a minimal turnover.[178] Neuburger, *et al.*[179] injected rats with C^{14}-labeled glycine and determined the rate of incorporation of this amino acid in different collagen fractions obtained from subcutaneous tissues and tail tendon; their results indicate that there is almost no collagen synthesis and, therefore, no metabolic turnover, and that the little there is can be explained on the basis of animal growth (Fig. 6–12). Other workers have confirmed these results with the same technique,[151] while Robertson has found a similar metabolic inertia of collagen in guinea pigs injected with N^{15}-labeled glycine.[180] It is not easy to believe that such an abundant structure as collagen

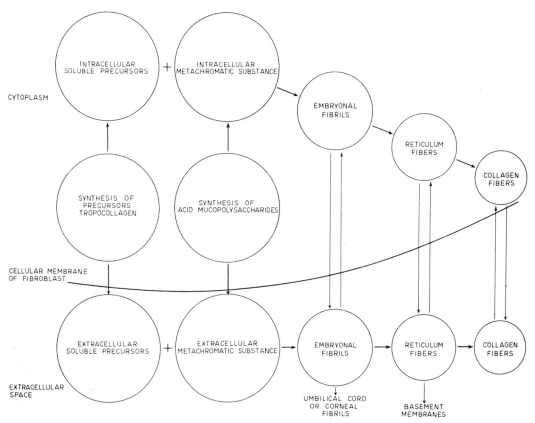

FIG. 6–11. Schematic representation of Fitton Jackson's hypothesis of fibrogenesis, which attempts to explain findings compatible with both intra- and extracellular formation of collagen.

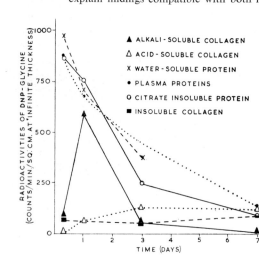

FIG. 6–12. Time/activity curves of proteins from the skin and plasma of rabbit. Alkali-soluble collagen shows a rapid rise and fall of radioactivity, compatible with its alleged role as precursor, whereas insoluble collagen has negligible incorporation of radioactive glycine. Other proteins are shown for comparison. (Courtesy of Dr. R. D. Harkness and the Editor, Lectures on the Scientific Basis of Medicine, vol. 5, The Athlone Press, London.)

should fail to participate in the rather generalized metabolic exchange of the rest of the organism, and perhaps the answer to this paradox lies in the study of other areas of connective tissues, where a more active turnover may be encountered.[136] On the other hand, Orekovitch,[153] Harkness et al.[151] Jackson,[152] and others, have found that soluble collagen fractions (procollagen, tropocollagen) show a rather rapid turnover of labeled amino acids, which fits with their suggested role as precursors of the insoluble form; indeed, many data favor tropocollagen as the simplest unit, probably secreted by the fibroblast (see above).

The metabolism of acid mucopolysaccharides may be examined from two different angles: the metabolism of the main components of the repeat unit, hexosamines and glucuronic acid, and the biochemical fate of formed acid mucopolysaccharides. The first aspect has been extensively dealt with by Dorfman,[181, 182] as follows. Glucosamine is derived from glucose without molecular breakdown, but the mechanism of amination is not very clear and perhaps the amino group is provided by the amido group of glutamine. Glucosamine, galactosamine and N-acetyl-glucosamine are oxidized in many tissues and the process liberates ammonia; glucosamine is transformed into glucosamine-6-phosphate with the participation of a phosphorylase, and then into glucosamine-1-phosphate with the influence of a phosphoglucomutase. Acetylation of glucosamine occurs after phosphorylation. On the other hand, glucuronic acid also derives from glucose without molecular breakdown and in the synthesis of this compound a liver thermostable factor with uridin diphosphate and glucuronic acid participates; in the rat, glucuronic acid is an intermediary product of the synthesis of ascorbic acid starting from glucose. The significance of glucose as a precursor of mucopolysaccharides has been clearly shown by Dorfman[183] in experimental diabetes. This author induced diabetes in rats with alloxan and measured the rate of incorporation of C^{14} in skin hyaluronic acid, and C^{14} and S^{35} in skin chondroitin sulfate. Untreated animals showed a considerably slower turnover of these mucopolysaccharides, while those receiving insulin showed a normal or even faster turnover, which was attributed to hypoglycemia. The conclusion was that the metabolism of acid mucopolysaccharides is impaired in diabetic animals and is restored to normal by the action of insulin.

The metabolic turnover of acid mucopolysaccharides is more active than that of collagen. It has been studied by means of S^{35}, which is incorporated into chondroitin sulphate,[184] or with carboxyl labeled with C^{14} in the acetyl group or in hexosamine;[185] Böstrom,[186] and Schiller and associates,[185] have found that the half-life of hyaluronic acid is approximately 48 hours while chondroitin sulphate has a slower turnover, with a half-life of approximately 6 days. In young animals the rate of exchange is greater than in adults, and S^{35} incorporation is faster in wound healing than in neighboring, normal tissues.[187]

Therefore, from a metabolic standpoint connective tissue is formed by two different phases: intercellular fibers, which are relatively inert, and ground substance (acid mucopolysaccharides) which conforms to the dynamic state of the rest of the organism. During connective tissue deposition, be it by normal growth or in wound healing, the metabolic turnover is accelerated. No doubt these data will play a fundamental role in the elucidation of the pathology of extracellular substances.

c. Connective Tissue Reabsorption. The mechanisms of deposition of connective tissues, examined in the preceding paragraphs, are not well known; the stimuli for fibroblastic and vascular proliferation have not been identified, nor is detailed information available concerning collagen or acid mucopolysaccharide metabolism. Nevertheless, something is known of these processes, which in addition to pathologic observations may provide a frame of reference for further investigations and interpretations. On the other hand, there is a very important aspect of the physiology of connective tissue which until very recently was not only abandoned but also dogmatically considered as closed, and this is the reabsorption of intercellular substances. The idea that a scar is something permanent is deeply ingrained in medicine, but recent observations have shown that it need not be necessarily so. This is of great interest since in many diseases, such as cirrhosis of the liver, chronic glomerulonephritis, pulmonary tuberculosis, atherosclerosis, etc., scarring or extensive proliferation of connective tissues is a constant and disabling feature. If means are found not only of preventing the proliferation of connective tissues, but also of eliminating them once they have been deposited, the final outcome of the diseases mentioned, as well as that of many others, might very well be different. Defeatism in this field is no longer justified in view of the data summarized below.

The first significant observation was made in 1936 by Cameron and Karunaratne,[188] during a study of experimental cirrhosis of the liver produced by CCl_4; these authors established that a certain number of injections of CCl_4 were necessary to produce cirrhosis in rats, and that if when the disease has been established, the administration of the toxic substance is discontinued, cirrhosis

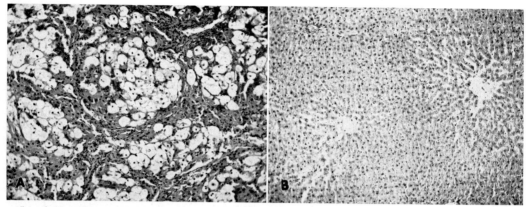

FIG. 6–13. Regression of experimental cirrhosis of the liver in the rat. *A*, Advanced stage of CCl₄ cirrhosis, showing hydropic degeneration of liver cells, nodular regeneration and fibrosis. *B*, The same liver seven months after discontinuation of CCl₄ and normal diet.

will disappear in some of the animals and the liver will show a normal structure in a few weeks (Fig. 6–13). Obviously, for the liver to return to normal there must be not only liver cell regeneration and architectural growth, but also reabsorption of connective tissue. The phenomenon will not occur in all animals and the number of those showing it will decrease when an additional number of CCl₄ injections are given, so it may be concluded that there is a certain threshold beyond which reversibility is not possible. Whether this is due to a loss of ability to reabsorb connective tissue, or to regenerate liver cells, or to both processes, is a matter of conjecture. Cameron and Karunaratne's studies were purely morphologic, but have been confirmed by Steinberg and Martin,[189] with a combination of radiologic and histologic techniques and with other types of experimental toxic cirrhosis, as well as by Morrione,[190] who made quantitative biochemical determinations of collagen together with histologic observations. In addition, Morrione[191] found that the reversibility of experimental cirrhosis of the liver was inhibited by protein-deficient, fatty diets. Cirrhosis of the liver produced by CCl₄ is accompanied by both relative and absolute increase of connective tissue, as shown both by histologic and biochemical means, so reversibility is not just a matter of architectural rearrangement.

Not only may toxic experimental cirrhosis be reversible, but also dietary cirrhosis has been shown to regress entirely with replacement of the cirrhogenic for a normal diet. Patek, *et al.*[192] placed rats on a 4 per cent casein diet for six months, performed liver biopsies and then gave the cirrhotic rats a commercial chow diet for 10 months. Histologic studies and collagen determinations were compared. It was found that cirrhosis disappeared entirely and that collagen values, which were twice as high in the livers of cirrhotic rats, returned to normal. It has been mentioned (see p. 117) that even cases of irreversible experimental cirrhosis may disappear entirely after partial hepatectomy. Furthermore, Ungar and Feldman[193] have shown that normal liver has the ability to reabsorb collagen, although they used catgut implanted within the hepatic substance; when autogenous tail tendon is used for the same experiment it is seen to remain essentially unchanged within the liver for as long as a year.[194]

Another technique for the study of reabsorption of connective tissue is the subcutaneous injection of carrageenin, a very toxic sulphated polysaccharide which induces an intense proliferation of connective tissue during the first 12 to 14 days after application, and then curiously enough there is slow reabsorption of all extracellular substances until at the end of 40 to 45 days little or nothing remains[195] (Fig. 6–14). Such process involves not only the neoformed connective tissue, but also the normal dermis of the animal, which is replaced by fatty tissue.[196] Jackson[152] found that during reabsorption there appear high concentrations of soluble collagens in the granulation tissue, and Slack has shown that the

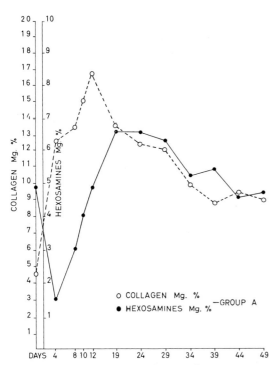

FIG. 6–14. Collagen and hexosamine concentration in the carrageenin granuloma. Observe that immediately after injection of the toxic material there is a rapid deposition of collagen, but that from the twelfth day onward this substance is reabsorbed, although in this experiment at the end of 49 days it is still higher than collagen in normal skin.

acid mucopolysaccharides are also reabsorbed.[197] The reversibility of experimental cirrhosis and of the carrageenin granuloma are instances of reabsorption of connective tissue deposited under pathologic stimuli. It could be supposed then, that extracellular substances formed under abnormal conditions might be different and carry in their own structure the germ of their transitorness; the reabsorption of normal dermis at the site of carrageenin injection, however, militates strongly against this possibility, and it has been shown that an autogenous tail tendon implanted within a progressive carrageenin granuloma is also reabsorbed.[198] But there are other situations in which the stimulus for deposition of connective tissue is not as definitely abnormal as the administration of CCl_4 or carrageenin and at least one of them may be considered as physiologic. Most of them have been observed with hormones, and in Table 37 some of the data are summarized.

When the drinking water of a group of rats is saturated with thiouracil there will be marked hyperplasia of the thyroid, which involves not only epithelium but also connective tissue; if thiouracil is eliminated from the water, the thyroid hyperplasia will regress. Harkness, *et al.*[199] have shown by means of chemical analysis that this process

Table 37. Conditions in Which There Is Connective Tissue Reabsorption.

ANIMAL	ORGAN	METHOD	TECHNIQUE OF STUDY
		1. Physiologic conditions	
Guinea pig	Symphysis	Relaxin	Histologic (Talmage, Storey)
Mouse	pubis		Chemical (Frieden)
Rat			
Rat	Uterus	Pregnancy	Chemical (Harkness, Hurley)
		Estrogen and progesterone	Histologic (Maibenco)
Human	Placenta	Delivery	Histologic (Hamperl)
		2. Pathologic conditions	
Rat	Liver	CCl_4 cirrhosis	Histologic (Cameron)
			Chemical (Morrione)
Rat	Liver	Toxic cirrhosis	Radiologic and histologic (Steinberg)
Rat	Liver	Dietary cirrhosis	Histologic and chemical (Patek)
Rat	Liver	Implantation of catgut and tendon	Histologic (Ungar)
Rat	Thyroid	Thiouracil	Chemical (Harkness)
Guinea pig	Skin	Carrageenin	Chemical (Robertson, Jackson, Slack)
			Histologic (Williams)

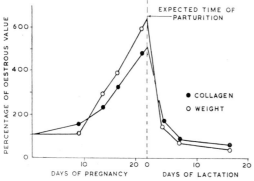

FIG. 6–15. Fresh weight, and total collagen, of uterine horns and cervix during pregnancy as a percentage of the value at estrus. The very rapid fall in collagen is apparent. (Courtesy of Dr. R. D. Harkness and the Editor, Lectures on the Scientific Basis of Medicine, vol. 5, The Athlone Press. London.)

involves disappearance and reabsorption of connective tissue. Such observations are suggestive of the same process wherever there is regression of some hyperplasia, but no studies are available in other systems.

In the pregnant rat, Harkness, et al.[200] have shown that there is a considerable increase of collagen content in wet weight, and that this increase is more marked in the more distended areas of the uterus, while at the sites of placentation and in the cervix the increase is less pronounced. After delivery the collagen content of the uterus decreases very rapidly, so the half-life of collagen is 2 days (Fig. 6–15). The same group of investigators has found that collagen is not shed into the lumen of the uterus and lost through the vagina, since plugs of cotton wool and gauze placed in the vagina of rats during postpartum uterine involution absorb material which is very poor in hydroxyproline.[201] Collagen increases in the uterus of virgin rats with the administration of α-estradiol sulphate or chorionic gonadotropin, but not with progesterone.[202] A histologic study of connective tissue changes in postpartum uterine involution in the albino rat[203] revealed no striking modifications in structure which could be correlated with the chemical variations in collagen content; since the latter have not discriminated between soluble and insoluble fractions, it is possible that the increase and reabsorption of collagen might be due to soluble precursors and not to insoluble, pre-

cipitated fibers. The marked softening of the symphysis pubis in guinea pigs observed with the administration of relaxin, was considered by Talmage[204] as due to splitting and dissolution of connective tissue fibrils, while chemical studies of relaxed symphyses indicate that there is an absolute loss of collagen from the symphyseal ligament[205] and the histologic survey of the effect of relaxin in mice by Storey suggests that it is due only to edema.[206] The peculiar intracellular, "collagen-like" formations described by Hamperl within decidual cells at the time of delivery in women[207] could also represent an instance of reabsorption of connective tissue, but no quantitative studies have been made.

In view of the preceding data it is permissible to suggest that the organism may have means to reabsorb connective tissue deposited under both abnormal as well as normal conditions; the nature of such mechanisms as well as the conditions under which they operate are not known, but their elucidation would contribute greatly to a better understanding of the regulation of extracellular substances in health and disease.

d. Hormonal Influence on Connective Tissues. Reference has been made to the effect of some hormones on proliferating connective tissues in the discussion of wound healing (p. 108) and many data can be found in the reviews by Iversen,[208] Asboe-Hansen,[209,210] and Ihnen and Pérez Tamayo.[211] Cortisone lowers the acid mucopolysaccharide content of ground substance and increases the polymerization of hyaluronic acid in synovial fluid.[212] Local application of cortisone acetate to rat skin is followed by a reduction of ground substance, a denser accumulation of collagen bundles and thickening of the skin;[213] ACTH decreases the amount of mucinous material in the subcutaneous tissues of myxedematous patients.[214] In thyroidectomized guinea pigs, systemic administration of a thyrotropic anterior pituitary extract causes mobilization of fat from the normal depots which is replaced by a mucinous substance with a high content of acid mucopolysaccharides; when stimulation is continued exophthalmos appears, which is caused by accumulation of mucinous material in the

Table 38. Hormonal Influence on Connective Tissue

ORGAN	ANIMAL	HORMONE	CHANGES IN CONNECTIVE TISSUES		
			CELLS	FIBERS	GROUND SUBSTANCE
Sex skin	Monkey	Estrogens	Increase in size and number	Thinner	Intense metachromasia
Comb	Cock	Estrogens	Proliferation of fibroblasts	Thinner	Intense metachromasia
Symphysis pubis	Guinea pig	Relaxin	Proliferation of fibroblasts	Thinner and dissociated	?
Retro-orbital and retroperitoneal tissue	Guinea pig	Thyroidectomy and TSH	None	Dissociation of collagen fibers	Intense metachromasia
Uterus, cervix and vagina	Rat	Estrogens	Change from round to spindle-shaped	Change from reticulum to collagen	Weak metachromasia
Breast fibro-adenoma	Human	Menstrual cycle	Occasionally large fibroblasts	Change from reticulum to collagen and vice versa	Cyclic metachromasia

(modified from Ihnen and Pérez Tamayo [211])

retrobulbar space.[215] In many respects the effect of thyrotropin on connective tissues is the opposite to that of the glucocorticoids, since generalized stimulation of the mucinous system and of mast cells results from its administration. On the other hand, thyroxine opposes all the effects of thyrotropin and is therefore a general inhibitor of connective tissues.[216] The effect of sex hormones on connective tissues varies from species to species, as well as between the two sexes. Estrogens increase the acid mucopolysaccharide content of connective tissues and, therefore, decrease their permeability.[217] This effect is particularly apparent in the sex skin of monkeys[218] and has been studied autoradiographically in the mucus membranes of uterus, Fallopian tubes and vaginal wall by means of S^{35}.[219] A similar study has been published showing that the effect is the same in guinea pig eye and skin connective tissues.[220] Pregnancy increases the amount of collagen in the rat uterus, an effect reproduced by α-estradiol (p. 274); relaxin influences the pelvic connective tissue, and especially the symphysis pubis. Testosterone stimulates the accumulation of hyaluronic acid in the cock's comb and the formation of collagen in the skin of capons[221] (Table 38).

e. Ascorbic Acid and Other Substances. Ascorbic acid has a profound influence on the deposition and maintenance of connective tissues, as shown first in the classic studies of Wolbach.[222] Wound healing in the scorbutic animal proceeds up to the accumulation of metachromatic ground substance and fibroblasts, but these cells show no parallel arrangement and there is no deposition of fibers; the addition of vitamin C to the diet will bring about the disappearance of metachromatic material and the formation of extracellular fibers.[223] Furthermore, if wounds are produced in normal animals and allowed to heal for a certain period, and then ascorbic acid is removed from the diet, the scars formed will disappear and the wounds may open again.[224] In the study by Pirani and Levenson[225] the effect was observed up to 30 days after wounding, but beyond this period neoformed connective tissue was not affected by the lack of vitamin C, while Abt, et al.[226] found that wounds could be disrupted even after 76 or more days of healing and 33 days of scurvy. In addition, they also observed that ascorbic acid was higher in scar tissue than in normal connective tissue.

Although the requirement of ascorbic acid in collagen formation is adequately documented, the mechanism involved is not clearly defined. It has been suggested that vitamin C is necessary for the formation of hydroxyproline from bound proline in a precollagen peptide,[149, 195] although no such peptide has been isolated from growing connective tissue; it has also been contended that ascorbic acid is required for the incorporation of "active" hydroxyproline to the collagen molecule.[148] Gross has suggested that vitamin C participates in the synthesis of new collagen (neutral salt-extractable) or that it is necessary for the preservation of this fraction immediately after being formed.[227] Mitoma and Smith found that in scurvy the incorporation into collagen of both proline and hydroxyproline is decreased, while the hydroxylation of proline appears to be unaffected;[228] such decreased incorporation of amino acids was not the result of a decreased protein synthesis. These results of *in vivo* experiments contrast with the lack of effect of vitamin C deficiency in tissue cultures of fibroblasts observed by Woessner and Gould.[229]

Other substances with an interesting influence on connective tissue are derived from amino-aceto-nitrile. Ponsetti and Baird[230] found that newly born rats fed with seeds of *Lathyrus odoratus* for a few weeks showed marked skeletal deformities, hernias and dissecting aneurysms of the aorta. The active principle was identified by Dupuy and Lee[231] as β-amino-aceto-nitrile; it has been mentioned that wound healing is inhibited by this substance, as well as some closely related compounds, and that this inhibition is not influenced by ascorbic acid.[232] Other observations are suggestive of a defect in collagen deposition, evidenced histologically as faulty formation of connective tissue fibers and chemically by low hydroxyproline values.[233, 234] There is some histochemical evidence pointing to a disturbance in acid mucopolysaccharide metabolism in experimental lathyrism[235] which has been observed to increase cholesterol atherosclerosis in rabbits.[236] A review of recent observations in experimental lathyrism has been published by Gardner.[237]

2. Functions. In spite of the fact that connective tissues are the most abundant structures in the organism, knowledge of their functions is in its infancy, and this situation is probably due to various causes: first, since connective tissues are formed mostly by intercellular substances, their study was considered unimportant in the era of cellular pathology; second, technical difficulties are very great and some of the classic physiologic methods of study cannot be applied, such as removal of the organ

and observation of the effects; third, the chemical nature of the components of connective tissues is very complex and it was necessary to wait for the recent advances in chemistry of proteins and other substances, such as acid mucopolysaccharides; fourth, it was necessary to think of the connective tissues as an integrated system in order to search for their participation in homeostasis. For these and other reasons most of what can be said regarding the functions of connective tissues must remain as speculation.

For a long time the only recognized function of connective tissue in the organism was that of support.[238] It is admitted that such mechanical function is not rigid and unchanging; on the contrary, support is elastic and adaptable to the needs created by different types of activities, and is modified by age and various diseases. Not only the skeleton is involved in this function, but also loose connective tissues forming capsules and stroma of parenchymatous organs, the surrounding atmosphere of blood vessels and nerves, the padding and cushioning in tissue spaces and in the neighborhood of organs such as eyes, kidneys, etc. Indeed, the connective tissues provide support to the organism, but the relation between parenchyma and stroma is so close that with the same propriety it might be said that the organism provides support to the connective tissues.

Another function of connective tissues is probably related to their massive bulk and their interstitial position; they are depots of energy, proteins and other elements in the organism. Energy is stored as fat, a very economic and easily accessible way of doing it since there is less water and the capacity for storage is increased. It has been mentioned that approximately half of the circulating proteins can be found in the interstitial space at a given moment, and that the proportions of albumin and globulins are different from those in plasma, which may indicate some form of selective storage. The physical properties of acid mucopolysaccharides suggest their role as polyelectrolytes and, therefore, their participation in water and electrolyte balance in the organism.[239] In addition, hyaluronic acid, being a highly hydrated structure easily deformed by changes in water content, may act as a lubricant or cushion to protect more delicate tissues from trauma or violent changes in pressure.[240] Blumberg, *et al.*[241] showed that changes in the electrolyte concentration of the surrounding environment will modify the molecular hydration of hyaluronic acid, probably widening the spaces between the turns of the coil, which might help to "fix" extracellular water and be of some significance in the pathogenesis of edema (*see* Chapter IX). On the other hand, chondroitin sulphates are found in areas of low aqueous content, and Boyd and Neuman,[242] and others,[243] have shown that they function in a manner similar to ionic exchange resins, thus regulating the electrolytic equilibrium in the interstitial spaces.[244]

Connective tissues must be passed by all substances leaving or entering capillaries and this simple fact provides the opportunity for an enormous influence on interstitial circulation and the control of the true "milieu interne." How far this is accomplished is not known, but the following observations suggest that connective tissues may play a more important role in homeostasis than that of simple passageway. Mucoproteins are viscous substances opposing a certain degree of resistance to diffusion in interstitial spaces, which can be demonstrated by lowering their viscosity with hyaluronidase.[245] This viscosity is under hormonal control[246, 247] and no great effort of imagination is necessary to envision a self-regulated mechanism for control of interstitial circulation by means of viscosity changes in the ground substance, brought about by hormones.

The presence of mast cells in connective tissues permits the inclusion of their functions, which are not only storage of heparin, histamine and 5-hydroxytryptamine, but also all the effects of these substances. Benditt[248] has provided an impressive list of the effects of heparin other than those in coagulation, observed by means of administration of this substance, but it is not known how many of them occur in the normal subject; the same considerations apply to histamine and 5-hydroxytryptamine. Two other "functions" of connective tissue would be inflammation and repair, discussed in other pages of this book, although the former can be considered only as such by adopting a finalistic position and the latter is present only under pathologic conditions.

3. Conclusion. The foregoing résumé of the organization, physiology and functions of connective tissues has been presented taking into account those features that are common to most or all areas of loose, relatively undifferentiated structure; specialized connective tissues such as muscle, bone or blood were not considered since they depart a great deal from less differentiated mesenchymal derivatives. Reviewing the common features of loose connective tissues in health, it appears permissible to consider them as a unitary system within the organism; structure, chemistry and functions are welded together in identical fashion in many different and apparently unrelated areas. Klemperer's demand for an integrated anatomicophysiologic unit to serve as the substrate for specific pathologic changes[8] is thus fulfilled, although admittedly many gaps in knowledge are patched up with speculations and others lay bare and uncovered. The connective tissue system is an heuristic concept which has survived many attacks; as a hypothesis it has proved of great value, providing a general frame of reference for adequate understanding of the massive amount of information accumulated in recent decades, but if a better hypothesis is presented (which appears unlikely) the concept of connective tissue as an organ would have to be abandoned or modified accordingly. Still, the most important data in favor of this concept are derived from pathology; indeed, it was from pathologic observations that the first attempts at presenting a synthesis were made, and it was from their observations in disseminated lupus erythematosus that Klemperer, *et al.*[7] suggested that the connective tissues should be considered as a "seat of disease," in the best of Morgagni's tradition. Two important lessons have been learned from the evolution of this concept: first, that anatomy, chemistry and physiology, which are sciences of the "normal," have much to learn from pathology; and second, that combined and multidisciplinary studies of single problems are often conducive to wider and more complete understanding of phenomena than isolated and unilateral efforts.

III. ELEMENTARY LESIONS OF CONNECTIVE TISSUES

In keeping with the rest of the organism, connective tissues have a limited capacity for morphologic reaction. When stimulated by any of a great variety of pathogenic agents, the resulting structural lesions always lie within a relatively small and stereotyped group in which intercellular substances and blood vessels are predominantly involved. It must be remembered that anatomic changes are only one aspect of pathologic processes, which may be manifested also by functional, biochemical or metabolic aberrations. Disease is the sum total of all these changes, not only morbid anatomy or histology. Nevertheless, histologic changes serve to localize the topography of diseases and to classify them in some general groups, as well as to point out similarities and differences among them. Morphologic resemblance, however, is no proof of etiologic or pathogenetic unity in diseases with different topographic distribution; in order to establish the etiology and pathogenesis of a given pathologic process it is necessary to approach them with adequate techniques, which are seldom anatomic. No claim as to the infectious nature of a certain disease can be considered more than a mere suggestion if adequate microbiologic methods have not been used; by the same token, generalizations concerning the nature of diseases involving the connective tissues as a system are valid only for the specific method of study used. There are only very few diseases with specific morphologic changes, and their meaning as to etiology and pathogenesis is understood because structural lesions have been correlated with microbiologic, serologic or epidemiologic studies. To generalize on the causes of disease from morbid anatomy is to repeat the same sterile extrapolation of Morgagni; in him, it was a sign of genius and a very valiant posture, considering the extent of knowledge in his time, but to do it at present is only revealing of an immoderate degree of technique worship.

These remarks must serve as introductory to a discussion of the elementary lesions of connective tissues, which at different times

Table 39.   Elementary Lesions of Connective Tissues

1. Mucinous edema
2. Fibrinoid necrosis
3. Granuloma formation
4. Sclerosis
5. Hyalinization

have been endowed with etiologic and pathogenic meaning; the number of changes observed in intercellular substances is indeed limited, while the array of possible causal agents is impressive. In the list appearing in Table 39 many structural abnormalities of the connective tissue are not included because they do not involve it in a systemic fashion or because they are not observed in "collagen diseases." To extend that list, in an effort to achieve completeness, would be to defeat the purpose of these paragraphs, which is a brief review of histologic changes usually present in some or all diseases involving the connective tissues as a system.

The elementary, systemic lesions of connective tissues are not mutually exclusive. On the contrary, they frequently coexist next to each other or even mingled in the same area, and they have been listed in a certain chronologic sequence which is possible to observe on some occasions, starting with mucinous edema and ending in hyalinization. Nevertheless, tissue changes may become apparent without any preceding alteration, remain unmodified for long periods, and resolve without necessarily passing into the following stage. Some of them, however, do follow a well defined life cycle, as Aschoff's bodies or the subcutaneous nodular lesions of rheumatoid arthritis. In addition to describing each one of the elementary lesions of connective tissues, a few remarks are presented on the role of hypersensitivity in their production, which has been repeatedly invoked as the major pathogenetic mechanism.

A. ELEMENTARY LESIONS

1. Mucinous Edema. Mucinous edema was described by Talalajeww[249] as the first change appearing in the perivascular or interstitial connective tissue of the myocardium in acute rheumatic fever. It is also found early in the beginning of other generalized disease, such as disseminated lupus or scleroderma; in the former, mucinous edema has been observed in the loose, sub-epicardial connective tissue, in the medi-astinum, in the perivascular atmosphere and occasionally away from blood vessels,[250] while in the latter it is present between col-lagen bundles in the dermis and better still in the intima of renal arterioles, where it serves as a diagnostic histologic sign.[251] It may also be seen in the stroma of synovial membranes in rheumatoid arthritis or in rheumatic fever.[252] Mucinous edema is the most important change in the group of cases published by Becker, *et al.*[253] as "familial collagenosis," with predominant cardiovas-cular manifestations. Experimentally, it may be reproduced by the same methods used for the induction of fibrinoid necrosis, which are mentioned below; in addition, Geschick-ter, *et al.*[254] observed mucinous edema with the administration of N,N'-dimethyl-p-phenylenediamine to rats and believed that it was important for the ulterior develop-ment of other connective tissue lesions.

The lesion appears as an interstitial, in-terfibrillary deposit of a basophilic, amor-phous and finely granular material which separates structures and is accompanied by little cellular infiltrate (Fig. 6–16); its properties have been studied by Lannigan[255] in auricular appendages removed during mitral commissurotomy. Although some-times it may have an irregular and fine fibrillary structure, this is considered to be an artifact produced by dehydration and precipitation during histologic processing. Histochemical studies have led some authors to consider mucinous edema as due to an increase in ground substance, especially acid mucopolysaccharides,[256] while others believe that it is the result of collagen dis-integration.[257] It seems more likely that the first possibility is true, although the origin of increased mucoproteins in tissues (fibro-blasts, mast cells, capillary filtration, etc.) is not known. A very similar picture is ob-served in the subcutaneous tissues in myx-edema,[258] either generalized or pretibial, where it has been chemically shown that there is an increase in acid mucopolysac-charides,[259] but in this case mucinous edema is not accompanied by cellular infiltration and is not followed by fibrinoid necrosis or other changes, as seems to be the case in collagen diseases. It is highly probable that many areas of mucinous edema are reab-sorbed as the acute phase of the disease in which it occurs subsides.

2. Fibrinoid Necrosis. The terms "fibrin-oid degeneration" and "fibrinoid necrosis" were introduced by Neuman in 1800, to describe a vascular or interstitial change characterized by the presence of an aci-dophilic, homogeneous and refractile ma-terial with some of the staining properties of fibrin.[260] That both "degeneration" and "ne-crosis" were used is indicative of some dif-ferences of opinion on the nature of the material, which were expressed at the time the lesion was described and which are still held by different authors; nevertheless, most investigators agree at present that whenever there is fibrinoid material there is also tis-sue necrosis (p. 44).

Fibrinoid necrosis is one of the most characteristic lesions of the acute, active

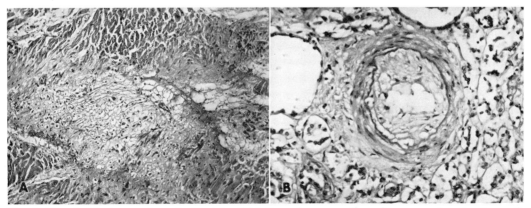

FIG. 6–16. *A*, Mucinous edema in the interstitial tissue in myocardium, in a case of acute rheumatic fever. *B*, Mucinous edema of the intima in a renal arteriole in scleroderma.

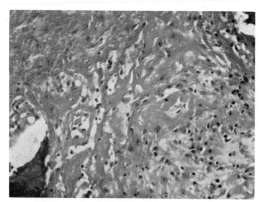

FIG. 6–17. Fibrinoid necrosis in subcutaneous rheumatic nodule.

stages of most collagen diseases;[261] it appears in all of them, although it is less frequently seen in dermatomyositis. It is especially prominent in the periarticular tissues in rheumatoid arthritis,[262] in the heart valves and the interstitial tissue of the myocardium in rheumatic fever,[263] in the blood vessels in polyarteritis nodosa,[264] and in the loose retroperitoneal, pericardial and subcutaneous tissue in disseminated lupus.[265] Microscopically it appears as an intensely eosinophilic and amorphous material, with irregular but well defined limits, refractile and with few accompanying cells (Fig. 6–17). It is also present in diseases definitely not acceptable as involving the connective tissues as a system, such as peptic ulcer,[266] certain inflammatory processes,[267] atherosclerosis,[268] thromboangiitis obliterans,[269] hygromas and other tumors.[270] Experimentally it has been reproduced by means of trauma, radiation or chemical injury of connective tissue,[271] orthostatic hypertension,[273] acute bacterial infection,[273] prolonged passive congestion,[272] experimental hypertension,[274] Arthus' phenomenon,[275] anaphylactic hypersensitivity,[276] administration of large doses of desoxycorticosterone,[277] etc.

The nature of fibrinoid necrosis has been discussed ever since it was first described; Neuman[278] believed it originated in diseased connective tissue, while Marchand[279] suggested it was fibrin infiltrating interstitial spaces. Most of the opinions held on the nature of fibrinoid necrosis are only variations of these two; those believing that this lesion derives from abnormal connective tis-

sue have implicated collagen,[280] ground substance[256] or smooth muscle,[281] while authors supporting the hypothesis that fibrinoid material originates in the blood have suggested fibrin[282, 283] or gamma globulin[284] as the main component. Chemical determinations in areas with abundant fibrinoid necrosis, as in subcutaneous nodules in rheumatoid arthritis,[285, 286] have shown that the composition is very different from collagen, while histochemical studies have suggested that nucleoproteins are present in high concentrations.[287] In view of the preceding data, some authors believe that fibrinoid material is not a homogeneous substance with the same chemical composition but that there are several different "fibrinoids," sharing only the morphologic aspect.[288, 289] A high concentration of gamma globulins in fibrinoid necrosis has been demonstrated in lupus, rheumatic fever and experimental serum sickness, while fibrinogen and/or fibrin predominate in thrombotic thrombocytopenic purpura, generalized Shwartzman phenomenon and premature placenta.

3. Granulomas. This lesion is a form of chronic inflammation (p. 75) characterized by a change in morphology of inflammatory cells, mainly macrophages, which become epithelioid and giant elements, and by the arrangement of these cells in nodules or groups more or less characteristic of the disease in which they occur. Granulomas are frequent in three collagen diseases, namely rheumatic fever, rheumatoid arthritis and polyarteritis nodosa; other entities of the same group may occasionally show them, but these are infrequent and not very characteristic.

There are four different types of nodules in rheumatic fever. Aschoff's nodules or bodies, which appear during acute attacks and last for variable (and probably prolonged) periods, are exclusively seen in the heart and in the adventitia of the great vessels and are formed in the center by granular fragmentation of collagen bundles with peripheral accumulation of large mononuclear and multinuclear cells with basophilic and irregular cytoplasm; the nuclei may be rounded or elongated, with the chromatin arranged as a central, serrated band (Anitschkow's myocytes) (Fig. 6–18). Some of

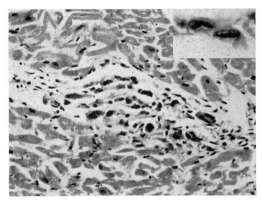

FIG. 6–18. Aschoff body in the myocardium in acute rheumatic fever. The inset shows two Anitschkow myocytes.

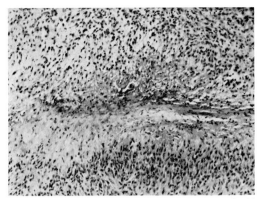

FIG. 6–19. Subcutaneous nodule in rheumatoid arthritis, with fibrinoid necrosis and palisading of epithelioid cells.

the cells may be multinucleated and occasionally show eosinophilic clumps of material resembling fragmented collagen fibers[290] in the cytoplasm. Gross and Ehrlich[291] described Aschoff's bodies passing through different stages of development, although it is not possible to predict the time required for each stage by the histologic appearance of the lesion. Three stages are recognized, which are the early or alterative, where there is mucinous edema and swelling of collagen fibers with little cellular infiltration; the second stage is known as granulomatous and corresponds with the fully developed Aschoff's body, while the third is the healing stage and shows mainly fibrosis. There is no definite evidence regarding the duration of each stage, but the entire cycle is believed to last approximately 6 months; some authors suggest that healing may follow the early or alterative phase without the process passing through the granulomatous stage.

The second type of nodule was described by Murphy with the name of the "myofiber Aschoff body." Found both in experimental animals[292] and in the myocardium of children dying from acute rheumatic fever,[293] it is a circumscribed area of myofiber necrosis about which Anitschkow and occasional giant cells accumulate. Saphir questions the wisdom of including these lesions under the term "Aschoff body."[294]

The third type of nodule, found in the brains of children dying from acute rheumatic fever with clinical manifestations of severe cerebral involvement, was described by Costero, et al.[295, 296] These nodules are formed by microglial elements and appear mainly in the neighborhood of blood vessels, although they may also occur at some distance from them.

The fourth type is also present in acute attacks of the disease and is characterized by subcutaneous periarticular nodules composed of a central zone of fibrinoid necrosis surrounded by epithelioid elements.[297] In rheumatoid arthritis periarticular nodules are also present with a similar histologic structure (Fig. 6–19), although they tend to be larger and to last longer than in rheumatic fever.[298] Granulomas may also appear in polyarteritis nodosa, although their presence near blood vessels or even in the interstitial tissues has caused Churg and Strauss[299] to separate different types of this disease with the names of allergic granulomatosis or allergic angiitis; according to these authors, true polyarteritis nodosa would never show granulomas. Granulomas have also been described in lupus erythematosus, but they occur more rarely (see below).

4. Fibrosis. Two different forms of fibrosis may be distinguished in collagen diseases, namely cicatricial and progressive. In the first form, connective tissues are deposited in areas of necrosis or destruction of tissue, as in the scarring of old Aschoff's bodies or in the healing of valvular lesions (Fig. 6–20); this type of fibrosis is wound healing and seems to have all the features of such process. The second form is a progressive deposit of connective tissue which is not associated with a previous lesion but appears primary, as in scleroderma, which has been called "progressive systemic sclerosis"[300] (Fig. 6–21). In all types of collagen

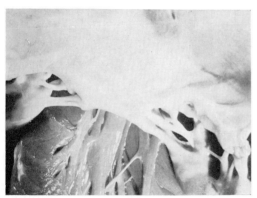

Fig. 6–20. Fibrosis of mitral valve in chronic rheumatic heart disease.

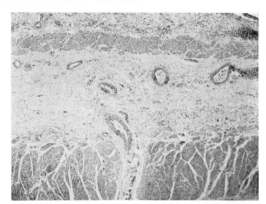

Fig. 6–21. Submucosal fibrosis of the esophagus in scleroderma. The thick band of connective tissue appears between the muscularis mucosae and the muscular layer.

diseases both forms of fibrosis are encountered, often in different areas, but the cicatricial form is more prominent in rheumatic fever, rheumatoid arthritis, disseminated lupus and polyarteritis nodosa, while the progressive form is characteristic of scleroderma and dermatomyositis.

5. Hyalinization. Extensive hyalinization of neoformed or even normal connective tissue is frequently observed in systemic collagen diseases, especially in old scars of granulomas or diffuse inflammation, as in the cardiac valves in rheumatic fever, and it is prominent in the subcutaneous tissues in scleroderma.

In addition to the elementary lesions described, each type of collagen disease shows different changes which are more or less characteristic, such as Libman-Sacks endocarditis in disseminated lupus or the renal lesions in scleroderma (*vide infra*); it is also of interest to point out that blood vessels are frequently involved in most diseases, although they are predominantly affected in polyarteritis nodosa.

B. HYPERSENSITIVITY AND THE CONNECTIVE TISSUES

Reference has been made to the influence of hypersensitivity on the inflammatory process (p. 80), and in Chapter VIII a more extended discussion of the role of hypersensitivity in disease is presented. Only a few remarks are included here on the effect of hypersensitivity in the connective tissues, which will serve as an introduction to the study of the etiology and pathogenesis of collagen diseases.

Blood vessels and interstitial substances are frequently the main shock organs in different forms of hypersensitivity, especially in the immediate type. When this occurs, lesions are generalized and reproduce quite closely those described in the preceding paragraphs. Repeated injections of antigen will bring about fibrinoid necrosis, especially in blood vessels, and granuloma formation; with healing there is fibrosis and, in time, even hyalinization of the neoformed connective tissue is present. Comparison of these studies with tissue changes of human collagen diseases has led several investigators to conclude that the elementary lesions of connective tissues are produced by hypersensitivity mechanisms, although the type of immune response involved varies according to different authors, since some of them believe it is similar to serum sickness;[301] others suggest a form of generalized Shwartzman reaction[302] and others favor the Arthus phenomenon.[303] Costero, *et al.*[304] contend that the triad: fibrinoid substance + epithelioid cells + primary fibrogenesis, is specific for the fibroblastic system and is the morphologic basis of hypersensitivity phenomena. Goldgraber and Kirsner[305] believe that the presence of granulomas and giant cells should arouse the suspicion of a hypersensitivity mechanism; and Movat and More[306] conclude that tissue changes characteristic of immune processes feature intense inflammation with vascular thrombosis, proliferation of macrophages and maturation and infiltration of plasma cells. Other opinions could be quoted but they would only increase the variety of tissue changes that at one time or another have been held to be either specific or highly suggestive of hypersensitivity. In a very informative paper, Dammin[307] reviews the tissue reactions patterns observed in states with a certain immune pathogenesis and compares them with others suspected of resulting from similar mechanisms, as well as with some lesions without recognized relationship to immunity; it is clearly brought out that morphologic similarity cannot be used alone to accept pathogenetic unity.

So far, defenders of the concept that hypersensitivity results in specific connective tissue lesions base their argument on two facts and one inference. The facts are that fibrinoid connective tissue changes and necrotizing arteritis can be provoked experimentally by allergic means, and that the same changes are present in human serum sickness. The inference is that such changes are present *only* in hypersensitivity; i.e., that they are specific, and therefore their recognition in a given disease is reason enough to classify it as due to hypersensitivity. Demonstration of this inference is not available at present, and there is some evidence questioning the proposed specificity of fibrinoid necrosis;[271] indeed, it is more and more apparent that "fibrinoid" is not a single, homogeneous substance but rather there are several different types with the same staining features.[288] Finally, it cannot be expected that the demonstration of hypersensitivity as the main pathogenetic mechanism responsible for the elementary lesions of connective tissues will be derived from purely morphologic observations; rather, it will probably result from the combined efforts of immunologists, biochemists, pathologists and other specialists, working with more elaborate methods, such as the fluorescent antibody technique or immunohistochemistry.

IV. DIFFUSE COLLAGEN DISEASES

A. CONCEPT

The concept of diffuse collagen disease has been expressed by Klemperer[7] as follows: "The term diffuse collagen disease was originally applied to acute and chronic maladies which are characterized anatomically by generalized alterations of the connective tissues, particularly by abnormalities of its extracellular components." According to this definition, the term diffuse collagen disease implies an anatomic synthesis and has no etiologic or pathogenetic connotations. This is the main difference with the group of "allergic diseases" postulated previously by Klinge,[308] which incidentally encloses the same entities but accepts a specific mechanism. The main contribution of such anatomic synthesis has been summarized by Klemperer: ". . . We did question Klinge's generalization. That was the reason why we advocated what might be called, in military parlance, a strategic retreat. The area to which retreat was suggested was the connective tissue. We believed that it was necessary to call attention to the significance of systemic changes of the collagenous tissue in human disease, specifically, of its intercellular components."[309] Furthermore, the term collagen disease has no clinical value as a diagnosis, or perhaps it would be better to state that it has as much value as "renal disease" or "pulmonary disease"; it is purely topographic, indicating the general area of suffering, the seat of disease. The degree of diagnostic accuracy achieved with the diagnosis of "collagen disease" in a given patient can be appreciated from the general features of these diseases: unknown etiology, obscure pathogenesis, diffuse pathology, variable symptomatology, progressive course, poor prognosis and ineffective treatment.[310] Devoid of etiologic meaning, of pathogenetic significance and of clinical specificity, the group of collagen diseases remains as a bold anatomic synthesis and has served not only to stimulate a great amount of work but also to support the concept of connective tissues as an integrated system within the organism.

The majority of authors accept the following entities as collagen diseases: *disseminated* or *visceral lupus erythematosus, rheumatic fever, rheumatoid arthritis, polyarteritis nodosa, scleroderma and dermatomyositis.* Other diseases mentioned have been thrombotic thrombocytopenic purpura, serum sickness, malignant hypertension, Loeffler's pneumonia, erythema nodosum, erythema multiforme, thromboangiitis obliterans, anaphylactoid purpura, pemphigus, etc. This deluge was due to two sets of circumstances that may be described as follows. (a) Many generalized diseases of unknown etiology were included because they involve the connective tissues, which is obviously not the purpose of the group in which only those entities with *primary* interstitial changes are admitted. (b) In view of the prompt adoption of an allergic pathogenesis for collagen diseases, entities in which this mechanism is recognized were also listed. The six diseases considered above show a series of common features which may serve to better establish the limits of the concept of collagen disease. These features may or may not be always present in all six entities, and sometimes some of them predominate to the exclusion of others; nevertheless, their review will probably serve to illustrate the great variability of anatomic, functional, biochemical and clinical manifestations of collagen diseases.

B. GENERAL PATHOLOGY

Most of the common features of diffuse collagen diseases may be encompassed in the following six points. (1) Collagen diseases show generalized and primary changes in the connective tissues. (2) The anatomic lesions, predominantly involving intercellular substances and small blood vessels, are mucinous edema, fibrinoid necrosis, granuloma formation, fibrosis and hyalinization. (3) There is a different and usually distinctive topographic distribution of each one of the elementary lesions in the various collagen diseases. (4) There are important, highly characteristic changes in the plasma proteins, and especially in the gamma globulins. (5) Most collagen diseases show signs of hypersensitivity of different types. (6) Most collagen diseases respond dramatically to steroid therapy. Each one of these six major common features of collagen diseases is separately discussed.

1. Generalized Changes in Connective Tissues. It is a condition *sine qua non* for collagen diseases that they show generalized or diffuse involvement of connective tissues.

Inflammation was described as the local reaction to injury of vascularized connective tissue, and is therefore not acceptable in this group. Similar reasons prevent the listing of morphea, discoid lupus, colloid millium, temporal arteritis and other ailments which might well be considered as localized collagen diseases. But in addition to the involvement being diffuse, it is also necessary that it be primary in the connective tissues. The meaning of this is not very clear, since the pathogeneses of the various collagen diseases are not known. Nevertheless, a definite difference seems to exist between myxedema, which is a generalized disturbance of intercellular substances characterized by accumulation of large amounts of mucoproteins due to hypothyroidism, and the more active lesions of connective tissues in collagen diseases. In all probability, increasing knowledge will permit a better definition of the mechanisms of production of connective tissue lesions.

2. Morphologic Reactions. The elementary lesions of connective tissues mentioned before summarize the variety of morphologic reactions in this area of the organism. Mucinous edema, fibrinoid necrosis, inflammation with granuloma formation, fibrosis and hyalinization, involving intercellular substances and small blood vessels, constitute the essential pathology of collagen diseases. But since connective tissues are limited to those patterns of reaction, other diseases such as serum sickness, drug reactions, bacterial infections, etc., will present the same changes. Therefore, characterization of collagen diseases cannot be only on the basis of histopathologic findings, which of necessity they must share with many processes, but must take into account all the other features which are being discussed.

3. Distribution of Elementary Lesions. The pattern of distribution of elementary lesions varies in the different collagen diseases;[311] a summary of it is presented in Table 40. Some specific changes serve to distinguish among the different entities, but in general skin, the cardiovascular structures, joints and kidneys are almost always involved. A brief description of the salient pathologic features of each of the six collagen diseases follows.

Table 40. Tissue Changes Characteristic of Connective Tissue Disease

	INCREASE IN GROUND SUBSTANCE (OR EDEMA)	FIBROPLASTIC PROLIFERATION	INFLAMMATORY REACTION (MONONUCLEAR)	FIBRINOID NECROSIS	PRESENCE OF		
					Vasculitis	Endocarditis	Pericarditis
Rheumatoid arthritis							
Subcutaneous nodules	++	+++	+++	+++	+	+	++
Synovitis	++	+++	++	+			
Rheumatic fever							
Subcutaneous nodules	++	+++	+++	+			
Aschoff bodies	+	+	+++	+	+	+++	+++
Valvulitis	+++	+	+	+++			
Polyarteritis nodosa							
Adventitia	+	+++	+++	+			
Media	0	+	+	+++	+++	0	0
Intima	+	+	++				
Dermatomyositis	+	++	++	+	+	0	0
Lupus erythematosus	++	+	+	++	++	++	++
Scleroderma	++	+ (fibroblast) +++ (collagen)	0	0 (pie) + (vessels)			

(Bunim and Black [311])

a. Disseminated Lupus Erythematosus. The skin lesions are characterized by erythema of the face and the exposed areas of the surface of the body; the most typical lesion is an elevated, sharply marginated erythematous area on the malar eminences and the bridge of the nose, which may produce the familiar "butterfly" picture. Petechiae or even large hemorrhages may be found, as well as occasional vesicular or bullous lesions; the skin of the fingertips and that around the nailbeds tends to swell and turn red or purple.[312] Skin lesions are no index of the extent of visceral involvement and may even be entirely absent throughout the course of the disease.[313] Microscopically, lesions are found in the connective tissue and blood vessels of the dermis; collagen bundles show intense acidophilia and increased thickness and refractility, and in acute cases they may appear fragmented and basophilic;[314] blood vessels may show fibrinoid necrosis of the wall and infiltration by lymphocytes and macrophages.[315] Other changes are hyperkeratosis with plugging of hair follicles and sweat gland ducts, parakeratosis, alternating acanthosis and atrophy of the epithelium with basal cell vacuolation and pigment mobilization (Fig. 6–22).

The cardiovascular system shows three distinctive lesions in disseminated lupus, which are atypical verrucous endocarditis (Libman-Sacks), hematoxylin bodies and necrotizing arteritis. Atypical endocarditis is characterized by the presence of single or multiple vegetations in the valvular edge, chordae tendineae or papillary muscles, where vegetations caused by other diseases are seldom, if ever, found.[316] Lupus vegetations are small and friable, but in the last stages of the disease they may increase in

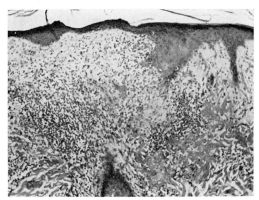

Fig. 6–22. Skin in acute disseminated lupus erythematosus. There is patchy atrophy of epithelium alternating with acanthosis, fibrinoid necrosis of connective tissue and diffuse inflammatory infiltration. (Courtesy of Dr. Edmundo Rojas.)

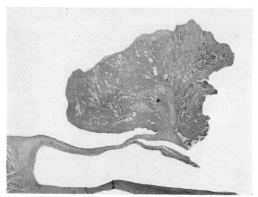

FIG. 6-23. Low power photomicrograph of Libman-Sacks endocarditis in disseminated lupus erythematosus.

size and become infected with pyogenic microorganisms; microscopically they show extensive fibrinoid necrosis of the valvular body with infiltration by polymorphonuclear leukocytes and monocytes (Fig. 6–23).[317] Hematoxylin bodies are not only encountered in the heart but also in renal glomeruli, serous membranes, synovia, lymph nodes, spleen and the connective tissues in general.[318] It is now certain that hematoxylin bodies are the tissue counterpart of the L.E. cell appearing in marrow aspirates or in the peripheral blood, and are formed by isolated or fused, swollen, amphophilic mesenchymal cell nuclei which appear as irregular and bluish masses (Fig. 6–24). Klemperer, et al.[319] believed that the L.E. body, whether in tissues or in vitro blood preparations, was produced by depolymerization of desoxyribonucleic acid in the nuclei of mesenchymal cells, but the brilliant and systematic cytochemical studies of God-

man, et al.[320] have shown that the phenomenon is better accounted for by the penetration of protein into the nucleus which displaces histone and combines with DNA. At the same time it was suggested by immunohistochemical techniques that gamma globulin was fixed to L.E. bodies,[321] and orthodox complement fixation methods have revealed that sera of patients with disseminated lupus and the L.E. phenomenon react in vitro with homologous and heterologous nuclei and with various DNA's.[322]

Most patients with disseminated lupus have arthralgias at one time or another; it is frequently the first symptom and may be accompanied by a certain degree of stiffness, especially of the fingers and knees.[323] Articular deformities are present in no more than 30 per cent of the cases, and then it may be difficult to decide if the patient has lupus plus rheumatoid arthritis, or only one disease; in addition, joint manifestations may resemble fibrositis, or the migrating polyarthritis of rheumatic fever.[324] The pathology of involved joints has not been extensively studied, but in the three cases published by Bennett and Dällenbach[252] there was fibrinoid necrosis surrounded by mucinous edema and mononuclear cell infiltration with some palisading; hematoxylin bodies have also been described.

The kidneys are very often involved in disseminated lupus,[325] and this is a very important complication because of its refractoriness to treatment, even by steroids, and because it is a frequent cause of death.[326] The patient may show the picture of nephrotic syndrome with proteinuria, hypoproteinemia, hyperlipemia and generalized edemas, only to later develop renal insufficiency, with uremia and hypertension.[327] The pathologic picture is that of nephrosclerosis with extensive vascular lesions, glomerular and tubular atrophy and interstitial fibrosis[328] (Fig. 6–25); the characteristic change is present in some glomerular loops which appear rigid, thickened and intensely eosinophilic (the "wire-loop" lesion)[329] (Fig. 6–26). Although this change is not specific for lupus, it is one of the lesions most frequently found and may suggest the diagnosis in otherwise obscure cases.[330]

Many other organs and tissues may show

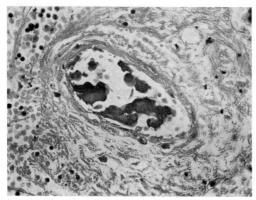

FIG. 6–24. Hematoxylin bodies in lupus erythematosus.

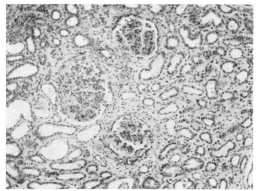

FIG. 6–25.   Kidney in disseminated lupus erythematosus. There are fibrinoid thrombi in glomerular capillaries, increased cellularity of glomerular tufts, vascular hyalinization and slight tubular atrophy.

lesions in disseminated lupus. Lymph nodes contain focal areas of necrosis and infiltration with macrophages and giant cells.[331] There may be splenomegaly and under the microscope there is perivascular concentric fibrosis, a lesion considered highly specific for this disease.[332] Striated muscles reveal interstitial inflammation similar to that encountered in rheumatoid arthritis,[333] and rarely there may be clumps of hematoxylin bodies with histiocytes and epithelioid cells resembling granulomas.[334] There are serous effusions and pleuritis seems to be a frequent finding.[335] Focal changes in the lung parenchyma are said to resemble those seen in rheumatic pneumonia, with hyaline membrane formation, capillary thromboses and necrosis of alveolar walls.[336] The endocrine glands have failed to reveal anatomic changes.[337]

A very important aspect of the pathology of disseminated lupus is the lack of correlation between anatomic changes and clinical severity; indeed, this seems to hold true for most collagen diseases. It is not rare to perform an autopsy of a patient who had advanced manifestations of diffuse involvement in many organs and find few or no anatomic lesions. On the other hand, extensive morphologic changes may be present without having produced any clinical manifestations.

b. Rheumatic Fever. As in disseminated lupus erythematosus, in rheumatic fever the cardiovascular system, the joints, the skin and the kidneys may be involved, but in contrast with lupus the lesions are more frequent and severe in the heart and articular tissues. The incidence of rheumatic fever varies in different countries. It is very frequent and severe in Boston and Mexico[338] and rare in England and Germany. A familial tendency has been demonstrated by Wilson,[339] and the influence of streptococcal infections of the upper respiratory tract is well established, although the exact role played by this microorganism in the pathogenesis of rheumatic fever is not known.[340]

The three layers of the heart are involved, which is very clearly seen in acute attacks. The pericardium shows acute, fibrinous inflammation and the gross picture may be quite similar to that seen in uremic, and even tuberculous, pericarditis; microscopically there is diffuse infiltration of the subepicardial tissues by lymphocytes and mononuclear cells, although occasionally there may be some polymorphonuclear leukocytes, and the surface is covered by a more or less thick layer of fibrin (Fig. 6–27).

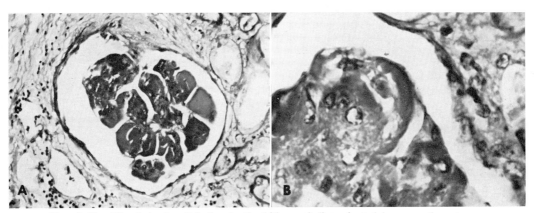

FIG. 6–26.   The "wire-loop" lesion in the kidney of disseminated lupus erythematosus.

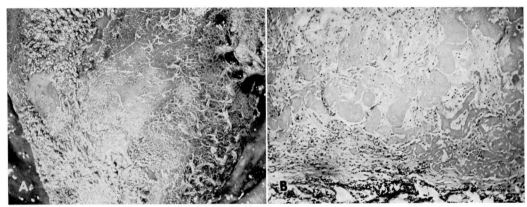

FIG. 6–27.   Acute fibrinous pericarditis in rheumatic fever. *A*, Close-up view of the gross aspect of pericardium. *B*, Microscopic aspect of fibrinous pericarditis.

The myocardium is soft and flabby, with irregular and poorly outlined areas of reddish discoloration; there is an interstitial myocarditis with surprisingly little damage in the myocardial fibers, but with perivascular Aschoff bodies and diffuse infiltration by lymphocytes and mononuclear cells.[341] In very early stages mucinous edema is very apparent, whereas such a lesion tends to disappear with time and in chronic cases only perivascular scars remain as the sole stigmata of old attacks.[342]

The most important lesions, however, are seen in the endocardium, and are characterized by endothelial swelling and exfoliation, fibrin deposition, fibrinoid necrosis of the valvular body surrounded by epithelioid cells with some palisading, or even true granulomas (Fig. 6–28). With the passage of time there is penetration of fibroblasts and organization of fibrin with deposition of collagenous bundles with a great tendency to hyalinization.[343] Vascular proliferation is also prominent, with formation of "musculo-elastic" arterioles which may be found at any distance from the base of the valve.[344] Grossly, the result of this process is a thick, opaque, hard and distorted valve, with disappearance of commissures which become fused and transform the valvular opening into an inextensible ring with a central, more or less elongated orifice (Fig. 6–29). Since fibrosis and hyalinization may also involve the chordae tendineae and result in shortening and fusion of these structures, in the end the hemodynamic conditions are drastically altered. Commissural fusion is responsible for stenosis while thickening and retraction of the valves result in insufficiency. Anatomically it is extremely difficult to speak of "pure" lesions, producing only stenosis or insufficiency, but clinically this

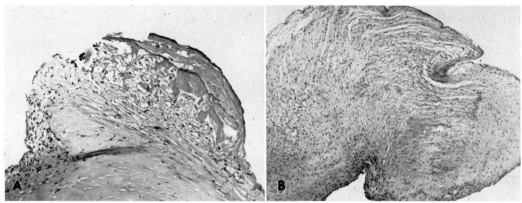

FIG. 6–28.   Rheumatic valvulitis. *A*, Acute verrucous lesion showing fibrinoid necrosis of valvular body with slight inflammation and subendothelial edema. *B*, Scarring of the valve with deposition of collagenous bundles.

differentiation is not only possible, but of great practical significance, since it may decide if the patient is a candidate for surgical correction of the lesion or not. The four valves of the heart may be involved in rheumatic fever, but the mitral valve is the most frequently affected, followed in decreasing order of frequency and severity by the aorta, the tricuspid and the pulmonary valves. The reason for this sequence is not known, although mechanical factors as well as differences in chemical composition have been postulated to explain it.

The skin may show erythematous eruptions, purpura or periarticular nodules, but all these lesions are transitory and occur mainly in children during acute attacks.[345] Renal lesions are infrequent and mild, and most of the times are represented by glomerulitis;[346] occasionally, however, glomerulonephritis may be present.[347] Joint in-

volvement is clinically important because of its frequency and diagnostic significance, but the lesion has not been extensively studied under the microscope. Other tissues that may be altered are the brain,[296] the lung[348] and the iris.[349]

c. *Rheumatoid Arthritis.* The predominant areas involved in this disease are the joints, especially those distally located in the extremities, although the sacroiliac joints or the vertebral column may also be affected producing well defined clinical pictures such as Strümpell-Marie's disease. The fundamental change is chronic synovitis, with early edema, congestion and thickening of the synovial membrane, papillary proliferation of the lining with formation of villi and focal areas of ground substance surrounded by epithelioid cells (Fig. 6–30); the latter are quite similar to subcutaneous nodules.[350] With further development of the lesion degenerative changes appear in the articular

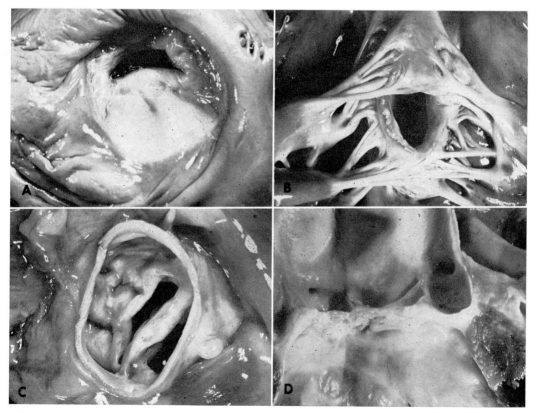

FIG. 6–29. Chronic rheumatic valvulitis. *A,* Mitral stenosis viewed from above, showing the diaphragm-like structure of the valve. *B,* Fusion of leaflets and chordae tendineae in the mitral valve viewed from below, in a case of chronic and acute rheumatic fever. *C,* Thickening and fusion of aortic valves. *D,* Fusion of comissures of aortic valves.

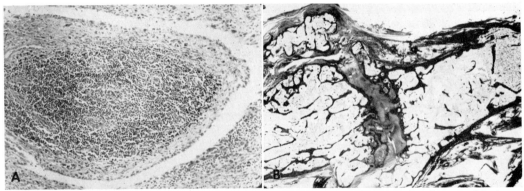

FIG. 6–30. Articular changes in rheumatoid arthritis. *A*, Chronic inflammation in synovial tissues with vascular proliferation and fibrosis. *B*, Osteophyte formation in metaphysis of phalanx. (Courtesy of Dr. Edward S. Murphy.)

cartilage, which is reabsorbed in some localized areas while in others it is invaded by vascularized connective tissue deriving from the inflamed synovia. In addition, there is rarefaction of bone in areas subjacent to the zones of cartilaginous reabsorption, which gives a characteristic radiologic picture.[351] Subcutaneous nodules show a similar picture in this disease to the one observed in rheumatic fever nodules.[352] Biopsy of calf muscles has been used to study the arteritis in rheumatoid arthritis, which is very frequent although unspecific[353]; in addition, such studies have revealed the presence of interstitial myositis with focal inflammation and degenerative changes in the striated muscle fibers.

Cardiovascular lesions similar to those found in rheumatic fever but less intense have been described in this disease; i.e., thickening and retraction of the mitral valve and aortic valves, which may cause hemodynamic changes and give rise to clinical manifestations.[354] Focal necrosis in lymph nodes is also present.[355]

A special form of rheumatoid arthritis is Still's disease, which occurs in children and is accompanied by hepatomegaly, splenomegaly and increase in size of lymph nodes, in addition to advanced and disabling joint changes;[356] splenomegaly in this disease may be accompanied by hypersplenism[357] (Felty's syndrome).

d. Polyarteritis Nodosa. Vascular lesions predominate in this disease, involving medium-sized and small muscular arterioles in any part of the body, so the clinical manifestations will be varied and bizarre;[358] the most frequently involved organs are kidney, heart, liver, digestive tract, pancreas, striated muscles, peripheral and central nervous system.[359] Grossly, the blood vessels appear irregular, with small and localized aneurysmatic dilations corresponding to the most severely damaged areas, where the wall is permanently weakened, and gives way to

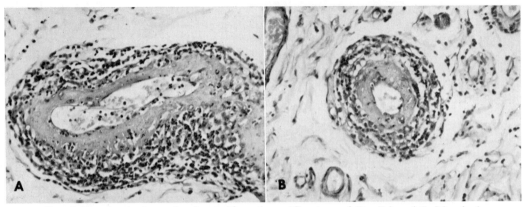

FIG. 6–31. Acute stage of polyarteritis nodosa. (Courtesy of Dr. Edward S. Murphy.)

the arterial pressure; the uninvolved or less intensely damaged areas may appear normal to the unaided eye, but under the microscope they are seen to suffer chronic inflammation with some destruction of the wall.[360]

Several stages may be distinguished in the evolution of the lesions. The acute stage is characterized by intense inflammatory infiltration of the entire thickness of the vascular wall by polymorphonuclear leukocytes, lymphocytes and macrophages; occasionally, there may be a predominance of eosinophilic leukocytes. In addition, in this stage there is mucinous edema and fibrinoid necrosis of the entire thickness of the vascular wall (Fig. 6–31). In the subacute stage there is a combination of healing with necrosis and inflammation, proliferation of fibroblasts and deposition of collagen fibers, but fibrinoid necrosis is still quite prominent.[361] In the chronic stage, the vascular wall is destroyed and replaced by a fibrous scar with very little inflammation.[362] All stages may coincide in the same case in different arteries or even in the same blood vessel, which indicates the recurrent character of this disease.

e. Scleroderma. The main system involved in scleroderma is the skin, but there is also progressive fibrosis in many other organs of the body, such as the heart, striated muscles, the digestive tract, the lungs, etc.[363] Indeed, it has been mentioned that progressive fibrosis is so characteristic of this disease that a synonym is "progressive systemic sclerosis."[364] When the pathologic tissue is limited to a small, localized area of the skin it is known as morphea, and if the distal portions of head and face are involved (tip of the nose, ears) together with Raynaud's syndrome, the disease is known as acrosclerosis.[365]

The skin lesions go through several stages, beginning with hard edema and a brownish-yellowish discoloration; later on there is induration and thickening of the epidermis, which becomes adherent to the subjacent dermal structures. In the last stages there is atrophy of the skin and subcutaneous tissues, which gives the skin its glistening and homogeneous aspect. There is also loss of hair follicles and disappearance of skin glands (Fig. 6–32), and with retraction and loss of elasticity the joint

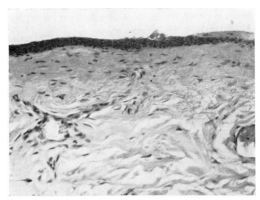

Fig. 6–32. Extreme atrophy and sclerosis of skin in scleroderma.

movements are made difficult or impossible, the face shows sharp features and inability to convey expression or emotions.[366] In advanced cases there are ulcers in the skin, especially of the fingers, and the hands may take the appearance of claws because of joint immobility and stretching of skin. Frequently there is calcification of subcutaneous soft tissues, a form of dystrophic calcification sometimes referred to as Thibierge-Weissenbach syndrome.[367]

In the heart the lesions are mainly found in the myocardium, where there is an increase of interstitial fibrous tissue separating the muscular bundles,[368] although occasionally there may also be pericardial fibrosis.[369] Blood vessels are frequently involved, especially those of small caliber, and the lesions belong to two general types. The first type is indistinguishable from malignant hypertension, with extensive fibrinoid necrosis and inflammation, sometimes suggestive of polyarteritis nodosa[370] of the entire wall, while the other type is more characteristic and consists of intimal proliferation, fibrosis and mucinous edema, and is clearly seen in the kidney.[371] Both types of lesions may occur in the same patient and even in the same artery, and their effects on the kidney are glomerular and tubular[372] atrophy and fibrosis (Fig. 6–33). Rarely, well developed "wire-loop" lesions may be seen in the glomeruli.

In the digestive tract, the lesions are more frequent and severe in the esophagus, which is involved in all advanced cases[373] and which radiologically shows decrease or absence of peristaltic movements with pro-

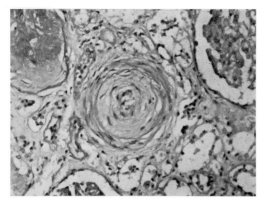

FIG. 6–33. Vascular lesion in the kidney in scleroderma.

longation of the emptying time, and alternating areas of constriction and dilation.[374]
Histologic study reveals proliferation of
connective tissue in the submucosa with
formation of a dense collagenous band
without signs of inflammation[375] (Fig.
6–21). Atrophy of the muscular layers is
often seen in the lower portion of the organ. Similar but less intense lesions have
been described in the stomach and the small
intestine.[376] The lungs show changes of variable radiologic appearance,[377] but the morphologic substrate is fibrosis with formation
of subpleural and basal cystic cavities
("bronchiolar cystic hyperplasia"). A less
frequent type is characterized by the progressive deposition of connective tissue in
the alveolar walls which transforms the
lungs into a dense mass of collagen fibers.[378]

f. Dermatomyositis. The organs principally involved in dermatomyositis are skin
and striated muscles, although the heart,
blood vessels and joints also suffer.[379] This
disease is often more acute than scleroderma and has an irregular course, with
exacerbations and almost complete remissions of all symptoms.[380] Approximately 20
per cent of all cases have been associated
with some form of malignant tumor and
there is no predilection for any specific
type.[381] Chronic cases show swelling of striated muscle fibers with hyaline degeneration and coagulative necrosis, interstitial
inflammation with mucinous edema, fibrinoid necrosis of arterioles and fibrosis. Vascular changes may resemble those seen in
scleroderma and lupus; the microscopic picture of the muscular biopsy is not specific

and should be interpreted in the light of
clinical data.[382] In the skin there is chronic
nonspecific inflammation in the dermis with
some atrophy of the epithelium; during exacerbations there may be epithelial desquamation and formation of bullae. Other
organs, such as the heart and synovial membranes, may show changes similar to scleroderma, but in general are less severe.[383]

4. Changes in the Plasma Proteins. Collagen diseases are also characterized by
changes in the plasma proteins, especially
gamma globulins. In an extensive review
Ehrich[384] summarized the data favoring the
idea that plasma cells produce abnormal
gamma globulins which are responsible for
damaging the connective tissues, and proposed the general term of "disgammaglobu-
linemias" for this group of diseases. This
illustrates the frequency and importance of
the changes in blood chemistry, especially
in gamma globulins, although it is doubtful
that such modifications may have pathogenetic meaning in collagen diseases.

In 1948, Hargraves, *et al.* described the
presence of L.E. (lupus erythematosus)
cells in the bone marrow of patients with
disseminated lupus.[385] These cells are polymorphonuclear leukocytes containing a
large deep purple or red cytoplasmic inclusion, which is formed by nuclear material
derived from lymphocytes or leukocytes.[386]
L.E. cells appear when the plasma of a
patient with disseminated lupus is mixed
with leukocytes of a normal subject, and
the humoral factor responsible for this phenomenon is thought to reside in the gamma
globulins.[387] Furthermore, in disseminated
lupus there may be hyperglobulinemia, hy-
perfibrinogenemia, increased sedimentation
rate and positive flocculation tests, which
indicate severe disturbances in protein metabolism; other abnormal proteins that have
been encountered are autoagglutinins, cryo-
agglutinins, cryoglobulins and C reactive
protein.[388] Abnormal proteins have also
been found in rheumatic fever, some of
them related to streptococcal infection such
as M protein, gamma globulins, antistreptolysin, etc.[389] Similar findings are of diagnostic significance in rheumatoid arthritis,
in which the Hageman factor and the serum
latex factors are of protein nature.[390] Lepow,
et al.[391] investigated a protein which pre-

cipitated spontaneously in cold serum at 24 hours in several cases of polyarteritis nodosa. All these data suggest that in collagen diseases there is a profound disturbance in the intermediary metabolism, which goes beyond any possible surmise from purely morphologic studies.

5. Hypersensitivity. Closely related to abnormal proteins is another common feature of collagen diseases, which is the frequent existence of hypersensitivity phenomena. Allergic manifestations may be nonspecific or apparently unrelated to the disease, and are often encountered either in the past history or as part of the clinical picture of the patient. Since they are the basis for one of the most popular hypotheses on the pathogenesis of collagen diseases, hypersensitivity phenomena are further discussed below.

6. Response to Steroid Therapy. Finally, the spectacular response of most collagen diseases to steroid therapy has been mentioned as an additional common feature which permits their grouping together.[392] It is true that most patients with disseminated lupus show excellent responses to steroids during the acute phases, but the same treatment is less favorable in the more chronic periods of the disease.[393] The effect of ACTH, cortisone and aspirin on acute rheumatic fever was found to be equally beneficial by an international survey,[394] but with different doses. MacCue[395] found that the incidence of late sequelae of rheumatic fever is decreased to one-half with the use of cortisone during the acute attack. In a series of papers, Costero, et al.[396, 397, 398] published their experience in the pathology of acute rheumatic fever in patients treated with cortisone; it was found in 30 autopsied cases that little change was produced by steroid treatment in cardiac and pulmonary lesions, but that cerebral and joint changes were much decreased. Delayed organization of endocardiac verrucae, abundant fibrinoid both in the heart structures and blood vessels and morphologic modifications of Aschoff bodies led these authors to conclude that cortisone seems to enhance the lesions when it is administered during the acute stage of rheumatic fever; on the other hand, healing is favored since it tends to produce less deformity. Patients with rheumatoid arthritis are greatly benefited by steroids especially in the early stages, but there are many problems involved in the chronic use of such hormones in more advanced cases.[399] Dermatomyositis and polyarteritis nodosa can be much alleviated with steroids;[393] in the latter, healing is accelerated and there is less tendency to formation of aneurysms.[400] Scleroderma is the exception to the general rule that patients with collagen diseases are benefited by the use of steroids in therapy;[401] there is evidence that cortisone or ACTH accelerates cardiovascular and renal complications.[402]

Since none of the collagen diseases is caused by an endocrine disturbance, the use of ACTH and cortisone in treatment is based on unspecific effects. The ability of steroids to suppress inflammatory symptoms in collagen diseases, especially pain, goes much beyond this particular group of ailments and is observed (and used) in many other diseases which are totally unrelated. Therefore, the rationale for quoting the response to steroid therapy as one of the features common to collagen diseases may be doubted; when considered together with the other five features mentioned above, however, favorable response to treatment may also contribute in characterizing the group as a whole.

C. ETIOLOGY AND PATHOGENESIS

To discuss the etiology and pathogenesis of collagen diseases as a group is not the result of their having similarities in causation and mechanism, but rather of the profound ignorance prevailing in this field. At the risk of tiring repetition it should be emphasized once again that the concept of collagen diseases is purely anatomic, that it represents a synthesis based on morphologic similarities without any implication of etiologic or pathogenetic relatedness. Some sweeping generalizations have been made, but since they lack the support of objective data they must remain as purely speculative; one danger of accepting any idea of uniformity in the etiology of collagen diseases is the closing, or at least slowing, of investigations aimed at unraveling causation and understanding of the pathologic mechanisms responsible for the lesions. The truth is that the etiology of each one of the diseases under discussion is not known and that their pathogenesis, which includes satisfactory explanations not only for the development of anatomic and biochemical abnormalities, but also for their topographic distribution, is far from being adequately understood. Nor is there any immediate hope of achieving clarity in these respects until more is known about the organization and composition of connective tissues, and especially of the differences existing in various areas, which will probably account for the peculiar distribution of lesions in each disease. These considerations must precede the following brief review of the two main theories of the nature of collagen diseases, namely Selye's endocrine theory and Klinge's allergic theory.

1. Endocrine Theory. According to Selye, collagen diseases (and many others) are the result of disturbances in the normal mechanisms of adaptation to stress; diseases of adaptation have been defined as follows.[403] "We conclude that the pathogenicity of many systemic and local irritants depends largely on the function of the hypophysis-adrenocortical system. The latter may either enhance or inhibit the body's defense reactions against stressor agents and we think that derailments of this adaptive mechanism are the principal factor in the production of certain maladies which we therefore consider to be essentially diseases of adaptation." The list of diseases of adaptation is impressive enough, and includes those under discussion. The concept developed from observations made in experimental animals exposed to nonspecific noxious agents such as cold and fatigue; it was found that many of those animals developed arterial hypertension and nephrosclerosis. Since at the same time it was observed that there was adrenal hypertrophy, it was postulated that an increase in the amount of adrenocorticotropic hormones might be responsible for hypertension and renal changes. Additional observations revealed that DOCA and somatotrophic hormone were capable of inducing both arterial hypertension and nephrosclerosis, together with myocardial, vascular and joint lesions; microscopic examination of these organs showed changes comparable to those seen in collagen diseases.[277]

Theoretically, the mechanisms responsible for diseases of adaptation would be as follows: (a) absolute deficiency or excess of corticoids and somatotrophic hormones produced during stress; (b) a relative disproportion between the secretion of ACTH and glucocorticoids, on one hand, and of somatotrophic hormone and mineralocorticoids, on the other; (c) the production by stress of metabolic disturbances resulting in abnormal tissue reactivity to normal amounts of ACTH, somatotrophic hormone and corticoids; (d) participation of additional organs, such as the central nervous system, liver and kidneys, in the abnormal response to stress.

These speculations were met with great enthusiasm, which is now being transformed into skepticism; today, they have lost the air of daring generalizations that they had when first propounded and very little is left of them that is not free of criticism. Those related to collagen diseases were based on morphologic similarities between lesions produced experimentally and those observed in human disease, but the degree of resemblance of experimental lesions to Aschoff bodies, polyarteritis nodosa and joint changes is certainly not great; indeed, many pathologists deny that they have more than a very superficial similarity and even if the experimental and human lesions were identical it would still be no proof of a unique cause or mechanism. Finally, several clinical studies have failed to reveal any endocrine disturbance in some of the collagen diseases.[337, 404] For all these reasons, the idea that connective tissues may be injured as a system by aberrations of the endocrine organs, and that they represent diseases of adaptation, is no longer entertained with any firmness, the same as with most or all the other diseases originally listed by Selye.

2. Allergic Theory. This is the favorite theory of the etiology and pathogenesis of collagen diseases, in spite of Klemperer's repeated efforts[405, 406] to avoid premature generalizations which would only prolong ignorance. Klinge's observations were published in 1931 and since that time knowledge of the different types of hypersensitivity has become quite complex, so that now it is necessary to be more specific when ascribing a given tissue change to an immune response; the different opinions may be listed in reference to the various types of immune mechanisms as follows:

a. Without reference to any specific type of immune response, Aegerter and Long,[407] and Costero, *et al.*[304] defend the idea that hypersensitivity is the expression of abnormal tissue metabolism, giving rise to antigenic globulins and altering also the connective tissues, which then would become the shock-organ. The distribution and morphology of the lesions are quoted in favor of such a hypothesis, in addition to the similarity of experimentally produced tissue changes and the existence of a clinical history of allergy in many human cases.

b. Klinge,[308] Rich,[408] and others,[409] believed that hypersensitivity in collagen diseases is of the anaphylactic type; i.e., lesions similar to those of collagen diseases are produced in experimental animals by means of repeated injections of antigen, usually egg albumin.

c. Weintraud,[110] Rich,[301] and others[306] suggest that the immune response in some forms of collagen diseases may also correspond to the serum sickness type, which is characterized by the administration of a single dose of antigen and takes some days in appearing.

d. Brunson and Davis[302] have postulated that collagen diseases are due to a generalized Shwartzman reaction, based on the frequency of appearance of fibrinoid changes in this experimental situation; indeed, they suggest the term "systemic fibrinoid diseases."

e. Some type of autoimmunity has been postulated almost simultaneously by several authors, although the nature of the antigen has not been agreed upon; thus, some believe it is a glycoprotein derived from connective tissues,[411] others suggest a nucleoprotein[412] and still others incriminate a combination of foreign substances introduced by pathogenic microorganisms and tissue proteins.[413]

In a fascinating study, Bardawil, *et al.*[414] showed that in several collagen diseases there is hypersensitivity to nuclear material, probably desoxyribonucleic acid, which fixes gamma globulin and requires no complement for the *in vitro* reaction (Fig. 6–34); furthermore, hypersensitivity to nuclear material was reproduced experimentally in rabbits,[415] thus adding further support to the hypothesis that similar mechanisms may be operative in some human cases.

Data favoring hypersensitivity in the etiology and pathogenesis of collagen diseases are not limited to morphologic and experimental observations; epidemiologic and clinical features of some diseases have also been considered as supporting some sort of allergic background. Thus, patients with disseminated lupus erythematosus show hypersensitivity to light and other nonspecific stimuli, and the same has been observed in scleroderma and dermatomyositis.[416] Although clinical data are against the presence

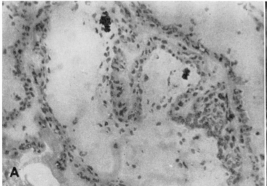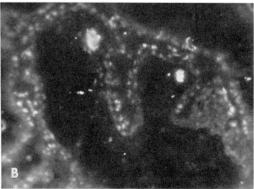

FIG. 6–34. Affinity of serum protein constituent of a patient with diffuse scleroderma for intranuclear nucleoproteins. *A*, Normal immature human placenta, showing general topography of a single villus in cross section. *B*, Same section as in *A* after direct staining with conjugate of serum proteins of patient with scleroderma to fluorescein isocyanate. Note positive nuclear binding reaction. (Courtesy of Dr. W. A. Bardawil and the Editor, American Journal of Pathology.)

of hypersensitivity in rheumatoid arthritis, the serum of some of these patients will agglutinate hemolytic streptococcus type A and other bacteria, collodion particles and sheep red cells.[417] This appears, however, to be a nonspecific agglutination dependent on the increased serum gamma globulins,[418] and therefore cannot be considered in support of an immune response.

In polyarteritis nodosa and in rheumatic fever there seem to be more data favoring hypersensitivity as important in etiology and/or pathogenesis. Vascular changes in polyarteritis nodosa are very similar to those of serum sickness[307] and of certain hypersensitivity reactions to drugs such as sulfonamides,[419] iodine[420] and similar compounds.[421] Furthermore, some types of diffuse vasculitis are associated with asthma and marked eosinophilia, as in the allergic granulomatosis of Churg and Strauss.[299] Rheumatic fever is associated with an infection by hemolytic streptococcus type A,[422] a fact clearly shown by (1) the frequency of preceding attacks of scarlet fever, (2) epidemics due to this microorganism which are followed by an increase in the incidence of rheumatic fever,[423] (3) the effectiveness of prophylactic treatment with penicillin immediately after streptococcal infection in the prevention of rheumatic fever,[424] (4) the presence of antibodies such as antistreptolysin, antistreptohyaluronidase and antistreptokinase, in the serum of patients with active rheumatic fever,[425] etc. Not all types of hemolytic streptococci are capable of inducing an attack or an exacerbation of rheumatic fever. Types 4 and 22 have not been found in the upper respiratory tract of these patients, and in a hospital for rheumatic children an epidemic of laryngitis produced by hemolytic streptococcus type A group 4 was found to have no influence on the natural course of the disease.[426] Finally, in favor of hypersensitivity is the fact that bacteria have not been found in the lesions of rheumatic fever and that there is a latent period of 10 to 14 days between the streptococcal infection and the appearance of the rheumatic attack.

It cannot be denied that this is an impressive array of facts incriminating hypersensitivity in rheumatic fever, but most if not all data quoted above point simply to the association of streptococcus and rheumatic fever, and not to an immune response. The only ones that could be interpreted as such are the evidence of antibody formation, which of course is also present in patients with streptococcal infections and no rheumatic fever, and the latent period between the infection and the attack or exacerbation of the disease. The latent period has been interpreted as the time needed by the organism to synthesize enough antibody to cause the tissue changes, but it cannot be accepted as such since a second infection will result in a second attack of rheumatic fever separated by the same latent period, and not by a shorter lapse, as would be expected from the anamnestic reaction.[427] That the streptococcus need not damage the connective tissues only by its presence or by an immune response has been shown experimentally by Sharp, *et al*.[428, 429] who extracted from C polysaccharide of the capsule of this microorganism a substance capable of producing the same type of tissue changes in the connective tissues without recourse to antigen-antibody reactions, but simply as a toxic substance.

From the foregoing discussion it seems reasonable to conclude that there are no data supporting the concept that collagen diseases have the same etiology and/or pathogenesis, that the different theories suggested are in urgent need of objective support, and that it does not serve any useful purpose to adopt a unitary explanation for such widely different phenomena. Perhaps the acceptance of ignorance is not pleasing, but in this case it is more realistic.

V. HERITABLE DISORDERS OF CONNECTIVE TISSUES

In his scholarly monograph "Heritable Disorders of Connective Tissue," McKusick[430] attempts a synthesis of a series of rare conditions having in common that they involve the connective tissues in a more or less diffuse manner and that they are heritable, even if not inherited in the particular instance. These disorders are not considered congenital malformations in the conven-

Table 41. Heritable Disorders of Connective Tissue in Man. A Synopsis of Symptoms

DISORDERS	SKIN	JOINTS	EYE	BONE	CARDIOVASCULAR SYSTEM	FASCIA	INHERITANCE	FUNDAMENTAL DEFECT
Ehlers-Danlos syndrome	Fragility; hyperelasticity	Hyperextensible	Ectopia lentis; microhemorrhages of retina		Dissecting aneurysm?	Eventration of diaphragm, hernia	Autosomal dominant (low penetrance)	In formation of collagen wicker-work?
Pseudoxanthoma elasticum	Dystrophy in wear and tear areas		Bruch's membrane, crazing of: angioid streaks		Peripheral arteries, medial sclerosis of; hemorrhages		Autosomal recessive; occasionally? dominant	Dystrophy of collagen?
Osteogenesis imperfecta	Thin; abnormal scar formation	Hyperextensible	Sclera, thinning of: blue sclerotics	Brittle bones; otosclerosis (deafness)		Hernia	Autosomal dominant	Maturation of collagen?
Marfan's syndrome		Hyperextensible	Suspensory ligament of lens: ectopia lentis	Excessive length of long bones: dolichostenomelia (long, thin extremities)	Aortic media: Aneurysm	Hernia	Autosomal dominant	Defect of elastic tissue?
Hurler's syndrome	Roughening; nodular thickening	Limitation of mobility	Clouding of cornea	Dwarfism; dysostosis multiplex	Intimal deposits in coronary arteries; valvular lessions	Hernia	Autosomal recessive	Qualitative and/or quantitative abnormality in formation of mucopolysaccharide or structural polysaccharide

(McKusick[430])

tional sense, although it is true that certain malformations do seem to occur with greater frequency in association with some of them. Although all five diseases included by Mc-Kusick in this group are very rare, they represent extremely useful tools for the study of the normal biology of connective tissues and they add support to the concept of connective tissue as a system. It is for this reason that these five diseases are briefly reviewed here.

The five diseases considered as heritable disorders of connective tissue are Marfan's syndrome, Ehlers-Danlos syndrome, osteogenesis imperfecta, pseudoxanthoma elasticum and Hurler's syndrome. A summary of clinical findings, type of inheritance and fundamental defect appears in Table 41. These diseases are considered the result of a single mutant gene which controls some basic enzymatic process because of the unlikelihood of several genes undergoing repeated and simultaneous mutations causing the same defects once and again with such exactitude; furthermore, in some of these diseases, and especially in osteogenesis imperfecta and the Ehlers-Danlos syndrome, most if not all pathologic changes can be ascribed to a single defect, namely in the formation and maturation of collagen. The clinical pictures are not always complete; i.e., some components of one syndrome may not be entirely developed or be missing, as with the ocular or skeletal manifestations of Marfan's syndrome, which then appears as a "forme fruste" with aortic changes, usually in the form of aneurysm. On the other hand, many individual manifestations occur in more than one of these syndromes. For instance, blue sclerae are characteristic of osteogenesis imperfecta, but may also be seen in Marfan's syndrome, or aortic lesions and ectopia lentis are important components of Marfan's syndrome, but may also appear in the Ehlers-Danlos syndrome. These overlaps are indicative of the failure of some function of connective tissue, which may be brought about by defects in any of the extracellular components or in various combinations of them.

A. MARFAN'S SYNDROME

This is an uncommon disease characterized by involvement of the eyes, the skeleton and the aorta and pulmonary artery; although the sexes are equally affected, aortic complications seem to be more frequent in males.[431] Inheritance follows the pattern of a single Mendelian autosomal dominant, although rarely it may also be recessive. Ectopia lentis, almost always bilateral, is the most telling ocular lesion in this syndrome, which is frequently accompanied by myopia and by retinal detachment.[432] The suspensory ligaments of the lens may be broken or attenuated, and there may be complete dislocation of the lens into the anterior chamber. The skeleton shows a tendency to dolichomorphism, with long extremities and arachnodactyly; height may be exaggerated, but true gigantism is not frequent. Skeletal deformities such as pectum excavatum, dolichocephaly, highly arched palate, kyphoscoliosis, etc., may dominate the picture and appear more prominent because of redundancy of joint capsules, ligaments and tendons, and because of muscular underdevelopment and hypotonia.[433]

The aorta and the pulmonary artery may show the only positive pathologic findings in autopsied cases. The media shows fragmentation and sparsity of elastic fibers, slight increase in the amount of smooth muscle fibers and increased vascularity; by far the most impressive finding is the presence of cystic spaces filled with metachromatic material.[434] These spaces may be few and widely separate, or else may replace almost the entire medial layer of the blood vessel; in the latter case, the wall may be thicker than normal. This picture is known as Erdheim's disease or idiopathic cystic necrosis of the media and is probably due to many different causes, some hereditary (like Marfan's syndrome) and some acquired.[435] The result of the aortic lesion is dilation, which may reach truly aneurysmatic proportions, dissection of the media and aortic regurgitation. Both the pulmonary artery and the aorta show medial changes which predominate in the main pulmonary artery and in the ascending portion of the aorta, although complications are by far more frequent in the latter, probably because of hemodynamic conditions.[436]

It has been postulated that the basic defect in Marfan's syndrome is in the elastic fiber.[430] The relation of the suspensory ligament of the lens with the aorta and the skeleton is not known, and the low hydroxyproline content of elastin is not in favor of such a suggestion, considering the findings of Sjoerdsman, *et al.*[437] of an increased urinary excretion of hydroxyproline, nor is the finding of normal elastic tissue in trachea, skin, intervertebral disks and other areas in patients with Marfan's syndrome.[438]

B. EHLERS-DANLOS SYNDROME

In this syndrome the changes are located in the skin, the skeleton, the eyes and some internal organs such as the respiratory and digestive tracts, and the heart; it is more frequent in males (2:1) and may become apparent at an early age. The disorder is probably inherited as a simple autosomal dominant.[439] The skin is usually very light and velvety in appearance and feel; it fits the underlying structures very well, but can be extended in a truly remarkable fashion, only to return to its normal position upon cessation of pull. Therefore, it is better described as hyperextensible and not as lax. In addition, the skin is fragile and brittle, bruises easily and bleeds more than normal; in knees, shins and elbows it becomes shiny, thin and hyperpigmented, and the scars are known as "cigarette paper" or "papyraceous." Microscopically there is an increase in elastic fibers in the dermis,[440] although some authors believe the change is not quantitative but qualitative, and others even described elastic fibers as decreased; collagen may be decreased and the arrangement is disorderly.[441] Working with the electron microscope, Tunbridge *et al.* failed to find any lesions in either collagen or elastic fibers.[442] Hemorrhages undergo calcification or even ossification, and this may represent a radiologic clue for the diagnosis of the Ehlers-Danlos syndrome.[443] Hyperextensibility of the joints is characteristic and sometimes extraordinary; habitual dislocation of the hip and other articulations is frequently seen, together with muscular hypotonicity and underdevelopment. Eye changes are variable from strabismus to blue sclerotics and ectopia lentis. Hiatal hernia, gastrointestinal diverticuli, spontaneous pneumothorax and other internal signs of connective tissue involvement have been reported but appear to be rather infrequent; more rarely there may be dissecting aneurysms of the aorta.

The basic defect in the Ehlers-Danlos syndrome seems to be in the collagen fibers, and Jansen[441] considers that the increase in elastic fibers is only a reparative phenomenon; according to this author the main disorder is not so much in the synthesis of collagen, but in its organization in bundles and networks; this facilitates disruption of subcutaneous tissue and provides little support to blood vessels.

C. OSTEOGENESIS IMPERFECTA

In this disease the main organs involved are bones, eyes, skin, ears and occasionally the cardiovascular system. Several types have been distinguished clinically, such as congenital and tarda, van der Hoeve's syndrome (the triad of brittle bones, blue sclerae and deafness), a "slender bone type" and a "thick bone type," etc., but they seem to be variable clinical expressions of the same fundamental disorder of connective tissues.[430] Inheritance is autosomal dominant and there seems to be a slight predominance of females.[444] In the congenital form the child is frequently stillborn and shows a poorly developed skeleton; the skull may be very thin and on x-ray shows a mosaic pattern due to the presence of numerous Wormian bones. If the child survives the mosaic pattern persists throughout life and is almost specific to the disease.[445] Micromelia or short extremities are also encountered in the congenital form, which may lead to confusion with achondroplasia; there may be multiple fractures which have occurred *in utero* from minimal trauma, and fragility of the skeleton is manifested later by the extreme triviality of trauma necessary for causing fractures. The bones are poorly formed and on x-ray appear extremely radiolucent, with very thin cortices, so sometimes it may be difficult to distinguish bone structure from surrounding soft tissues. In less severe cases the bones are not shortened and fractures heal normally and rapidly or there may even be hypertrophic callus formation, which is composed mainly of cartilage with insufficient production of a healthy bony union.[446] Microscopically the picture varies in severity according to the nature and duration of the case, but in all there is the same fundamental disorder— lack of deposition of bone matrix.[447] The little there is is normally calcified, but most areas where bone trabeculae should exist show only fibroblasts in a more or less dense stroma; the epiphyseal line is normal but the cartilaginous bars are coated only by thin layers of osteoid tissue.[448] Microfractures are common in those thin and poorly formed bone trabeculae.

The joints are characteristically excessively mobile, as in Marfan's syndrome and the Ehlers-Danlos syndrome. The reason for this is the presence of weak, stretched tendons and joint capsules, as well as the deformity and maladaptation of the bony surfaces of the joints, but muscular hypotonia and underdevelopment may also play a role. Blue sclerae are very frequent in this disease, but rarely they may not be present in otherwise typical instances. The sclerae appear blue because of their thinness and the showing through of the underlying choroid pigment; often the part of the sclera immediately around the cornea is whiter, resulting in the so-called "Saturn's ring." Other ocular changes have been embryotoxon (a congenital opacity in the periphery of the cornea), hypermetropia, keratoconus and ectopia lentis.

The skin is usually thin and translucent, bruises and bleeds easily and the scars formed may be wider than normal. Deafness is not always present, but when found it has all the clinical pattern of otosclerosis; it may be aggravated by middle-ear infections and sometimes begins with pregnancy. Calcification of the large peripheral arteries has been described, which may also involve pulmonary and cerebral vessels; associated rheumatic fever may be confused with inherited developmental anomalies, but congenital heart disease seems to occur with some frequency in these patients.

D. PSEUDOXANTHOMA ELASTICUM

The clinical manifestations of pseudoxanthoma elasticum involve the skin, the eyes and the cardiovascular system. It is inherited as an autosomal recessive and predominates in females; most of the manifestations become apparent more or less late in life. Skin changes consist of yellowish or orange-colored mottling or streaks with loss of elasticity of the skin of the sides of the neck, axillae, groins and extensor surfaces of the elbows and knees; the face, scalp, palms and soles are entirely spared, but the oral mucosa, as well as the rectum and vagina, may be involved.[449] In approximately half of the cases there is angioid streaking of the eye fundus; the streaks are brownish or gray and are much wider than veins but their course resembles vessels. There may also be proliferative changes and hemorrhages from the retinal vessels, and loss of vision, though severe, is usually incomplete.[450] Arterial hypertension occurs with sufficient frequency to make it worthy of inclusion in the clinical picture, together with arterial calcification, especially of the arms and legs.[451] Aortic dilation and cerebral vascular changes have also been reported, the latter in association with the high frequency of psychiatric disorders observed in these patients.

Hemorrhage, usually gastrointestinal, is the main problem in many cases, and although it may originate from a peptic ulcer, in most instances the source is not apparent;[452] such hemorrhages may prove fatal, or else they may also appear in other locations including subarachnoid, retinal, renal, uterine and nasal bleeding. The microscopic changes have been better studied in the skin, since the number of autopsied cases is still very meager. Histologic sections show a mid-dermal zone of curlicues of small, compactly massed, basophilic elastic fibers which are diagnostic of the condition; basophilia is partly caused by calcium incrustations. Elastic fibers may appear ruptured and degenerated throughout the cardiovascular system, including the aorta and the pulmonary artery; McKusick[430] reports two autopsies, one with definite elastic changes in the endocardium.

Although on first view the main defect would seem to be in the elastic fibers, a number of very cogent reasons are given by McKusick[430] in favor of the hypothesis of a primary defect in collagen fibers. For instance, elastic fibers are normally present in the upper dermis, whereas the lesion in pseudoxanthoma elasticum appears much deeper. Furthermore, the arteries predominantly involved are the so-called muscular arteries, which have much collagen and little elastic tissue in the medial layer. Finally, electron microscope studies have shown that the dystrophic fibers, although abnormal in other respects, have the characteristic 650 Å periodicity of collagen.[442] The fact that abnormal fibers stain with elastic stains is explained, by suggesting that "collagen may undergo dystrophic, chemical or physicochemical changes, with resulting acquisition of the tinctorial characteristics of elastic fibers." Moran and Lansing,[453] however, have reported microincineration, enzymatic and electron microscopic observations on the skin in one case and concluded that they are all suggestive of elastic fibers. The subject requires additional studies before a final decision is reached, since the same authors found an increase in collagen fibers.

E. HURLER'S SYNDROME

Also known as lipochondrodystrophy or gargoylism, this syndrome is characterized by disturbances in skeletal growth with irregularities in endochondral ossification and consequent grotesque deformities of the axial skeleton, extremities and skull. There is also limitation of joint motion, deafness, hepatosplenomegaly, cardiac abnormalities, clouding of the cornea and mental deficiency. There is a predominance in males and the disease is usually inherited as an autosomal recessive trait, less commonly as a sex-linked recessive.[454]

The patient may appear normal at birth, but with the passage of the first year the syndrome becomes manifest. The head is large and bulging; the nose has a saddle appearance with a broad tip and wide nostrils; the eyes are widely separated and there is scaphocephalia with frontal hyperostosis. The shape of the sella turcica on x-rays of the skull is characteristically elongated and shallow ("shoe-shaped"). The general features of the face, with thick lips, open mouth and prominent tongue, suggest cretinism; the neck is short and the chest may show kyphosis or other deformities. The extremities are short and claw-hands are present in patients more than a few years old; radiologically the long bones show expansion of the medullary cavity with swelling of the shaft. The abdomen is prominent, partly because of hepatosplenomegaly, which may be pronounced; diastasis recti and umbilical hernia are the rule.[455]

The endocrine glands are normal, including the pituitary gland, which is of normal size in spite of the enlarged sella turcica.[456] Peripheral leukocytes may show inclusions known as Alder bodies, but they are more frequent in the bone marrow, especially in cells classified as histiocytes; histochemical studies of these inclusions suggest that they are formed by the same material stored in reticuloendothelial cells of other areas of the organism.[457] Deafness is partly the result of middle-ear infections, which are particularly frequent in these patients because of the deformity of the nasopharynx. Clouding of the cornea has been described in over two thirds of cases, those inherited as sex-linked recessive being spared. Mental development is normal during the first few months or years, but it becomes progressively slower and in many cases there is deterioration of mental faculties.[458]

Microscopically the essential lesion is the presence of cells with large cytoplasm containing a finely granular or vacuolated material in cartilage, fasciae, tendons, periosteum, blood vessels, heart valves, meninges, cornea, liver, spleen, lymph nodes, etc.; even epithelial cells such as in the pituitary may contain the material. Similar material balloons the nerve cells of both the central nervous system and the peripheral ganglia, and the nerve cells in the nuclear layer of the retina. Histochemical studies of the intracytoplasmic material are suggestive of a glycoprotein,[459] while chemical analyses of liver and spleen have rendered at least two distinct compounds, one a complex polysaccharide and the other a glycolipid, which have been named fractions P and S, respectively.[460] Meyer, et al.[461] found large amounts of heparitin sulphate and chondroitin sulphate B in the tissues and urine of a patient. As suggested by Meyer, the basic defect in Hurler's syndrome is a genetic error in the differentiation of the fibroblasts, which produce excessive amounts of mucopolysaccharides. The result is accumulation of these substances, not only in fibroblasts but in many other cells of the organism, including the reticuloendothelial system; in this view, Hurler's syndrome is both a generalized disorder of the connective tissues and a storage disease.

REFERENCES

1. Schade, H.: Die Physikalische Chemie in der Inneren Medizin ed. 3, Dresden, Theodor Steinkopf. 1923.
2. Schade, H.: Untersuchungen zur Organfunktion des Bindegewebes, Ztschr. f. exper. Path. u. Ther. *11:*369, 1912.
3. Jäger, E.: Zur pathologischen Anatomie der Thromboangiitis obliterans bei juveniler Extremitätgangrän, Virchows Arch. path. Anat. *284:*526, 584, 1932.
4. Rössle, R.: Die Rheumatische Formenkreiss, Verchows Arch. path. Anat. *288:*780, 1933.
5. Klinge, F.: Der Rheumatismus, Ergebn. allg. Path. *27:*1, 1933.
6. Klemperer, P., Pollack, A. D., and Baehr, G.: Diffuse collagen disease, J.A.M.A. *119:*331, 1942.
7. Klemperer, P.: Concept of collagen diseases, Am. J. Path. *26:*505, 1950.
8. Klemperer, P.: The role of connective tissues in diseases of the cardiovascular system, Bull. New York Acad. Med. *28:*204, 1952.
9. Klemperer, P.: The significance of the intermediate substances of the connective tissues, in human disease, Harvey Lect. *49:*100, 1954.
10. Costero, I.: Caracterización del sistema fibroblástico. I. Bases doctrinarias, Arch. Inst. cardiol. México *24:*237, 1954.
11. Costero, I., Barroso-Moguel, R., Pomerat, C. M., and Chévez, A.: Caracterización del sistema fibroblástico. II. Fibrogénesis intracelular en tejido conectivo cultivado, Arch. Inst. cardiol. México *24:*337, 1954.
12. Costero, I., Barroso-Moguel, R., and Chévez, A.: Caracterización del sistema fibroblástico. III. Histogénesis de las lesiones reumáticas, Arch. Inst. cardiol. México *24:*437, 1954.
13. Costero, I.: Barroso-Moguel, R., Chévez, A., and Pomerat, C. M.: Caracterización del sistema fibroblástico. IV. Fibrocitos reticulares, Arch. Inst. cardiol. México *24:*539, 1954.
14. Costero, I., Chévez, A., Barroso-Moguel, R.: Caracterización del sistema fibroblástico. V. Cultivo in vitro de válvulas cardíacas, Arch. Inst. cardiol. México *25:*1, 1955.
15. Costero, I., Chévez, A., Barroso-Moguel, R., and Pomerat, C. M.: Caracterización del sistema fibroblástico. VI. Morfología de las células mesenquimatosas *in vitro*, Arch. Inst. cardiol. México *25:*125, 1955.
16. Ragan, C. (ed.): Transactions of Conferences on Connective Tissues, 1 to 5, New York, Macy Foundation, 1950–1954.
17. Randall, J. T. (ed.): Nature and Structure of Collagen, London, Butterworth, 1953.
18. Asboe-Hansen, G. (ed.): Connective Tissues in Health and Disease, Copenhagen, Eijnar Munksgaard, 1954.
19. Tunbridge, R. E., Keech, M., Delafresnaye, J. F., and Wood, G. C. (eds.): Connective Tissues, A symposium, Springfield, Charles C Thomas, 1957.
20. Ragan, C.: The physiology of the connective tissue (loose areolar), Ann. Rev. Physiol. *14:*51, 1952.
21. Baker, B. L., and Abrams, G. D.: The physiology of connective tissue, Ann. Rev. Physiol. *17:*61, 1955.

22. Bunim, J. J., and Black, R. L.: Connective tissue (collagen) diseases, Ann. Rev. Med. *8:*389, 1957.
23. Maximow, A. A., and Bloom, E.: A Textbook of Histology, Philadelphia, W. B. Saunders, 1957.
24. Edwards, L. C., and Dunphy, J. E.: Wound healing, New Eng. J. Med. *259:*224, 275, 1958.
25. Novack, C. R., and Paff, G. H.: Localization of acid phosphatase in fibroblast, Anat. Rec. *109:*71, 1951.
26. Bangle, R. J.: The occurrence and distribution of glycogen in hemangioma, dermatofibrosarcoma protuberans, hemangiopericytoma, and Kaposi's sarcoma, Am. J. Path. *28:*1027, 1952.
27. Davidson, J. N., and Leslie, I.: The changing cell number and composition of chicken heart explants growing *in vitro*, Exper. Cell Res. *2:*366, 1952.
28. Fisher, A., Fisher, G., Landschütz, C., Ehrenswärd, G., Rafelson, M., Jr., and Stgernholm, R.: Amino acid formation from C14 labeled glucose in culture of fibroblasts from embryonic chicken heart tissue, Acta physiol. scandinav. *27:*247, 1952.
29. Bouceck, R. J., and Noble, N. L.: Biochemical studies on cholesterol in in vivo cultivated connective tissue, Circulation Res. *5:*27, 1957.
30. Asboe-Hansen, G.: On the Structure and Functions of the Mast Cells, in Tunbridge, R. E., *et al.* (eds.): Connective Tissue, A Symposium, Springfield, Charles C Thomas, 1957.
31. Ehrlich, P.: Beiträge zur Kenntnis der granulierten Bindegewebszellen und der eosinophylen Leukocyten, Arch. Anat. u. Physiol. *3:*166, 1879.
32. Holmgren, H., and Wilander, O.: Beitrag zur Kenntnis der Chemie und Funktion der Ehrlichschen Mastzellen, Ztschr. mikr. anat. Forsch. *42:*242, 1937.
33. Michels, N. A.: The Mast Cells, in Downey, H. A. (ed.): Handbook of Hematology, New York, Paul B. Hoeber, 1938.
34. Benditt, E. P., Arase, M., and Roeper, M. E.: Histamine and heparin in isolated rat mast cells, J. Histochem. *4:*419, 1956.
35. Riley, J. F., and West, G. B.: The presence of histamine in tissue mast cells, J. Physiol. *120:*528, 1953.
36. Hedbom, A., and Snellman, O.: Isolation and analysis of the large cytoplasmic granules of the tissue mast cells, Exper. Cell Res. *9:*148, 1955.
37. Benditt, E. P., Wong, R. L., Arase, M., and Roeper, E.: 5-Hydroxytryptamine in mast cells, Proc. Soc. Exper. Biol. & Med. *90:*303, 1955.
38. Asboe-Hansen, G.: The origin of synovial mucin: Ehrlich's mast cell—a secretory element of the connective tissue, Ann. Rheumat. Dis. *9:*149, 1950.
39. Riley, J. F.: The Mast Cells, Edinburgh, E. & S. Livingstone, 1959.
40. Higginbotham, R. D.: The Mast Cell, in Springer, G. F. (ed.): Polysaccharides in Biology, Tr. 4th Conf., New York, Macy Foundation, 1959.
41. Sylvén, B.: On the Topographical Cytochemistry of Tissue Mast Cells, in Tunbridge, R. E., *et al.* (eds.): Connective Tissue, A Symposium, Springfield, Charles C Thomas, 1957.
42. Spector, W. G.: Substances which affect capillary permeability, Pharmacol. Rev. *10:*475, 1958.
43. Riley, J. F.: The effects of histamine liberators on the mast cells of the rat, J. Path. & Bact. *65:*471, 1953.
44. Asboe-Hansen, G.: The mast cell, Internat. Rev. Cytol. *3:*399, 1954.
45. Benditt, E. P.: An enzyme in mast cells with some

properties resembling chymotrypsin, Fed. Proc. *15:*507, 1956.

46. Montagna, W.: Histology and cytochemistry of human skin. XI. The distribution of β-glucuronidase, J. Biophys. Biochem. Cytol. *3:*343, 1957.

47. Gustavson, K. H.: The Chemistry and Reactivity of Collagen, New York, Academic Press, 1956.

48. Gross, J.: Behavior of collagen units as model in morphogenesis, J. Biophys. Biochem. Cytol. Suppl. *2* (Part 2) 261, 1956.

49. Jackson, D. S.: Some biochemical aspects of fibrogenesis and wound healing, New Eng. J. Med. *259:*814, 1958.

50. Robb-Smith, A. H. T.: The riddle of reticulin, J. Mt. Sinai Hosp. *24:*1155, 1957.

51. Robb-Smith, A. H. T.: What is reticulin? in Tunbridge, R. E., *et al.* (eds.): Connective Tissue, A Symposium, Springfield, Charles C Thomas, 1957.

52. Lillie, R. D.: The allochrome procedure: a differential method segregating the connective tissues: collagen, reticulum, and basement membranes into two groups, Am. J. Clin. Path. *21:*484, 1951.

53. Kramer, H., and Little, K.: Nature of Reticulin, in Randall, J. T. (ed.): Nature and Structure of Collagen, London, Butterworth, 1953.

54. Robb-Smith, A. H. T.: The Nature of Reticulin, in Ragan, C. (ed.): Tr. 3rd Conf. Connective Tissues, New York, Macy Foundation, 1952.

55. Fullmer, H. M., and Lillie, R. D.: The oxytalan fiber: a previously undescribed connective tissue fiber, J. Histochem. *6:*425, 1958.

56. Fullmer, H. M.: The peracetic-orcein-Halmi stain: a stain for connective tissues, Stain Technol. *34:* 81, 1959.

57. Weiss, J.: The nature of the reaction between orcein and elastin, J. Histochem. *2:*21, 1954.

58. Lillie, R. D.: Histochemistry of connective tissue, Lab. Invest. *1:*30, 1952.

59. McManus, J. F. A.: Histochemistry of connective tissues, in Asboe-Hansen, G. (ed.): Connective Tissue in Health and Disease, Copenhagen, Munksgaard, 1954.

60. Bowes, J. H., Elliot, R. G., and Moss, J. A.: The composition of collagen and acid soluble collagen of bovine skin, Biochem. J. *61:*143, 1955.

61. Eastoe, J. E.: Amino acid composition of mammalian collagen and gelatin, Biochem. J. *61:* 589, 1956.

62. Neuman, R. E., and Logan, M. A.: The determination of collagen and elastin in tissues, J. Biol. Chem. *186:*549, 1950.

63. Zacharidés, P. A.: Recherches sur la structure du tissu conjonctif, sensibilité du tendon aux acides, Compt. rend. Soc. Biol. *52:*182, 1900.

64. Nageotte, J.: Action des sels neutres sur la formation du caillot artificiel de collagene, Compt. rend. Soc. Biol. *96:*828, 1927.

65. Jackson, D. S., Leach, A. A., and Jacobs, S.: Amino acid composition of collagen fractions of rabbit skin, Biochim. et Biophys. acta *27:* 418, 1958.

66. Wyckoff, R. W. G., and Corey, R. B.: X-ray diffraction patterns from reprecipitated connective tissue, Proc. Soc. Exper. Biol. & Med. *34:*285, 1936.

67. Bahr, G.: Reconstitution of collagen fibrils as revealed by electron microscopy, Exper. Cell Res. *1:*603, 1950.

68. Orekhovitch, V. N., Stanowski, A. A., and Plonitkova, N. E.: Isolation of crystalline proteins of a new type (procollagen) from various organs of the vertebrates, Chem. Abst. *43:*259, 1949.

69. Gross, J., Highberger, J. H., and Schmitt, F. O.: Extraction of collagen from connective tissue by neutral salt solution, Proc. Nat. Acad. Sc. *41:*1, 1955.

70. Jackson, D. S., and Bentley, J. P.: On the significance of the extractable collagens, J. Biophys. Biochem. Cytol. *7:*37, 1960.

71. Jackson, D. S.: Chemistry of the Fibrous Elements of Connective Tissue, in Page, I. H. (ed.): Connective Tissue, Thrombosis, and Atherosclerosis, New York, Academic Press, 1959.

72. Jackson, D. S., and Williams, G.: Nature of reticulin, Nature *178:*915, 1956.

73. Windrum, G. M., Kent, P. W., and Eastoe, J. E.: The constitution of human renal reticulin, Brit. J. Exper. Path. *36:*49, 1955.

74. Partridge, S. M., and Davies, H. F.: Composition of the soluble proteins derived from elastin, Biochem. J. *61:*21, 1955.

75. Lansing, A. I., Roberts, E., Ramasarma, G. B., Rosenthal, T. B., and Alex, M.: Changes with age in amino acid composition of arterial elastin, Proc. Soc. Exper. Biol. & Med. *76:*714, 1951.

76. Partridge, S. M., Davis, H. F., and Adair, G. S.: The chemistry of connective tissue. II. Soluble proteins derived from partial hydrolysis of elastin, Biochem. J. *61:*11, 1955.

77. Burton, D., Hall, D. A., Keech, M. K., Reed, R., Saxl, H., Tunbridge, R. E., and Wood, M. J.: Apparent transformation of collagen into "elastin." Nature *176:*966, 1955.

78. Keech, M. K.: Transformation of collagen to elastin in dermal collagens with varying sensitivity towards collagenase, Ann. Rheumat. Dis. *17:*23, 1958.

79. Partridge, S. M.: Elastin-like Structures from Collagen, in Stainsby, G. (ed.): Recent Advances in Gelatin and Glue Research, New York, Pergamon Press, 1958.

80. Grassmann, W., Hanning, K., Endres, H., and Riedel, A.: Amino-acid Sequences of Collagen, in Tunbridge, R. E., *et al.* (eds.): Connective Tissue, A Symposium, Springfield, Charles C Thomas, 1957.

81. Hall, D. A., Lloyd, P. F., Saxl, H., and Happey, F.: Mammalian cellulose, Nature *181:*470, 1958.

82. Rich, A., and Crick, F. H. C.: The structure of collagen, Nature *176:*915, 1955.

83. Gustavson, K. H.: The function of hydroxyprolines in collagens, Nature *175:*70, 1955.

84. Schmitt, F. O.: The Macromolecular Basis of Collagen Structure, in Page, I. H. (ed.): Connective Tissue, Thrombosis, and Atherosclerosis, New York, Academic Press, 1959.

85. Bear, R. S.: X-ray diffraction studies on protein fibers. I. The large fiber-axis period of collagen, J. Am. Chem. Soc. *66:*1297, 1944.

86. Kellgren, J. H., Ball, J., Astbury, W. T., Reed, R., and Beighton, E.: Biophysical studies of rheumatoid connective tissue, Nature *169:*493, 1951.

87. Gross, J., and Schmitt, F. O.: The structure of human skin collagen as studied with the electron microscope, J. Exper. Med. *88:*555, 1948.

88. Wyckoff, R. W. G.: The Fine Structure of Connective Tissues, in Ragan, C. (ed.): Tr. 3rd Conf. Connective Tissue, New York, Macy Foundation, 1952.

89. Porter, K. R.: Repair Process in Connective Tissues, in Ragan, C. (ed.): Tr. 2nd Conf. Connective Tissue, New York, Macy Foundation, 1951.

90. Bear, R. S.: The structure of collagen fibrils, Advances in Protein Chemistry 7:69, 1952.

91. Schwarz, W.: Morphology and Differentiation of the Connective Tissue Fibers, in Tunbridge, R.

E., *et al.* (eds.): Connective Tissue, A Symposium, Springfield, Charles C Thomas, 1957.

92. Vanamee, O., and Porter, K. R.: Observations with electron microscope on solvation and reconstitution of collagen, J. Exper. Med. *94:*255, 1951.

93. Highberger, J. H., Gross, J., and Schmitt, F. O.: Interaction of mucoprotein with soluble collagen; an electron microscope study, Proc. Nat. Acad. Sc. *37:*286, 1951.

94. Gale, J. C.: Electron microscopic studies of collagen from normal and diseased tissues, Am. J. Path. *26:*707, 1950.

95. Keech, M. K.: The percentage of tapered fibril ends in skin collagen from cases with and without collagen disease, Yale J. Biol. & Med. *26:* 527, 1954.

96. Wolpers, C.: Elektronenmikroskopische Untersuchungen zur Pathologie kollagenen Fasern, Frankfurt Ztschr. Path. *61:*417, 1950.

97. Rich, A. R., Voisin, G. A., and Bang, F. B.: Electron microscopic studies of the alteration of collagen fibrils in the Arthus phenomenon, Bull. Johns Hopkins Hosp. *92:*222, 1953.

98. Watson, R. F., Rothbard, S., and Vanamee, P.: The antigenicity of rat collagen, J. Exper. Med. *99:*535, 1954.

99. Hill, A. G. S., and Cruickshank, B.: A study of antigenic components of kidney tissue, Brit. J. Exper. Path. *34:*27, 1953.

100. Milazzo, S. S.: A study of the immunological properties of reticulin, J. Path. & Bact. *73:*527, 1957.

101. Cruickshank, B., and Hill, A. G. S.: The histochemical identification of a connective tissue antigen in the rat, J. Path. & Bact. *34:*27, 1953.

102. Duran-Reynals, F.: Introduction, in Duran-Reynals, F. (ed.): The ground substance of the mesenchyme and hyaluronidase, Ann. New York Acad. Sc. *52:*946, 1950.

103. Dorfman, A.: The effects of adrenal hormones on connective tissue, Ann. New York Acad. Sc. *56:*698, 1953.

104. Moore, R. D., and Schoenberg, M. D.: Studies on connective tissue. I. The polysaccharides of the human umbilical cord, Arch. Path. *64:*39, 1957.

105. Bondareff, W.: Submicroscopic morphology of connective tissue ground substance with particular regard to fibrillogenesis and aging, Gerontologia *1:*222, 1957.

106. Chase, W. H.: Extracellular distribution of ferrocyanide in muscle, Arch. Path. *67:*525, 1959.

107. Dennis, J. B.: Effects of various factors on the distribution of ferrocyanide in ground substance, Arch. Path. *67:*533, 1959.

108. Joseph, N. R., Engel, M. B., and Catchpole, H. R.: Interaction of ions and connective tissue, Biochim. et biophys. acta *8:*575, 1952.

109. Gersh, I., and Catchpole, H. R.: The nature of ground substance of connective tissue, Perspect. Biol. & Med. *3:*282, 1960.

110. Gersh, I., and Catchpole, H. R.: The organization of the ground substance and basement membrane and its significance in tissue injury, disease and growth, Am. J. Anat. *85:*457, 1949.

111. Slack, H. G. B.: Some notes on the composition and metabolism of connective tissue, Am. J. Med. *26:*113, 1959.

112. Meyer, K., Hoffman, P., and Linker, A.: The Acid Mucopolysaccharides of Connective Tissue, in Tunbridge, R. E., *et al.* (eds.): Connective Tissue, A Symposium, Springfield, Charles C Thomas, 1957.

113. Meyer, K., Davidson, E., Linker, A., and Hoffman, P.: The acid mucopolysaccharides of connective tissue, Biochem. & Biophys. Acta *21:*506, 1956.

114. Meyer, K.: Chemical structure of hyaluronic acid, Fed. Proc. *17:*1075, 1958.

115. Davidson, E. A., and Meyer, K.: Chondroitin, a new mucopolysaccharide, J. Biol. Chem. *211:* 605, 1954.

116. Meyer, K., and Rapport, M. M.: The mucopolysaccharides of the ground substance of connective tissue, Science *113:*596, 1951.

117. Hoffman, P., Linker, A., and Meyer, K.: Chondroitin sulfates, Fed. Proc. *17:*1078, 1958.

118. Jeanloz, R. W.: Structure of heparin, Fed. Proc. *17:*1082, 1958.

119. Balasz, E. A.: Physical chemistry of hyaluronic acid, Fed. Proc. *17:*1086, 1958.

120. Michaelis, L., and Granick, S.: Metachromasy of basic dyestuffs, J. Am. Chem. Soc. *67:*1212, 1945.

121. Levine, A., and Schubert, M.: Metachromasy of thiazine dyes produced by chrondroitin sulfate, J. Am. Chem. Soc. *74:*91, 1952.

122. Lison, L.: La signification histochimique de la métachromasie, Compt. rend. Soc. Biol. *118:* 821, 1935.

123. Sylvén, B.: Ueber das Vorkommen von Hochmolekulären Esterschwechselnsäuren in Granulationgewebe und bei der Epithelregeneration, Acta chir. Scandinav. *86:* (Suppl. 66), 1, 1945.

124. Kramer, H., and Windrum, G. M.: The metachromatic staining reaction, J. Histochem. *3:* 227, 1955.

125. Wagner, B.: Hypersensitivity. The Role of Connective Tissue, in Mellors, R. C. (ed.): Analytical Pathology, New York, McGraw-Hill, 1957.

126. DiFerrante, N.: Quantitative colorimetric assay of acid mucopolysaccharides, J. Biol. Chem. *209:* 579, 1954.

127. Immers, J.: Chemical and histochemical demonstration of acid esters by acetic iron reagent, Exper. Cell Res. *6:*127, 1954.

128. Wagner, B. M., and Tedeschi, C. G.: Studies in rheumatic fever. II. Origin of cardiac giant cells, Arch. Path. *60:*423, 1955.

129. Lillie, R. D.: Factors influencing periodic acid-Schiff reaction of collagen fibers, J. Histochem. *1:*353, 1953.

130. Bangle, R., Jr., and Alford, W. C.: The chemical basis of the periodic acid-Schiff reaction of collagen fibers with reference to periodate consumption by collagen and insulin, J. Histochem. *2:*62, 1954.

131. Benditt, E. P., and French, J. E.: Histochemistry of connective tissue. I. The use of enzymes as specific histochemical reagents, J. Histochem. *1:*315, 1953.

132. Meyer, K., and Rapport, M. M.: Hyaluronidases, Advances Enzymol. *13:*199, 1952.

133. French, J. E., and Benditt, E. P.: Histochemistry of connective tissue. II. The effect of proteins on the selective staining of mucopolysaccharides by basic dyes, J. Histochem. *1:*321, 1953.

134. Follis, R. H., Jr.: Effect of proteolytic enzymes and fixation on metachromasia of skin collagen, Proc. Soc. Exper. Biol. & Med. *76:*272, 1951.

135. Wagner, B. M.: Histochemical studies of fibrinoid substances and other abnormal tissue proteins. II. Effect of fibrinolytic enzymes, Arch. Path. *59:*63, 1955.

136. Neuberger, A.: The proteins of connective tissue and their metabolism, Ann. Rheumat. Dis. *19:* 1, 1960.

137. Jackson, D. S.: The Formation and Breakdown of Connective Tissue, in Tunbridge, R. E., *et al.* (ed.): Connective Tissue, A Symposium, Springfield, Charles C Thomas, 1957.

138. Humphrey, J. H., Neuberger, A., and Perkins, D. J.: Observations on the presence of plasma proteins in skin and tendon, Biochem. J. *66:*390, 1957.

139. Cohen, S., Holloway, R. C., Matthews, C., and McFarlane, A. S.: Distribution and elimination of I131 and C14 labeled plasma proteins in the rabbit, Biochem. J. *62:*143, 1956.

140. Shatton, J., and Schubert, M.: Isolation of a mucoprotein from cartilage, J. Biol. Chem. *211:*565, 1954.

141. Partridge, S. M., and Davis, H. F.: The chemistry of connective tissues. IV. The presence of a non-collagenous protein in cartilage, Biochem. J. *68:*298, 1958.

142. Schubert, M.: Chondromucoprotein, Fed. Proc. *17:*1099, 1958.

143. Schwann, T.: Microscopical Researches into the Accordance in the Structure and Growth of Animals and Plants, London, Syndenham Society, 1847.

144. Virchow, R.: Die Cellularpathologie in ihre Begründung auf physiologische und pathologische Geweblehre, Berlin, A. Hirschwald, 1848.

145. von Ebner, V.: Die Chorda dorsalis der niederen Fische und die Entwicklung des fibrillären Bindegewebe, Ztschr. wiss. Zool. *62:*469, 1896.

146. Baitsell, G. A.: A study of the clotting of the plasma of frog's blood and the transformation of the clot into fibrous tissue, Am. J. Physiol. *44:*109, 1917.

147. Delaunay, A., and Bazin, S.: Le métabolisme du collagene. I. L'anabolisme à la lumière des données biochimiques, Rev. franc. études clin. biol. *3:*896, 1958.

148. Robertson, W. van B., Hiwett, J., and Herman, C.: The relation of ascorbic acid to the conversion of proline hydroxyproline in the synthesis of collagen in the carrageenin granuloma, J. Biol. Chem. *234:*105, 1959.

149. Gould, B. G., and Woessner, J. F.: The influence of ascorbic acid on the proline, hydroxyproline, glycine, and collagen content of regenerating guinea pig skin, J. Biol. Chem. *226:*289, 1957.

150. Robbins, W. C., Watson, R. F., Pappas, G. D., and Porter, K. R.: Some effects of anticollagen serum on collagen formation in tissue culture: preliminary report, J. Biophys. Biochem. Cytol. *1:*381, 1955.

151. Harkness, R. D., Marko, A. M., Muir, H. M., and Neuberger, A.: Metabolism of collagen and other proteins of skin of rabbits, Biochem. J. *56:*558, 1954.

152. Jackson, D. S.: Connective tissue growth stimulated by carrageenin. I. Formation and removal of collagen, Biochem. J. *65:*277, 1957.

153. Orekhovitch, V. N., and Shpikiter, V. O.: Procollagens as Biological Precursors of Collagen and the Physicochemical Structure of these Proteins, in Tunbridge, R. E., *et al.* (eds.): Connective Tissue, A Symposium, Springfield, Charles C Thomas, 1957.

154. Gross, J.: Studies on formation of collagen. II. Influence of growth rate on neutral salt extracts of guinea pig dermis, J. Exper. Med. *107:*265, 1958.

155. Gross, J.: On the Significance of the Soluble Collagens, in Page, I. H. (ed.): Connective Tissue, Thrombosis, and Atherosclerosis, New York, Academic Press, 1959.

156. Stearns, M. L.: Studies on development of connective tissue in transparent chambers of rabbit's ear, Am. J. Anat. *66:*133, 1940; *67:*55, 1940.

157. Porter, K. R., and Pappas, G. D.: Collagen formation by fibroblasts of the chick embryo dermis, J. Biophys. Biochem. Cytol. *5:*153, 1959.

158. Wasserman, F.: Fibrillogenesis in the regenerating rat tendon with special reference to growth and composition of the collagenous fibrils, Am. J. Anat. *94:*399, 1954.

159. Costero, I., Barroso-Moguel, R., Pomerat, C. M., and Chévez, A.: Caracterización del sistema fibroblástico. II. Fibrogénesis intracelular en tejido conectivo cultivado, Arch. Inst. cardiol. México *24:*337, 1954.

160. Jackson, S. F.: The morphogenesis of avian tendon, Proc. Roy. Soc. London s.B *144:*556, 1956.

161. Grossfeld, H., Meyer, K., and Godman, G. C.: Differentiation of fibroblasts in tissue culture as determined by mucopolysaccharide production, Proc. Soc. Exper. Biol. & Med. *88:*31, 1955.

162. Grossfeld, H., Meyer, K., and Godman, G.: Mucopolysaccharides produced in tissue culture, J. Biophys. Biochem. Cytol. *3:*391, 1957.

163. Gaines, L. M., Jr.: Synthesis of acid mucopolysaccharides and collagen in tissue cultures of fibroblasts, Bull. Johns Hopkins Hosp. *106:*195, 1960.

164. Gersh, I.: Ground substance and the plasticity of connective tissues, Harvey Lect. *45:*211, 1950.

165. Mancini, R. E., and Bocarini, E.: Mucoproteína de tejido conectivo adulto y embrionario, Rev. Soc. argent. biol. *27:*1951.

166. Pérez Tamayo, R., and Ihnen, M.: Effect of methionine in experimental wound healing. A morphologic study, Am. J. Path. *29:*233, 1953.

167. Meyer, K.: Chemistry of Connective Tissue, in Ragan, C. (ed.): Tr. 1st Conf. Connective Tissue, New York, Macy Foundation, 1950.

168. Kirby, J.: Discussion of Physical and Chemical Problems of Fiber Formation, in Randall, J. T. (ed.): Nature and Structure of Collagen, New York, Academic Press, 1953.

169. Moss, J.: The carbohydrate of collagen, Biochem. J. *61:*151, 1955.

170. Grossman, W., Hoffman, V., Kühn, K., Hörmann, H., Endres, H., and Wolf, K.: Electron Microscope and Chemical Studies of the Carbohydrate Groups in Collagen, in Tunbridge, R. E., *et al.* (eds.): Connective Tissue, A Symposium, Springfield, Charles C Thomas, 1957.

171. Arguedas, J. M., and Pérez Tamayo, R.: The pattern of wound healing of skin autografts and skin homografts in the rat, Surg. Gynec. & Obst. *106:*671, 1958.

172. Grillo, H. C., Watts, T., and Gross, J.: Studies in wound healing. I. Contraction and wound contents, Ann. Surg. *148:*145, 1958.

173. Jackson, D. S.: Some biochemical aspects of fibrogenesis and wound healing, New Eng. J. Med. *259:*814, 1958.

174. Jackson, S. F.: Fibrogenesis in connective tissues, Nature *173:*950, 1954.

175. Jackson, S. F.: The formation of connective and skeletal tissues, Proc. Roy. Soc. London s.B *142:*536, 1954.

176. Jackson, S. F.: Cytoplasmic granules in fibrogenic cells, Nature *175:*39, 1955.

177. Jackson, S. F.: Structural Problems Associated with the Formation of Collagen Fibrils *in vivo,* in Tunbridge, R. E., *et al.* (eds.): Connective Tissue, A Symposium, Springfield, Charles C Thomas, 1957.

178. Harkness, R. D.: Metabolism of collagen, in Lecture on the Scientific Basis of Medicine *5:*183, 1956.

179. Neuberger, A., Perrone, J. C., and Slack, H. G. B.: The relative metabolic inertia of tendon collagen in the rat, Biochem. J. *49:*199, 1951.

180. Robertson, W. van B.: Influence of ascorbic acid on N^{15} incorporation into collagen *in vivo*, J. Biol. Chem. *197:*495, 1952.

181. Dorfman, A.: Metabolism of the mucopolysaccharides of the connective tissue, Pharmacol. Rev. *7:*1, 1955.

182. Dorfman, A.: The biochemistry of connective tissue, J. Chron. Dis. *10:*403, 1959.

183. Dorfman, A.: Studies on the biochemistry of connective tissue. Pediatrics *21:*576, 1958.

184. Boström, H., and Gardell, S.: Uptake of sulphates in mucopolysaccharides esterified with sulfuric acid in the skin of adult rats after intraperitoneal injection of S^{35}-labeled sodium sulfate, Acta chem. scandinav. *7:*216, 1953.

185. Schiller, S., Matthews, M. B., Cifonelli, J. A., and Dorfman, A.: The metabolism of mucopolysaccharides in animals. III. Further studies on skin utilizing C^{14}-glucose, C^{14}-acetate, and S^{35}-sodium sulfate, J. Biol. Chem. *218:*139, 1956.

186. Boström, H.: Biosynthesis of Sulfated Polysaccharides, in Springer, G. F. (ed.): Polysaccharides in Biology, Tr. 4th Conference, New York, Macy Foundation, 1959.

187. Upton, A. C., Odell, T. T., and Gude, W. D.: Incorporation of sulfur^{35}-labeled sulfate in healing wounds and in platelets of normal and scorbutic guinea pigs, Fed. Proc. *14:*421, 1955.

188. Cameron, G. R., and Karunaratne, W. A.: Carbon tetrachloride cirrhosis in relation to liver regeneration, J. Path. & Bact. *42:*1, 1936.

189. Steinberg, B., and Martin, R. A.: Absorption of scar tissues in experimental nodular cirrhosis of the liver, Arch. Path. *41:*1, 1946.

190. Morrione, T. G.: Quantitative study of collagen content in experimental cirrhosis, J. Exper. Med. *85:*217, 1947.

191. Morrione, T. G.: Factors influencing collagen content in experimental cirrhosis, Am. J. Path. *25:*273, 1949.

192. Patek, A., Jr., Oken, D. E., Sakamoto, A., de Fritsch, N., and Bevans, M.: Recovery from dietary cirrhosis of the liver in the rat. Changes in hepatic collagen and microscopic appearance, Arch. Path. *69:*168, 1960.

193. Ungar, H., and Feldman, J. D.: The absorption of collagen in the liver. I. Histologic changes accompanying the absorption of implanted surgical gut in the liver, Am. J. Path. *29:*963, 1953.

194. Ungar, H.: The absorption of collagen in the liver. II. Observations on the absorption of implanted surgical gut under various dietary conditions, Am. J. Path. *29:*973, 1957.

195. Robertson, W. van B., and Schwartz, B.: Ascorbic acid and formation of collagen, J. Biol. Chem. *201:*689, 1953.

196. Williams, G.: A histological study of the connective tissue reaction to carrageenin, J. Path. & Bact. *73:*557, 1957.

197. Slack, H. G. B.: The metabolism of sulphated mucopolysaccharides in carrageenin-induced granuloma, Biochem. J. *64:*7, 1956.

198. Rojkind, M.: Estudios sobre la reabsorción del tejido conjuntivo. Tésis Recepcional, Facultad de Medicina de la Universidad Nacional Autónoma de México, 1960.

199. Harkness, M. L. R., Harkness, R. D., and Stamler, J.: Changes in the collagen content of the thyroid in rats treated with thiouracil, J. Physiol. *125:*51, 1954.

200. Harkness, M. L. R., and Harkness, R. D.: The collagen content of the reproductive tract of the rat, during pregnancy and lactation, J. Physiol. *123:*492, 1954.

201. Harkness, R. D., and Moralee, B. C.: The time-course and route of loss of collagen from the rat uterus during post-partum involution, J. Physiol. *132:*502, 1956.

202. Hurley, S. L., and Herrman, H.: Effect of estrogen and progesterone on collagen content of the rat uterus, heart, and skeletal muscle, Fed. Proc. *14:*230, 1955.

203. Maibenco, H. G.: Connective tissue changes in post-partum uterine involution in the albino rat, Anat. Rec. *136:*59, 1960.

204. Talmage, R. V. N.: Changes produced in symphysis pubis of guinea pigs by sex steroids and relaxin, Anat. Rec. *99:*91, 1947.

205. Frieden, E. H., and Hisaw, F. L.: The mechanism of symphyseal relaxation. The distribution of reducing groups, hexoseamine, and proteins in symphyses of normal and relaxed guinea pigs, Endocrinology *48:*88, 1951.

206. Storey, E.: Relaxation in the pubic symphysis of the mouse during pregnancy and after relaxin administration, with special reference to the behavior of collagen, J. Path. & Bact. *74:*147, 1957.

207. Hamperl, H.: Ueber "Kollageneinschlüsse" in Deciduazellen, Klin. Wchnschr. *20:*939, 1958.

208. Iversen, K.: Hormonal Influence on Connective Tissue, in Asboe-Hansen, G. (ed.): Connective Tissue in Health and Disease, Copenhagen, Eijnar Munksgaard, 1954.

209. Asboe-Hansen, G.: Hormonal effects on connective tissue, Physiol. Rev. *38:*446, 1958.

210. Asboe-Hansen, G.: Endocrine control of connective tissue, Am. J. Med. *26:*470, 1959.

211. Ihnen, M., and Pérez Tamayo, R.: Breast stroma. A morphological and histochemical study, Arch. Path. *56:*46, 1953.

212. Sundblad, L., Egelius, N., and Jonsson, E.: Action of hydrocortisone on hyaluronic acid of joint fluids in rheumatic arthritis, Scand. J. Clin. & Lab. Invest. *6:*295, 1954.

213. Castor, W. C., and Baker, B. L.: The local action of adrenocortical steroids on epidermis and connective tissue of the skin, Endocrinology *47:*234, 1950.

214. Werner, S. C., Hamilton, H., and Frantz, V. K.: Some effects of ACTH in chronic thyroiditis and myxedema, Proc. 2nd Clin. ACTH Conf. *2:*521, 1951.

215. Asboe-Hansen, G., and Iversen, K.: Influence of thyrotrophic hormone on connective tissue. Pathogenetic significance of mucopolysaccharides in experimental exophthalmos, Acta endocrinol. *8:*90, 1951.

216. Iversen, K., and Asboe-Hansen, G.: Studies on the fat mobilizing factor of the anterior pituitary gland. Suppressive action of thyroxine, Acta endocrinol. *11:*111, 1952.

217. Warren, G. H., and Fagan, R.: Accumulation of dermal mucopolysaccharides in animals following injection of estradiol benzoate, Proc. Soc. Exper. Biol. & Med. *103:*786, 1960.

218. Rienits, K. G.: The acid mucopolysaccharides of the sexual skin of apes and monkeys, Biochem. J. *74:*27, 1960.

219. Zachariae, F.: Autoradiographic (S^{35}) and histochemical studies of sulfomucopolysaccharides in the rabbit uterus, oviducts and vagina. Variations under hormonal influence, Acta endocrinol. *29:*118, 1958.

220. Larsen, G.: Effect of hormones on S^{35}-labeled sulfate uptake in guinea pig eye and skin connective tissues, Arch. Ophth. *63:*761, 1960.

221. Schiller, S., Benditt, E. P., and Dorfman, A.: Effect of testosterone and cortisone on the hexo-

samine content and metachromasia of chick combs, Endocrinology *50:*504, 1952.

222. Wolbach, S. B.: Controlled formation of collagen and reticulum. A study of the source of intercellular substance in recovery from experimental scorbutus, Am. J. Path. *9:*689, 1933.

223. Dunphy, J. E., Udupa, K. N., and Edwards, L. C.: Wound healing: new perspective with particular reference to ascorbic acid deficiency, Ann. Surg. *144:*304, 1956.

224. Hunt, A. H.: Role of vitamin C in wound healing, Brit. J. Surg. *28:*436, 1941.

225. Pirani, C. L., and Levenson, S. M.: Effect of vitamin C deficiency on healed wounds, Proc. Soc. Exper. Biol. & Med. *82:*95, 1953.

226. Abt, A. F., Schuching, S. V., and Roe, J. H.: Connective tissue studies. II. The effect of vitamin C deficiency on healed wounds, Bull. Johns Hopkins Hosp. *105:*67, 1959.

227. Gross, J.: Studies on the formation of collagen. IV. Effect of vitamin C deficiency on the neutral salt-extractible collagen of skin, J. Exper. Med. *109:*557, 1959.

228. Mitoma, C., and Smith, T.: Studies on the role of ascorbic acid in collagen synthesis, J. Biol. Chem. *235:*426, 1960.

229. Woesner, J. F., and Gould, B. S.: Collagen biosynthesis: tissue culture experiments to ascertain role of ascorbic acid in collagen formation, J. Biophys. Biochem. Cytol. *3:*685, 1957.

230. Ponsetti, I. V., and Baird, W. A.: Scoliosis and dissecting aneurysm of the aorta in rats fed with Lathyrus odoratus seeds, Am. J. Path. *28:*1059, 1952.

231. Dupuy, H. P., and Lee, J. G.: The isolation of a material capable of producing experimental lathyrism, J. Am. Pharm. A. *43:*61, 1954.

232. Enzinger, F. M., and Warner, E. D.: Wound healing in experimental lathyrism, Lab. Invest. *6:* 251, 1957.

233. Hurley, J. V., and Ham, K. N.: The nature of the connective tissue defect produced by the aminonitriles, Brit. J. Exper. Path. *40:*216, 1959.

234. Enzinger, F. M., and Warner, E. D.: Experimental lathyrism. Effect of aminoacetonitrile on connective tissue formation in adult rats, Arch. Path. *69:*333, 1960.

235. Pyörälä, K., Punsar, S., Seppälä, T., and Karlsson, K.: Mucopolysaccharides of the aorta and epiphyseal cartilage in lathyric growing rats and rat fetuses, Acta path. et microbiol. scandinav. *41:* 497, 1957.

236. Schwartz, C. J.: The nature of the ground substance changes in experimental lathyrism and their effect on atherogenesis in cholesterol fed rabbits, Brit. J. Exper. Path. *40:*44, 1959.

237. Gardner, A. F.: Experimental lathyrism: review of literature, Am. J. Clin. Nutrition *7:*213, 1959.

238. Villamil, M. F., and Mancini, R. E.: Tejido Conectivo y Enfermedades del Colágeno. Ed. López & Etchegoyen, S. R. L., Buenos Aires, 1959.

239. Farbers, S. J.: Mucopolysaccharides and sodium metabolism, Circulation *21:*941, 1960.

240. Kulonen, E.: On the relation of hyaluronic acid to the water and electrolyte metabolism, Acta physiol. scandinav. *27:*82, 1952.

241. Blumberg, B. S., Oster, G., and Meyer, K.: Changes in the physical characteristics of the hyaluronate of ground substance with alterations in sodium chloride concentration, J. Clin. Invest. *34:*1454, 1955.

242. Boyd, E. S., and Neuman, W. F.: Surface chemistry of bone: ion-binding properties of cartilage, J. Biol. Chem. *193:*1953.

243. Joseph, N. R., Engel, M. B., and Catchpole, H. R.: Homeostasis of connective tissues; potassium-sodium relations, Arch. Path. *58:*40, 1954.

244. Joseph, N. R., Catchpole, H. R., Laskin, D. M., and Engel, M. B.: Titration curves of colloidal surfaces. II. Connective tissues, Arch. Biochem. *84:*224, 1959.

245. Duran-Reynals, F.: Tissue permeability and the spreading factor, Bact. Rev. *6:*197, 1942.

246. Opsahl, J. C., White, A., and Duran-Reynals, F.: Effect of adrenocortical hormone on the dermal spreading of India ink in normal and adrenalectomized mice, Ann. New York Acad. Sc. *52:*1061, 1950.

247. Seifter, J., Baeder, D. H., and Derviris, A.: Alteration in permeability of some membranes by hyaluronidases and inhibition of this effect by steroids, Proc. Soc. Exper. Biol. & Med. *72:* 136, 1949.

248. Benditt, E. P.: Actions of heparin other than those of coagulation, Ann. Rev. Med. *8:*407, 1957.

249. Talalajew, W. T.: Der akute Rheumatismus, Klin. Wchnschr. *8:*124, 1929.

250. Klemperer, P. P., Pollack, A. D., and Baehr, G.: Pathology of disseminated lupus erythematosus, Arch. Path. *32:*569, 1941.

251. Moore, H. C., and Sheehan, H. L.: The kidney of scleroderma, Lancet *1:*68, 152.

252. Bennett, G. A., and Dällenbach, F. D.: Synovial membrane changes in disseminated lupus erythematosus, Mil. Surgeon *109:*531, 1951.

253. Becker, B. J. P., Chatgidakis, C. B., and van Lingen, G.: Cardiovascular collagenosis with parietal endocardial thrombosis. A clinicopathologic study of forty cases, Circulation *7:*345, 1953.

254. Geschickter, C. F., Athanasiadou, P. A., and O'Malley, W. E.: The role of mucinolysis in collagen disease, Am. J. Clin. Path. *30:*93, 1958.

255. Lannigan, R.: The rheumatic process in the left auricular appendage, J. Path. & Bact. *77:*49, 1959.

256. Altschuler, C. F., and Angevine, D. M.: Histochemical studies on the pathogenesis of fibrinoid, Am. J. Path. *25:*1061, 1949.

257. Klinge, F.: Das Gewebsbild des fieberhaften Rheumatismus. I Mitteilung. Das rheumatische frühinfiltrat (Akut degenerativ-exudatives Stadium), Virchows Arch. path. Anat. *278:*438, 1930.

258. Gabrilove, J. L., and Ludwig, A. W.: The histogenesis of myxedema, J. Clin. Endocrinol. *17:* 1925, 1957.

259. Beierwaltes, W. H., and Jay, A. B.: Mucopolysaccharide content of skin in patients with pretibial myxedema, J. Clin. Invest. *38:*945, 1959.

260. Neuman, E.: Die Picrocarminfärbung und ihre Anwendung auf die Entzündungslehre, Arch. mikr. Anat. *18:*130, 1880.

261. Klemperer, P.: Ueber fibrinoide Substanzen, Wien. klin. Wchnschr. *65:*713, 1953.

262. Raven, R. W., Weber, F. P., and Price, L. W.: The necrobiotic nodules of rheumatoid arthritis, Ann. Rheumat. Dis. *7:*63, 1948.

263. Barroso-Moguel, R., and Costero, I.: Lesiones valvulares en el reumatismo, Arch. Inst. cardiol. México *19:*663, 1949.

264. Zeek, P. M.: Periarteritis nodosa: a critical review, Am. J. Clin. Path. *22:*777, 1952.

265. Klemperer, P.: The pathogenesis of lupus erythem·

atosus and allied conditions, Arch. Int. Med. *28:*1, 1948.

266. Askanazy, M.: Ueber Bau und Enstehung des chronisches Magengeschwür, sowie soorpitzenbefunde in chron, Virchows Arch. path. Anat. *234:*111, 1921.

267. Schosning, F.: Das Gewebsbild des fieberhaften Rheumatismus. Das Verhaltern der Fasern des kollagenen Bindegewebes bei Rheumatismus und anderen Entzündungen, Virchows Arch. path. Anat. *286:*291, 1932.

268. Jucker, P.: Ueber die Nekrosen in der athero-Sklerotischen Platte und ihre Beziehung zum Atherom, Virchows Arch. path. Anat. *295:*301, 1935.

269. Jäger, E.: Zur pathologischen Anatomie der Thromboangiitis obliterans bei juveniler Extremitätgrangrän, Virchows Arch. path. Anat. *284:*526, 584, 1932.

270. Ricker, G.: Die Verflüsigung des Bindegewebsfasern zugleich ein Beitrag der Kenntniss der Fibrinoiden Degeneration, Virchows Arch. path. Anat. *163:*44, 1901.

271. Movat, H. Z., More, R. H., and Wolochow, D.: Cellular and intercellular changes in mechanical, chemical and radiation injury of connective tissue, Brit. J. Exper. Path. *41:*97, 1960.

272. Meesen, H.: Ueber Coronarinsufiziens nach Histamincollaps und nach Orthostatischencollaps, Beitr. path. Anat. *99:*327, 1937.

273. Clawson, B. J.: Experimental endocarditis with fibrinoid degeneration in the heart valves of the rat, Arch. Path. *50:*68, 1950.

274. Montgomery, P. O'B., and Muirhead, E. E.: Similarities between the lesions of human malignant hypertension and the hypertensive state of the nephrectomized dog, Am. J. Path. *29:*1147, 1953.

275. Opie, E. L.: Pathogenesis of the specific inflammatory reaction of immunized animals (Arthus phenomenon), J. Immunol. *9:*259, 1924.

276. Gerlach, W.: Studies ueber hyperergische Entzündung, Virchows Arch. path. Anat. *247:*294, 1923.

277. Selye, H.: The general adaptation syndrome and the diseases of adaptation, J. Clin. Endocrinol. *6:*117, 1946.

278. Neuman, E.: Zur Kenntnis der fibrinoiden Degeneration des Bindegewebes bei Entzündungen, Virchows Arch. path. Anat. *144:*201, 1896.

279. Marchand, F.: Zur Kenntnis der fibrinösen exsudation bei Entzündungen, Virchows Arch. path. Anat. *145:*279, 1896.

280. Glynn, L. E., and Loewi, G.: Fibrinoid necrosis in rheumatic fever, J. Path. & Bact. *64:*329, 1952.

281. Booth, E., Muirhead, E. E., and Montgomery, P. O'B.: The "fibrinoid" of renal cortical necrosis due to Shwartzman reaction. Evidence for its origin from smooth muscle, Arch. Path. *61:*169, 1956.

282. Movat, H. Z., and More, R. H.: The nature and origin of fibrinoid, Am. J. Clin. Path. *28:*331, 1957.

283. Gitlin, D., Craig, J. M., and Janeway, C. A.: Studies on the nature of fibrinoid in the collagen diseases, Am. J. Path. *33:*55, 1957.

284. Vazquez, J. J., and Dixon, F. J.: Immunohistochemical analysis of lesions associated with fibrinoid change, Arch. Path. *66:*504, 1958.

285. Kantor, T., Sokoloff, L., Smith, A., and Ziff, M.: Chemical and histological studies of the fibrinoid material of the subcutaneous rheumatoid nodule, Ann. Rheumat. Dis. *10:*471, 1951.

286. Ziff, M., Kantor, T., Bien, E., and Smith, A.: Studies on the composition of the fibrinoid

material of the subcutaneous nodule in rheumatoid arthritis, J. Clin. Invest. *32:*1253, 1953.

287. Gueft, B., and Laufer, A.: Further cytochemical studies in lupus erythematosus, Arch. Path. *57:*201, 1954.

288. Wolman, M., and Laufer, A.: Study of different "fibrinoids" by histochemical means, Proc. Soc. Exper. Biol. & Med. *92:*325, 1956.

289. Wagner, B. M.: Histochemical studies of fibrinoid substances and other abnormal tissue proteins. III. Proteolysis of fibrinoids, J. Mt. Sinai Hosp. *24:*1323, 1957.

290. Baggenstoss, A. H., and Saphir, O.: Rheumatic Disease of the Heart, in Gould, S. E. (ed.): Pathology of the Heart, ed. 2., Springfield, Charles C Thomas, 1960.

291. Gross, L., and Ehrlich, J. C.: Studies on the myocardial Aschoff body; descriptive classification of lesions, Am. J. Path. *10:*467, 1934.

292. Murphy, G. E., and Swift, H. F.: The induction of rheumatic-like cardiac lesions in rabbits by repeated focal infections with group A streptococci, J. Exper. Med. *91:*485, 1950.

293. Murphy, G. E.: Evidence that Aschoff bodies of rheumatic myocarditis develop from injured myofibers, J. Exper. Med. *95:*319, 1952.

294. Saphir, O.: The Aschoff nodule, Am. J. Clin. Path. *31:*534, 1959.

295. de Gortari, A., Pellón, R., and Costero, I.: Encefalopatía del reumático. I. Frecuencia insospechada de los accidentes cerebrales en el curso de la fiebre reumática y su papel como factores determinantes de la muerte en 107 casos, con el estudio correspondiente de necropsia, Arch. Inst. cardiol. México *17:*193, 1947.

296. Costero, I., Barroso-Moguel, R., de Gortari, A., and Pellón, R.: Encefalopatía del reumático. II. Cuadro histopatológico del encéfalo jugoso, Arch. Inst. cardiol. México *17:*488, 1947.

297. Cardona Lynch, E.: Arquitectura e histogénesis de los nódulos subcutaneos en el reumatismo, Arch. Inst. cardiol. México *19:*129, 1949.

298. Sokoloff, L.: The vascularity of the early subcutaneous nodules of rheumatoid arthritis, Bull. New York Acad. Med. *29:*733, 1953.

299. Churg, J., and Strauss, L.: Allergic granulomatosis, allergic angiitis and periarteritis nodosa, Am. J. Path. *27:*277, 1951.

300. Orabona, M. L., and Albano, O.: Systemic progressive sclerosis (or visceral scleroderma), Acta med. scandinav. *160:* Suppl. 333, 1958.

301. Rich, A. R.: Hypersensitivity in disease with special reference to periarteritis nodosa, rheumatic fever, disseminated lupus erythematosus, and rheumatoid arthritis, Harvey Lect. *42:*106, 1947.

302. Brunson, J. G., and Davis, R. L.: Systemic fibrinoid disease, Arch. Path. *60:*593, 1955.

303. More, R. H., and Movat, H. Z.: Cellular and intercellular phenomena in the Arthus phenomenon, Arch. Path. *67:*679, 1959.

304. Costero, I., Barroso-Moguel, R., and Chévez, A.: Las llamadas enfermedades de la colágena y el sistema fibroblástico, Principia Cardiol. *5:*44, 1958.

305. Goldgraber, M. B., and Kirsner, J. B.: Granulomatous lesions, an expression of a hypersensitive state: an experimental study, Arch. Path. *66:*618, 1958.

306. More, R. H., and Movat, H. Z.: Character and significance of the cellular response in the collagen diseases and experimental hypersensitivity, Lab. Invest. *8:*873, 1959.

307. Dammin, G. J.: Serum Sickness and Related States,

in Lawrence, H. S. (ed.): Cellular and Humoral Aspects of the Hypersensitive States, New York, Paul B. Hoeber, 1959.

308. Klinge, F.: Der Rheumatismus. Ergebn. allg. Path. 27:1, 1933.

309. Klemperer, P.: Discussion of MacLeod, C. M.: Hypersensitivity and Disease, in Lawrence, H. S. (ed.): Cellular and Humoral Aspects of the Hypersensitive States, New York, Paul B. Hoeber, 1959.

310. Talbott, J. H., and Moleres, R. F.: Collagen Disease, New York, Grune and Stratton, 1956.

311. Bunim, J. J., and Black, R. L.: Connective tissue (collagen) diseases, Ann. Rev. Med. 8:389, 1957.

312. Jarcho, S.: The Clinical Features of Systemic Lupus Erythematosus, in Baehr, G., and Klemperer, P. (eds.): Systemic Lupus Erythematosus, New York, Grune and Stratton, 1959.

313. Bille, B. S. V.: Lupus erythematosus disseminatus with and without skin eruption, Acta med. scandinav. 140:280, 1951.

314. Chévez, A.: Contribución a la histopatología del lupus eritematoso, Arch. Inst. cardiol. México 24:175, 1954.

315. Barroso-Moguel, R.: Lesiones vasculares en el lupus eritematoso, Arch. Inst. cardiol. México 27:167, 1957.

316. Libman, E., and Sacks, B.: A hitherto undescribed form of valvular and mural endocarditis, Arch. Int. Med. 33:701, 1924.

317. Gross, L.: Cardiac lesions in Libman-Sacks disease with consideration of its relationship to acute diffuse lupus erythematosus, Am. J. Path. 16: 375, 1940.

318. Pollack, A. D.: Some Observations on the Pathology of Systemic Lupus Erythematosus, in Baehr, G., and Klemperer, P. (eds.): Systemic Lupus Erythematosus, New York, Grune and Stratton, 1959.

319. Klemperer, P., Gueft, B., Lee, S. L., Leuchtenberger, C., and Pollister, A. W.: Cytochemical changes in acute lupus erythematosus, Arch. Path. 49:503, 1950.

320. Godman, G. C., Deitch, A. D., and Klemperer, P.: The composition of the L. E. and hematoxylin bodies of systemic lupus erythematosus, Am. J. Path. 34:1, 1958.

321. Holman, H. R., and Kunkel, H. G.: Affinity between the lupus erythematosus serum factor and cell nuclei and nucleoprotein, Science 126:162, 1957.

322. Robbins, W. C., Holman, H. R., Deicher, H., and Kunkel, H. G.: Complement fixation with cell nuclei and DNA in lupus erythematosus, Proc. Soc. Exper. Biol. & Med. 96:575, 1957.

323. Friedman, H. H., Schwartz, A., Trubek, M., and Steinbrocker, O.: The pararheumatic arthropathies, Ann. Int. Med. 38:732, 1953.

324. Harvey, A. M., Shulman, L. E., Tumulty, P. A., Conley, C. L., and Schoenrich, E. H.: Systemic lupus erythematosus: review of the literature and clinical analysis of 138 cases, Medicine 33:291, 1945.

325. Haserick, J. R.: Modern concepts of systemic lupus erythematosus; a review of 126 cases, J. Chron. Dis. 1:317, 1955.

326. Muehrcke, R. C., Kark, R. M., Pirani, C. L., Pollack, V. E., and Steek, I. E.: Histological and clinical evolution of lupus nephritis, Ann. Rheumat. Dis. 14:371, 1955.

327. Muehrcke, R. C., Kark, R. M., Pirani, C. L., and Pollack, V. E.: Lupus nephritis: a clinical and pathologic study based on renal biopsies, Medicine 36:1, 1957.

328. Smith, J. F.: The kidney in lupus erythematosus, J. Path. & Bact. 70:41, 1955.

329. Klemperer, P., Pollack, A. D., and Baehr, G.: Pathology of disseminated lupus erythematosus, Arch. Path. 32:569, 1941.

330. Churg, J., and Grishman, E.: Phase microscopy studies of renal glomeruli. Glomerular deposits of hyaline substances, Am. J. Path. 29:199, 1953.

331. Moore, R. D., Weisberger, A. S., and Bowerfind, E. S.: Histochemical studies of lymph nodes in disseminated lupus erythematosus, Arch. Path. 62:472, 1956.

332. Kaiser, J. H.: The specificity of periarterial fibrosis of the spleen in disseminated lupus erythematosus, Bull. Johns Hopkins Hosp. 71:31, 1943.

333. Lowman, E. W.: Muscle, nerve, and synovial changes in lupus erythematosus, Ann. Rheumat. Dis. 10:49, 1951.

334. Teilum, G.: Miliary epithelioid cell granulomas in lupus erythematosus disseminatus, Acta path. et microbiol. scandinav. 22:73, 1945.

335. Winslow, W. P., Ploss, L. N., and Loitman, B.: Pleuritis in systemic lupus erythematosus: its importance as an early manifestation in diagnosis, Ann. Int. Med. 49:70, 1958.

336. Purnell, D. C., Baggenstoss, A. H., and Olsen, A. M.: Pulmonary lesions in disseminated lupus erythematosus, Ann. Int. Med. 42:619, 1955.

337. Mortensen, V., and Gormsen, H.: Lupus erythematosus disseminatus; Libman-Sacks disease, Acta med. scandinav. 266:743, 1952.

338. Salazar Mallén, M., and Rulfo, J. F.: On some features of rheumatic fever and rheumatic heart disease as seen in the National Cardiological Institute of Mexico, Ann. Int. Med. 42:607, 1955.

339. Wilson, M. G., and Schweitzer, M.: Pattern of hereditary susceptibility in rheumatic fever, Circulation 10:699, 1954.

340. McCarthy, M.: Present state of knowledge concerning pathogenesis and treatment of rheumatic fever, Bull. New York Acad. Med. 28: 307, 1952.

341. Saphir, O., and Langendorf, R.: Non-specific myocarditis in acute rheumatic fever, Am. Heart J. 46:432, 1953.

342. Hall, E. M., and Anderson, L. R.: The incidence of rheumatic stigmas in hearts which are usually considered nonrheumatic, Am. Heart J. 25:64, 1943.

343. Barroso-Moguel, R., and Costero, I.: Lesiones valvulares en el reumatismo, Arch. Inst. cardiol. México 19:663, 1949.

344. Gross, L., and Friedberg, C. K.: Lesions of the cardiac valves in rheumatic fever, Am. J. Path. 12:855, 1936.

345. Burke, J. B.: Erythema marginatum, Arch. Dis. Child. 30:359, 1955.

346. Pérez Tamayo, R.: Alteraciones renales en la fiebre reumática, Tésis Recepcional, Escuela Nacional de Medicina, México, 1950.

347. Hartman, S. A., and Bland, E. F.: Rheumatic fever and glomerulonephritis, Am. J. Med. 10:47, 1951.

348. Cuéllar, A., and Pérez Tamayo, R.: Estudio anatomoclínico de la neumonitis reumática, Arch. Inst. cardiol. México 21:594, 1951.

349. Godtfredsen, E.: Ophthalmological signs and symptoms of mesenchymal diseases, Acta ophth. 32: 717, 1954.

350. Kulka, J. P., Bocking, D., Ropes, M. W., and Bauer, W.: Early joint lesions of rheumatoid arthritis, Arch. Path. 59:129, 1955.

351. Collins, D. N.: Is there a pathological definition of

rheumatoid arthritis? Acta med. scandinav. *341* Suppl. 5, 1957.

352. Fawns, H. T., and Landells, J. W.: Histochemical studies in rheumatic conditions. II. The nodule of rheumatoid arthritis, Ann. Rheumat. Dis. *13:* 28:1954.

353. Cruickshank, B.: The arteritis of rheumatoid arthritis, Ann. Rheumat. Dis. *13:*136, 1954.

354. Clark, W. S., Kulka, J. P., and Bauer, W.: Rheumatoid aortitis with aortic regurgitation, Am. J. Med. *22:*580, 1957.

355. Bunim, J. J., Sokoloff, L., Williams, R. R., and Black, R. L.: Rheumatoid arthritis: a review of recent advances in our knowledge concerning pathology, diagnosis and treatment, J. Chron. Dis. *1:*168, 1955.

356. Norcross, B. M., Lockie, M. L., and McLeod, C. C.: Juvenile Rheumatoid Arthritis, in Progress in Arthritis, New York, Grune and Stratton, 1959.

357. Talkov, R. H., Bauer, W., and Short, C. L.: Rheumatoid arthritis associated with splenomegaly and leukopenia, New Eng. J. Med. *227:*395, 1942.

358. Blankehorn, M. A., and Knowles, H. C.: Periarteritis nodosa: recognition and clinical symptoms, Ann. Int. Med. *41:*887, 1954.

359. Nuzum, J. W., Jr., and Nuzum, J. W.: Polyarteritis nodosa; statistical review of one hundred seventy-five cases from the literature and report of a "typical" case, Ann. Int. Med. *94:*942, 1954.

360. Griffith, G. C., and Nural, I. L.: Polyarteritis nodosa: a correlation of clinical and postmortem findings in 17 cases, Circulation *3:*481, 1951.

361. Rose, M. H., Littmann, D., and Houghton, J.: Polyarteritis nodosa; a clinical and pathological study and report of six cases, Ann. Int. Med. *32:*1114, 1950.

362. Blaisdell, E., and Porter, J. E.: Healed stage periarteritis nodosa, New Eng. J. Med. *214:*1087, 1941.

363. Piper, W. N., and Helwig, E. B.: Progressive systemic sclerosis; visceral manifestations in generalized scleroderma, Arch. Dermat. & Syph. *72:*535, 1955.

364. Goetz, R. H.: The pathology of progressive systemic sclerosis (generalized scleroderma) with special reference to the changes in the viscera, Clin. Proc. *4:*337, 1945.

365. Ramsey, A. S.: Acrosclerosis, Brit. M. J. *2:*877, 1951.

366. O'Leary, P. A., and Montgomery, G. H.: Dermatohistopathology of various types of scleroderma, Arch. Dermat. & Syph. *75:*78, 1957.

367. Leinwand, I., Duryee, A. W., and Richter, M. N.: Scleroderma (based on a study of over 150 cases), Ann. Int. Med. *41:*1003, 1954.

368. Goldman, I. R., Young, J. M., and Knox, F. H.: Myocardial involvement in generalized scleroderma, Dis. Chest *25:*94, 1954.

369. Mustakallio, K. K., and Sarajas, S. S.: Some aspects of scleroderma heart disease, Am. Heart J. *47:* 437, 1954.

370. Lewis, T.: Notes on scleroderma (dermatomyositis), Brit. J. Dermatol. *52:*233, 1940.

371. Bartels, E. D., Christensen, L. K., and Ohlsen, A. S.: Renal affection complicating scleroderma, Acta path. et microbiol. scandinav. *105* Suppl. 174, 1955.

372. Rodnan, G. P., Schreiner, G. E., and Black, R. L.: Renal involvement in progressive systemic sclerosis (generalized scleroderma), Am. J. Med. *23:* 445, 1957.

373. Dornhorst, A. C., Pierce, J. W., and Whimster, I. W.: The esophageal lesion in scleroderma, Lancet *1:*698, 1954.

374. Boyd, J. A., Patrick, S. J., and Reevers, R. J.: Roentgen changes observed in generalized scleroderma; report of sixty three cases, Arch. Int. Med. *94:*248, 1954.

375. Goldgraber, M. B., and Kirsner, J. B.: Scleroderma of the gastrointestinal tract, Arch. Path. *64:*255, 1957.

376. Abrahms, H. L., Carnes, W. H., and Eaton, J.: Alimentary tract in disseminated scleroderma with emphasis on small bowel, Arch. Int. Med. *94:*61, 1954.

377. Traquada, R. E., Simmons, D. H., and Miller, J. H.: Pulmonary fibrosis in scleroderma, Arch. Int. Med. *105:*607, 1960.

378. Getzowa, S.: Cystic and compact pulmonary fibrosis in progressive scleroderma, Arch. Path. *40:*99, 1945.

379. Dowling, G. B.: Scleroderma and dermatomyositis, Brit. J. Dermat. *67:*275, 1955.

380. Domzalski, C. A., and Morgan, C. V.: Dermatomyositis: diagnostic features and therapeutic pitfalls, Am. J. Med. *19:*370, 1955.

381. Williams, R. C., Jr.: Dermatomyositis and malignancy: a review of the literature, Ann. Int. Med. *50:*1174, 1959.

382. Wallace, S. L., Lattes, R., and Ragan, C.: Diagnostic significance of muscle biopsy, Am. J. Med. *25:*600, 1958.

383. O'Leary, P., and Waisman, M.: Dermatomyositis: a study of forty cases, Arch. Dermat. & Syph. *41:*1001, 1940.

384. Ehrich, W. C.: Nature of collagen diseases, Am. Heart J. *43:*141, 1952.

385. Hargraves, M. M., Richmond, H., and Morton, R.: Presentation of two bone marrow elements: the "Tart" cell and the "L. E." cell, Proc. Staff Meet. Mayo Clin. *23:*25, 1948.

386. Godman, G. C.: The Nature and Pathogenetic Significance of the L. E. Cell Phenomenon of Systemic Lupus Erythematosus, in Baehr, G., and Klemperer, P. (eds.): Systemic Lupus Erythematosus, New York, Grune and Stratton, 1959.

387. Haserick, J. R., and Lewis, L. A.: Blood factor in acute disseminated lupus erythematosus. II. Induction of specific antibodies against L. E. factor, Blood *5:*718, 1950.

388. Lee, S. L., and Davis, B. J.: The Blood in Systemic Lupus Erythematosus, in Baehr, G., and Klemperer, P. (eds.): Systemic Lupus Erythematosus, New York, Grune and Stratton, 1959.

389. Stollerman, G. H., Lewis, A. J., Schults, I., and Taranta, A.: Relationship of immune response to group A streptococci to the course of chronic and recurrent rheumatic fever, Am. J. Med. *20:* 163, 1956.

390. Vaughan, J. H.: Serum responses in rheumatoid arthritis, Am. J. Med. *26:*596, 1959.

391. Lepow, H., Rubinstein, L., Woll, F., and Greisman, H.: A spontaneously precipitable protein in human sera, with particular reference to the diagnosis of polyarteritis nodosa, Am. J. Med. *7:*310, 1949.

392. Hench, P. S.: Discriminate use of cortisone and corticotropins in general medicine, with special reference to collagen diseases, Acta med. scandinav. *154:*274, 1956.

393. Stillman, J. S.: Current status of steroid therapy in rheumatic disorders, New Eng. J. Med. *259:*820, 1958.

394. United Kingdom and United States Joint Report. Treatment of acute rheumatic fever in children:

cooperative clinical trial of ACTH, cortisone, and aspirin, Circulation *11:*343, 1955.

395. McCue, C. M.: Steroid therapy for rheumatic fever, J. Pediat. *51:*255, 1957.

396. Costero, I., Barroso-Moguel, R., Chévez, A., Monroy, G., and Contreras, R.: Las lesiones de la fiebre reumática de los enfermos tratados con cortisona. I. Consideración especial de la miocarditis, Arch. Inst. cardiol. México *28:*155, 1958.

397. Costero, I., Barroso-Moguel, R., Chévez, A., Monroy, G., and Contreras, R.: Las lesiones de la fiebre reumática en los enfermos tratados con cortisona. II. Participación visceral más frecuente, Arch. Inst. cardiol. México *28:*294, 1958.

398. Costero, I., Barroso-Moguel, R., Chévez, A., Monroy, G., and Contreras, R.: Las lesiones de la fiebre reumática de los enfermos tratados con cortisona. III. La respuesta general del organismo. Discusión general y conclusiones, Arch. Inst. cardiol. México *28:*427, 1958.

399. Howell, D. S., and Ragan, C.: Course of rheumatoid arthritis during four years of induced hyperadrenalism (IHA), Medicine *35:*83, 1956.

400. Baggenstoss, A. H., Schick, R. M., and Polley, H. F.: The effect of cortisone on the lesions of periarteritis nodosa, Am. J. Path. *27:*537, 1951.

401. Sommervielle, J.: Scleroderma and dermatomyositis, Practitioner *173:*151, 1954.

402. Hannigan, C. A., Hannigan, H. M., and Scott, E. Z.: Scleroderma of the kidneys, Am. J. Med. *20:*793, 1956.

403. Selye, H.: The General Adaptation Syndrome and Diseases of Adaptation, in Karsner, H. T. (ed.): Year Book of Pathology and Clinical Pathology, Chicago, Year Book Publishers, 1950.

404. Robles Gil, J.: Clinical study of visceral lesions and endocrine disturbances in eight cases of scleroderma, Ann. Int. Med. *34:*862, 1951.

405. Klemperer, P.: General considerations of collagen diseases, Acta med. scandinav. *154:* Suppl. 261, 1956.

406. Klemperer, P.: Pathology of Systemic Lupus Erythematosus, in McManus, J. F. A. (ed.): Progress in Fundamental Medicine, Philadelphia, Lea and Febiger, 1952.

407. Aegerter, E. E., and Long, J. H.: Collagen diseases, Am. J. Med. Sc. *218:*324, 1949.

408. Rich, A. R., and Gregory, J. E.: Experimental anaphylactic lesions of coronary arteries of the "sclerotic" type, commonly associated with rheumatic fever and disseminated lupus erythematosus, Bull. Johns Hopkins Hosp. *81:*312, 1947.

409. Rössle, R.: Die Rheumatische Formenkreis. Virchows Arch. path. Anat. *288:*780, 1933.

410. Weintraud, O.: Der Rheumatismus. Ergebn. allg. Path. *27:*1, 1933.

411. Mellors, R. C., Ortega, L. G., and Holman, H. R.: Role of gamma globulin in pathogenesis of renal lesion in systemic lupus erythematosus and chronic membranous glomerulonephritis, with an observation on the lupus erythematosus cell reaction, J. Exper. Med. *106:*191, 1957.

412. Dameshek, W.: Systemic lupus erythematosus; a complex autoimmune disorder, Ann. Int. Med. *48:*707, 1958.

413. Cavelti, P. A.: Autoimmunologic disease, J. Allergy *26:*95, 1955.

414. Bardawil, W. A., Toy, B. L., Galins, N., and Bayles, T. B.: Disseminated lupus erythematosus, scleroderma, and dermatomyositis as manifestations of sensitization to DNA-protein. I. An immuno-histochemical approach, Am. J. Path. *34:*607, 1958.

415. Bardawil, W. A., Toy, B. L., and Galins, N.: Hypersensitivity to histone induced experimentally in rabbits, Lancet *1:*988, 1958.

416. Banks, B. M.: Is there a common denominator in scleroderma, dermatomyositis, lupus erythematosus, the Libman-Sacks syndrome, and polyarteritis nodosa? New Eng. J. Med. *225:*433, 1941.

417. Vaughan, J. H., and Waller, M. V.: Specificity of the rheumatoid factor. Arthritis & Rheumat. *1:* 262, 1958.

418. Heller, G., Jacobson, A. S., Kolodny, M. H., and Schuman, R. L.: The hemagglutination test for rheumatoid arthritis. I. An immunological analysis of the factors involved in the reaction, J. Immunol. *69:*27, 1952.

419. Gelfand, M. L., and Aronoff, S.: Periarteritis nodosa—possible relation to the increased usage of sulphonamides, Ann. Int. Med. *30:*919, 1949.

420. Rasmussen, H.: Iodide hypersensitivity in the etiology of periarteritis nodosa, J. Allergy *26:*394, 1955.

421. Waugh, D.: Myocarditis, arteritis, and focal hepatic, splenic and renal granulomas apparently due to penicillin sensitivity, Am. J. Path. *28:* 437, 1952.

422. Waksman, B. H.: Etiology of rheumatic fever: review of theories and evidence, Medicine *28:* 143, 1949.

423. Catanzaro, F. J., Stetson, C. A., Morris, A. J., Chamovitz, R., Rammelkamp, C. H., Jr., Stolzer, B. L., and Perry, W. D.: The role of the streptococcus in the pathogenesis of rheumatic fever, Am. J. Med. *17:*749, 1954.

424. Miller, J. M.: Prophylaxis of rheumatic fever and rheumatic heart disease, New Eng. J. Med. *260:* 220, 1959.

425. Quinn, R. W., and Liao, S. J.: A comparative study of antihyaluronidase, antistreptolysine "O," antistreptokinase, and streptococcal agglutination titers in patients with rheumatic fever, acute hemolytic streptococcal infections, rheumatoid arthritis, and non-rheumatoid forms of arthritis, J. Clin. Invest. *29:*1156, 1950.

426. Kutter, A. G., and Krumwiede, E.: Observations on the effect of streptococcal upper respiratory infections in rheumatic children: a three year study, J. Clin. Invest. *20:*273, 1941.

427. MacLeod, C. M.: Hypersensitivity and Disease, in Lawrence, H. S. (ed.): Cellular and Humoral Aspects of the Hypersensitive States, New York, Hoeber-Harper, 1959.

428. Schwab, J. H., and Cromartie, W. J.: Immunological studies on a C polysaccharide complex of Group A streptococci having a direct toxic effect on connective tissue, J. Exper. Med. *111:* 295, 1960.

429. Cromartie, W. J., Schwab, J. H., and Craddock, J. G.: The effect of a toxic cellular component of Group A streptococci on connective tissue, Am. J. Path., *37:*79, 1960.

430. McKusick, V. A.: Heritable Disorders of Connective Tissue, ed. 2, St. Louis, C. V. Mosby, 1960.

431. MacLeod, M., and Williams, W. A.: The cardiovascular lesions in Marfan's syndrome, Arch. Path. *61:*143, 1956.

432. Hudson, J. R.: Marfan's syndrome with retinal detachment, Brit. J. Ophth. *35:*244, 1951.

433. Sinclair, R. J. G.: The Marfan syndrome, Bull. Rheumat. Dis. *8:*153, 1958.

434. Tung, H. L., and Liewbow, A. A.: Marfan's syndrome. Observations at necropsy with special reference to medio-necrosis of the great vessels, Lab. Invest. *1:*382, 1952.

435. Burman, S. O.: Medial degeneration and its relation to dissecting aneurysms, Surg. Gynec. & Obst. *110:*1, 1960.

436. Thomas, J., Brothers, G. B., Anderson, R. S., and Cuff, J. R.: Marfan's syndrome. A report of three cases with aneurysm of the aorta, Am. J. Med. *12:*613, 1952.

437. Sjoerdsma, A., Davidson, J. D., Undefriend, S., and Mitoma, C.: Increased excretion of hydroxyproline in Marfan's syndrome, Lancet *2:*994, 1958.

438. Roark, J. W.: Marfan's syndrome. Report of one case with autopsy, special histological study and review of the literature, Arch. Int. Med. *103:*123, 1959.

439. Saedmundsson, J.: Ehlers-Danlos syndrome; a congenital mesenchymal disorder. Acta med. scandinav. *154:* (Suppl. 312) 399, 1956.

440. Robinson, H. M., Jr., and Ellis, F. A.: Cutis laxa, Arch. Dermat. & Syph. *77:*656, 1958.

441. Jansen, L. H.: The structure of the connective tissue, an explanation of the symptoms of the Ehlers-Danlos syndrome, Dermatologica *110:*108, 1955.

442. Tunbridge, R. E., Tattersall, R. N., Hall, D. A., Astbury, W. T., and Reed, R.: The fibrous structure of normal and abnormal human skin, Clin. Sci. *11:*315, 1952.

443. Katz, I., and Steiner, K.: Ehlers-Danlos syndrome with ectopic bone formation, Radiology *65:*352, 1955.

444. Hills, R. G., and McLanahan, S.: Brittle bones and blue scleras in five generations, Arch. Int. Med. *59:*41, 1937.

445. Ruth, E. B.: Osteogenesis imperfecta. Anatomic study of a case, Arch. Path. *36:*211, 1943.

446. Scott, D., and Stiris, G.: Osteogenesis imperfecta tarda. A study of three families with special reference to scar formation, Acta med. scandinav. *145:*237, 1953.

447. Follis, R. H., Jr.: Osteogenesis imperfecta congenita; a connective tissue diathesis, J. Pediat. *47:*713, 1952.

448. Follis, R. H. Jr.: Histochemical studies on cartilage and bone. III. Osteogenesis imperfecta, Bull. Johns Hopkins Hosp. *93:*386, 1953.

449. McKusick, V. A.: Hereditary disorders of connective tissue, Bull. New York Acad. Med. *35:* 143, 1959.

450. Levy, G., and Brewer, R. L.: Pseudoxanthoma elasticum. Report of a case, Am. J. Med. *26:*157, 1959.

451. Wolff, H. H., Stokes, J., and Schlesinger, B.: Vascular abnormalities associated with pseudoxanthoma elasticum, Arch. Dis. Child. *27:*82, 1952.

452. Kaplan, L., and Hartman, S. W.: Elastica disease; case of Grönblad-Strandberg syndrome with gastrointestinal hemorrhage, Arch. Int. Med. *94:* 489, 1954.

453. Moran, T. J., and Lansing, A. I.: Studies on the nature of the abnormal fibers in pseudoxanthoma elasticum. Arch. Path. *65:*688, 1958.

454. Halperin, S. L., and Curtis, G. M.: The genetics of gargoylism, Am. J. Ment. Deficiency *46:*298, 1942.

455. Straus, R., Merliss, R., and Reiser, R.: Gargoylism. Review of the literature and report of the sixth autopsied case with chemical studies. Am. I. Clin. Path. *17:*671, 1947.

456. Smith, E. B., Hempelmann, T. C., Moore, S., and Barr, D. P.: Gargoylism (dysostosis multiplex): two adult cases with one autopsy, Ann. Int. Med. *36:*652, 1952.

457. Jermain, L. F., Rohn, R. J., and Bond, W. H.: Studies on the role of the reticuloendothelial system in Hurler's disease, Clin. Res. *7:*216, 1959.

458. Jervis, G. A.: Gargoylism: study of 10 cases with emphasis on the formes frustes, Arch. Neurol. & Psychiat. *63:*681, 1950.

459. Lindsay, S., Reilly, W. A., Gotham, T. J., and Skahen, R.: Gargoylism. II. Study of the pathologic lesions and clinical review of 12 cases, Am. J. Dis. Child. *76:*239, 1948.

460. Uzman, L. L.: Chemical nature of the storage substance in gargoylism, Arch. Path. *60:*308, 1955.

461. Meyer, K., Grumbach, M. M., Linker, A., and Hoffman, P.: Excretion of sulfated mucopolysaccharides in gargoylism (Hurler's syndrome) Proc. Soc. Exp. Biol. Med. *97:*275, 1958.

Chapter VII

GENERAL PATHOLOGY OF

THE HOST-PARASITE RELATION

I. INTRODUCTION

Struggle for survival among different biologic species is determined by two main factors: their close vicinity, and their use of the same elements for metabolism. The result is a continuous contest in which species with more adequate conditions survive, while those less fortunate die and disappear or are used as means for survival by the

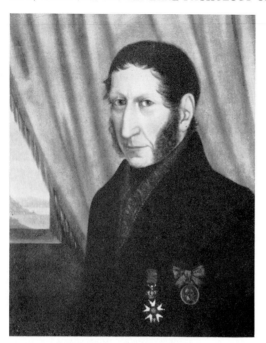

FIG. 7–1. Agostino Bassi.

nomenon, the nomenclature used for different aspects of such a relation has a strong teleologic flavor. For instance, metabolic (or other) processes which accidentally inhibit or make difficult the establishment of parasitic organisms in man are referred to as "defense mechanisms," while those constitutional or metabolic features of parasites which facilitate their entry and proliferation in the host are known as "aggressive mechanisms." Surely, if medical literature were written by animal parasites with finalistic inclinations, what are now "defense" mechanisms would become means of "aggression," and vice versa.

In 1546 Fracastorius published a small booklet entitled *De Contagione,* in which the idea that some diseases may be produced by "insensible and small particles" is clearly expressed; although this was purely imaginative, the doctrine followed from some sagacious observations in human

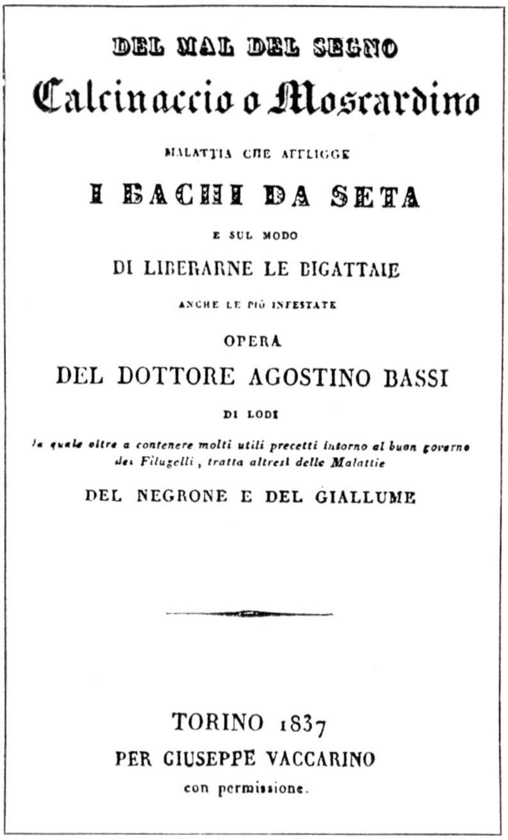

former. A constant drama is played in Nature, in which different species forever strive to gain the elements necessary for growth, maintenance and reproduction, both from the surrounding environment as well as from other organisms. Close contact between different organisms results in various types of relations, such as commensalism, where one individual is benefited, while the other is unaffected, and symbiosis, where both parties of the relation are benefited from their association. Of special interest here is the relation known as parasitism, which ". . . is in a sense a compromise or truce between two living things, accompanied by predatory processes whenever the opportunity is offered one or the other party."[1] From a biologic standpoint parasitism is a normal, or even better a natural, relation between two or more living organisms. The idea that parasitism is pathologic arises from man's preoccupation in maintaining his privileged position in Nature; in fact, human parasitism is considered only when, actually or potentially, the nonhuman party of the relation is capable of producing anatomic and/or functional changes in man. Perhaps because of a tendency to ignore the fact that parasitism is a natural biologic phe-

DEL MAL DEL SEGNO

Calcinaccio o Moscardino

MALATTIA CHE AFFLIGGE

I BACHI DA SETA

E SUL MODO

DI LIBERARNE LE BIGATTAIE

ANCHE LE PIÙ INFESTATE

OPERA

DEL DOTTORE AGOSTINO BASSI

DI LODI

la quale oltre a contenere molti utili precetti intorno al buon governo
dei Filugelli, tratta altresì delle Malattie

DEL NEGRONE E DEL GIALLUME

TORINO 1837

PER GIUSEPPE VACCARINO

con permissione.

FIG. 7–2. Title-page of Bassi's celebrated work, in which appears the description of the first experimental demonstration of contagion.

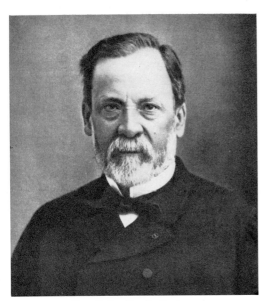

FIG. 7–3. Louis Pasteur.

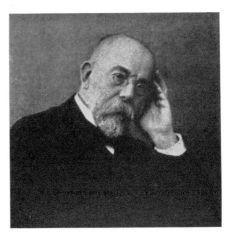

FIG. 7–4. Robert Koch.

disease. It was not until 1835, however, that Agostino Bassi (Fig. 7–1), an Italian lawyer with great interest in scientific research, described the causal agent of muscardine, a disease of silkworms, and showed experimentally that it is transmissible. In his own words,[2] "The many observations and experiences undertaken throughout long years have shown me that mark disease or muscardine does not arise spontaneously in the silkworm or in other insects; it is always derived from an external organism which penetrates into the animal and in developing generates disease and death. This is an organized being, living and vegetable; it is a parasite plant, a fungous production. This cryptogram plant will not develop, grow or regenerate but in the living animal, and will fail to do it in the dead animal . . ." (Fig. 7–2).

With a red-hot needle Bassi transferred white filaments from one silkworm to another and observed that the second worm became sick and died. For approximately 25 years or more beginning apparently in 1817, Bassi worked on these and other observations, and although afflicted by a conjunctivitis (attributed by Bassi himself to a contamination with the parasite of the silkworm) which decreased his vision a great deal, was able to prove experimentally

Fracastorius' speculation of 289 years' standing.[3] Louis Pasteur (Fig. 7–3) contributed the next fundamental step in the knowledge of the host-parasite relation when he suggested that well defined disease entities were caused by specific germs, but his main contribution was to demolish the theory of heterogenesis or spontaneous generation, thus making possible the parasitic theory of disease. To deny the possibility of spontaneous generation was to universalize Bassi's experimental demonstration that muscardine was transmissible. The field was fertile for the monumental work of Robert Koch (Fig. 7–4), who created modern bacteriology and definitively established the role of microorganisms in infectious diseases with his observations on *Bacillis anthracis*. On the basis of this contribution and his subsequent work on tuberculosis, a series of principles have developed under the name of Koch's postulates,[4] which represent the ideal conditions to be fulfilled in order to consider a parasite as the cause of a given disease.

Koch's principles may be summarized as follows.[5] (1) The microorganism should be present in all cases of the disease in question, in sufficient numbers and adequate distribution to account for the symptoms. (2) The microorganism should be cultured outside the patient in order to determine its ability for independent life. (3) Inoculation of the microorganism into a healthy subject should reproduce the disease with all its manifestations, and the microorganism should be again isolated from this new patient with all its characteristics. These three postulates are ideal and, therefore, are not completely fulfilled in many diseases with a certain infectious etiology; furthermore, they were enunciated at a time when immunology was in its beginnings and the aggressive mechanisms of parasites were not explored. An additional postulate might be added, which is the appearance of antibodies specific against the germ, or the presence of a high degree of immunity in the convalescing subject. A very complete analysis of these and other related problems can be found in Topley and Wilson's book.[6]

In little over a century extraordinary progress in knowledge of the etiology of infectious diseases has permitted the development of effective means to fight them. Prophylactic measures have wiped out endemic diseases in different areas, as malaria from the Panama Canal Zone, and rabies in England; in other instances, the natural history of the disease has been drastically modified, as with onchocercosis in Mexico. *Onchocerca volvulus* will produce irreversible lesions in the eyes causing blindness, and before the introduction of chemotherapeutic agents such as Hetrazan there were many individuals so afflicted, but campaigns of prophylaxis and treatment of early cases have decreased the number of blind patients so that at present only those already blinded at the time the campaign was started remain.[7]

The general pathology of the host-parasite relation may be conveniently examined by first reviewing those characteristics of the host which are beneficial in the struggle for survival, i.e., defense mechanisms, followed by a summary of factors determining pathogenicity of parasites, or aggressive mechanisms, and finally an analysis of changes occurring in both host and parasite when the relation is established, which is the infectious disease. This is the sequence followed in this chapter, to which some remarks on chemotherapy have been added with special emphasis on mechanisms and effects, both in the host and in the parasite. The importance of such therapeutic methods is sufficient justification, if any were necessary, to include such a section in a book on general pathology.

II. DEFENSE MECHANISMS OF THE HOST

It is convenient to point out once more that the finalistic flavor of the term "defense mechanisms" should not obscure the true nature of these processes. As will be seen in the following paragraphs, defense mechanisms are not specifically designed to impede entry or development of parasites in the organism. Rather, this effect constitutes an accident or collateral product of physiologic processes carrying out different functions; throughout the course of biologic evolution, however, the existence of "accidental" protective mechanisms has favored survival of the fittest. This favorable effect is comparable to inflammation (p. 88) and just as in the local reaction to injury of vascular connective tissues, defense mechanisms may turn against the host and reveal that their "defensive" role is an interpretation *a posteriori,* acceptable only at the level of the species and without any individual purpose.

Defense mechanisms are different in various parts of the organism. From a general standpoint, they may be considered in two groups: (a) local mechanisms, the main role of which is to inhibit penetration of pathogenic agents within the body, and which are therefore to be found in areas of contact with the surrounding environment such as skin, digestive system, etc. and (b) systemic mechanisms, which constitute the second line of defense and come into play once parasites have penetrated the first line, represented by the local mechanisms. The functions of systemic defense mechanisms are the elimination of pathogenic agents and the blocking of their toxins. Defense mechanisms may also be classified as specific and nonspecific;[8] most local mechanisms are nonspecific while some systemic defenses are among the most specific of biologic phenomena.

A. LOCAL DEFENSE MECHANISMS

Whatever the site of the organism where local defense mechanisms are considered, they always fall within one of the following four groups:[9]

1. *Mechanical or Physical Mechanisms.* Instances of this group are desiccation, tem-

perature, cellular desquamation and the intermittent or continuous elimination of organic secretions such as saliva, gastrointestinal juices, urine, etc.

2. *Biochemical Mechanisms.* Certain fatty acids and local pH values will act as protective mechanisms of a biochemical nature.

3. *Biologic Mechanisms.* These may be humoral, as lysozyme, other enzymes and antibodies in secretions; or cellular, as phagocytosis occurring in local inflammation.

4. *Bacterial Mechanisms.* Some saprophytic bacteria may inhibit the establishment and growth of pathogenic organisms, and this effect may result from the production of antibiotic substances or metabolic competition.

The limits between the foregoing groups are obviously not clear, and on some occasions it may be found that one mechanism will protect the body in more than one way. Furthermore, they rarely if ever act in isolation, but rather as a group and showing some synergistic effects. The peculiarities of local defense mechanisms in each of the areas in contact with the environment are summarized in the following paragraphs.

1. Skin and Conjunctivae. Comparison of the bacterial flora encountered at a given moment on the skin with that of the environment will show two main differences: (1) There are fewer germs on the cutaneous surface than in the environment, and since the skin is in direct contact with the environment there must be some decontaminating mechanisms. (2) The vast majority of microorganisms present on the cutaneous surface are saprophytes, so decontamination is selective in nature. Pillsbury and Kligman[10] have studied the normal bacterial flora of the skin in many areas and their results appear in Table 42.

The integrity of the skin represents a formidable mechanical barrier to the penetration of many microorganisms, but a skin entirely free of cuts or bruises is very rare. The defense mechanisms of the skin (inadequately referred to as "autosterilizing") have been summarized by Burtenshaw[11] in the following five groups: (1) cellular desquamation; (2) desiccation; (3) acidity

Table 42. Resident Flora of Normal Human Skin

I. AEROBIC	
A. Bacteria	B. Lipophilic fungi
1. Micrococci (Staphylococci):	1. Pityrosporon
M. epidermidis	*P. ovale*
M. albus	*P. orbiculare*
M. candidus	
M. flavus	
2. Corynebacteria:	
Lipophilic *Corynebacterium*	
(*Corynebacterium tenuis* in axilla)	

II. ANAEROBIC
A. *Propionibacterium acnes*
B. *M. saccharolyticus*

(Pillsbury and Kligman[10])

of the skin; (4) secretion of certain fatty acids; and (5) others less well known. The effectiveness of these groups has been studied by Arnold, *et al.*[12] who contaminated the skin of the palms with 8 different germs and then determined the percentage of survival of the inoculum at 10, 20 and 30 minutes. Their results appear in Table 43, where the efficiency of self-decontaminating mechanisms is apparent for some strains but not for others.

Cellular desquamation and desiccation are constant phenomena but their intensity varies according to the area of the body surface under study; it can be shown that in skin folds these processes are less intense than in exposed surfaces. Nevertheless, in a very complete study Hellat[13] concluded that desiccation is the most important of all defense mechanisms mentioned above. Skin

Table 43. Effectiveness of Defense Mechanisms of the Skin

(per cent of recovery of primary inoculum)

BACTERIAL STRAIN	TIME OF CULTURE		
	10′	20′	30′
B. coli	100		
B. typhosus	100		
B. enteritidis	100		
B. prodigiosus	98	100	
B. pyocyaneus	98	100	
S. albus (air)	95	98.2	99.5
S. epidermidis albus	82	92	96
S. aureus	82	94	97

(Arnold, *et al.*[12])

pH has been investigated by means of cutaneous electrodes by Marchionini, et al.,[14] and their results show that although in some sites it may reach values as acid as 5 and even 3, in others it is alkaline, as in the axilla, in the inguinal folds and between the toes; alkaline pH favors establishment and survival of bacteria. Sweating lowers the skin pH and enhances the bactericidal efficiency of the cutaneous surface. Marchionini's ideas gained great popularity, perhaps because of the attractiveness of the term "acid mantle" (Säuremantel) used to describe acid pH in the skin, but others believe that it is not the alkaline pH that explains bacterial survival in skin folds, but humidity, and have also shown that both "resident" and pathogenic strains can survive at pH 5 or 6, which is characteristic of the skin surface.[6] Rapid disappearance of staphylococcus from the skin has been attributed to the presence of oleic acid.[15] Lysozyme has also been isolated from the skin but in very low concentrations. Antibiosis remains an intriguing possibility considering the variety of the "resident" flora, but more studies are necessary.

Local defense mechanisms in the conjunctiva are mainly two: the mechanical action of tears, which creates a continuous flow towards the lacrimal duct and carries away bacteria and other particles into the nasal fossae, and the biologic action of tears which is due to lysozyme.[16] This enzyme was described by Flemming in 1922 in tears, nasal secretions and many tissues of the body, including the skin; lysozyme destroys many saprophytic bacteria through hydrolysis of certain surface polysaccharides. The effect is particularly clear with *Micrococcus lysodeikticus* (lysis indicator), also described by Flemming. Tears possess the highest concentration of lysozyme in the organism,[17] and this enzyme doubtlessly contributes to decontamination of the conjunctivae; avitaminosis A causes a marked decrease in the concentration of lysozyme in tears and it is well known that in this condition there is often a purulent infection of the eye (xerophthalmia purulenta).

2. Respiratory Tract. Nasal fossae and nasopharynx are important filters since with inspired air many pathogenic agents could reach the intimacy of the organism; their efficiency is manifested not only by the scarce number of bacteria normally present in the posterior half of the nasopharynx, but also by the few particles of the same size which penetrate the lower respiratory tract, such as dust, carbon, etc. The size of the external opening of the nose and vibrissae are the first obstacles to the free passage of particles much larger than bacteria, but which carry vast numbers of germs in the air.[18] Irregularity and tortuosity of the nasal fossae, with formation of air currents and whirls, favor contact between inspired particles and mucosa with other filtering mechanisms and may also be considered defense mechanisms, since if the nasal fossae were straight tubes there would be no change in the speed of the air current and the number of penetrating particles would be much greater.[19] Nevertheless, the most important defense mechanisms of the upper respiratory tract are the secretion of mucus, the ciliary movement and the presence of bactericidal substances such as lysozyme, neutralizing antibodies, and others less well known. Bowman's glands produce approximately one liter of mucus every 24 hours, which extends as a film on the surface in contact with air and traps most of the particles. Nasal secretion has a circulation of its own which leads from any point in the mucosa towards the hypopharynx, and from there to the esophagus and the rest of the digestive tract. Therefore, the destination of bacteria trapped in the nasal mucus is the stomach. Such mucus circulation is provided by the movement of the cilia of the mucosa. Proetz,[20] who has studied these structures extensively, believes they are the most important defense mechanism of the body. They appear in lower animals; they are very vigorous and function under very unfavorable conditions and in extremes of temperature; their activity continues after death; they regenerate with great rapidity, and only one or two drugs of common use affect them. Cilia are approximately 7 μ long and are arranged as the hair of a rug, covering almost the entire inner surface of the nasal fossae with the exception of the olfactory area and a smaller portion facing the middle turbinate.[21] Their movements are undulatory, rapid and energetic when directed towards the nasopharynx ("effective" hit), slow and weak when aimed towards the opening of the nasal fossae ("recovery" hit); the frequency of such movements is 8 to 12 per second. Ciliary movement is important because it provides the force to move the film of mucus covering the nasal mucosa, which displaces at a speed of 2.5 to 7.5 mm. per minute; therefore, the entire mucus film is renewed approximately every half hour. The most effective inhibitor of ciliary movement is desiccation.[22]

In addition to mucus secretion and ciliary movement, the upper respiratory tract receives an important amount of lysozyme through the lacrimal duct and this enzyme probably acts as bacteriostatic agent in the nasal fossae.[23] There is evidence that lysozyme is not the only humoral defense in this area since some authors have described neutralization of the influenza virus[24, 25] and probably of poliomyelitis virus by the nasal mucus. The relation of these substances to the resistance of certain individuals during epidemics of upper respiratory infections is not known, but possibly they play an important role in defense. The efficiency of mechanisms described above may be judged from the interesting study of Cralley,[26] who showed that more than 96 per cent of bacteria (*Serratia marcescens*) inhaled by the rabbit are retained in the upper respiratory tract.

Trachea and bronchi possess three main defense mechanisms, namely mucus secretion, ciliary movement and the cough reflex. The first two function in a manner similar to that described for the nasal fossae, except that the direction of mucus circulation promoted by ciliary movement is towards the larynx. Conditions influencing the activity of cilia were studied by Hill using horse trachea;[27] the effect of temperature is of great significance, since cold decreases ciliary movement and it is well known that infections of the lower respiratory tract are particularly frequent after exposures to low temperatures. Cough is an additional defense mechanism which eliminates large numbers of particles and bacteria accumulated in the mucus secreted by bronchioles, bronchi and trachea. Collection of the mucus in the higher portion of the trachea, especially below the vocal cords, stimulates the cough reflex and completes elimination of many filtered microorganisms and other particles.

The lower respiratory tract, formed by alveolar ducts, atria and alveoli, are protected mainly by phagocytosis. Some aspects of this phenomenon have been discussed (p. 68); Cralley[26] showed that in the rabbit, 90 per cent of bacteria reaching the alveoli disappear in 3 hours, and none can be found at the end of 12 hours. Bacteria that are not destroyed *in situ* are carried away to the intrapulmonary, hilar and mediastinal lymph nodes, where they are retained and finally eliminated.[28] This is a very important mechanism because in spite of all the other filtering and defense mechanisms of the upper respiratory tract there can be no doubt that some particles and bacteria continuously reach the distal air spaces, as witnessed by the finding of anthracotic pigment in the hilar and mediastinal lymph nodes of all normal adults.

3. Digestive Tract. Through the digestive tract the organism comes in contact with many pathogenic parasites, so the number and efficiency of its defense mechanisms must be high. The oral surface is lined by a thick multistratified epithelium which serves as a barrier to the penetration of microorganisms, and this becomes apparent when there are breaks in it. For instance, the epithelium of the tonsillar crypts becomes very thin or may even be absent in small areas known as "Stöhr pores," where the lymphoid tissue is directly in contact with bacteria penetrating within the crypts, and this may be part of the explanation for the frequency of tonsillar infections.[29] Another instance is found in the breaks produced by removal of teeth, which is frequently accompanied by bacteriemia;[30] according to Hobson and Juel-Jensen, after teeth extractions the penetration of bacteria to the circulation may represent a potential danger for the patient, especially in the presence of cardiac valvular lesions, which may result in bacterial endocarditis.[31] Saliva has bacteriostatic and even bactericidal properties against some microorganisms, such as *Corynebacterium diphtheria,* and some intestinal pathogens. Dold[32] described a thermolabile bactericidal factor in saliva of a protein nature with the name of "inhibin," but other authors believe that it is

H_2O_2 produced by streptococci which acts against other bacteria.[6] If this is true it would be an instance of bacterial antagonism, where the metabolic products of one strain make impossible the establishment of another.

The continuous flow of saliva through the excretory ducts of salivary glands provides mechanical and chemical protection to the glands, and this becomes more apparent when there is dehydration, hemorrhage or any other process interfering with secretory activity, since salivary gland infections are more frequent under these conditions. Salivary secretion, together with suction movements of lips, tongue and cheeks, creates a current detailed in the classical studies of Bloomfield,[33, 34] who deposited carbon particles and bacteria in different areas of the oral mucosa and observed that they always moved towards the pharynx and the digestive tract. Since the tonsils are protected by the anterior folds, Bloomfield recovered only few particles and bacteria from them. A complete summary of the defense mechanisms of the oral mucosa is presented by Simmons.[35]

The gastric pH plays a very important role as a defense mechanism since large numbers of bacteria filtering through the oral defenses and reaching the stomach are destroyed or their reproduction is inhibited in acid medium; these microorganisms include some intestinal pathogens such as salmonella, shigella and brucella. Garrod[36] studied the sensitivity to gastric secretions of several microorganisms and found that the more sensitive the germ the less its ability to produce infections via the digestive tract. A general principle was proposed, namely that "infectivity of intestinal pathogens varies with their resistance to gastric bactericidal effect." Although the study has not been amplified, the principle is correct; unfortunately, there are large individual variations in secretion and pH of gastric juice, not only from one person to another, but also in the same individual at different hours and under various conditions, so the "gastric germicidal barrier" is frequently passed by intestinal pathogens. In addition, some parasites are provided with capsules resistant to the action of gastric secretion, as *Entamoeba histolytica,*

which represent a passport to the intestines. Mucus secretion and cellular desquamation hinder the penetration of bacteria through the wall of the stomach.

There are several mechanisms of disinfection (also known as "autodisinfection") in the intestine, which control the "resident" flora and keep it constant. At the time when the child is exclusively breast fed the intestinal flora is formed only by *Lactobacillus bifudus* which produces large amounts of lactic acid and keeps the pH very low, thus inhibiting establishment and growth of other microorganisms. With changes in the variety of foods the intestinal "resident" flora is modified but remains very susceptible to pH changes. Working with dogs, Arnold[37] found that by increasing the alkalinity of the contents of the upper intestine the "resident" flora became similar to that of the lower intestine. Furthermore, it was also shown that changes in gastric secretion are not the only factors determining pH of intestinal contents, but that modifications in temperature are also effective, whether by fever or environmental influences. "Autodisinfection" mechanisms seem to depend on the presence of neutralized acid in the lower intestine (ileum, cecum), and when acid is missing the cecum contains bacteria usually found in the duodenum; furthermore, a protein-rich meal has the same effect, which lasts several hours.

In addition to mechanisms inhibiting the establishment of pathogenic agents in the intestine, there are others related to the permeability of the intestinal wall to bacteria. Arnold[37] has found that the lymph of the thoracic duct of dogs is free of germs, but when the normally acid duodenal content is neutralized or alkalinized there appear bacteria in the thoracic duct; similar effects are obtained with protein-rich meals or with temperature changes. Mucus secretion is another important factor in intestinal protection;[38] lysozyme is found in variable amounts in intestinal secretions of some animal species, but its role in defense has not been determined. Finally, as in the stomach, irritability of the intestinal wall favors the elimination of many bacteria through diarrhea, since simultaneously with transit acceleration there is increased intestinal secretion, appearance of many macrophages, etc.

4. Genitourinary Tract. The foregoing discussions of epithelial resistance, cellular desquamation, pH, "resident" bacterial flora, etc., are applicable to the genitourinary tract. Urine has both pH and mechanical effects, but the rarity of infections in the urethra in cases of anuria or with shunting of urinary flow suggests that there must be other defense mechanisms in this area.[29]

A clear instance of the "accidental" nature of defense mechanisms is provided by the female genital tract. Estrogens stimulate deposition of glycogen in the epithelial lining of the vagina, which upon desquamation provides abundant substrate for proliferation of *Lactobacillus acidophilus;* this microorganism, in the same fashion as *L. bifidus,* produces large amounts of lactic acid and lowers the pH beyond the possibility of establishment and survival of other germs. Therefore, the ages of greatest susceptibility to vaginal infection are those without an important estrogenic secretion, i.e., before puberty and after the menopause; gonorrheal vulvovaginitis in children and chronic cervicitis in older women bear witness to the efficiency of this defense mechanism, as well as the improvement of such conditions with the use of hormones.[39]

In summary, local defense mechanisms are found in areas in contact with the surrounding environment and are nonspecific. Very often their effect is synergistic, although which will predominate depends not only on the area of contact with microorganisms, but also on the nature of the germs. Their efficiency, although not measurable, is surely extraordinary; many infectious diseases occur when local defense mechanisms fail.

B. SYSTEMIC DEFENSE MECHANISMS

Systemic or general defense mechanisms come into play when local defenses have been insufficient to inhibit penetration of parasites within the organism. For didactic reasons they may be considered in two groups, humoral and cellular, but this division is artificial and in the end cells are responsible for both. The separation is not new. From the very beginning of their study a controversy existed on the role played by humoral and cellular mechanisms in the defense of the organism. The extraordinary vigor and perseverance of Metchnikoff[10] are responsible for the acceptance of phagocytosis as a fundamental defense mechanism, and it is not without significance that the same cells involved in this process have been held to play an important role in the synthesis of antibodies, the carriers of humoral defense.

1. Humoral Defense Mechanisms. There are two large groups of humoral substances involved in systemic defense against parasites: antibodies and other compounds whose protective effect follows different mechanisms. Several aspects of the immune response are discussed in Chapter VIII, while here only those referring to its role in defense are reviewed.

a. Antibodies. ". . . among those whom in the country I was frequently called upon to inoculate, many resisted every effort to give them the smallpox. These patients I found had undergone a disease they called the Cow Pox contracted by milking cows affected by a peculiar eruption on their teats. On enquiry, it appeared that it had been known among the dairies [from] time immemorial and that vague opinion prevailed that it was a preventive of the smallpox . . . I was struck with the idea that it might be practicable to propagate disease [cowpox] by inoculation, after the manner of the smallpox, first from the cow and finally from one human being to another. I anxiously waited some time for an opportunity of putting this theory to the test. At length the period arrived. The first experiment [May 14, 1796] was made upon a lad of the name of Phipps, in whose arm a little vaccine virus was inserted taken from the hand of a young woman who had been accidentally infected by a cow. Notwithstanding the resemblance which the pustule thus excited on the boy's arm bore to variolous infection, yet as the indisposition attending it was barely perceptible, I could scarce persuade myself the patient was secure from the smallpox. However, on being inoculated some months [July 1] afterwards, it proved that he was secure."[41]

With these words Jenner described his first observations, started in 1775 and published 14 years later. The nature of the effect of vaccination (antibody production) was not suspected for a long time, even by Pasteur, who used the very same principle in his work on fowl cholera, anthrax and rabies, and who baptized the procedure with the name of "vaccination" in Jenner's honor. It was not until von Behring and Kitasato used the serum of animals injected with detoxified cultures of *Clostridium tetani* to protect others against the effects of tetanic toxin that the presence of special substances in the serum was accepted. In his second paper, published a week later, von Behring showed that the same effect could be obtained with diphtheric toxin and that it was specific; i.e., tetanic antitoxin will not protect against diphtheria toxin and vice versa. Many investigations followed, especially those of Ehrlich, which established the phenomenon of antibody production as a general biologic principle and laid the foundations of modern immunology.

"Antibody is defined as a humoral globulin produced by the body in response to an antigen, and capable of reacting with the antigen in some observable way."[42] This definition has important exceptions, but may be accepted for practical purposes since it covers most of the antibodies involved in defense. Exceptions refer to the so-called "natural," "normal," "physiologic," or "nonspecific" antibodies, which were first known as opsonins, alexin and complement. They were observed for the first time by Nuttall in 1888,[43] who described the bactericidal property of defibrinated serum, while other authors showed that serum would prepare bacteria for phagocytosis. Their origin is not known, but Boyd[44] has summarized the three following hypotheses: (a) A "normal" antibody is really the response to an antigen that was unobserved or that penetrated into the organism through an unusual route. Obviously, this hypothesis denies the existence of this group of antibodies and would consider all antibodies as acquired. (b) "Normal" antibodies are produced not against the organism with which they react but against another organism, closely related or not, with similar or identical antigens. There are many instances of this type of antibody, which would not be "natural" but acquired; nevertheless, the differences between "normal" and ordinary antibodies are not explained by this theory. (c) "Natural" antibodies are a genetic character, independent of previous stimuli and comparable in their inheritance to blood groups; an instance would be the blood agglutinins.

There are some differences between the antibodies produced against bacteria, viruses and parasites, and although they are more apparent than real they will be used to systematize the following description.

A. ANTIBODIES AGAINST BACTERIA. When a microorganism comes in contact with serum containing specific antibody a series of changes observable grossly and microscopically may occur which depend more on the medium in which they appear and on the method used to study them than on the nature of the antibody. This unitary theory of antibodies[45] has many adherents; it does not mean that a single pure antigen will give rise to only one variety of antibody, but that reactions between antigen and antibody are fundamentally the same, although they may differ in appearance and there are some observations indicating that antibody molecules in an immune serum are rather heterogeneous. Almost all reactions participating in defense fall in one of the following types.

I. Agglutination. As indicated by its name, agglutination is the clumping of bacteria in masses or groups, probably due to a modification in electrical charges on the bacterial surface, since the phenomenon is influenced by electrolyte concentration, pH and the amount of antibody. Its protective effect is partly due to the fact that agglutination contributes to the localization of bacteria at the site of entry into the organism. This was clearly shown by Cannon and Pacheco,[46] who inoculated staphylococci in the subcutaneous tissues of previously immunized and control animals and observed that in the latter there was a violent inflammation with wide dissemination of bacteria in the subcutaneous space, while in the former there was a localized abscess where staphylococci were agglutinated and failed to disseminate.

II. Neufeld phenomenon. This is the swelling (Quellung) of the capsule of some microorganisms, which increases several times in diameter and appears darker. The Neufeld phenomenon is probably due to imbibition of water in the capsule and its result in immunity is the same as in agglutination.

III. Bacterial lysis (Pfeiffer phenomenon). This reaction, the result of which is much more spectacular and theoretically ideal for protection, is unfortunately limited to a few bacteria (*Vibrio comma, Hemophilus influenzae,* brucella, and some gram-negative intestinal strains. It is probably due to the combined effect of antibody and a complement. The administration of large amounts of antibody to an animal infected with susceptible organisms showing the Pfeiffer phenomenon results in the rapid destruction of many bacteria and the release of toxic substances which may kill the animal; this is not the case when vaccination is prophylactic because the infecting dose is small and antibody opposes bacterial proliferation.

IV. Opsonization. It has been observed that the destruction of bacteria by phagocytes is greatly increased in the presence of immune serum from either normal or immunized animals. The factors facilitating phagocytosis have been called "bacteriotropins," "opsonins," "alexin," "complement," etc.; most of these factors were at first considered to be different substances, but at present the consensus is almost unanimous that they are identical.[45] Serum opsonins seem to consist of two components: thermostable antibody and a thermolabile substance to be found also in normal serum, but the antibody concentration is greater in immune serum. Opsonization represents the coating of bacteria with a fine protein fiber which greatly enhances phagocytosis; the mechanism by which ingestion of microorganisms is facilitated is not known. Howard and Wardlaw have shown that the phagocytic activity of the reticuloendothelial system of the liver is dependent on serum opsonins, so that even in this instance the separation of humoral from cellular immunity is obscured.[47]

V. Antitoxic effect. Antitoxic sera are usually effective against exotoxins. In spite of the antigenic capacity of endotoxins, antibodies usually fail to neutralize their toxic effects. This is probably due to the complexity of antigens, as in the case of salmonella and shigella. It has been shown that the antigenic compounds of these bacteria are formed by carbohydrates, lipids and proteins, and that while the most antigenic fraction is the carbohydrate, the most toxic fraction is the protein; therefore, antibody would be formed against the least toxic fraction of the antigen and would leave the protein free to exert its noxious action on the cells.

B. ANTIBODIES AGAINST VIRUSES. For a long time it was thought that humoral defense mechanisms against viruses were basically different from those conferring bacterial immunity. With advancing knowledge about viruses, however, these differences have been vanishing so that at present it is generally admitted that, considering the size of the particles and their predominantly intracellular position, humoral defense mechanisms against viruses are the same as against bacteria.[48] The action of antibodies on viruses is not known. In a recent experiment with a mixture of virus and antibody it was easily demonstrated that they are not combined since they may be separated by dilution, centrifugation or decreasing the amount of material injected into the test animal.[49] If a certain period is allowed to elapse, however, the combination between virus and antibody is completed and sometimes is irreversible.[50] This peculiarity is responsible for the name "neutralizing" which is usually attached to viral antibodies, but it has also been demonstrated in some bacteria. Furthermore, under special circumstances it is possible to demonstrate that the typical *in vitro* serologic reactions for bacterial antibodies (precipitation, agglutination, complement fixation, etc.) are also obtained with viral antibodies.[47]

Another interesting phenomenon is that of interference.[51] It has been shown that intramuscular inoculation of neurotropic virus of yellow fever into monkeys will not produce disease, whereas the viscerotropic virus is fatal to 100 per cent of experimental animals; the injection of neurotropic virus, however, protects against the viscerotropic virus, and the injection can be made simultaneously or even 20 hours after inoculation of the viscerotropic virus. It is accepted that this phenomenon does not depend on the appearance of antibodies but on the competition of the two viruses for the same intracellular enzymatic systems or the production by the infected cell of a nonsedimentable factor which renders it resistant to infection by a different virus.[52] Such a factor was discovered by Isaacs[53] and named interferon. It has been suggested that interfering viruses stimulate the cell to elaborate protein-like substances of nonviral origin that prevent superinfection with homologous or heterologous viruses. Finally, it has been said that "cellular" immunity would explain certain cases of resistance to viral infection, but all those mentioned so far can be accounted for by different mechanisms.[54]

C. ANTIBODIES AGAINST ANIMAL PARASITES. According to Taliaferro,[55] all data at hand seem to indicate that humoral defense mechanisms against animal parasites are identical to those involved against other living agents of disease such as bacteria, rickettsiae and viruses. The study of antibodies against animal parasites has certain advantages over the study of other antibodies, such as the inability of many animal parasites to multiply within the organism, which facilitates a quantitative appreciation of the infective dose and, therefore, of the effect of antibodies. Furthermore, the size of animal parasites provides abundant material for the study and preparation of antigens.[56] Using these and other advantages it has been found that antibodies inhibit the reproduction of animal parasites by at least three different methods.[57] (1) Nematodes show a marked decrease of all metabolic processes, including those necessary for multiplication. A good example is *Nippostrongylus muris,* a nematode parasite in the rat and similar to ancylostoma; when the rat recovers from an infection with *N. muris* it acquires relative resistance to a second infection due to a precipitin-like antibody which *in vivo* forms a precipitate with the secretions and excretions coming from the different orifices of the parasite such as mouth, excretory pore and anus. Sometimes the mouth is filled with the precipitate which may reach the entire intestine and, with disintegration of the parasite, the antibody reacts with the entire organism.[58] The mechanism of action of this antibody has been much discussed and at present it is believed that the destruction of the parasite is caused either by mechanical obstruction of the nat-

ural orifices or by an antagonistic action of the antibody against enzymes necessary for digestion and assimilation of proteins. A similar phenomenon was observed by Oliver González[59] in the case of *Ascaris lumbricoides* var. *suum,* which is of special interest since this parasite may infest man as well as pigs.

(2) In some forms of infections by plasmodia there is a synergistic effect on the parasite, brought about both by the antibody and by the physiologic effects of the antigen-antibody complex on the host. This double effect has been postulated by several authors since it occurs when there is intense agglutination and phagocytosis of the parasite in the reticuloendothelial system, and because it appears associated with degenerated forms of the parasite in the peripheral blood, which predominate during crises. No circulating antibody has been demonstrated in this type of immunity.

(3) Some nonpathogenic trypanosomes and *Trypanosoma lewisi,* which does not infect man, induce the formation of an antibody which specifically blocks reproduction without influencing any of the other metabolic functions of the parasite. Chandler[60] has summarized a series of observations indicating that the effect of this antibody, known as "ablastin," depends on its concentration; when it is abundant the parasites are agglutinated and their reproduction is inhibited, but when the concentration is low the only result will be inhibition of multiplication. This effect has been shown to result from inhibition of nucleic acid and protein synthesis in the parasite.[61]

b. Other Humoral Mechanisms. For years it has been known that serum and tissues contain a series of ill-defined, unspecific substances with variable degrees of bactericidal or bacteriostatic activity. They have received many different names; Skarnes and Watson[62] offer the classification given in Table 44. An instance of a humoral defense mechanism which cannot be called antibody is the serum factor (bactericidin) conferring resistance against *Bacillus subtilis,* which may be passively transmitted but is not adsorbed to the antigens of the microorganism nor to living bacteria.[63] Other examples would be the antivirus substances extracted from tissues of animals infected

Table 44. **Tissue Antimicrobial Substances**

NAME	COMMON SOURCE	HEAT STABILITY	CHEMICAL CLASS
1. Gram-negative			
Complement	Serum	Labile	Euglobulin-carbohydrate-albumin
Properdin (normal) antibody	Serum	Labile to relatively stable	Euglobulin
Phagocytin	Neutrophilic leukocytes	Relatively stable	Globulin fraction
Lysozyme (special case)	Ubiquitous distribution	Stable	Small basic protein
2. Gram-positive			
beta-Lysin	Serum	Relatively stable	Protein (?)
Lysozyme	Ubiquitous distribution	Stable	Small basic protein
Histone	Lymphatics (nucleoprotein)	Stable	Small basic protein
Protamine	Sperm cells (nucleoprotein)	Stable	Small basic protein
Tissue polypeptides	Lymphatics (nucleoprotein)	Stable	Linear basic peptides
Leukin	Neutrophilic leukocytes	Stable	Basic peptides (protamine)
Plakin	Blood platelets	Relatively stable	Peptide (?)
Hematin, mesohematin	Red blood cells	Stable	Iron prophyrins
Spermine, spermidine	Pancreas, prostate	Stable	Basic polyamines
Lactenin	Milk	Relatively stable	Protein (?)

(Skarnes and Watson[62])

with several viruses such as Newcastle,[64] mumps,[65] etc. Recently, the interest in "natural" humoral defense mechanisms, which are all those that cannot be called antibodies, has increased greatly,[66] and one of the most important reasons has been Pillemer's discovery of the properdin system. In several publications Pillemer, et al.[67, 68] described and studied a system composed of a serum euglobulin, complement and ionic Mg^{++}; the name properdin derives from the Latin voice *perdere,* to destroy. This system participates in the destruction of bacteria, protozoons, viruses and abnormal red blood cells, and in addition it is related to resistance of experimental animals to shock and radiation.[69] Properdin differs from antibody in that it is nonspecific; it does not require antigen for its existence (it is present in normal serum and even in the serum of rats born and kept germfree); it is found in fraction III-1 of plasma, while antibody is in both fractions II and III, and requires Mg^{++} and fractions C_1 and C_4 of complement in order to be effective, while antibody requires no complement. Fraction C_3 is specifically inactivated by the properdin system, while the antigen-antibody compound inactivates fractions C_1, C_2 and C_4, and has no effect whatsoever on fraction C_3.[70] Pillemer[68] has remarked that, ". . . properdin may be a primordial type of 'antibody.' More highly developed and specific substances (antibodies) may have been formed during the process of evolution." Another natural humoral defense mechanism would be lysozyme, which has recently been found to act against certain encapsulated anthrax strains in the presence of high levels of HCO_3^- and CO_2.[71]

2. Cellular Systemic Defenses. Cellular defense mechanisms of systemic distribution are essentially the same as those participating in local defense, described in Chapter II and comprised almost entirely under the process of phagocytosis. This process is a function of the reticuloendothelial system, and most of the humoral mechanisms operate only to facilitate phagocytosis. Many types of particles, including bacteria, are rapidly "cleared" from the blood when introduced into the circulation by intravenous route. Contrary to popular belief, most microorganisms are less capable of causing disease when injected intravenously than when administered by any other route.[72] Although the pattern of clearance varies with the particular animal species and the specific microorganism under study, certain general characteristics of the removal proc-

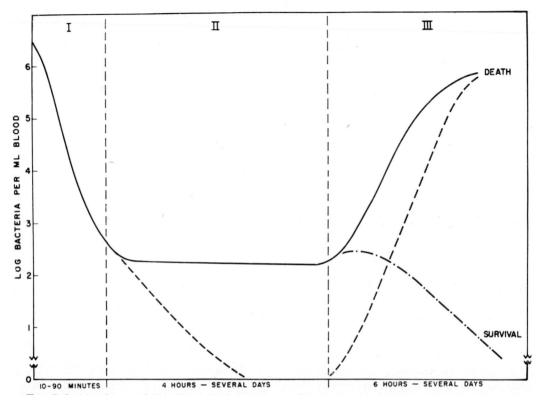

FIG. 7–5. A schema of blood stream clearance as reflected by blood cultures. In phase I, bacteria disappear rapidly from the circulation. During phase II, bacteremia may disappear or persist at low levels. Depending on the virulence of the bacterium under study, resurging bacteremia or sterilization of the blood stream may be observed in phase III. (Courtesy of Dr. D. E. Rogers and the Editor, Bacteriological Reviews.)

ess seem to hold for most cases; they have been reviewed by Rogers,[73] who separates them into three phases (Fig. 7–5). In the first phase, clearance is rapid, with 90 to 99 per cent of circulating bacteria disappearing during this period, which varies from 10 minutes to several hours. In the second phase microorganisms persist in the circulation at lower concentrations or continue to be removed at slower rates for several hours to several days. The third phase is related to the final outcome of infection, since animals surviving will show complete disappearance of all bacteria while in those with fatal infections bacteria reappear in the peripheral blood in increasing numbers and remain there until the death of the animal. Most of the microorganisms cleared from the circulation are trapped in vascular organs containing large numbers of cells of the reticuloendotheial system, such as liver and spleen, although other organs may also be important.[74] Using *Escherichia*

coli infections in rabbits, Rogers and Melly[75] showed that blood emerging from the splanchnic area (liver, spleen and intestines) was the only blood showing any significant decrease in the number of bacteria, and Beeson, *et al.*[76] made similar observations in patients with bacterial endocarditis. Immunization will increase the clearing power of splanchnic organs to a varied but always important degree, and this effect can be shown in the isolated and perfused liver.[77]

The reticuloendothelial system seems to have an almost infinite capacity for removing bacteria from the circulation, as shown by measuring the clearing of microorganisms from the blood after repeated injections of the same [78] or different bacteria;[79] when this work is done using particulate matter such as carbon or colloidal substances in amounts comparable to those used in bacteriologic experiments the same results are obtained.[80] But if massive doses of particulate matter are administered then the capacity for trapping of the splanchnic tissues may be exceeded.[81] Nevertheless, striking disappearance of circulating microorganisms may still be observed, revealing the existence of other factors at play in the clearing of blood. One such factor is the circulating polymorphonuclear leukocyte, which competes with fixed macrophages for the ingestion of bacteria,[82] and another would be the leukocyte sequestered in capillary beds which remains active in removing bacteria from the circulating blood.[83] The lung is also involved in the process, as well as the bone marrow, lymph nodes, etc.

Many factors have been tested in search for possible effects on this clearing mechanism of the blood, such as starvation, irradiation, shock, diabetes, splenectomy, corticotropins, adrenal steroids, etc., and none has been found to influence the first phase of swift removal of bacteria from the circulation. On the other hand, the maximal capacity of the reticuloendothelial system is depressed immediately after administration of endotoxin or overwhelming infection, or increased with estrogens. Intracellular destruction of bacteria, judged by the likelihood of resurging bacteremia and death in the later phases of the clearance process, is inhibited by several factors such as starvation, shock, irradiation, endotoxins, etc.; there is no known way to enhance intracellular destruction of microbes.[73]

Phagocytosis and destruction of bacteria is only one way in which the reticuloendothelial system participates in defense. Biozzi, et al.[84] have shown by means of a quantitative technique that the reticuloendothelial system protects the organism against some gram-negative endotoxins and that this effect may be partially blocked by giving the experimental animals massive doses of particulate matter or carbon.

C. CONCEPT OF IMMUNITY

The Romans used the word "immune" to designate those persons exempt from taxation and other obligations to the state; the meaning was later extended to protection granted the early Christian church and its officers ("papal immunity"). The general concept of "exemption" was extended to "render free," and usage implied that such protection was innate. Immunity was later defined as that state in which the individual may come in contact with a pathogenic agent without showing the clinical manifestations of disease. Physiologically, the organism has learned to defend itself, either through previous contact with the agent or by less well known means related to its genetic constitution. It seems that previous experience has only enhanced and made more specific mechanisms which were there before and which have many other functions different from "defense." Even the exquisite specificity of some antibodies, the speed of the clearing mechanisms of the blood and the almost infinite capacity for phagocytosis of the reticuloendothelial system fail often enough; indeed, the present trend is to consider infectious disease not as the result of invasion by pathogenic microorganisms, but as the failure of local and systemic defense mechanisms.[85] The degree of immunity conferred by previous experience with pathogenic bacteria and/or their products is rarely absolute or permanent. Sometimes antibodies are unable to block the effects of toxins, as in salmonellosis; at other times, phagocytosis occurs but cells are unable to destroy ingested bacteria, which are protected in this position from both antibodies and therapeutic agents, as in brucellosis, tuberculosis and many viral diseases; finally, immunity may be high but short-lived, and in time it will reach levels below those necessary to be of any protective value to the organism. For all these reasons immunity is not an absolute concept; several types must be considered, which should cover most of the mechanisms discussed in the previous paragraphs. The most widely accepted forms of immunity are listed in Table 45.

As any biologic process, immunity is influenced by many factors, which may be considered in two groups according to their origin, namely extrinsic and intrinsic. Very rarely is immunity absolute and permanent, as in measles or poliomyelitis; more often it shows variations caused by the following extrinsic factors:

1. Starvation. Natural or acquired resistance to infection is usually decreased by malnutrition, as witnessed by the increase in many infectious diseases during epochs

Table 45. Types of Immunity

I. Natural immunity
   A. Specific
   B. Nonspecific

II. Acquired immunity
   A. Nonspecific
   B. Specific
      1. Active
         a. Natural
         b. Artificial
      2. Passive
         a. Natural (congenital)
         b. Artificial

of famine and/or war, although some authors believe that this situation is complicated by other factors such as poor sanitary conditions.[86] Experimentally it has been shown that various dietary deficiencies of protein or certain vitamins facilitate the development of infections, measured by survival time or percentage of survival of experimental animals.[87] Schneider has argued against considering these two different outcomes as representatives of the same "resistance;"[88] some viral infections may even be less frequent in starved, vitamin-deficient animals, and host-resistance to malaria is probably enhanced by a deficiency of p-aminobenzoic acid.[89] Antibodies are less adequately formed in malnourished subjects.[90]

2. Fatigue. It has been suggested that physical fatigue decreases resistance to infections, especially during the incubation period, but objective experimental data are not sufficient to draw an acceptable conclusion.

3. Temperature. Pasteur's classical demonstration of increased susceptibility of fowl to anthrax by submerging their feet in cold water is indicative of the significance of temperature in infection. That this effect is more complicated than initially considered is shown by the fact that frogs, which are cold blooded animals, are resistant to anthrax but become susceptible when their temperature is increased to 37° C. Temperature changes are important in infections of the respiratory tract; the influence of temperature on ciliary movement has been mentioned, and the effect of fever in antibody synthesis and other defense mechanisms is referred to below (p. 339).

4. Irradiation. Small doses of x-rays and other radiant sources may increase resistance to infection,[91] but large doses will depress antibody synthesis and phagocytosis.[92]

5. Drugs and Chemical Compounds. Alcohol decreases resistance to infections not only because it depresses the local inflammatory reaction and interferes with antibody synthesis during vaccination, but also because chronic alcoholism is usually accompanied by malnutrition. All substances depressing the bone marrow, such as barbiturates, sulphonamides, thiouracil, benzol, etc., depress the reticuloendothelial system and favor the development of infections.[93]

6. Intercurrent Infections. The synergystic action of two or more pathogenic agents has greater effects on resistance than those caused by isolated microorganisms. Experimentally, influenza virus A will induce slight changes in monkeys characterized by leukopenia, while hemolytic streptococcus C produces minimal disturbances when administered intranasally, but if both pathogenic agents are introduced into the monkey at the same time the result will be streptococcal pneumonia, probably as a consequence of the leukopenia produced by the virus.[94] Something similar happened in the pandemic of influenza in 1918, with the association of the influenza virus with *Hemophilus influenzae*.

7. Other Factors. Diabetes mellitus is frequently accompanied by infections, especially of the skin and of the urinary tract, and some metabolic bases for this increased susceptibility have been suggested by Dubos.[95] Despite some criticism, experimental animals with alloxan diabetes have been shown to be easy prey of mucormycosis, a fungus which otherwise is unable to invade the rabbit.[96] Hypofunction of the pituitary and adrenal glands permits smaller numbers of infectious agents to multiply than would do so in a normal host, and hypoadrenalism increases susceptibility to bacterial toxins; indeed, either a deficiency or an excess of adrenal steroids has been repeatedly shown to alter defense mechanisms of the host and favor infection.[97] This, however, is an inference based on end results and no definite pattern of influence on defense mechanisms has emerged from the voluminous literature accumulated on the effect of adrenal secretions in infection.[98] Perhaps the inhibition of the inflammatory response (p. 87), a reduction in the formation of antibodies and in the functions of the reticuloendothelial system are the only well documented effects.[99] Differences in sex ratio in many infectious diseases might also be due to hormonal influence of defense mechanisms, but attempts to reproduce these effects in experimental animals have not always met with success. Additional data are presented below.

To summarize, resistance to infection belongs to two general types, namely natural and acquired. Natural resistance is genetically determined[100] and most of the mechanisms involved are obscure, although many of them are the result of anatomic and metabolic features of the host. Acquired immunity is a function of the reticuloendothelial system and of all cells involved in protein synthesis, and the mechanisms are phagocytosis and antibody formation. "Resistance" of the organism is, within present day knowledge, limited to these functions, so that interpretation of the ways in which different factors influence the evolution and final outcome of infections should always be attempted within their general frame. To speak of resistance without specific reference to them is to invoke an empty concept to fill in areas of ignorance.

III. AGGRESSIVE MECHANISMS OF THE PARASITE

Only a small fraction of living beings can parasitize man and the upper mammals, and it is of this fraction that knowledge is less incomplete, although immense gaps are yet to be filled before adequate understanding of the mechanisms of infectious disease is possible. The existence of a parasite depends on several conditions, enumerated by Cameron[101] as follows:

1. *Penetration into the Host.* If this condition is to be fulfilled the host should be in the same environment as the parasite and come in immediate contact with it; further-more, local defense mechanisms of the host should be ineffective against the parasite.

2. *Adequate Conditions of the Host.* Once inside the host, the parasite should find adequate conditions for survival.

3. *Protective Mechanisms of the Parasite Against Defenses of the Host.* Successful counteraction of the host's general defense mechanisms by the parasite is another *sine qua non* condition of parasitism.

4. *Absence of Effective Reaction of the Host.* If the host can build up defenses such as specific antibodies, the parasite should be able to remain unaffected by them.

When these four general conditions are fulfilled parasitism is possible. Those related to transportation of the parasite from one host to another fall in the category of communicability or transmissibility; conditions of penetration into, and persistence within, the host, are known as invasiveness. The capacity of parasites to produce disease is referred to as pathogenicity, while virulence represents the degree of pathogenicity of a given strain (see below). It is easy to understand that none of the features defined depends exclusively on the parasite, but rather they are more or less determined by the interaction between parasite and host. Anyway, discussions on how microorganisms produce disease are very apt to follow a circular course and end in platitudinous conclusions. In order to avoid this ever-present danger it may be convenient to concentrate as much as possible upon some special attributes of parasites—those appearing as immediately responsible for disease—and group them under the general term of "aggressive mechanisms." Discussion of other conditions necessary for the existence of parasitism may be conveniently postponed until the study of the interaction between host and parasite is undertaken.

A. PATHOGENICITY AND VIRULENCE

There seems to be general agreement in considering pathogenicity as the capacity of parasites to produce disease, and virulence as the measure of this capacity. Therefore, a given biologic agent cannot have virulence without being pathogenic, and it is inconceivable to have a pathogen of which some idea of virulence is not available, even of the crudest nature. But in his masterly discussion on the meaning of pathogenicity, Miles[102] appears to give different meaning to both this term and to virulence. According to this author, *"Pathogenicity* is best regarded as an attribute of a species, a genus, or some other grouping of parasites. . . . *Virulence,* on the other hand, is conveniently reserved for the pathogenicity of a given stable homogeneous strain of a microbe, as determined by observation of its action on the host in relation to which the statement about virulence is made." Therefore, pathogenicity becomes a predictable, but not necessarily demonstrable, potentiality of a bacterial species, while virulence is the observed capacity to produce disease of a given strain of such species. There is really no basic opposition between these uses of the terms; if anything, Miles' concepts are more operational and, therefore, more applicable to specific instances.

Pathogenicity has been associated with the ability of parasites to multiply within the organism and although in many instances this is true, there are important exceptions which must be taken into account, especially with some animal parasites. In human cysticercosis the parasite, once inside the host, does not reproduce, but rather reaches a terminal stage in its evolution, a dead-end alley. The same thing occurs with trichinosis. Furthermore, it does not seem adequate to limit pathogenicity to proliferation in tissues in the cases of tetanus, botulism and diphtheria, where bacterial multiplication is minimal and the symptoms are caused by the production of strong toxins. Pathogenicity has only two degrees in bacteria; bacteria are pathogens or nonpathogens. On the other hand, virulence, the degree to which microorganisms are capable of inducing disease, shows an almost infinite variation. Furthermore, virulence depends more specifically on the aggressive mechanisms of the parasite and cannot be reduced to the expression of one or a few characteristics. "Virulence is not a permanent, intrinsic property of a given species. It expresses only the ability of a given strain of the infective agent, in a certain growth phase, to produce a pathological state in a particular host when introduced into that host under well defined condi-

tions."[103] In the case of *Clostridium tetanii,* virulence can be translated as the capacity of a given strain to produce tetanic toxin in greater or lesser amounts and with more or less toxic effects when compared with another strain, while in *Mycobacterium tuberculosis* virulence is probably due to the ability of this microorganism to proliferate and resist the defense mechanisms of the host.

Both pathogenicity and virulence are not immutable properties of parasites. On the contrary, they may be modified in the laboratory and, in all probability, they show variations of a more "spontaneous" nature. BCG and $H_{37}Ra$ are strains of *Myco. tuberculosis* of experimentally lowered virulence, by means of repeat cultures; on the other hand, virulence may be augmented by means of successive inoculations. Such changes are probably due to selection of bacterial mutants and not to a modification of metabolism of all members of the colony. A similar phenomenon lies at the basis of specificity in pathogenicity; no parasite is pathogenic for all animal species and some of them show an exquisite degree of specificity, as *Myco. leprae* which until recently had been found to be pathogenic only in man, but the studies of Binford have shown that the golden hamster will present granulomatous inflammation when infected with this microorganism.[104] Specificity is obviously not due only to the parasite but also, and to a very great degree, to the conditions of the host. This is demonstrated by the development of pathogenicity in a parasite by merely changing the features of the host, or by increases in virulence obtained through the same mechanisms. For instance, guinea pigs treated with cortisone become susceptible to the poliomyelitis virus; rabbits die of tuberculosis when inoculated with human strain of *Myco. tuberculosis,* if at the same time they are receiving the same steroid,[105] etc.

Variations in virulence encountered in strains isolated from a given animal species cannot be extrapolated to other species. An excellent instance of this is the isoniazid-resistant strains of *Myco. tuberculosis* obtained by Middlebrook[106] from human cases of the disease after prolonged chemotherapy, and shown by the same author to have a substantial decrease in virulence for guinea pigs. This important observation cannot be extrapolated to man and used as a proof of decreased virulence of isoniazid-resistant tubercle bacilli because, among other reasons, such strains are frequently isolated from patients with progressive and extensive disease; obviously, the experimental method cannot be used in this instance to solve the problem.

Although virulence is considered dependent on the aggressive mechanisms of parasites, this statement requires some qualifications. First, virulence can only be shown by its effect on the host, i.e., by disease, which is not only composed of the effects of aggressive mechanisms, but also of the reactions of the organism and of the interactions which make up the host-parasite relation; therefore, interpreting the different mechanisms of pathogenicity one must be careful to discriminate between that belonging to the parasite and that corresponding to the host. Second, although in some instances the mechanisms of virulence (aggression) are well known, in many others they are purely hypothetical and lack specific demonstration. This means that in many infectious diseases, although the etiologic agent is known, the actual mechanisms of injury are ignored. It is important to emphasize this ignorance not only because it exists, but also because it tends to be minimized in discussions of infectious disease. To know that the etiologic agent of tuberculosis is *Myco. tuberculosis* is extremely important, not only from a scientific viewpoint, but also because it permits prophylactic measures which have eliminated this scourge from several enlightened communities. But in spite of sustained efforts by some of the best scientific brains in the world for over 70 years the mechanisms by which Koch's bacilli induce disease are yet to be uncovered; *Myco. tuberculosis* produces no toxins; colossal amounts of bacillary fractions are required to produce lesions, and the role of hypersensitivity is a subject of controversy.[107] There is a gap filled with ignorance between the *in vitro* properties of biologic agents of disease and their effects on the host, and the only way to bridge this gap is by continuous investigation of the aggressive mechanisms of pathogenic agents and their interactions with the host. But before this can be done we must recognize that there is such a gap.

B. AGGRESSIVE MECHANISMS OF BACTERIA, RICKETTSIAE, VIRUSES AND FUNGI

The parasite that has invaded the host and is proliferating within the tissues may produce damage by interfering with metabolism and the functions of different organs in several possible ways: the production of toxic substances, interference with nutrition or with detoxifying mechanisms of the host, stimulation of the inflammatory reaction and/or hypersensitivity, mechanical disturbances, etc. Some of the available information is summarized in the following paragraphs.

1. Toxins. Toxins are substances produced by bacteria which affect the host as chemical poisons, or favor invasion of microorganisms, or both. Some of the most potent toxicants are among them, as the toxin produced by *Clostridium botulinum*.[108] Ideally, the criteria for accepting that a toxin is responsible for some or all the harmful effects of an infectious disease are fulfilled when the organism is known to produce a toxin; virulent variants produce the toxin and avirulent ones do not; injection of the toxin separately from the germs produces symptoms that mimic the disease; the infecting organism produces the disease without multiplying profusely or spreading extensively; the blood is sterile, and organs at a distance from the seat of infection are affected; finally, the disease can be prevented by immunization against the toxin.

There are two general types of toxins, namely endo- and exotoxins, according to the mechanism by which they are released to the surrounding environment; endotoxins require death and disintegration of the microorganism, while exotoxins are released by living bacteria. Chemically, toxins may also be considered in two general groups; one is formed by proteins, the other by polymolecular compounds containing proteins, phospholipids and polysaccharides. Chemical differences are reflected in various properties of these two groups of substances which appear summarized in Table 46. Toxins are antigenic and stimulate for-

Table 46. Differences Between the Two Chemical Types of Bacterial Toxins

PROTEINS	POLYMOLECULAR COMPOUNDS
Almost all derive from gram-positive bacteria Endotoxins and exotoxins	Somatic antigens O of gram-negative germs
	Endotoxins
High toxicity	Less toxic
Specific pharmacologic action	The effect is independent of the causal agent
Very thermolabile	Less thermolabile
Neutralized by antibody in stoichiometric proportions	Partially neutralized by antibody, even in the presence of excess antigen
Toxoid may be prepared	Toxoid may not be prepared

mation of antibodies; neutralization of toxic effects, however, is not always the result of combination with specific antibodies, possibly because the antigenic fraction is not the only one responsible for symptoms, as is the case with enteric pathogens. An extensive review of these and many other properties of toxins has been published by van Heyningen.[109]

The mechanism of action of most bacterial toxins is not understood in detail. Diphtheria toxin has been isolated as a pure crystalline protein containing only those amino acids normally found in the body.[110] The selective effect on myocardium and central nervous system suggests some interference with oxidative metabolism, since these two are the tissues most sensitive to oxygen lack. Pappenheimer[111] has found that the concentration of iron in the culture medium is critical for the production of toxin by the bacteria. In an iron-free medium, no toxin is produced; at low concentrations of iron toxin is produced and, in addition, porphyrins appear in the culture filtrate; at higher concentrations of iron, neither toxin nor porphyrins are found, but cytochrome b is synthesized by the bacteria. From these findings Pappenheimer[112] has suggested that the toxin is the protein moiety of bacterial cytochrome b, and that at low concentrations of iron it cannot be linked with the porphyrins and iron to form cytochrome b; furthermore, Pappenheimer proposed that diphtheria toxin acts by specifically blocking synthesis of one or more components of the host's cytochrome sys-

tem. This would result in inhibition of oxidative phosphorylation and would account very well for the selective action on the central nervous system and heart. Nevertheless, the situation is perhaps more complicated since, as pointed out by Pappenheimer, no direct demonstration of any impressive decrease in the cytochrome b content of intoxicated tissues is available, and mitochondria isolated from poisoned animals fail to show any abnormalities.[113]

Both botulinum and tetanus toxins act directly upon nerve cells, the former on the cholinergic nerve endings of the peripheral somatic and autonomic fibers, the latter on neurons of the cerebrospinal axis; the exact mechanism is not known, although the immunity of adrenergic fibers of the autonomic nervous system to both toxins suggests that it may be closely related to the metabolism of choline in nerve cells.[114] Culture filtrates of *Clostridium perfringens* have been found to contain a number of toxic proteins, the chief one being known as "alpha" toxin. This is a very active lecithinase, splitting the phospholipid lecithin to yield phosphoryl choline and the diglyceride; other clostridia have also been found to produce lecithinase.[115] Since lecithin occurs in cell membranes it is to be expected that a toxic lecithinase will have a widespread effect in the body in addition to a hemolytic effect. Animals injected with alpha toxin show edema, hemorrhage, local necrosis and shock, which can be reasonably ascribed to the effect of lecithinase on cellular and capillary permeability. Macfarlane and Datta[116] treated isolated mitochondria with alpha toxin and found that the phospholipid present was rapidly broken down and that the phosphatase activity was increased; the latter effect can be attributed to rupture of the mitochondrial membrane with release of the enzyme, since normal mitochondria will show no phosphatase activity. Additional data on the mechanism of action of these and other bacterial toxins have been presented by Dawkins and Rees.[117]

2. Antigens. Although toxins are antigenic some bacteria possess nontoxic antigenic substances which serve as aggressive mechanisms against the host. For instance, *Bacillus anthracis* has a capsular polypeptide (polyglutamic acid) which acts by neutralizing a bactericidal substance present in normal serum, but there must also be an extracellular factor for full effectiveness. In addition, *B. anthracis* has been shown by Smith and Keppie[118] to produce a specific lethal factor *in vivo* but not *in vitro*. The capsule of pneumococcus interferes with phagocytosis, especially when the germ is within exudates and away from surfaces or many polymorphonuclear leukocytes which might favor Wood's phenomenon of surface phagocytosis[119] (*see* Chapter II). Nevertheless, the presence of superficial antigens related to virulence in some bacteria bears no relation to pathogenicity in other microorganisms, which are only rarely agents of disease[120] although they may have the same antigenic structure; for this reason, other factors must be taken into account to explain pathogenicity in addition to capsular antigens.

3. Other Substances. These are usually nonantigenic and they are not considered toxins. Rather, their role is to aid in invasion of the host or to lower some of the defense mechanisms, favoring establishment and proliferation of parasites. Streptococci, staphylococci, some strains of diphtheria bacillus and other microorganisms produce hyaluronidase, an enzyme acting on hyaluronic acid, which is one of the major components of connective tissue ground substance and a determinant of its viscosity. Hydrolysis of hyaluronic acid will decrease resistance to spreading in the interstitial tissues and will favor bacterial dissemination;[121] a similar role may be postulated for streptokinase and other proteolytic enzymes. Some capsular polysaccharides, as well as endotoxins and lipopolysaccharides, decrease the concentration of properdin in the serum and, therefore, the animal's resistance to experimental infection.[122] This effect, however, depends on the doses of bacteria, since it has been shown that the same substances used in lower amounts may stimulate properdin formation and increase resistance. Finally, some bacterial components will induce an elevation of temperature, changing the living conditions of both host and parasite in the manner discussed below.

4. Metabolic Competence. This hypothetical mechanism of virulence is almost entirely limited to viruses. It is accepted that viruses are incomplete metabolic systems which require intracellular enzymes to carry out their functions. When viruses penetrate within cells they "kidnap" the enzymes from the systems where they are found and produce disturbances which are manifested as clinical symptoms. In this particular case, competition is for a specific enzyme or group of enzymes and occurs within the cell. In other cases the virus carries an enzyme, the substrate of which is to be found on the cellular surface and is known as "receptor"; for instance, the influenza virus has the capacity to agglutinate erythrocytes and this capacity may be blocked by a serum mucopolysaccharide which may also serve as substrate for the viral enzyme.[123] If it is accepted that union between viral enzyme and "receptor" is a necessary step for penetration of the virus, then the enzyme is an aggressive mechanism.

C. AGGRESSIVE MECHANISMS OF ANIMAL PARASITES

The production and utilization of toxins as aggressive agents, clearly defined as an important feature of some bacteria, has not been shown to exist in infections by animal parasites.[124] Aggressive mechanisms of such disease agents are better considered as mechanical, despoiling, anoxic, hypersensitivity, enzymatic, and others.

1. Mechanical. Many animal parasites damage the host by mechanical means, interfering with patency of preformed ducts, compressing vital organs, etc. A mass of *Ascaris* may produce obstruction of the intestine in children or the worms may climb from the duodenum into the bile ducts and give rise to obstructive jaundice which may be mistaken for calculi in the gallbladder; cerebral cysticercosis will produce neurologic symptoms mainly on the basis of pressure and irritation of the nervous substance;[125] the clinical and pathologic features of malignant malaria are probably due to massive occlusion of visceral capillaries by parasitized and abnormal red blood cells which form small thrombi.[126]

2. Despoliation. This is the destruction of normal constituents of the host's organism beyond the possibilities of adaptation, which brings about clinical disturbances. *Ancylostoma* feed on the intestinal blood of the host; trypanosomes and schistosomes require glucose for their metabolism and use the one present in blood;[127] several intracellular protozoons use the protoplasm of the parasitized cell for nutrition, etc.

3. Anoxic. Oxygen lack may be the result of several aggressive mechanisms, but it represents the fundamental disturbance in malaria, where it is due to decrease in the number of red blood cells through hemolysis of parasitized erythrocytes,[127] and also to a decrease in oxygen saturation of hemoglobin.

4. Antigenicity. Hypersensitivity is an important aggressive mechanism of animal parasites, which has been mistaken for a toxic effect. It is a humoral and/or cellular reaction appearing in previously sensitized hosts.

Sprent[128] has described the presence of granulomatous inflammation in animals infected with larvae of *Ascaris lumbricoides,* as long as the host was previously sensitized with an antecedent infection; similar lesions may be encountered in toxoplasmosis and in cutaneous leishmaniasis. Several parenteral helminth infections (fascioliasis, trichinosis and onchocercosis) reveal in the first months various manifestations of hypersensitivity, but after a few months some form of "habituation" to antigens develops and such manifestations disappear. Nevertheless, in the case of onchocercosis, when many microfilarias die as the result of treatment with Hetrazan, hypersensitivity reappears. Any helminthiasis capable of passing beyond the intestinal tract, even only during certain stages of migration, may give rise to eosinophilia. Hydatid cyst fluid and extracts of some helminths may give rise to anaphylactic shock both in experimental animals and in human patients as long as they have been previously sensitized. In Chagas' myocarditis it has been postulated that an important factor in destruction of myocardial fibers is sensitization against partially demolished, parasitized myocardial fibers.[129] Experimental amebic abscess of the liver in guinea pigs can be produced only by intracecal injection of ameba in animals that have suffered previous intestinal amebiasis.[130] Many other instances

might be quoted in support of hypersensitivity as an important aggressive mechanism in animal parasites. In his excellent review, Hawking ends by saying,[124] ". . . the most serious disturbances usually arise from the host's own immunological reactions. Either the host becomes allergic to products of the parasite, or its parasiticidal antibodies kill off many parasites at one time and thus liberate innumerable distintegration products which excite the usual reactions to foreign proteins and similar substances. A potential host with ambition to survive should learn how not to admit parasites and how, if they gain entry, to get rid of them without disturbance."

5. Enzymatic. Recently, the presence of proteolytic enzymes in *E. histolytica*[131] has been shown beyond any reasonable doubt. Similar enzymes have been described in helminth larvae of schistosomes,[132] and oncospheres of taeniae.[133] These enzymes aid the parasite in invading and migrating within the host and play some role in their own protein digestion.

6. Others. Interference with protein nutrition of the host has been described in animals infected with *A. lumbricoides,* thus adding one more factor to the explanation of malnutrition in parasitized subjects.[134] In the same parasite, Oliver-González and Torregrosa isolated a substance similar to the human isoagglutinogen α-2, and suggested that anemia in patients parasitized by *Ascaris* might be due to agglutination of circulating red blood cells.[135]

D. PARASITIC ASSOCIATIONS

There is no doubt that the combined effects of two or more biologic agents of disease will bring about more severe complications than those due to each one in isolation, although some exceptions were noted when "interference" was discussed. Only one of the many instances of deleterious effect of parasitic association will be mentioned, which is the combined effect of bacteria and *E. histolytica*. Experimentally it has been shown that intracecal inoculation of virulent *E. histolytica* after complete sterilization of the intestine of guinea pigs will fail to produce any lesions, while inoculation of experimental animals with normal bacterial flora in the intestine will result in the typical lesions of amebiasis.[136]

IV. THE HOST-PARASITE RELATION

Penetration and establishment of the parasite within the host are complex phenomena in which many of the factors so far mentioned play a role. But once this relation is established the fate of both members, host and parasite, is ruled by the changing equilibrium between defensive mechanisms of the host, aggressive mechanisms of the parasite and all the factors influencing either or both. The resulting dynamic process is the host-parasite relation, an ever-changing (or potentially ever-changing) interaction which at any moment may shift in one direction, causing severe disease, or in the other, inducing complete disappearance of any abnormality. Equilibrium between the forces of host and parasite has been described as "a state of neutrality, although this neutrality may be of an armed nature with the likelihood of frontier incidents."[137]

A. TYPES OF HOST-PARASITE RELATION

According to the nature of the equilibrium between host and parasite several types of relation have been distinguished, of which only the following three will be mentioned because of their significance in pathology: infection, the status of the "healthy carrier" and disease. It should be recognized that these three relations differ only in degree, and that even such differences are more apparent than real. From a biologic standpoint, they represent different aspects of the same form of host-parasite relation, namely parasitism.

1. Infection. The presence of biologic pathogenic agents in the organism is known as infection. It matters little whether this presence is momentary, transitory or permanent; what is significant is that disease agents come in contact and remain, for whatever period of time, with a given subject. There are no fundamental differences between infection and infestation, except that the second term is more frequently used when the relation is established with animal parasites.

Not all infections are clinically manifest; the process is the same although host and parasite are capable of peaceful coexistence for variable periods. Frequently (although the exact, or even approximate, frequency is not known) pathogenic agents that come in contact with the organism are rapidly eliminated through the local and/or systemic defense mechanisms, and disease is averted. At other times, pathogenic bacteria such as staphylococci are found in high proportions in otherwise healthy subjects;[138] fungi like *Actinomyces bovis* are known to be present in the tonsils of normal people;[139] a break in local defense mechanisms, which for the first instance may be a fall in temperature and for the second a rupture in the continuity of the lining epithelium, may result in penetration within the organism of such pathogenic agents and the production of the clinical symptoms of disease.

Focal infections are very frequent and most probably they play a dominant role in diseases such as rheumatic fever, glomerulonephritis and bacterial endocarditis. In these instances, bacteria are lodged in the tonsils or in a dental caries, and either by sensitization of the organism, by a sudden invasion of the blood through a break in the epithelium or by other less well known mechanisms they are capable of initiating severe diseases as the ones mentioned.[140]

2. The "Healthy Carrier." The status of perfect equilibrium between host and parasite is known as the "healthy carrier." Quotation marks are used to indicate that the term refers to the clinical appearance of the host and not to the reality of the biologic phenomenon. Such a situation has important epidemiologic implications since through the continuous elimination of pathogenic agents the "healthy" subject may represent a serious danger for the community. An instance of this is the convalescing, or even the completely recovered, typhoid fever patient, who keeps *Salmonella typhi* in the gallbladder and is continuously eliminating this bacteria with the feces. Sometimes the "healthy carrier" is a transitory status, as in diphtheria, where microorganisms take longer to disappear than the clinical manifestations of the disease, but on some occasions the status may be permanent, as is possible in typhoid fever and some viral infections. Febrile herpes in childhood may disappear, but the patient becomes a permanent carrier of the virus, which becomes manifest whenever there is high fever due to any cause;[141] another instance is the high frequency with which *E. histolytica* is found in the stools of the population in Mexico, while only few subjects show any clinical manifestations of disease.[142]

The equilibrium between host and parasite may come to an end through different mechanisms which depend mainly on the nature of the parasite. Some instances were pointed out above, in reference to pneumococci and *A. bovis;* another clear case is that of *Bartonella muris,* which with few exceptions is found in many different strains of rats which otherwise appear completely healthy. Nevertheless, after splenectomy this parasite proliferates within the red blood cells and destroys them, producing a profound anemia which ends with the life of the rat in 4 to 6 days. In this case a defense mechanism of the host has been eliminated, although the exact mechanism of action is unknown. In other cases it is possible that the parasite may gain in virulence through the appearance of mutants with more potent aggressive mechanisms; the host-parasite equilibrium is broken and the "healthy carrier" becomes ill.

3. Disease. Infectious disease is that type of host-parasite relation where the equilibrium has been lost to the detriment of the host. It gives rise to two different types of manifestations: those related to disturbed defense mechanisms and metabolic changes in the host, which are nonspecific and occur in most or all infections, and those secondary to the effect of the aggressive mechanisms of the parasite, which are specific for the particular biologic agent of disease involved. Fever and leukocytosis appear in many infectious processes and although their pathogenesis is not clearly defined (see below) they may have some beneficial consequences for the host. On the other hand, the neurotoxic effect of tetanus toxin and the hemolytic effect of some toxins of *Cl. perfringens* depend on the specific activities of these two poisons. By the same token, anemia and eosinophilia in ancylostomiasis result from the despoliating and hypersensi-

tive effects of the parasite. In each particular case the etiologic agent will modify the picture of infectious disease, providing a profile which may serve the informed physician to establish a diagnosis and guide treatment.

B. ESTABLISHMENT

The conditions necessary for a parasite to leave its habitual reservoir, reach the potential host, pass through the body surface and become established within the organism, represent epidemiologic problems of great significance. When the biologic cycle of a given parasite is known, it becomes possible to break it at some point and thus eliminate the disease. Obviously, such conditions will vary according to almost every different pathogen, but some general concepts may still be reviewed under three separate headings: transmissibility or communicability factors, invasiveness or penetration through the body surface and means of dissemination, migration and localization within the organism of the host.

1. Transmissibility. With the exceptions of endogenous infections and food poisoning by botulinum or toxins of enteric pathogens, all parasites require to be carried from some reservoir or source of infection to the new host. Mechanisms are very variable and are not limited to pathogenic organisms. They permit a distinction between transmissible and contagious diseases, although such difference is more a matter of degree and incidental to the manner in which the germ will reach the host. A contagious disease is produced by parasites which pass directly from one person to another, for instance, Koch's bacillus in pulmonary tuberculosis. On the other hand, a transmissible disease is produced by a germ requiring special manipulations, usually through special vectors, in order to reach the new host; for instance, plasmodia in malaria. Without the mosquito the plasmodium has no means of reaching another victim; therefore, antimalaria campaigns have been directed against this intermediary vector. It is easy to understand that although not all infectious diseases are contagious all must be transmissible, since otherwise they would not exist.

Communicability depends on two types of factors, which are extrinsic and intrinsic.[143] Of these two, the former are better known while the latter are only vaguely understood. The most important extrinsic factors are as follows: (1) The first is an adequate reservoir, which is usually a patient and/or a place where bacteria survive more easily, exist in sufficient numbers and are able to leave readily. The upper respiratory tract is an adequate reservoir for pneumococci, the soil for spores of *B. anthracis,* the wall of the intestine for *E. histolytica,* etc. (2) The number of parasites is important, especially when transmission occurs from one animal species to another, since conditions of survival will vary and when there are few microorganisms the probability of development of adequate mutants is low. (3) The possibility of dissemination is another obvious extrinsic factor for communicability. McLeod and Pappenheimer[144] quoted plague in man as an instance. This disease occurs in two clinical forms called "bubonic" and "pneumonic," respectively. The bubonic form is spread from rats to man through the bite of the rat flea; buboes form near the bite of the flea and although there is widespread hematogenous dissemination no secondary cases occur since the infection is "closed." On the other hand, pneumonic plague is contagious to those in proximity to the sufferer who expels enormous numbers of plague bacilli during coughing and in discharges from the respiratory tract. (4) The vehicle used by the pathogenic agent to pass from a host or another reservoir to the new host is another fundamental factor in communicability. Transmission may occur through direct contact (contagion), through the placental circulation, through objects handled by a patient or fomites, through water, milk or food, through animal vectors or through the air. (5) Finally, germs should be capable of remaining on the surface of the organism as long as may be necessary before penetration is possible, and for this they need adequate countermeasures against local defense mechanisms or simple insusceptibility to them.

Intrinsic factors in communicability depend on the germs themselves and are related to their ability to survive outside the host's organism, which may be very great in some instances, as with *Cl. tetani,* or very small in others, as with streptococci. It has also been observed that, under certain circumstances, some strains of a given microorganism are more transmissible than others, without any apparent explanation, although such difference may occasionally be associated with other changes, as demonstrated by Schwentker, *et al.*[145]

2. Invasiveness. This is the ability of some parasites to overcome the local defense mechanisms of the host and penetrate beyond its external barriers. Most of the substances involved in this process have been discussed as aggressive mechanisms of parasites, but another interesting instance may be cited. Recently, Lewert and Lee[146] found that larvae or cercariae of *Schistosoma mansoni* and other skin-penetrating helminths produce proteolytic enzymes similar to collagenase from *Cl. perfringens.* If skin and subcutaneous tissues are considered as a mechanical barrier against infection, then these enzymes are clear examples of mechanisms of invasiveness of the parasites mentioned.

3. Dissemination, Migration and Localization. These phenomena occur with many parasites, sometimes with an exquisite degree of specificity, but the actual mechanisms ruling them are so obscure that perhaps the only thing that can be said is that they occur. In some instances dissemination appears to be passive, the parasites being carried away by blood or lymph, or else they fall into a serous cavity such as the meninges and are disseminated by the cerebrospinal fluid. Other parasites have a perfectly well defined cycle within the organism, as *Plasmodium vivax* or *S. mansoni,* hypothetically due to the presence of better conditions of survival in the involved areas of the organism. Still others manifest their effect only in certain organs or tissues, as the poliomyelitis virus or the hepatitis virus. To solve this problem by stating that such viruses are "neurotropic" and "hepatotropic" is to use circular language, which fails completely to explain the reasons for this peculiar organic preference.

C. FACTORS INFLUENCING THE HOST-PARASITE RELATION

At the risk of tiring repetition it is convenient to review some of the factors influencing the host-parasite relation, whatever the type and evolution of such relation may be. In the first place, the number of parasites is of great significance and on many occasions it will be the factor deciding the direction in which the equilibrium will be displaced, while in other instances a very small number of parasites suffices to cause a fatal disease. In the second place, the development of immunity after the first attack of infectious disease will on many occasions modify the host's response to a second infection, so that if immunity is absolute there will be no other disease although the parasite may reside in the host, or the disease will be much milder. On the other hand, immunity is frequently developed parallel to hypersensitivity, which may be responsible for many severe complications or different features which otherwise would not appear. An instance of the influence of previous contact with a causal agent is tuberculosis. During the first contact with tubercle bacilli the lesion heals in the vast majority of instances leaving a small calcified nodule in the lung and another one in the hilar or mediastinal lymph nodes. A second exposure to tubercle bacilli, when adequate in number of microorganisms and acting in a susceptible host, will produce the usual pulmonary disease with destructive caseous lesions, cavity formation and fibrous reaction. The difference between the host's reaction to the first, when compared to the second infection, is probably due in part to the development of hypersensitivity.[107]

The general conditions of the host, such as age, sex, nutritional status, physical fatigue, etc., have been mentioned as important in determining the effectiveness of defense mechanisms. Variations in virulence of different bacterial strains are also significant factors influencing the outcome of the host-parasite relation. Of no less significance is the effect of medical treatment, which is aimed at two fundamental goals: the blocking of toxic effects of parasites and their destruction, either directly or by facilitating the action of systemic defense mechanisms, and the improvement of the general conditions of the host, which in itself results in an increase in defense mechanisms.

The host-parasite relation is closer when parasitism is intracellular. The greatest obstacle in the analysis of physiologic factors participating in the host-parasite relation resides in the enormous complexity and variability of the environment *in vivo*. Thus, much is known of the composition and characteristics of the extracellular fluids of the body, and this knowledge has partly facilitated the study of extracellular infections. Unfortunately, the analysis of factors determining behavior and fate of microbial agents during their residence within the cells is much more difficult, perhaps because so little is known of the intracellular environment. Some isolated observations, however, may be mentioned to illustrate the peculiar nature of the intracellular relation of host and parasite. For instance, an intracellular microorganism is frequently found within a vacuole with a very acid pH, probably due to accumulation of lactic acid. Since many bacteria are highly susceptible to the toxic action of this acid, it is possible that this substance may bring about their destruction. Anoxia will reinforce the effect of lactic acid on microorganisms, and anoxia is the rule in the inflammatory focus (*see* Chapter II); in the center of the tuberculous granuloma the oxygen concentration is practically zero, and this modifies metabolism from aerobic to anaerobic, changing also intracellular biochemical conditions. These and many other aspects of the host-parasite relation are admirably discussed in Dubos' monograph.[95]

D. NONSPECIFIC REACTIONS OF THE HOST

The rupture of equilibrium between host and parasite often results in a series of different and apparently unconnected reactions of the host. Some may be quite specifically directed against the parasite, as antibody synthesis, while others are nonspecific and may also appear as response to many other stimuli such as trauma, burns, surgical operations, intense physical fatigue, psychologic tension, etc. In this section only those reactions commonly seen in infections are discussed, the remainder being more properly elaborated as part of the metabolic response to injury (*see* Chapter X). Here it may suffice to point out that all such reactions represent part of the protective or adaptive mechanisms which come into play after any type of stress and that result in maintenance of the constancy of the *milieu intérieur*. They are, therefore, homeostatic mechanisms working towards reintegration of physiologic equilibrium.

1. Fever. The elevation of the body temperature above normal limits resulting from disease is known as fever. The organism has delicate mechanisms which regulate its temperature within narrowly variable limits (36.0 to 40.0° C) depending on the site, age, sex and metabolic status of the subject.[147] These mechanisms were represented by DuBois[148] in his well-known scheme (Fig. 7–6). Heat is produced in the organism from the metabolism of carbohydrates, fat and proteins, and may increase through the specific dynamic action of foods, by disease, by elevation of the basal metabolic rate, by muscular exercise and by chills. On the other hand, heat is lost by increase in air movement, in radiation surface or in insensible loss of water by evaporation, by a low environmental temperature, by sweating, by an increase in skin circulation, etc.;

indeed, all factors increasing conduction, radiation and evaporation will be accompanied by heat loss. The equilibrium between heat production and loss is regulated by the central nervous system, more specifically by the hypothalamus.[149]

Other than the fever present in some cases of central nervous system lesion, the pathogenesis of the other types of fever is unknown. Menkin isolated a substance from exudates produced by injection of turpentine which, when injected into the experimental animal, will produce fever. This substance was named "pirexin."[50] Menkin's work has been criticized because of the possible presence of impurities in his preparations,[151] but more recent work and theories on the pathogenesis of fever are only variations of his "humoral" approach; the only differing point seems to be the source of the pyrogen.[152] It is well known that many bacteria possess substances capable of increasing the temperature of experimental animals

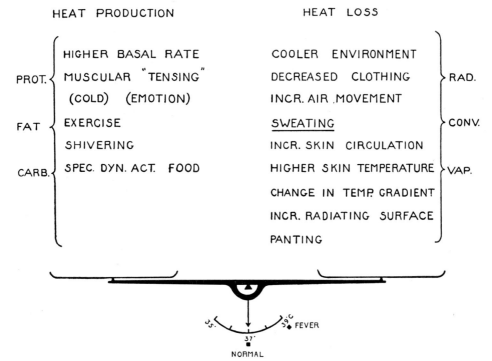

FIG. 7–6. Diagram showing the more important factors which increase heat production on the one hand and heat loss on the other. Those which increase heat production do so through an increased metabolism of protein, fat and carbohydrate in varying proportions. The factors which increase heat loss do so by increasing radiation, convection and vaporization. The diagram of the balance indicates that heat production and heat loss are almost always in equilibrium, so that a normal body temperature is maintained at an average of 37° C. (From Du Bois, E., The Mechanism of Heat Loss and Temperature Regulation. Stanford University Press.)

and man,[153] and some have been used therapeutically, as in the case of typhoid vaccine. Beeson isolated a pyrogenic substance from polymorphonuclear leukocytes,[154] and Atkins and Wood have shown that immediately before elevation of temperature in experimental animals given intravenous typhoid vaccine there is leukopenia.[155] Bennett, *et al*[156] showed that the formation of endogenous pyrogen, following the injection of bacterial endotoxin, is markedly depressed in animals previously made leukopenic with nitrogen mustard. In view of these and other findings, Wood[157] has postulated the following mechanism for endotoxin induced fever:

Injected pyrogen→ (exogenous)	Injury of cells→ (leukocytes)	Release of endogenous→ pyrogen	Stimulation of thermoregulatory→ centers in brain	Fever

An important reason to believe that a "humoral" pathogenesis of fever is likely to be true is that fever appears almost always when there is tissue destruction; according to such a hypothesis, dying cells would release substances which would act in the hypothalamus, setting the regulation of temperature at a higher level. When there is no tissue destruction fever may be ascribed to some disturbance in heat production, as in hyperthyroidism or the administration of dinitrophenol, where there is increased metabolism,[158] or in sunstroke, heart failure or gastrointestinal hemorrhages, where there is decreased heat loss.

Fever is accompanied by important physiologic changes in the organism, especially in the respiratory and circulatory systems. There is hyperventilation, due perhaps to influence of the thermoregulator center on the pneumotaxic center in the hypothalamus, and the result may be alkalosis. In the circulation there is peripheral vasodilation, hypotension and tachycardia.[159] It has been mentioned that fever inhibits the "autodisinfection" mechanism of the intestine and also favors the appearance of herpes in subjects with previous histories of similar attacks. On the other hand, fever has been considered as beneficial to the organism, although this contention has never been substantiated. That fever therapy is of help in the treatment of gonorrhea and neurosyphilis is established beyond reasonable doubt, but here it is no more a defense mechanism than the administration of penicillin in pneumococcal pneumonia. Many studies are reviewed in Bennet and Nicastri's recent paper on fever as a mechanism of resistance,[160] and the conclusion reached by these authors is that there is no evidence in favor of the two possible ways in which fever might serve as a defense mechanism, namely by direct thermal effects upon microorganisms and their products, or by increasing one or more of the various humoral and cellular mechanisms that are responsible for resistance to infection.

2. Leukocytosis and Leukopenia. Although infections may produce leukocytosis and leukopenia, there are many other conditions that share this ability, such as physical exercise, convulsions, pain, hemorrhage, and the effect of many drugs and toxic substances. Sometimes it is possible to distinguish these forms of leukocytosis and leukopenia by the absence of immature elements in the circulating blood, since most of them are due to a redistribution of mature leukocytes which are normally stored in different organs, caused by adrenaline.[161] Changes in white blood cells encountered in different infectious diseases vary widely and possibly cannot be explained on the basis of a single mechanism.[162] There may be elevation of polymorphonuclear neutrophilic leukocytes, lymphocytes, monocytes, eosinophiles, isolated or in all possible combinations. Furthermore, the peripheral count of white blood cells varies not only in different patients, but also in the same patient in different days. Menkin[163] isolated from exudates produced in the pleural cavity of dogs by injection of turpentine two substances of protein nature which he called "leukocytosis promoting factor" and "leukopenic factors," and postulated that they would act directly on the bone marrow, the first one stimulating and the other inhibiting it. Although these studies indicate in a general way the probable mechanisms of production of leukocytosis and leukopenia in the particular instance of turpentine-induced abscesses, they are quite far from being an acceptable explanation of all the other types of changes in the white cell blood count in infection or in other situations; for instance, Polak and Némec believe that the ACTH-induced leukocytosis is due to increased mobility of leukocytes.[164]

The most commonly observed change is an elevation in the total number of leukocytes with neutrophilia, which appears to be influenced by at least three factors, namely the infectious agent, the extent of tissue damage and the virulence of the microorganism. Almost all the so-called pyogenic organisms produce leukocytosis with neutrophilia: streptococcus, staphylococcus, gonococcus, pneumococcus, meningococcus, etc.; the same response is present with infections produced by some fungi as actinomycetes, parasites like *E. histolytica* (especially in the so-called amebic hepatitis) and viruses as in poliomyelitis, rabies and cowpox. The extent of tissue damage is of great significance since in small and superficial infections the elevation in circulating leukocytes will be slight or nonexistent, while large lesions with abundant pus show high leukocytosis and neutrophilia. Peripheral white blood cell counts are also dependent on the virulence of the causal agent. In other types of infections the elements increasing are mainly lymphocytes, and this is clearly seen in typhoid fever, tuberculosis and infectious mononucleosis; in this last instance there is not only an increase in circulating lymphocytes, but also some of them show characteristic nuclear changes which are qualified as "atypical" and suggest the diagnosis.[165] Some viral diseases may also show lymphocytosis, as whooping cough and lymphocytic choriomeningitis. Leukopenia is a bad omen, especially in the course of massive infections by highly virulent microorganisms, since it indicates an inability of the organism to mobilize its systemic defenses; in other instances such as typhoid fever, influenza and measles, leukopenia is only part of the usual clinical picture.

Eosinophilia, which frequently occurs in infections produced by animal parasites, has been associated with the development of hypersensitivity, but neither the mechanism nor the significance in defense of this phenomenon is known.

3. Acceleration of Sedimentation Rate.

The observation that normal blood placed in a receptacle undergoes uniform coagulation, while that obtained from a subject with an infectious disease shows distinct sedimentation of four different layers, is as old as history; in fact, it served as a basis for a classification of "humors" affected in different diseases. This differential layering is due to the sedimentation of red blood cells in plasma, which is determined by the density of the latter.[166] Since the resistance caused by viscosity of the plasma is proportional to the radius of particles (assuming that they were spherical) while the weight of red blood cells is proportional to the cube of their radius, any increase in the size of sedimenting particles will be accompanied by an increase in the speed of displacement. The usual mechanism of increase in size of red blood cells is the formation of rouleaux. Nevertheless, rouleaux formation is explained by modifications in plasma, since red blood cells with increased sedimentation rate have a normal speed of displacement when they are placed in the plasma of a normal subject.[167] Modifications related to increased sedimentation rate are found in the plasma proteins, especially in the concentration of alpha and gamma globulins, which is proportional to the viscosity of plasma. Therefore, measurements of plasma viscosity or density are equivalent to determinations of red blood cell sedimentation rates.[168]

Normal figures for sedimentation rate are 0 to 15 mm. per hour (Wintrobe). Accelerations occur when there is tissue destruction and increased fibrinogen and plasma globulins; therefore, all infections causing tissue necrosis will show acceleration of the sedimentation rate. This simple clinical test is very useful for determining the presence and activity of infectious diseases, or of any other type of ailment that fails to give other clinical manifestations. On the other hand, the test is entirely nonspecific and is commonly used to study the evolution of known diseases, such as rheumatic fever or tuberculosis. It may even be positive in normal conditions such as pregnancy, for which incidentally it was first popularized as a clinical test by Fahraeus.[169]

4. Fibrinolysis. In 1903 Morawitz[170]

demonstrated that the blood of some cadavers that remained fluid for a long time contained an agent capable of dissolving fibrin, and this agent was later identified as an enzyme and baptized fibrinolysin. In 1937, McFarlane observed that fibrinolysis was not limited to the blood of cadavers but that it also occurred in recently operated subjects, although it appeared to be better related to the nervous tension associated with surgery.[171] The same phenomenon, but much more intense and dramatic, is known as "acute fibrinolysis" and has become a well known, although fortunately rare, cause of operative or postoperative death.[172] The plasma contains a precursor of the fibrinolytic enzyme called profibrinolysin which may be activated by streptokinase. It is of interest in this section because streptokinase may be produced by certain bacteria such as streptococci and pneumonococci, which are therefore capable of activating the system. Fibrinolysis is usually discrete in infections, and it may even prevent the formation of thrombi in areas of injury or the formation of further thrombi beyond such areas of tissue destruction.

V. CHEMOTHERAPY*

Early in the nineteenth century several chemical compounds were used in the treatment of various infectious diseases, such as quinine in malaria or emetine in amebiasis. Nevertheless, the science of chemotherapy begins with Paul Ehrlich, who envisaged the idea that certain substances could exist that would attack microorganisms without damaging the host's tissues. This was the first mention of selective toxicity, one of the basic principles of modern chemotherapy. Ehrlich's experiments led to the discovery of arsphenamine, the first success of rational chemotherapy. The development of sulfonamides by Domagk marks a new era in the rapid development of chemotherapy, and the finding of the therapeutic effect of penicillin led many research workers to look for antimicrobial substances produced by mi-

* This section was contributed by Luis F. Bojalil, Q.B.P.

croorganisms and even higher plants. Such agents are known as antibiotics.[173]

A. DEFINITION

The word "chemotherapy" literally means the treatment of disease with chemical agents. The acceptance of such wide meaning would force the inclusion of a very large number of compounds in therapy, and the classification as chemotherapeutic agents of substances such as sodium bicarbonate or aspirin, and also vitamins, hormones, antitoxins, antisera, etc. Therefore, the term should be used according to Ehrlich's original idea, "the treatment of infectious diseases with chemical agents." Substances acting through stimulation of the host's defense mechanisms, either directly (antisera, enzymes) or indirectly (vitamins, hormones), are also outside the realm of chemotherapeutic agents.

B. SELECTIVE TOXICITY

Selective toxicity is one of the fundamental conditions for a substance to be considered as a chemotherapeutic agent. This simply means that such a compound should have a lethal or inhibitory effect on pathogenic agents without damaging the host's tissues, at least in therapeutic doses. Antiseptic or disinfecting agents may be highly active against microorganisms *in vitro,* but their high toxicity for tissues prevents their inclusion in the group of compounds with selective activity. Accordingly, not all antibiotics are chemotherapeutic agents; many cannot be used because of their toxic effects on the host.[174]

Antiseptic substances are general protoplasmic poisons, which would serve to explain their lack of selective activity; on the other hand, it is not at all clear why some compounds considered as chemotherapeutic agents fail to injure the host's tissues, when their effect on a given parasite involves the blocking or inhibition of an enzyme present also in the host's cells.[175]

In general, it may be accepted that some chemotherapeutic substances are bacteriostatic while others are bactericidal; however, there is no sharp division, since by varying the conditions of observation the same substance may inhibit bacterial multiplication in one case and kill the microorganisms in another. Bacteriostatic agents stop bacterial growth, so that the number of viable microorganisms remains constant for hours and even days; later, the number of bacteria decreases, an observation attributed to autolysis. The bacteriostatic effect is lost if the culture is diluted beyond the effective concentration of the drug, in which case bacterial reproduction is reassumed. Bactericidal agents exert an irreversible effect, since microorganisms fail to multiply when they are removed from the presence of effective concentrations of the drug. Nevertheless, the separation of chemotherapeutic agents into bacteriostatic and bactericidal is arbitrary, considering that it depends more on quantitative than on qualitative factors. The same holds for substances active against fungi (fungistatic and fungicidal agents) and other microorganisms.

C. MECHANISM OF ACTION

Much work has been done on the mechanism of action of chemotherapeutic agents, especially on those used more frequently in medical practice. Although the results are encouraging and a vast amount of information is being accumulated, it is not easy to decide which is the primary locus of action of each of the substances so far analyzed in different organisms. The difficulties seem to stem from two main sources. In the first place, the inhibition of growth of a susceptible microorganism by a given substance is accompanied by the blocking of many metabolic reactions, while others continue to be active. One important problem is to find precisely which of the involved metabolic pathways is directly responsible for the inhibition of growth, and once this is established, which are the links between such metabolic pathways and the others similarly injured. In the second place, most studies on the mechanism of action of chemotherapeutic agents have been carried out *in vitro,* and although it is quite possible that the same conditions are operating *in vivo,* it is equally possible that some factors in the host are influencing the activity of the drugs on microorganisms. With these two limitations in mind, some instances of the mechanisms by which chemical substances inhibit bacterial growth or kill microorganisms will be examined.

1. Antimetabolites. In 1940, Woods[176] observed that the bacteriostatic effect of sulfonamides was completely and competitively reverted by p-aminobenzoic acid. It was then suggested that the bacteriostatic effect of sulfonamides was due to their ability to create in the bacterial cell a deficiency of an essential metabolite, p-aminobenzoic acid, which was necessary for multiplication. Such action is attributed to the structural similarity between metabolite (p-aminobenzoic acid) and antimetabolite (sulfonamides).

Most antimetabolites, including perhaps some antibiotics such as chloromycetin and cycloserin, have a low molecular weight and relatively simple structural formulas, when compared with most other antibiotics, which have high molecular weights and act in ways other than metabolic competition. The antibiotic effect of some groups of compounds with structures similar to amino acids, purines and pyrimidines, and with antimetabolite activity, has not been fully explored. Such antimetabolites may replace several substances during the synthesis of nucleic acids and proteins, thus rendering the final product useless for metabolic activity within bacterial cells. For instance, the growth curve of *E. coli* grown in an adequate medium containing p-fluorophenylalanine is linear arithmetic and not linear exponential. In this case, p-fluorophenylalanine is incorporated in the protein instead of phenylalanine and tyrosine, with the consequent accumulation of these two amino acids in the medium; at the same time, the capacity of *E. coli* to synthesize protein (β-galactosidase) is considerably decreased.[177] It seems quite likely that some analogs of purines and pyrimidines used as antitumor agents, such as thioguanine and the antivirus thiouracil agent, follow, at least in part, a similar mechanism of action. Indeed, it has been shown that 5-fluorouracil, a promising antitumor substance, is exclusively incorporated within the ribonucleic acid of tumor cells,[178] and that 8-azoguanine, an effective antivirus compound, becomes a part of nucleic acid of tobacco mosaic virus.[179]

2. Permeability Factors. Although it was first believed that chemotherapeutic agents, and especially antimetabolites, should be designed to block metabolic reactions peculiar to parasites, some recent information suggests that such a condition need not be fulfilled. In some instances the antibiotic may not penetrate through the cell membrane of the parasite in order to exert its lytic action. A very clear case in point is that of polymyxins, which show a definite effect on the cytoplasmic membrane of parasites.[180] In other cases, the chemotherapeutic agent penetrates through the membrane of both parasite and host cells, but the effect is manifested only in the parasite; it has been shown by means of tissue cultures that penicillin G penetrates cells of mammals.[181] Therefore, it is permissible to suppose that the low toxicity of this antibiotic for man is due to the lack of reactive sites in human cells which are present in microorganisms, and not to permeability factors, as was believed at one time. Such supposition is supported by the finding that penicillin inhibits the synthesis of a polyphosphoglycerol compound which is present only in the cell wall of susceptible bacteria.[182] Penicillin has also been found to inhibit the synthesis of the cell wall, with the consequent accumulation of uridine pyrophosphate, hexosamine-amino acid complexes.[183] Permeability differences between host and parasite are of great significance since failure to penetrate within the host's cells will make the antibiotic effective only against extracellular bacteria. For this reason, intracellular brucella[184] and tubercle bacilli[185] are not reached by streptomycin.

3. Other Effects on the Parasite's Metabolism. In addition to the possible modes of action of chemotherapeutic agents discussed above, there are others that deserve brief mention. A large number of antimicrobial compounds are capable of reacting with thiol (SH) groups, which are abundant in biologic systems; this may be the explanation of the antitrypanosomal activity of arsenic derivatives. Chloromycetin seems to inhibit protein synthesis in susceptible bacteria, whereas such an effect is absent in most yeasts and protozoons, as well as in the cells of mammals.[186] It is well known that piperazine (diethylenediamine), used against ascariasis and oxyuriasis, will block the action of acetylcholine, which is related to the muscular activity of worms. Although paralysis of those parasites is surely followed by their death, piperazine may also interfere with other vital processes.[187]

D. RESISTANCE

Resistance is a general biologic phenomenon which may appear when any microorganism comes in contact with chemotherapeutic agents for a more or less prolonged period. Bacterial resistance tends to appear in patients treated with antibiotics when therapy fails to eliminate the infecting microorganisms rapidly. Once the parasite is drug-resistant it may retain this character for an indefinite time.[188]

1. Mechanisms of Drug-Resistance. Several theories have been advanced to explain the emergence of bacterial resistance, three of which are discussed in the following paragraphs.

a. Mutation. Bacterial populations contain some microorganisms (mutants) which are less sensitive to drugs than the remainder of the population, so that when the entire group comes in contact with the antimicrobial agent sensitive members are eliminated while resistant microorganisms survive and continue multiplying.[189] Resistant mutants appear spontaneously, so that the effect of the drug is simply to select them from sensitive bacteria.[190, 191]

b. Adaptation. This theory postulates that the drug is not only a selecting agent but also stimulates the development of resistance in the entire bacterial population.[192, 193] Probably, adaptation contributes less than mutation to the emergence of resistance.[194]

c. Recombination. It has been shown that the genetic material of one microorganism may be transferred to another; thus, the receptor cell acquires new properties. This interesting phenomenon has been observed in *E. coli* and other microorganisms.[195, 196] Through this mechanism drug-resistance may be transmitted from one bacterial strain to another, as has been done with penicillin- or sulfonamide-resistance between different strains of pneumococci,[197,198] and with streptomycin-resistance between different strains of *E. coli*. Therefore, the possibility exists that by recombination of genetic material the character of drug-resistance might be communicated to infecting microorganisms, but this possibility has yet to be documented.

2. Crossed Resistance. The emergence of bacterial resistance to a given drug may be accompanied by resistance to other chemotherapeutic agents, especially those with similar chemical structures. For instance, bacterial strains resistant to oxytetracyclines are usually also resistant to chlortetracycline and other tetracyclines.[199] Another instance occurs with streptomycin and dihydrostreptomycin.

3. Methods of Avoiding the Appearance of Bacterial-Resistance. *a. Combined Chemotherapy.* The use of combinations of drugs which prevents crossed resistance will delay the emergence of resistant strains of microorganisms. Such is the case with the simultaneous use of dihydrostreptomycin and p-aminosalicylic acid in the treatment of tuberculosis.[200] On the other hand, it is not always easy to select an adequate combination of antibiotics, especially since the nature of the antimicrobial effect varies with different combinations of drugs and with the specific microorganism. In the following scheme appear some of the most useful combinations.

GROUP I	GROUP II
Penicillin	Tetracyclines
Streptomycin	Chloramphenicol
Bacitracin	Erythromycin
Neomycin	Sulfonamides
Polymixin B	

Combinations among components of Group I are frequently synergistic or indifferent, but never antagonistic; combinations of Group II may have additive or indifferent effects, but they never oppose each other. Combinations between members of Groups I and II vary in their activity; when microorganisms are very sensitive to agents in Group I, there may be antagonism, while when bacteria are relatively resistant the rule is to observe additive effects.

b. Rapid Elimination. The rapid elimination of sensitive bacteria can only be obtained by maintaining a high concentration of the antibiotic wherever microorganisms are found in the body. In practice, however, this is rarely possible since doses required to reach high levels of the drug throughout the organism will cause toxic damage to the host.

4. Clinical and Epidemiologic Significance of Resistance. The problem of bacterial resistance and chemotherapy has been reviewed by several authors.[203, 204] From Finland's excellent survey[205] it may be concluded that the emergence of drug resistance in staphylococci and *Mycobacterium* represents one of the most important problems in medicine today. In other bacteria, the frequency of appearance of drug resistance *in vivo* is much lower. Among group A hemolytic streptococci it is rare to find strains resistant to any of the antibiotics used in treatment, and the same is true of meningococci and most strains of *Streptococcus viridans.* Many strains of gonococcus are resistant to sulfonamides, but it is difficult to encounter one strain resistant to penicillin or other antibiotics.

The emergence of drug-resistant strains is met more frequently during the treatment of chronic infections, of which tuberculosis is the most formidable instance. In tuberculosis resistant strains appear after 3 to 4 weeks of treatment with any of the antituberculous drugs in use (streptomycin, isoniazid, or para-aminosalicylic acid).[206, 209] Combined therapy, on the other hand, greatly diminishes the speed of development of bacterial resistance.[210] Some cases have been reported of bacterial endocarditis with isolation of penicillin-resistant strains of *Streptococcus,*[211, 212] and there may also occur a rapid increase of resistance to streptomycin in urinary tract infections due to coliform germs, or in meningitis caused by *H. influenzae.*[213] In general, it appears that streptomycin is the antibiotic responsible for more cases of resistance in the host's tissue.[205] Garrod[212] observed increased resistance to penicillin in a case of actinomycosis caused by *A. bovis* and believed it due more to habituation than to substitution; in mycetomas caused by *Nocardia,* increased resistance has been noticed after treatment with diamino-diphenyl-sulphone,[214, 215, 216] but the reason for this is not known.

5. Rupture of Biologic Equilibrium. A different category of resistant microorganisms is that replacing the original bacterial population during the course of treatment. It is not rare to observe that after a patient has responded well to treatment of an infectious disease there may be a recurrence of signs and symptoms of the disease; this phenomenon is usually attributed to elimination of the causal agent by the drug or drugs used and its replacement by another, resistant microorganism. Replacing bacteria are usually *Staphylococcus, Proteus, Pseudomonas, Escherichia* and several types of yeasts. For instance, instead of penicillin-resistant *Streptococcus pyogenes,* which used to be quite common in wounds and abscesses, nowadays it is more frequent to find naturally resistant germs such as *Proteus* and *Pseudomonas.*[217, 218] The appearance of *Monilia* (*Candida*) is more common in the body cavities of subjects treated with wide spectrum antibiotics such as the tetracyclines[219, 220, 221] than with other types of antibiotics.[222] Such organisms may be responsible for hospital infections, which are discussed below.

a. Infection by Staphylococcus. It has been observed that staphylococci isolated from hospital personnel (physicians, nurses, students and even patients) tend to be more and more resistant to penicillin.[223] Suppression of sensitive staphylococci and their replacement by resistant mutants has been suggested as an explanation of this finding, mainly because of the almost unlimited use of antibiotics in these institutions. Needham and Nichols[224] isolated 60 per cent of penicillin-resistant strains at the Mayo Clinic; Finland and Wilcox[225] obtained 85 per cent in one of Boston's hospitals and the situation in Mexico is not much different.[226, 227] Resistance of these bacteria to other chemotherapeutic agents is also high. Several hospital epidemics of staphylococcal infections in newborns have been reported; surely these children could have been infected with staphylococci derived from the respiratory tract or hands of other persons (physicians, nurses, patients).

Another important complication of staphylococcal infections is the so-called pseudomembranous enterocolitis, which has been associated with the use of tetracyclines. It seems that the intestinal bacterial flora is rapidly replaced by staphylococci, so that pure cultures of this germ can be obtained from the feces of such patients. It has been suggested[228] that staphylococci may damage the intestinal mucosa with locally produced enterotoxins, or that vascular lesions are the main pathogenetic factor. The latter opinion is of interest since it points out the possibility that staphylococci may be only one of various causes leading to pseudomembranous enterocolitis.[229]

b. Persistence. In many infectious processes, and especially in those of chronic course such as tuberculosis, it is extremely difficult to eliminate all infecting microorganisms by treatment. During the course of therapy many bacteria persist within the host despite their continued sensitivity to chemotherapeutic agents. Such persistence can be attributed to the low metabolic activity developed by some microorganisms when faced with antimicrobial drugs.[230] It has been established that many antibiotics are more effective when acting on actively multiplying bacteria; for instance, isoniazid is almost without effect on resting tubercle bacilli.[231] Persistence may be so prominent that even in experimental animals inoculated with tubercle bacilli and treated for prolonged periods it is difficult to avoid relapses after withdrawal of the antimicrobial drug. Sometimes this occurs immediately after discontinuation of treatment, although the infective agent could not be recovered during the period of treatment.[232]

Persistent bacteria may play a very important role in several chronic infectious diseases such as pyelonephritis, osteomyelitis or bacterial endocarditis, in which the drug may act exclusively as a transitory depressor, but not as a radical bactericidal agent. Modern chemotherapy is unable to cope with persistent germs once they gain that status, but their development may be avoided in many cases by the judicious use of various combinations of drugs.[233]

c. Dependence. Certain microorganisms not only become resistant to antibiotics, but may even use the drug for their multiplication. Emerson and Cushing[234] described a strain of *Neurospora* which could grow better in the presence of sulfanilamide than in its absence, and Miller and Bonhoff[235] isolated some strains of streptomycin-dependent meningococci. Dependence on antibiotics has been described in tubercle bacilli,[236] in *Cryptococcus neoformans,* in *Sporotrichum schenckii,*[237, 238] and in several other microorganisms. Obviously, in this curious situation treatment will not only fail to improve the condition of the patient, but may even lead to severe consequences.

E. CONTROL OF CHEMOTHERAPY IN THE LABORATORY

1. Sensitivity Tests. The value of testing the sensitivity of a given bacterial strain to several antibiotics *in vitro* should rest on the degree of correlation between results obtained in the laboratory and the patient's response to the treatment. It seems that *in vitro* sensitivity tests not only permit prediction of the outcome of infections when treated with different antibiotics, but may also give an idea of the most adequate doses of the preferred chemotherapeutic agent. Nevertheless, objective data in this respect are relatively scarce, although the degree of correlation in those available is quite high.[239] There is no dearth of discrepancies, however, between laboratory tests and clinical results; clinical improvement may follow the use of a given antibiotic despite the isolation of resistant bacteria, as is not infrequently the case with patients infected by penicillin-resistant *Staphylococcus aureus* and treated with penicillin. In this instance, however, the existence of penicillinase produced by the resistant microorganism makes the results of the *in vitro* test strongly dependent on the size of the inoculum used in testing.

In tuberculosis there may also be clinical and radiological improvement despite the isolation of resistant strains of tubercle bacilli in the laboratory. This paradox may be explained by the fact that tuberculosis is usually earmarked by multiple lesions, and the bacilli recovered from the sputum may be representative of one lesion caused by resistant bacteria while other lesions contain sensitive microorganisms; thus, the antibiotics would act on those areas with a sensitive population, giving rise to beneficial results for the patient.[240, 241]

2. Repeated Examinations. The need for repeated and careful microbiologic studies in cases of infectious diseases follows from the preceding discussion. Such studies will indicate if treatment is adequate or not, and the emergence of resistant strains that may force a change in the type of antibiotic used.

F. THE HOST-PARASITE RELATION

Chemotherapeutic agents may possess a strong antimicrobial activity *in vitro,* and yet fail to eliminate infection even with prolonged treatments. This fact indicates the existence within the host of a series of factors which affect the antibacterial activity of drugs in a profound manner. Starting from the very moment antibiotics are administered to the time they reach the site of the lesion they undergo a series of changes which decrease their antibacterial activity, so that their actual effect is only a fraction of what could be expected considering the dose administered. There are several possible causes for this phenomenon:[95, 242] (a) Many substances are partially or totally inactivated; thus, the pH of gastric secretions will inactivate penicillin when this drug is given *per os.* (b) Intramuscular injection is followed by precipitation of several antibiotics *in situ,* thus hindering their reabsorption. (c) Once antibiotics reach the circulation they are exposed to many different physiologic processes that may modify their structure and eliminate their activity; a case in point is acetylation of sulfonamides in the liver, which causes a considerable decrease in the antibacterial effect of the drug. (d) Other drugs are adsorbed to the serum proteins, especially albumins. This appears to be one of the most important mechanisms of loss of chemotherapeutic effect.[243] (e) Many antibiotics are unable to penetrate the cell membrane of phagocytes, and some that do penetrate are inactivated in the intracellular medium, limiting their usefulness to extracellular bacteria. For instance, streptomycin cannot pass through cell membranes, while isoniazid, penicillin and cycloserine will do it freely. (f) Tissue injury produced by bacteria is accompanied by radical changes in the physiologic and biochemical conditions of the local area, and these modifications will have a decisive influence on the activity of chemotherapeutic agents. For instance, streptomycin and penicillin show a marked decrease in activity in acid pH, which prevails in many inflammatory foci; ketoacids and pyridoxal, released from necrotic tissues, antagonize the effect of streptomycin and isoniazid, respectively. (g) Finally, metabolites released during inflammation may act as bacteriostatic agents, inhibiting bacterial growth and leaving without effect those antimicrobial agents active against multiplying bacteria.

REFERENCES

1. Smith, T.: Parasitism and Disease, Princeton, Princeton University Press, 1934.
2. Bassi, A.: Del Mal del Segmo, Calcinaccio o Moscardino, Malattia che Affligge i Bachi da Sota, e sur Modo di Liberarne le Bigattaje Anche le Piu Infestante, ed. 2, Milán, Paolo Andrea Molina, 1837.
3. Harant, H., and Théodorides, J.: Un pionnier de la parasitologie et un precurseur des doctrines pastoriennes, Agostino Bassi (1773–1856), Montpellier méd. 3:393, 1956.
4. King, L. S.: Dr. Koch's postulates, J. Hist. Med. & Allied Sc. 7:350, 1952.
5. Fildes, P., and McIntosh, J.: The etiology of influenza, Brit. J. Exper. Path. 1:119, 159, 1920.
6. Wilson, G. S., and Miles, A. A.: Topley and Wilson's Principles of Bacteriology and Immunity, ed. 5, Baltimore, Williams and Wilkins, 1946.
7. Ruiz Reyes, F.: Estado actual de las lesiones oculares oncocercosas, Medicina, México 37:573, 1957.
8. Nungester, W. J.: Nonspecific factors in immunity, Ann. Rev. Microbiol. 8:363, 1954.
9. Gladstone, G. P.: Pathogenicity and Virulence of Microorganisms. II. Communicability, in Florey, H. W. (ed.): General Pathology, Philadelphia, W. B. Saunders, 1958.
10. Pillsbury, D. M., and Kligman, A. M.: Some Current Problems in Cutaneous Bacteriology, in MacKenna, R. M. B. (ed.): Modern Trends in Dermatology, ed. 2, London, Butterworth, 1954.
11. Burtenshaw, J. M. L.: The Autogenous Disinfection of the Skin, in MacKenna, R. M. B. (ed.): Modern Trends in Dermatology, New York, Hoeber, 1948.
12. Arnold, L., Gustafson, C. J., Hull, T. G., Montgomery, B. E., and Singer, C.: The self-disinfecting power of the skin as a defense against microbic invasion, Am. J. Hyg. 11:345, 1930.
13. Hellat, A.: Studies on the self-disinfecting powers of the skin, Ann. med. exper. et biol. Fenniae 26 (Suppl. 8), 1948.
14. Marchionini, A., Schmidt, R., and Kiefer, J.: Säuremantel der Haut und Bacterien-Abwehr. II Mitteilung. Ueber die regionäre Verschiedenheit der Bakterien-abwehr und Desinfektionskraft der Hautoberfläche, Klin. Wchnschr. 17: 736, 1938.
15. Ricketts, C. R., Squire, J. R., and Topley, E.: Human skin lipids with particular reference to self-sterilizing power of skin, Clin. Sc. 10:89, 1951.
16. Thompson, R.: Lysozyme and the antibacterial properties of tears, Arch. Ophth. 25:491, 1941.
17. Salton, M. R. J.: The properties of lysozyme and its action on microorganisms, Bact. Rev. 21:82, 1957.
18. Van den Ende, M., Lush, D., and Edward, D. G.: Reduction of dust-borne bacteria by treating floors, Lancet 2:133, 1940.
19. Nungester, W. J., Wolf, A. A., and Jourdonais, L. F.: Consideration of the respiratory pattern as a predisposing factor in the etiology of pneumonia, J. Infect. Dis. 71:57, 1942.
20. Proetz, A. W.: Applied Physiology of the Nose, Philadelphia, W. B. Saunders, 1940.
21. Lucas, A. M., and Douglas, L. C.: Principles underlying ciliary activity in the respiratory tract, Arch. Otolaryng. 20:518, 1934.
22. Proetz, A. W.: Recent progress in nasal physiology, Proc. Roy. Soc. Med. 41:793, 1948.
23. Thompson, R.: Lysozyme and its relation to the antibacterial properties of various tissues and secretions, Arch. Path. 30:1096, 1940.
24. Francis, T., Jr., and Brightman, I. J.: Virus-inactivating capacity of nasal secretions in the acute and convalescent stages of influenza, Proc. Soc. Exper. Biol. & Med. 48:116, 1941.
25. Adrenies, C. H., Isoaes, A., and Marmion, B. P.: Neutralizing action of human nasal secretions on neurotropic influenza virus, Brit. J. Exper. Path. 35:264, 1954.
26. Cralley, L. J.: Factors affecting retention and rate of removal of bacteria from the tracheal tree and lungs, Am. J. Hyg. 36:303, 1943.
27. Hill, L.: The ciliary movement of the trachea studied in vitro. A measure of toxicity, Lancet 2:802, 1928.
28. Robertson, O. H.: Phagocytosis of foreign material in the lung, Physiol. Rev. 21:112, 1941.
29. Payling-Wright, G.: An Introduction to Pathology, ed. 2, London, Longmans and Green, 1958.
30. Schirger, A., Martin, W. J., Royer, R. Q., and Needham, G. M.: Bacterial invasion of blood after oral surgical procedures, J. Lab. & Clin. Med. 55:376, 1960.
31. Hobson, F. G., and Juel-Jensen, B. E.: Teeth, Streptococcus viridans, and subacute bacterial endocarditis, Brit. Med. J. 2:1501, 1956.
32. Dold, H.: Die Inhibition (Keimvermehrungshemmung) als Abwehrmittel die normalen Schleimhaut gegen Infektion, Ztschr. Hyg. 124:597, 1943.
33. Bloomfield, A. L.: The dissemination of bacteria in the upper air passages. I. The circulation of foreign particles in the mouth, Am. Rev. Tuberc. 5:903, 1922.
34. Bloomfield, A. L.: The dissemination of bacteria in the upper air passages. II. The circulation of bacteria in the mouth, Bull. Johns Hopkins Hosp. 33:145, 1922.
35. Simmons, N. S.: Studies on the defense mechanisms of the mucous membranes, with particular reference to the oral cavity, Oral Surg. 5:513, 1952.
36. Garrod, L. P.: The susceptibility of different bacteria to destruction in the stomach, J. Path. & Bact. 45:473, 1937.
37. Arnold, L.: Alterations in the endogenous enteric bacterial flora and microbic permeability of the intestinal wall in relation to the nutritional and meteorological changes, J. Hyg. 29:82, 1929.
38. Florey, H.: Mucin and the protection of the body, Proc. Roy. Soc. London s.B 143:147, 1955.
39. Brown, W. E.: Treatment of gonorrheal vulvovaginitis with estrogens, Am. J. Dis. Child. 64: 221, 1942.
40. Hirsch, J. G.: Immunity to infectious disease. Review of some concepts of Metchnikoff, Bact. Rev. 23:48, 1959.
41. Gladstone, G. P., and Abraham, E. P.: Acquired Immunity: the Serological Reactions of Bacteria, in Florey, H. (ed.): General Pathology, ed. 2, Philadelphia, W. B. Saunders, 1958.
42. Raffel, S.: Immunity. Hypersensitivity. Serology, New York, Appleton Century Crofts, 1953.
43. Nuttall, G.: Experiments üeber die bacterienfeindlichen Einflüsse des thierischen Körpers, Ztschr. Hyg. 4:353, 1888.
44. Boyd, W. C.: Fundamentals of Immunology, ed. 3, New York, Interscience Publishers, 1953.
45. Zinsser, H., Enders, J. F., and Fothergill, L. D.: Immunity: Principles and Application in Medi-

cine and Public Health, New York, Macmillan, 1939.

46. Cannon, P., and Pacheco, G. A.: Studies in tissue immunity. Cellular reactions of the skin of the guinea pig as influenced by local active immunization, Am. J. Path. *6:*749, 1930.

47. Howard, J. G., and Wardlaw, A. C.: The opsonic effect of normal serum on the uptake of bacteria by the reticulo-endothelial system, J. Immunol. *1:*338, 1958.

48. Bedson, S. P.: Immunity, in Bedson, S. P., Downie, A. W., MacCallum, F. O., and Stuart-Harris, C. H.: Virus and Rickettsial Diseases, ed. 2, London, Edward Arnold, 1955.

49. Maitland, H. B.: Immunity to viruses, in Lectures on the Scientific Basis of Medicine, *3:*259, 1954.

50. Salaman, M. H.: Further studies on combination of vaccinia with anti-vaccinial serum: action *in vitro* of neutralizing antibody on elementary bodies, Brit. J. Exper. Path. *19:*192, 1938.

51. Schlesinger, R. W.: Interferences Between Animal Viruses, in Burnet, F. M., and Stanley, W. M. (eds.): The Viruses: Biochemical, Biological, and Biophysical Properties, New York, Academic Press, 1959.

52. Wagner, R. R.: Viral interference, Bact. Rev. *24:*151, 1960.

53. Isaacs, A.: Viral interference, Symposium Soc. Gen. Microbiol. *9:*102, 1959.

54. Elberg, S. S.: Cellular immunity, Bact. Rev. *24:*67, 1960.

55. Taliaferro, W. H.: The mechanism of acquired immunity in infections with parasitic worms, Physiol. Rev. *20:*469, 1940.

56. Biagi, F. F., and Tay, J.: A precipitation reaction for the diagnosis of cysticercosis, Am. J. Trop. Med. *7:*63, 1958.

57. Taliaferro, W. H.: The inhibition of reproduction of parasites by immune factors, Bact. Rev. *12:*1, 1948.

58. Taliaferro, W. H., and Sarles, M.: The histopathology of the skin, lungs, and intestine of rats during passive immunity to *Nippostrongylus muris,* J. Infect. Dis. *71:*69, 1942.

59. Oliver González, J.: Antigenic analysis of the isolated tissues and body fluids in the round worm *Ascaris lumbricoides* var. *suum,* J. Infect. Dis. *72:*202, 1943.

60. Chandler, A. C.: Some considerations relative to the nature of immunity in *Trypanosoma lewisi* infections, J. Parasitol. *44:*129, 1958.

61. Taliaferro, W. H., and Pizzi, T.: The inhibition of nucleic acid and protein synthesis in *Trypanosoma lewisi* by the antibody ablastin, Proc. Nat. Acad. Sc. *46:*733, 1960.

62. Skarnes, R. C., and Watson, D. W.: Antimicrobial factors of normal tissues and fluids, Bact. Rev. *21:*273, 1957.

63. Myrvik, Q. N., and Weiser, R. S.: A serum bactericidin for *Bacillus subtilis,* J. Immunol. *74:*9, 1955.

64. Bang, F. B., Foard, M., and Karzon, D. T.: Mode of action of heat-labile serum inactivating substance in Newcastle disease virus, Bull. Johns Hopkins. *88:*83, 1951.

65. Leymaster, G. R., and Ward, T. G.: The effect of complement in the neutralization of mumps virus, J. Immunol. *61:*95, 1949.

66. Rowley, D.: Antibacterial systems of serum in relation to nonspecific immunity to infection, Bact. Rev. *24:*106, 1960.

67. Pillemer, L., Blum, L., Lepow, I. H., Ross, O. A., Todd, E. W., and Wardlaw A. C.: The properdin system and immunity: I. Demonstration and isolation of a new serum protein, properdin, and

its role in immune phenomena, Science *120:*279, 1954.

68. Pillemer, L.: The nature of the properdin system and its interactions with polysaccharide complexes, Ann. New York Acad. Sc. *66:*233, 1956.

69. Wedgwood, R. J.: Immunity, infection, and properdin, Arch. Int. Med. *104:*497, 1959.

70. Wedgwood, R. J.: Concerning the nature of the properdin system, Pediatrics *22:*991, 1958.

71. Gladstone, G. P., and Johnston, H. H.: The effect of cultural conditions on the susceptibility of *Bacillus anthracis* to lysozyme, Brit. J. Exper. Path. *36:*363, 1955.

72. Dutton, A. A. C.: The influence of the route of infection on lethal infections in mice, Brit. J. Exper. Path. *36:*128, 1955.

73. Rogers, D. E.: Host mechanisms which act to remove bacteria from the blood stream, Bact. Rev. *24:*50, 1960.

74. Bennett, I. L., Jr., and Beeson, P. B.: Bacteremia: a consideration of some experimental and clinical aspects, Yale J. Biol. & Med. *26:*241, 1954.

75. Rogers, D. E., and Melly, M. A.: Studies on bacteriemia. III. The blood stream clearance of *Escherichia coli* in rabbits. J. Exper. Med. *105:*113, 1957.

76. Beeson, P. B., Brannon, E. S., and Warner, J. V.: Observations on the sites of removal of bacteria from the blood in patients with bacterial endocarditis, J. Exper. Med. *81:*9, 1945.

77. Wardlaw, A. C., and Howard, J. G.: A comparative survey of the phagocytosis of different species of bacteria by Kupffer cells, Brit. J. Exper. Path. *40:*113, 1959.

78. Roberts, D. E.: Studies on bacteriemia. I. Mechanisms relating to the persistence of bacteriemia in rabbits following the intravenous injection of staphylococci, J. Exper. Med. *103:*713, 1956.

79. Martin, S. P., and Kerby, G. P.: The splanchnic removal in rabbits during fatal bacteriemias of circulating organisms and of super-imposed nonpathogenic bacteria, J. Exper. Med. *92:*45, 1950.

80. Biozzi, G., Benacerraf, B., and Halpern, B. N.: Quantitative study of the granulopoietic activity of the reticulo-endothelial system. II. A study of the kinetics of the granulopoietic activity of the R. E. S. in relation to the dose of carbon injected. Relationship between the weight of the organs and their activity, Brit. J. Exper. Path. *34:*441, 1953.

81. Biozzi, G., Benacerraf, B., Halpern, B. N., Stiffel, L., and Hillemand, B.: Exploration of the phagocytic system of the reticuloendothelial system with heat denatured human albumin labeled with I^{131} and application to the measurement of liver blood flow in normal man and some pathologic conditions, J. Lab. & Clin. Med. *51:*230, 1959.

82. Wood, W. B., Jr., Smith, M. R., Perry, W. D., and Berry, J. W.: Studies on the cellular immunology of acute bacteriemia. I. Intravascular leukocytic reaction and surface phagocytosis, J. Exper. Med. *94:*521, 1951.

83. Hollingsworth, J. W., Finch, S. C., and Beeson, P. B.: The role of transfused leukocytes in experimental bacteriemia of irradiated rats, J. Lab. & Clin. Med. *48:*227, 1956.

84. Biozzi, G., Benacerraf, B., and Halpern, B. N.: The effect of *Sal. typhi* and its endotoxin on the phagocytic activity of the reticuloendothelial system of mice, Brit. J. Exper. Path. *36:*226, 1955.

85. Dubos, R. J.: Infection into disease, Perspect. Biol. & Med. *1:*425, 1958.

86. Schneider, H. A.: Nutrition and resistance-susceptibility to infection, Am. J. Trop. Med. *31:* 174, 1951.

87. Schaedler, R. W., and Dubos, R. J.: Effect of dietary proteins and aminoacids on the susceptibility of mice to bacterial infections, J. Exper. Med. *110:*921, 1959.

88. Schneider, H. A.: Nutritional factors in host resistance, Bact. Rev. *24:*186, 1960.

89. Scrimshaw, N. S., Taylor, C. E., and Gordon, J. E.: Interactions of nutrition and infection, Am. J. Med. Sc. *237:*367, 1959.

90. Lisker, R., Chagoya, V., and Laguna, J.: Respuesta immunológica en la desnutrición, Rev. invest. clín. *6:*473, 1954.

91. Talmage, D. W.: Effect of ionizing radiation on resistance to infection, Ann. Rev. Microbiol. *9:* 335, 1955.

92. Benacerraf, B.: Influence of irradiation on resistance to infection, Bact. Rev. *24:*35, 1960.

93. Halpern, B. N.: The role and function of the reticuloendothelial system in immunological processes, J. Pharm. & Pharmacol. *11:*321, 1959.

94. Benacerraf, B.: Quantitative aspects of phagocytosis, in Symposium on Liver Function, Washington, Am. Inst. Biol. Sc., 1958.

95. Dubos, R. J.: Biochemical Determinants of Microbial Disease, Cambridge, Harvard University Press, 1954.

96. Sheldon, W. H., and Bauer, H.: The development of the acute inflammatory response to experimental cutaneous mucormycosis in normal and diabetic rabbits, J. Exper. Med. *110:*845, 1959.

97. Kass, E. H., and Finland, M.: Corticosteroids and infections, Advances Int. Med. *9:*45, 1958.

98. Kass, E. H.: Hormones and host resistance to infection, Bact. Rev. *24:*177, 1960.

99. Thomas, L.: Cortisone, ACTH, and infections, Bull. New York Acad. Med. *31:*485, 1955.

100. Gowen, J. W.: Genetic effects in nonspecific resistance to infectious disease, Bact. Rev. *24:* 192, 1960.

101. Cameron, T. W. M.: Parasites and Parasitism, New York, John Wiley and Sons, 1956.

102. Miles, A. A.: The meaning of pathogenicity. Symposium on Mechanisms of Microbial Pathogenicity, Cambridge, Cambridge University Press, 1955.

103. Dubos, R.: The Bacterial Cell, Cambridge, Harvard University Press, 1945.

104. Binford, C. H.: Histiocytic granulomatous Mycobacterial lesions produced in the golden hamster (*Cricetus auratus*) inoculated with human leprosy, Lab. Invest. *8:*901, 1959.

105. Shwartzman, G. (ed.): The Effect of ACTH and Cortisone upon Infection and Resistance, New York, Columbia University Press, 1953.

106. Middlebrook, G., and Cohn, M. L.: Some observations on the pathogenicity of isoniazid-resistant variants of tubercle bacilli, Science *118:* 297, 1952.

107. Rich, A. R.: The Pathogenesis of Tuberculosis, ed. 2, Springfield, Charles C Thomas, 1951.

108. van Heyningen, W. E.: The role of toxins in pathology, in Symposium on Mechanisms of Microbial Pathogenicity, Cambridge, Cambridge University Press, 1955.

109. van Heyningen, W. E.: Bacterial Toxins, Oxford, Blackwell Scientific Publications, 1950.

110. Pope, C. G., and Stevens, M.: Isolation of a crystalline protein from highly purified diphtheria toxin, Lancet *2:*1190, 1953.

111. Pappenheimer, A. M., Jr.: Diphtheria toxin. III. A reinvestigation of the effect of iron on toxin and porphyrin production, J. Biol. Chem. *167:* 251, 1947.

112. Pappenheimer, A. M., Jr., and Williams, C. M.: Effects of diphtheria toxin on the cecropia silkworm, J. Gen. Physiol. *35:*727, 1952.

113. Pappenheimer, A. M., Jr.: The pathogenesis of diphtheria, in Symposium on Mechanisms of Microbial Pathogenicity, Cambridge, Cambridge University Press, 1955.

114. Payling-Wright, G.: Botulinum and tetanus toxins, in Symposium on Mechanisms of Microbial Pathogenicity, Cambridge, Cambridge University Press, 1955.

115. MacFarlane, M. G.: On the biochemical mechanism of action of gas-gangrene toxins, in Symposium and Mechanisms of Bacterial Pathogenicity, Cambridge, Cambridge University Press, 1955.

116. MacFarlane, M. G., and Datta, N.: Observations on the immunological and biochemical properties of liver mitochondria with reference to the action of *Clostridium welchii* toxin. Brit. J. Exper. Path. *35:*191, 1954.

117. Dawkins, M. J. R., and Ress, K. R.: A Biochemical Approach to Pathology, London, Edward Arnold, 1959.

118. Smith, H., and Keppie, J.: Observations on experimental anthrax: demonstration of a specific lethal factor produced *in vivo* by *Bacillus anthracis*, Nature *173:*869, 1954.

119. Wood, W. B., Jr., Smith, M. R., and Watson, B.: Studies on the mechanism of recovery in pneumococcal pneumonia. IV. The mechanism of phagocytosis in the absence of antibody. J. Exper. Med. *84:*387, 1946.

120. Varela, G., Aguirre, A., and Carillo, J.: *Escherichia coli-Gómez.* Nueva especie aislada de un caso mortal de diarrea, Bol. med. Hosp. Infantil México *3:*3, 1946.

121. Duran-Reynals, F.: Tissue permeability and the spreading factors in infection: a contribution to the host-parasite problem, Bact. Rev. *6:*197, 1942.

122. Pillemer, L., Schoenberg, M.D., Blum, L., and Wurz, L.: Properdin system and immunity. II. Interaction of the properdin system with polysaccharides, Science *122:*545, 1955.

123. Burnet, F. M.: Principles of Animal Virology, New York, Academic Press, 1955.

124. Hawking, F.: The Pathogenicity of Protozoal and Other Parasites: General Considerations, in Symposium on Mechanisms of Microbial Pathogenicity, Cambridge, Cambridge University Press, 1955.

125. Haining, R. B., and Haining, R. G.: Cysticercosis cerebri, J.A.M.A. *172:* 2036, 1960.

126. Maegraith, B.: Pathological Processes in Malaria and Blackwater Fever. Oxford, Blackwell Scientific Publications, 1948.

127. Bueding. E.: Studies on the Glycolytic Enzymes of *Schistosoma mansoni*, in Cole, W. H. (ed.): Some Physiological Aspects and Consequences of Parasitism, New Brunswick, Rutgers University Press, 1955.

128. Sprent, J. F. A., and Chen, H. H.: Immunological studies in mice infected with the larvae of *Ascaris lumbricoides*. I. Criteria of immunity and immunizing effect of isolated worm tissues, J. Infect. Dis. *84:*111, 1949.

129. Laranja, F. S., Dias, E., Nobrega, G., and Miranda, A.: Chagas' disease. A clinical, epidemiologic, and pathologic study, Circulation *14:*1035, 1956.

130. Maegraith, B. G., and Harinasuta, C.: Experimental amebic infection of the liver in guinea

pigs. II. Abscess formation in animals with persistent intestinal lesions, Ann. Trop. Med. *48:*434, 1954.

131. Neal, R. A.: Proteolytic enzymes in *Endamoeba histolytica,* Nature *178:*599, 1956.

132. Lewert, R. M., and Lee, C. L.: Studies on the passage of helminth larvae through host tissues, J. Infect. Dis. *95:*13, 1954.

133. Silverman, P. H., and Maneely, R. B.: Studies on the biology of some tapeworms of the genus Taenia. III, Ann. Trop. Med. *49:*326, 1955.

134. Venkatachalam, P. S., and Pathwardan, V. N.: The role of *Ascaris lumbricoides* in the nutrition of the host; effect of ascariasis on digestion of protein, Tr. Roy. Soc. Trop. Med. & Hyg. *47:*169, 1956.

135. Oliver-González, J., and Torregrosa, M. V.: A substance in animal parasites related to the human isoagglutinogens, J. Infect. Dis. *74:*173, 1944.

136. Phillips, B. P., Wolfe, P. A., Rees, C. W., Gordon, H. A., Wright, W. H., and Reyniers, J. A.: Studies on the ameba-bacteria relationship in amebiasis, Am. J. Trop. Med. *4:*675, 1955.

137. Gladstone, G. P.: Pathogenicity and Virulence of Microorganisms. I. The germ theory of disease and the relationship between host and parasite, in Florey, H. W. (ed.): General Pathology, Philadelphia, W. B. Saunders, 1958.

138. Martin, W. J., Nichols, D. R., and Henderson, E. D.: The problem of management of nasal carriers of staphylococci, Proc. Staff Meet. Mayo Clin. *35:*282, 1960.

139. Peabody, J. W., Jr., and Seabury, J. H.: Actinomycosis and nocardiosis, J. Chron. Dis. *5:*374, 1957.

140. Simon, H. J.: Attenuated Infection. The Germ Theory in Contemporary Perspective, Philadelphia, J. B. Lippincott, 1960.

141. Scott, T. F. McN.: Infection with the virus of herpes simplex, New Eng. J. Med. *250:*183, 1954.

142. Flores Barroeta, F., Núñez, V., and Biagi, F. F.: Observaciones sobre amibiasis en material de autopsia. Estudio de 109 casos, Prensa méd. México *24:*141, 1959.

143. McLeod, C. M., and Pappenheimer, A. J., Jr.: Properties of Bacteria which Enable Them to Cause Disease, in Dubos, R. J. (ed.): Bacterial and Mycotic Infections of Man, Philadelphia, J. B. Lippincott, 1958.

144. Coburn, A. F., and Pauli, R.: The interaction of host and bacterium in the development of communicability by *Streptococcus hemolyticus,* J. Exper. Med. *73:*551, 1940.

145. Schwentker, F. F., Janney, J. H., and Gordon, J. E.: The epidemiology of scarlet fever, Am. J. Hyg. *38:*27, 1943.

146. Lewert, R. M., and Lee, C. L.: The collagenase-enzyme of skin-penetrating helminths, Am. J. Trop. Med. *6:*473, 1957.

147. Pickering, G.: Regulation of body temperature in health and disease, Lancet *1:*56, 1958.

148. DuBois, E. F.: Lane Medical Lectures, Stanford, Stanford University Press, 1937.

149. Beeson, P. B.: Fever, in McBryde, C. M. (ed.): Signs and Symptoms, ed. 2, Philadelphia, J. B. Lippincott, 1952.

150. Menkin, V.: Chemical basis of fever with inflammation, Arch. Path. *39:*28, 1945.

151. Bennett, I. L., Jr., and Beeson, P. B.: Studies on the pathogenesis of fever. II. Characterization of fever producing substances from polymorphonuclear leukocytes and from the fluid of sterile exudates, J. Exper. Med. *98:*493, 1953.

152. Petersdorf, R. G., and Bennett, I. L., Jr.: The experimental approach to the mechanism of fever, Arch. Int. Med. *103:*991, 1959.

153. Bennett, I. L., Jr., and Cluff, L. E.: Bacterial pyrogens, Pharmacol. Rev. *9:*427, 1957.

154. Beeson, P. B.: Temperature-elevating effect of substance obtained from polymorphonuclear leukocytes, J. Clin. Invest. *27:*524, 1948.

155. Atkins, E., and Wood, W. B., Jr.: Studies on pathogenesis of fever I. Presence of transferable pyrogen in blood stream following injection of typhoid vaccine, J. Exper. Med. *101:*519, 1955.

156. Bennett, I. L., Jr., Petersdorf, R. G., and Keene, W. R.: Pathogenesis of fever: evidence for direct cerebral action of bacterial endotoxins, Tr. A. Am. Physicians *70:*64, 1957.

157. Wood, W. B., Jr.: Studies on the cause of fever, New Eng. J. Med. *258:*1023, 1958.

158. Petersdorf, R. G., and Bennett, I. L., Jr.: Studies on the pathogenesis of fever. VIII. Fever-producing substances in the serum of dogs, J. Exper. Med. *106:*293, 1957.

159. Altschule, M. D., and Freedberg, A. S.: Circulation and respiration in fever, Medicine *24:*403, 1945.

160. Bennett, I. L., Jr., and Nicastri, A.: Fever as a mechanism of resistance, Bact. Rev. *24:*16, 1960.

161. Chatterjea, J. B., Dameshek, W., and Stefanini, M.: Adrenalin (epinephrine) test as applied to hematological disorders, Blood *8:*211, 1953.

162. Tullis, J. L.: Blood Cells and Plasma Proteins, New York, Academic Press, 1953.

163. Menkin, V.: Studies on inflammation. XVIII. On the mechanisms of leukocytosis in inflammation, Am. J. Path. *16:*13, 1940.

164. Polak, H., and Némec, J.: Notes on the mechanism of leukocytosis, Blood *14:*931, 1959.

165. Custer, R. P., and Smith, E. B.: The pathology of infectious mononucleosis, Blood *3:*830, 1948.

166. Wintrobe, M. M.: Clinical Hematology, ed. 4, Philadelphia, Lea and Febiger, 1956.

167. Macfarlane, R. G.: The Reactions of the Blood to Injury, in Florey H. W. (ed.): General Pathology, ed. 2, Philadelphia, W. B. Saunders, 1958.

168. Fahraeus, R.: The influence of the rouleaux formation of the erythrocytes on the rheology of the blood, Acta med. scandinav. *161:*151, 1958.

169. Fahraeus, R.: The suspension stability of the blood, Acta med. scandinav. *55:*1, 1921.

170. Morawitz, P.: Ueber einige postmortale Blutveränderungen, Beitr. chem. Physiol. u. Path. *8:*1, 1906.

171. MacFarlane, R. G.: Fibrinolysis following operation, Lancet *1:*10, 1937.

172. Cooper, J. F.: The surgical aspects of fibrinolysis, Surg. Gynec. & Obst. (Internat. Abstr. Surg.) *108:*417, 1959.

173. Waksman, S. A.: Microbial Antagonisms and Antibiotic Substances, ed. 2, New York, Commonwealth Fund, 1947.

174. Work, T. S., and Work, E.: The Bases of Chemotherapy, New York, Interscience Publications, 1948.

175. Jawetz, E., Melnick, J. L., and Adelberg, E. A.: Review of Medical Microbiology, ed. 4, Los Altos, California, Lange Medical Publications, 1960.

176. Woods, D. F.: The relation of p-aminobenzoic acid to the mechanisms of the action of sulphanilamide, Brit. J. Exper. Path. *21:*74, 1940.

177. Munier, R., and Cohen, G. N.: Incorporation d'analogues structuraux d'aminoacides dans les protéines bactériennes. Biochim. et biophys. acta *21:*592, 1956.

178. Heidelberger, C., Cahudhuri, N. K., Danneberg,

P., Mooreu, D., Griesbach, L., Duschinsky, R., Schnitzer, R. J., Pleven, E., and Scheiner, V.: Fluorinated pyrimidines, a new class of tumour inhibitory compounds, Nature *179:*663, 1957.

179. Matthews, R. E. F.: Effects of some purine analogues on tobacco mosaic virus, J. Gen. Microbiol. *10:*521, 1954.

180. Newton, B. A.: The properties and mode of action of the polymyxins, Bact. Rev. *20:*14, 1956.

181. Eagle, H., and Saz, A. K.: Antibiotics, Ann. Rev. Microbiol. *9:*173, 1955.

182. Mitchell, P.: Penicillin and the logic of chemotherapy, Gior. microbiol. *2:*440, 1956.

183. Park, J. T., and Strominger, J. L.: Mode of action of penicillin. Biochemical basis for the mechanism of action of penicillin and for its selective toxicity, Science *125:*99, 1957.

184. Magoffin, R. L., and Spink, W. W.: The protection of intracellular brucella against streptomycin alone and in combination with other antibiotics, J. Lab. & Clin. Med. *37:*924, 1951.

185. Mackaness, G. B. and Smith, N.: The bactericidal action of isoniazid, streptomycin and Terramycin on extracellular and intracellular tubercle bacilli, Am. Rev. Tuberc. *67:*322, 1953.

186. Gale, E. F.: Specific inhibitors of protein synthesis, Symp. Soc. Gen. Microbiol. *8:*212, 1958.

187. Bueding, E., and Swartzwelder, C.: Antihelminthics, Pharmacol. Rev. *9:*329, 1957.

188. Schnitzer, R. J., and Gramberg, E.: Drug Resistance of Microorganisms, New York, Academic Press, 1957.

189. Luria, S. E., and Delbrük, M.: Mutations of bacteria from virus sensitivity to virus resistance, Genetics *28:*491, 1943.

190. Demerec, M.: Origin of bacterial resistance to antibiotics, J. Bacteriol. *56:*63, 1948.

191. Lederberg, J., and Lederberg, E.: Replica plating and indirect selection of bacteria mutants, J. Bacteriol. *63:*339, 1952.

192. Jackson, S., and Hinshelwood, C. N.: An investigation of the nature of certain adaptive changes in bacteria, Proc. Roy. Soc. London s.B *136:*562, 1950.

193. Barer, G. R.: The action of Streptomycin on *Bacterium lactis aerogenes,* J. Gen. Microbiol. *5:*1, 1951.

194. Dean, A. C. R., and Hinshelwood, C. N.: Observation on bacterial adaptation. An adaptation in microorganisms, Symp. Soc. Gen. Microbiol. *3:*21, 1953.

195. Lederberg, J.: Recombination mechanisms in bacteria, J. Cell. & Comp. Physiol. *45:* (suppl. No. 2) 75, 1955.

196. Woolman, E. L., Jacob, F., and Hayes, W.: Conjugation and genetic recombination in *Escherichia coli* K-12, Cold Spring Harbor Symp. Quant. Biol. *21:*141, 1956.

197. Hotchkiss, R. D.: Transfer of penicillin resistance in pneumococci by the desoxyribonucleate derived from resistant cultures. Cold Spring Harbor Symp. Quant. Biol. *16:*457, 1951.

198. Hotchkiss, R. D., and Evans, A. H.: Analysis of the complex sulfonamide resistance locus of pneumococcus, Cold Spring Harbor Symp. Quant. Biol. *23:*85, 1958.

199. Fusillo, M. H., and Romansky, M. J.: The simultaneous increase in resistance of bacteria to aureomycin and terramycin upon exposure to either antibiotic, Antibiotics & Chemother. *1:* 107, 1951.

200. Steele, J. D.: Results of an international survey of pulmonary tuberculosis, Am. Rev. Tuberc. *73:* 128, 1956.

201. Jawetz, E., and Gunnison, J. B.: Studies on antibiotic synergism and antagonism. A scheme of combined antibiotic action, Antibiotics & Chemother. *2:*243, 1952.

202. Klein, M., and Schorr, S. E.: The role of bacterial resistance in antibiotic synergism and antagonism, J. Bacteriol. *65:*454, 1953.

203. Lepper, M. H.: Microbial resistance to antibiotics, Ann. Int. Med. *43:*299, 1955.

204. Pollock, M. R.: Drug resistance and mechanisms for its development, Brit. M. Bull. *16:*16, 1960.

205. Finland, M.: Emergence of antibiotic-resistant bacteria, New Eng. J. Med. *253:*909, 1955.

206. Muschenheim, C., McDermott, W., Hadley, S. J., Hull-Smith, H., and Tracy, A.: Streptomycin in the treatment of tuberculosis in humans. II. Pulmonary tuberculosis, Ann. Int. Med. *27:*989, 1947.

207. Steenken, W., Meade, G. M., and Coates, E. D.: Demonstration of increased drug resistance of tubercle bacilli from patients treated with hydrazines of isonicotinic acid, Am. Rev. Tuberc., *65:*754, 1953.

208. Bojalil, L. F., Monier, A., and Ramírez, P.: Determinación de la sensibilidad de *Myobacterium tuberculosis* a la isoniazida, Rev. mex. tuberc. *14:*291, 1953.

209. Cerbón, J.: La incidencia de cepas de *Mycobacterium tuberculosis* resistentes a los quimioterapéuticos en pacientes con tuberculosis recién descubierta, Rev. mex. tuberc. *18:*289, 1957.

210. Medical Research Council. Various combinations of isoniazid with streptomycin or with P.A.S. in the treatment of pulmonary tuberculosis, Brit. M. J. *1:*435, 1955.

211. Dowling, H. F., Hirsh, H. L., and O'Neil, C. B.: Studies on bacteria developing resistance to penicillin fractions X and G *in vitro* and in patients under treatment for bacterial endocarditis, J. Clin. Invest. *25:*665, 1946.

212. Garrod, L. P.: The reactions of bacteria to chemotherapeutic agents, Brit. M. J. *1:*953, 1951.

213. Alexander, H. E., and Leidy, G.: Mode of action of streptomycin of type b, *H. influenzae.* I. Origin of resistant organisms J. Exper. Med. *85:* 29, 1947.

214. González-Ochoa, A., Shiels, J., and Vázquez, P.: Acción de la 4-4′ diaminodifenilsulfona frente a *Nocardia brasiliensis,* Gac. méd. México *52:* 345, 1952.

215. Mackinnon, J. E., Artagaveytia-Allende, R. C., and García-Zorrón, N.: The inhibitory effect of chemotherapeutic agents on the growth of causal organisms of exogenous mycetomas and nocardiosis, Tr. Roy. Soc. Trop. Med. & Hyg. *52:*78, 1958.

216. Bojalil, L. F., and Medina, B.: Acción de diversos agentes quimioterapéuticos sobre el crecimiento de algunas especies de *Nocardia,* Rev. Latinoamer. Microbiol. *2:*33, 1959.

217. Pulaski, E. J.: Surgical Infections, in Principles and Practice of Antibiotic Therapy, New York, Medical Encyclopedia, 1954.

218. Lowbury, E. J. L.: Cross infection of wounds with antibiotic-resistant organisms, Brit. M. J. *1:*985, 1955.

219. Young, G., Krasner, R. I., and Yudkofsky, P. L.: Interactions of oral strains of *Candida albicans* and lactobacilli, J. Bacteriol. *72:*525, 1956.

220. Torack, R. M.: Fungus infections associated with antibiotic and steroid therapy, Am. J. Med. *22:* 872, 1957.

221. Pérez-Miravete, A., and Carrillo-López, J.: Estudios sobre flora vaginal. III. Alteraciones de la

flora vaginal inducidas por antibióticos y antagonismos bacterianos, Rev. Latinoamer. Microbiol. *1:*267, 1958.

222. González-Mendoza, A., and Bojalil, L. F.: The incidence of *Candida albicans* in the sputum of tuberculous patients, Am. Rev. Tuberc. *77:* 543, 1958.

223. Editorial: The antibiotic-resistant staphylococci, Antibiotics & Chemother. *5:*115, 1953.

224. Needham, G. M., and Nichols, D. R.: Recent changes in sensitivity of *Micrococcus pyogenes* to various antibiotic agents, J. Lab. & Clin. Med. *41:*150, 1953.

225. Finland, M., and Wilcox, C.: Antibiotic combinations and resistance to antibiotics: penicillin with other antibiotics against penicillin-resistant staphylococci, Proc. Soc. Exper. Biol. & Med. *83:*605, 1953.

226. Rodríguez, M. A., and Vizcaya, Z. R.: Sensibilidad a cuatro antibióticos de *Micrococcus pyogenes* coagulasa-positivos aislados de pacientes intra y extra-hospitalarios, Rev. Latinoamer. Microbiol. *1:*101, 1958.

227. Sánchez, L. E., Barocio, L., Bolaños, G., Brüggemann, C., and Velasco, N.: Epidemiología de las infecciones estafilocócicas. II. Estudio de los portadores de *Staphylococcus aureus* y sus diseminaciones en un servicio materno infantil, Rev. Latinoamer. Microbiol. *2:*63, 1959.

228. Surgalla, M. J., and Dack, G. M.: Enterotoxin produced by Micrococci from cases of enteritis after antibiotic therapy, J.A.M.A. *158:*649, 1955.

229. Brandt, H., and Luna Olivares, A.: Enterocolitis seudomembranosa, Prensa méd. México *24:*59, 1959.

230. McDermott, W.: Microbial persistence, Yale J. Biol. & Med. *30:*257, 1958.

231. Schaeffer, W. B.: The effect of isoniazid on growing and resting tubercle bacilli, Am. Rev. Tuberc. *69:*125, 1954.

232. Bojalil, L. F., Pérez Tamayo, R., and Bastarrachea, F.: Persistence of tubercle bacilli in the organs of guinea pigs under chemotherapy. Am. Rev. Tuberc. *77:*473, 1958.

233. Jawetz, E.: Antimicrobial Chemotherapy. Ann. Rev. Microbiol. *10:*85, 1956.

234. Emerson, S., and Cushing, J. E.: Altered sulphonamide antagonism in *Neurospora,* Fed. Proc. *5:* 379, 1946.

235. Miller, C. P., and Bohnhoff, M.: Two streptomycin-resistant variants of meningococcus, J. Bacteriol. *54:*467, 1947.

236. Spendlove, G. A., Cummings, M. M., Fackler, W. B., and Michael, M.: Enhancement of growth of a strain of *M. tuberculosis* (var. *hominis*) by streptomycin, Pub. Health. Rep. *63:* 1177, 1948.

237. González Ochoa, y Bojalil, L. F.: Actividades *in vitro* de complejos sulfa-cobre sobre algunos hongos patógenos, Rev. Inst. Salubr. Enf. Trop. *19:*1, 1950.

238. González Ochoa, A., Bojalil, L. F., y Soto Pacheco, R.: Acción estimulante de las sulfonamidas cobre y de la penicilina sobre el desarrollo de *Crytococcus neoformans* y *Sporotrichum schenki,* respectivamente, Rev. Soc. Mex. Hist. Nat. *9:* 35, 1950.

239. Gould, J. C.: The laboratory control of antibiotic therapy, Brit. M. Bull. *16:*29, 1960.

240. Turnbull, F. W. A., and Stewart, S. M.: Studies on the distribution of drug resistant tubercle bacilli within the lung, Am. Rev. Tuberc. *73:*406, 1956.

241. Bojalil, L. F., Bastarrachea, F., Cerbón, J., and Pérez Tamayo, R.: Distribution of tubercle bacilli resistant to streptomycin and isoniazid within the lung, Acta tuberc. scandinav. *35:*265, 1958.

242. McDermott, W.: Chemotherapy of Microbial Diseases, in Dubos, R. J. (ed.): Bacterial and Mycotic Infections of Man, ed. 3, Philadelphia, J. B. Lippincott, 1958.

243. Davis, B. D.: The binding of sulfonamide drugs by plasma proteins. A factor determining the distribution of drugs in the body, J. Clin. Invest. *22:*753, 1943.

CHAPTER VIII

GENERAL PATHOLOGY

OF THE IMMUNE RESPONSE

I. INTRODUCTION

It has been known for a long time that convalescing subjects, or those completely recovered from certain infectious diseases, become more resistant to new attacks of the same disease. Such an observation was the basis of Jenner's momentous discovery of vaccination in 1789, of Pasteur's studies on fowl cholera, carbuncle and rabies, and of von Behring and Kitasato's finding of antitoxins in 1890. Up to that time, however, all studies on the production of protective substances by the organism had been carried out with specific pathogenic agents or their toxins. But in 1891, Ehrlich showed that protective substances also developed when nonbacterial toxins, such as abrin and ricin, were used. Such a defensive mechanism was considered of great significance in survival, and perhaps this is the reason why this branch of science is known as immunology, and the formation of antibody is referred to as the immune response. Nevertheless, a new field was opened (or rather the limits of immunology were suddenly expanded) by Portier and Richet's publication in 1902[1] (Fig. 8–1) on the "toxicity" of *Actinaria* (sea anemone) extracts. These authors described their results as follows: "The poison obtained from tentacles of actinia provides a clear example of the anaphylactic effect. Intravenous injection of glycerinated solutions are fatal for the dog when the dose is greater than 0.15 cc. per kg.; when the dose is between 0.15 cc. and 0.30 cc., death supervenes in 4 to 5 days, and when it is more than 0.30 cc., the animal succumbs in a few hours. With doses below 0.15 cc. per kg. the dog, with few exceptions, survives after a period of illness lasting 4 to 5 days. But if instead of injecting normal dogs the animals used have received a non-fatal dose 2 or 3 weeks before, doses of 0.08 to 0.25 cc. per kg. become very rapidly fatal, demonstrating the anaphylactic effect after the first injection.

> *Mathurin* (had received 0.12 cc. 16 days before) 0.25 cc. Dead in three quarters of an hour.
> *Galatea* (had received 0.12 cc. 16 days before) 0.12 cc. Dead overnight.
> *Pierrot* (had received 0.08 cc. 15 days before) 0.16 cc. Dead in half hour . . ."

In their conclusions, Portier and Richet called attention to: "The analogy between this decreased immunity (anaphylaxis) to the injection of actinotoxin and the extremely decreased immunity of tuberculous animals to tuberculin." At the same time as Portier and Richet, Theobald Smith observed a similar phenomenon in guinea pigs during a study of diphtheria toxin. Many subsequent publications revealed that antibody formation, useful to the organism in some cases, was detrimental in others; slowly investigators became conscious that several diseases of obscure etiology and variable clinical manifestations could represent human instances of the phenomenon described by Portier and Richet. An obvious consequence of this idea was that the term "immunology" became inadequate to describe the general field of study in this science; certainly, anaphylactic shock, serum disease and other pathologic processes cannot be considered as instances of immunity (*senso stricto*), and it is even more paradoxical to label some diseases as "diseases of autoimmunity." Antibody synthesis is a general biologic phenomenon, common to many different species, sometimes useful in defense and at other times injurious to the organism, which refuses to conform to teleologic or narrow interpretations.

The central interest in this chapter is the pathology of the immune response, but it is convenient to review briefly some general concepts of antigens, antibodies and the antigen-antibody reaction in order to avoid repetitions in the following discussion of pathology; those interested in obtaining ad-

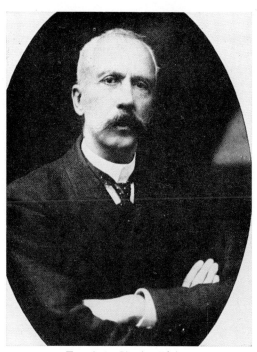

Fig. 8–1. Charles Richet.

ditional information on other physiologic aspects of this problem should consult specialized works.[2, 3, 4]

II. ANTIGENS AND ANTIBODIES

The vast majority of hypersensitivity reactions are due to the combination of one or several antigens with one or several antibodies; there are instances (some of which are mentioned below) where antibody has not been identified in the circulating blood with present day techniques. Nevertheless, the similarities of these reactions with others showing serum antibody justify their inclusion here, and their existence does not negate the usefulness of a brief review of the nature of antigen, antibody and their reactions.

A. NATURE OF ANTIGENS

An antigen is a substance capable of inducing antibody formation and of combining with it. Substances with the ability of combining with antibody but incapable of stimulating its synthesis are known as haptens, a term introduced by Landsteiner.[5]

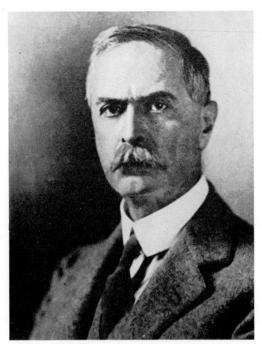

Fig. 8–2. Karl Landsteiner.

The nomenclature has become more complicated with the study of new properties of antigens, so that at present the following terms and definitions are currently used.

1. Complete or *functional antigen.* A substance capable of inducing antibody formation and of combining with it.

2. Incomplete or *haptenic antigen.* A substance which may combine with antibody but fail to stimulate its formation. There are two subtypes:

> *Complex hapten:* when combined with antibody it gives rise to the known immunologic reactions (precipitation, flocculation, etc.)

> *Simple* or *inhibitor hapten:* it can be demonstrated only by the prevention of antibody reaction with other antigens which would give visible serologic reactions.

1. Chemical Structure. Antigenic substances are of very varied chemical structure, frequently quite complex. The vast majority are proteins, so the same difficulties germane to the study and analysis of protein structure are applicable to antigens. There is an additional group of antigenic substances of great significance in pathology,

polysaccharides, with a less complicated structure, which occur mainly in bacterial capsules. Finally, a few antigens and many haptens have a relatively low molecular weight and their structure is better known.

There are a series of characteristics which seem to be necessary for most substances to be antigenic, and although some flagrant exceptions may be found for each one, it is of interest to review them.

(a) Antigens have a high molecular weight. The higher the molecular weight the greater the antigenic capacity. The minimal molecular weight compatible with antigenicity is 600, but this only occurs with haptens. The ability to stimulate antibody synthesis begins somewhere around a molecular weight of 10,000; serum albumin, one of the most potent antigens and the one that has been used most widely in experimental work has a molecular weight of 69,000, while the tobacco mosaic virus weighs more than 50 millions. On the other hand, a high molecular weight is not always accompanied by antigenicity, as is the case of some nucleoproteins with molecular weights of over 1 million, and gelatin, with a molecular weight of 100,000. Gelatin is, however, a denatured protein highly modified by chemical treatment (it is obtained by boiling collagen in acid or alkaline solutions), and some recent observations suggest that it may be slightly antigenic.[6]

(b) An antigenic protein should be foreign to the organism. In general, the body does not form antibodies against its own normal proteins (some exceptions are already known to this statement), and this observation led Ehrlich to postulate his rule of "horror autotoxicus." The more different is the protein to those normally found in the organism, the greater is its antigenic capacity.

(c) Antigens should remain in the circulation a sufficient period of time. It has been suggested that one of the reasons why substances with low molecular weight are not antigenic is that they escape rapidly from the blood vessels, before a sufficient amount has been fixed in the antibody-forming cells.

(d) Antigens should be assimilable by the organism. Certain substances of high molecular weight cannot be metabolized and are not antigenic, as gum acacia or methylcellulose; such observation suggests that antigens should be susceptible to the enzymatic action of the organism and that in some phase of their disintegration the true antigenic fragments are released.

(e) Antigens are usually naturally occurring substances. Synthetic haptens are numerous and polyvinyl pyrrolidone (a synthetic polymer) is antigenic,[7] but these are the exceptions; most of the known antigens are natural substances occurring in the environment, in microorganisms or in animals.

Almost all antigens are specific in their reactions with antibodies. Landsteiner's (Fig. 8–2) great contribution to immunology was to show, by means of synthetic antigens, that antibodies are formed against specific chemical groups. According to Boyd,[2] "The great significance of the work of Landsteiner on artificial antigens and of its confirmation and extension by others was this: it showed that antibodies could be directed towards groups of known chemical constitution in an antigen, and *could react with these groupings by themselves.*" Unfortunately, since most antigens are pro-

teins it is extremely difficult to determine the reactive groups; Table 47, taken from Cushing and Campbell,[4] lists some of the chemically characterized proteins that have been shown to behave as antigens.

For a long time it was thought that proteins were the only antigenic substances, but the work of Avery[8] and others showed that polysaccharides may also stimulate antibody synthesis. It is very difficult to obtain pure polysaccharides without any traces of protein, but fortunately at least one has been isolated from parasitic helminths as *Ascaris suum* and *Trichinella spiralis*,[9] without any nitrogen. These polysaccharides will induce antibody formation only in man and mice, they resemble glycogen, occur mainly in the capsule of microorganisms and are at least partly responsible for their virulence; furthermore, they are water soluble, non-dialyzable and optically active. Their molecular weight is not known but it is probably greater than 100,000. In many cases they serve to separate a species of bacteria into different types, as pneumococci, of which there are more than 70 types, and streptococci, of which there are more than 14 types.[10]

Table 47. Some Chemically Characterized Proteins Shown to be Antigenic

ANIMAL PROTEINS		VEGETABLE PROTEINS	BACTERIAL
Food	*Enzymes*	*General*	*General*
Hemoglobin	Pepsin	Edestin	Nucleoprotein
Albumin	Pepsinogen	Gliadin	Tuberculin
Various globulins	Trypsin	Zein	*Enzymes*
Fibrinogen	Chymotrypsin	Excelsin	Streptolysin
Fibrin	Catalase	Amandin	Fibrinolysin
Hemocyanin	Cytochrome	Nucleoproteins	Zymase
Egg	Ribonuclease	Gluten	Amylase
Albumin	Dehydrogenase	Hordein	*Toxins*
Mucins	Tyrosinase	*Enzymes*	Tetanus
Vitellin	Luciferase	Urease	Diphtheria
Lysozyme	Hyaluronidase	Papain	Botulism
Milk	Renin	*Toxins*	Staphylotoxin
Casein	*Hormones*	Ricin	Streptococcus
Lactoglobulin	Thyroglobulin	Abrin	(scarlet fever)
Lactalbumin	Pitressin		Clostridium
	Corticotrophin		
Special tissue proteins	*Toxins*		
Pig gastric mucin	Snake poisons		
Myoglobin	Scorpion poison		
Myosin	Sea anemones		
Keratin	Spiders		
Fibroma (silk)	*Synthetic proteins*		
Chrondromucoids	Proteins		
	Pitressin		

It has been said that lipids may be antigenic, but the preparations used have been impure or the lipid has been combined with heterophile serum. Other substances such as formalin, sulfonamides and penicillin, which may awake hypersensitivity reactions (*vide infra*), can only act as antigens when combined with plasma proteins. In this case it is accepted that the protein is changed in nature and becomes antigenic.

2. Cellular Antigens. Although one of the scientific goals of immunology is to know the intimate chemical structure of antigens, in practice they occur as parts of parasites, of cells such as erythrocytes or of complex formations such as hair, pollens, etc. Obviously not all components of the structures mentioned function as antigens, and in many cases it has been possible to separate them in a more or less pure form. But in actual experience an important group of antigens is associated with cells, so it may be wise to view them as such for the time being.

Cellular antigens may have a high degree of specificity, as for instance blood groups, while others are shared by many members of the same animal species or even of species widely separated in the zoologic scale, as is the case of Forssman's antigen. Some of the most common cellular antigens are the following.

a. Blood Groups. The chemical structure of blood groups is not known, but an excellent review of the present state of knowledge has been published by Kabat.[11] There are four major blood groups, known as A, B, AB and O. In addition, there are in the serum natural antibodies agglutinating groups A and B, and their existence is regulated by Landsteiner's rule, which establishes that the serum regularly contains natural antibodies against the absent antigens. When agglutinins are directed against antigens of the same species they are known as isoagglutinins. Antigens A and B stimulate the production of antibodies in man which, together with the existence of natural isoagglutinins, constitute some of the basic limitations of blood transfusions. In order to avoid untoward reactions blood transfusions should always be made with blood of the same group or group O, which is considered as universal donor because there are no natural isoagglutinins against

it. Blood groups are inherited as dominant mendelian characters. The fact that there are only 21 possible combinations between different blood groups has been used to solve some medicolegal problems of disputed paternity[12] or of other types;[13] Sussman has recently analyzed some of the problems inherent in this complex subject.[14] Blood groups are present not only in erythrocytes but in almost all cells and fluids of the organism; some exceptions are cerebrospinal fluid, testes, lens, hair, compact bone and cartilage, nails, etc. In addition to the four groups mentioned many others have been described, some of significance in blood transfusions as Rh, others of forensic interest as groups M and N; details of these groups may be found in specialized works.[15, 16]

b. Bacterial Antigens. These include a very heterogeneous group of substances usually found on the surface of microorganisms and used for taxonomic, diagnostic and therapeutic purposes. Some of the most important bacterial antigens are polysaccharides occurring in many microorganisms such as pneumococcus, meningococcus, klebsiella, carbuncle bacillus, cholera bacillus, diphtheria bacillus, rickettsia, clostridium, various spirochetes, etc.[10] The existence of capsular polysaccharides has permitted classification of pneumococci into more than 70 groups,[17] and it is known that virulence in this microorganism is associated with a substance known as SSS. Lancefield has classified streptococci by means of antigens extracted from them;[18] at least three such antigens have been isolated, which are M protein, an acid soluble nucleoprotein; C substance, a complex carbohydrate, and a group-specific antigen known as T. By means of these antigens streptococci have been classified in groups from A to N, but it is doubtful that the majority of these bacteria are already classified. These groups are important because some of them have been found associated with different diseases. For instance, all group A streptococci isolated from human infections are characterized by having C substance and are distinguished in groups by the presence of M protein, which is one of the factors determining virulence.[19] Types 8 and 12 are associated with glomerulonephritis,[20] and type 4 has no influence on rheumatic fever.[21] Salmonellas have two different antigens known as flagellar and somatic and distinguished as O and H, respectively;[22] O antigen is closely related to virulence. In *S. typhi* a surface antigen referred to as Vi is a determining factor in virulence.[23]

c. Antigens of Viruses and Animal Parasites. Many viruses are capable of stimulating antibody formation, but little or nothing is known of their antigens. Chickenpox virus induces the appearance of at least four substances: one is thermolabile (L), another one is thermostable (S), the third one is an agglutinin ("X") and the fourth is antibody directed against nucleoproteins.[24] It has been mentioned (p. 334) that parasites possess antigenic compounds of the polysaccharide group, and it is certain that there are many others that remain to be studied.

d. Heterophile Antigens (Forssman's Antigen). In 1911, Forssman[22] observed that injection of ground guinea pig organs into rabbits would stimulate the appearance of antibodies (lysins) against sheep erythrocytes. At present the designation Forssman's antigen is given to any substance that, injected into the rabbit, is capable of inducing formation of antibodies against sheep red blood cells. Usually, Forssman's antigens are thermostable and soluble in alcohol; they behave as complete haptens since by themselves they are unable to produce hemolysins. Combination with plasma proteins is necessary. Besides Forssman's antigens there are other systems in which crossed serologic reactions occur between two or more animal species, sometimes widely separated in the zoologic scale. Some of these systems are: man-dog-pig; man-rat-rabbit-guinea pig; man-pneumococcus 14.[2]

B. NATURE OF ANTIBODIES

It is customary to distinguish between two different types of antibodies, namely natural and acquired. Knowledge of antibodies is based almost exclusively on the acquired type, produced in man, horse and rabbit. These limitations should be remembered before accepting any definition of antibody, since careful and detailed study of natural or acquired types induced in other animal species might reveal facts that would demand its modification. For an acceptable working definition, ". . . we may then conveniently define antibody as specific proteins which appear in the body fluids (particularly the blood serum) in response to exposure to foreign antigens and which are characterized chiefly by affinity for the specific antigen."[4] Antibodies were first recognized by means of different serologic reactions and were named accordingly; thus, lysins, bacteriolysins, amboceptor, agglutinins, antitoxins, etc., were some of the terms in use. Later on it was believed that all these reactions depended more on the system used to determine the presence of antibody than on its nature, and the "unitary" theory of antibody developed, which held that the injection of a molecularly pure antigen would produce a single antibody, and that the latter would have the ability of giving different serologic reactions.[26] The most widely used example was the antibody against the capsular antigen of pneumococci, which precipitates the polysaccharide in solution, agglutinates the specific pneumococcus, produces complement fixation, favors phagocytosis and protects against infection by the specific pneumococcus. Nevertheless, more recent studies have revealed that the molecular population of antibody in a given serum is highly heterogeneous, even when strictly purified antigen is used to stimulate its formation.[27] Heterogeneity of antibodies is demonstrated by studies of "valence" (*vide infra*), by variations in the strength of combination with antigen and by differences in physical properties of several fractions of purified antibody which preserve specificity, such as solubility, molecular size and electrophoretic pattern.[28]

1. Chemical Structure. Antibodies are proteins with many resemblances to serum globulins, and especially to gamma globulins. Indeed, they differ only in their ability to combine with antigen. In electrophoresis they move with the peak of gamma globulins,[29] although some have been found associated with alpha globulins.[30] Combination of antibody with antigen will reduce the previously increased area of gamma globulins.[2] Sedimentation rates in ultracentrifugation are the same for antibodies and gamma globulins.[31] All data available on chemical structure of antibodies and gamma globulins are compatible with identity.[32] Patients with agammaglobulinemia are unable to form antibodies.[33] An immunologic cross reaction may be obtained between serum gamma globulin and antibody when both are used as antigens. For all these reasons it seems fairly certain that antibodies are a form of serum gamma globulin. The molecular weight of most antibodies is approximately 160,000; the shape of the molecule appears as asymmetric and resembles a cigar, measuring some 300 Å in longest diameter and 38 Å in the shortest diameter.[34]

2. "Valence." One molecule of antigen may combine with several molecules of antibody. By means of artificial antigens, however, it has been shown that they have a limit in size, and that when this size is exceeded antibodies are formed only against a fraction of the molecule. These findings suggest that there is also an upper limit for the size of the combining site of antibody, which is approximately 800 Å. This is not only a very small area, but additional data suggest that each antibody molecule has no more than two or three combining sites.[35] This point is important because it has been suggested that some of the properties of special antibodies such as "reagins" or "blocking" antibodies (anti-Rh) may be due to the fact that they are univalent, and therefore fail to precipitate antigen, etc.

3. Site of Formation. This interesting problem has been extensively reviewed by McMaster,[36] and Harris and Harris.[37] Early studies showed that reticuloendothelial elements would ingest bacteria and other antigenic particles, and this suggested the idea that the same cells participate in antibody synthesis; furthermore, previous "blocking" of the reticuloendothelial system by means of inert particles such as carbon or India ink would decrease the formation of antibody. Attempts to show that pure cultures of macrophages can form antibodies have failed systematically.[38] Recently, Stevens and McKenna[39] showed that diced spleens will produce antibody *in vitro,* and that monocytes from peritoneal exudates of rabbits synthesize antibody in tissue cultures for approximately 3 weeks.[40] The relation between such monocytes and the macrophagic system is not clear, but monocytic cells are unable to phagocytize. The role of lymphocytes in antibody synthesis has been

suggested on the basis of the following experiments: (1) Harris and Harris[41] gave subcutaneous injections of antigen to rabbits and isolated the draining lymph node; by an ingenious technique they were able to cannulate the efferent lymphatic vessel and separate the containing lymph and cells. Antibody titres were much higher in the cells than in lymph; 99 per cent of the cells were identified as lymphocytes. (2) Wesslén[42] injected animals with bacterial antigen twice, cannulated the thoracic duct and obtained pure lymphocytes which were shown to produce antibody *in vitro*. When antigen is injected into an animal, its lymph nodes obtained and the cells suspended and injected into another animal, it is possible to observe the appearance of antibody in the serum of the second animal. With this technique, Roberts and Dixon[43] found that the amount of antibody produced corresponded with one third of the wet weight of transplanted cells, of which 85 per cent were lymphocytes.

On the other hand, it has also been proposed that plasma cells are the elements chiefly involved in antibody synthesis, and the following studies may be mentioned in favor of this view: (1) Bjørneboe et al.[44] observed in rabbits with repeated injections of pneumococcal antigen that the fat of the renal pelvis contained a greater amount of antibody than other tissues; when this fat was examined under the microscope it was found that there was a cellular infiltrate composed of 90 per cent plasma cells and 10 per cent lymphocytes. (2) Fragments of splenic red pulp maintained *in vitro* and belonging to animals previously injected with antigen will produce antibody. In his experiments, Fagraeus[45] removed the splenic white pulp, where most of the lymphocytes are found, and used only red pulp, where a predominance of plasma cells is the rule. (3) Coons *et al.*[46] developed an ingenious method which permits intracellular localization of antigen or antibody, and which consists of placing histologic sections of tissue with antibody in contact with antigen. An antigen-antibody complex is formed which fixes antigen in sites rich in antibody. The slide is then submerged in a solution containing antibody coupled with a fluorescent compound which will combine with antigen and will reveal the original site of antibody production. With this technique it was shown that antibody was present in plasma cells. (4) Nossal has published a series of papers on antibody production by single cells. In addition to interesting data dealing with some theories of antibody formation, antibody-producing cells have been identified as plasmablasts and plasma cells.[47] (5) Suspensions of cells taken from animals immunized with bacteria, when mixed with suspensions of these bacteria, resulted in specific agglutination of bacteria with plasma cells.[48] (6) In patients with agammaglobulinemia, the failure of antibody and gamma globulin synthesis is associated with the absence of plasma cells in the tissues.[49]

The previous summary suggests that reticuloendothelial elements, monocytes, lymphocytes and plasma cells participate in antibody synthesis. In fact, Burnet and Fenner[50] proposed that the reticuloendothelial system would only modify antigen and pass it to other cells, which would then use it as a "template" for antibody synthesis. According to McMaster,[36] . . . "until the cytologists can convincingly demonstrate just which cells are plasma cells and which are not, which are lymphoid but not lymphocytes, what the life cycle of the lymphocyte really is, and what is the relationship of these cells to one another and to macrophages, polymorphonuclears, and fixed reticuloendothelial cells, we shall remain confused." A similar opinion is voiced by Harris and Harris.[37] It would seem, however, that this is more a semantic than a morphologic confusion, since what is required is not demonstration of which cells are plasma cells but simply a generally accepted definition of plasma cells. Identification of elements capable of antibody synthesis might well begin precisely there, and continue with a careful study of their morphologic features and interchanges, which could be related to different phases of protein formation. This is what is being attempted by Nossal[47] in isolated single cells with brilliant results, and what has been shown by Roberts et al.,[51] and Roberts.[52] In the latter study, rabbits were immunized by repeated intravenous and subcutaneous injections of bovine serum albumin, donors

were selected among those showing a good antibody response and sacrificed when the production of antibody was low. Mesenteric and popliteal lymph nodes were pooled and free cell suspensions obtained, washed and injected into recipient rabbits. These recipient animals had been previously given 400 r in whole body radiation to insure a temporary inhibition of immune response. Immediately after the injection of cells, they were stimulated with I^{131}-labeled bovine serum albumin. The recipient rabbits were sacrificed at various times and tissue from the injection sites was fixed and sectioned in order to study the nature of the cells present. It was determined that over 90 per cent of cells transferred were lymphocytes. On the basis of correlated immunologic and morphologic observations, Roberts concluded as follows:

"1. The transferred cells were responsible for the synthesis of antibody.
2. The lymphocytes in the transferred cells were probably the basic cells responsible for the process.
3. The lymphocytes metamorphosed during the synthesis of antibody to plasma cells, with intermediate cell types prominent during the most active phase of antibody synthesis."

These remarks refer to cells producing most of the antibody, since it has been shown that many others are also capable of antibody synthesis, although in smaller amounts.[53]

4. Theories of Formation. The first theory of antibody synthesis was proposed by Ehrlich and it was composed of two main parts. First, it was suggested that the organism possesses preformed receptors which would increase in number under the influence of specific antigens, but this part was abandoned with Landsteiner's demonstration of antibody production against synthetic arsanilic and tartranilic acids, since it would be impossible for the organism to have receptors for all possible antigenic substances. The second part of Ehrlich's hypothesis, adopted by Breinl and Haurowitz in 1930,[54] was the proposition that antigen

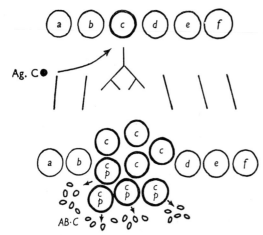

FIG. 8–3. Burnet's illustration of the clonal selection theory of immunity. Contact of the corresponding antigenic determinant *Ag.C.* with cells of clone *c* stimulates proliferation of antibody-producing plasma cells *cp* and non-antibody producing types *c*. (Courtesy of Dr. M. Burnet and Cambridge University Press.)

is used as a "template" by gamma globulin-synthesizing cells to modify the peptide chain by placing "complementary" amino acids on the reactive sites of antigen. Landsteiner showed that antigenic specificity is due to small chemical groups (determining groups) and these would serve as template for production of specific globulins. This theory requires the presence of antigen during the formation of antibody, a condition appearing inconceivable to Burnet and Fenner[50] since immunity to yellow fever and other viral diseases lasts many years, certainly longer than the usual duration of the parasite in tissues. In order to explain the continuous formation of antibody in absence of antigen, Burnet and Fenner proposed that antigen modifies an enzyme of the globulin-synthesizing system, the result being a different protease. This enzyme would become a hereditary character of the individual for the duration of his own life. Such theory takes into account antibody production for long periods without contact with antigen, but there is some evidence that antigens may persist for many months.[55] Pauling[56] suggested that the difference between gamma globulins and antibodies is the manner in which the peptide chain is folded; i.e., it resides in the spatial structure of the molecule and not in the chemical composition. This theory is in agreement with the idea of several valences in antibodies and with the study of terminal chains in gamma globulin and antibody, which have shown them to be identical.[57] Nevertheless, Stavitsky has advanced a series of very cogent arguments against Pauling's theory, including the experimental demonstration that little if any preformed protein is converted to antibody.[58]

Jerne[59] published in 1955 a new and quite different theory of antibody synthesis in which the idea of penetration of antigen into body cells as necessary for antibody production was altogether discarded. Jerne believed that circulating gamma globulins had all the reactive sites necessary to unite with any potential antigenic determinant except those already existing in accessible components of the body. The function of the antigen would be that of a carrier of spontaneously circulating antibody to a system of cells which can reproduce this antibody. With the liberation of more antibody a second injection of antigen would find many more antibody-producing cells and would give a secondary stimulus to antibody production. On the basis of this theory, Burnet[60] has elaborated the clonal selection theory of antibody synthesis, which is best presented in his own words. "It assumes that in the animal there exist clones of mesenchymal cells, each carrying immunologically reactive sites corresponding in appropriate complementary fashion to one (or possibly a small number of) potential antigenic determinants. This provides a population of cells which, when an appropriate stage of development has been reached, are capable of producing the population of globulin molecules which collectively provide the normal antibodies. When an antigen is introduced it will make contact with a cell of the corresponding clone, presumably a lymphocyte, and by so doing stimulate it to produce in one way or another more globulin molecules of the cell's characteristic type. The obvious way of achieving this is to postulate that stimulation initiates proliferation as soon as the cell in question is taken into an appropriate tissue niche, spleen, lymph node or subacute inflammatory accumulation." An elegant elaboration of this theory is to be found in Burnet's stimulating monograph,

"The Clonal Selection Theory of Acquired Immunity."[60]

5. Factors Influencing Formation. Many factors influence the capacity of the organism for antibody synthesis,[61] some of which have been mentioned in the discussion of defense mechanisms (p. 321). Nevertheless, there are others which might conveniently be summarized since they appear to be important in immunology.

a. Dose of Antigen. Within certain limits, the larger the doses of antigen the greater will be the immune response.[62] When these limits are surpassed antibody production is blocked (immunologic paralysis)[63] and may remain so for several months.[64, 65]

b. Chemical Composition of Antigen. Not much is known of this factor because of the complexity of most antigens, but it is considered as the explanation of differences in antigenic capacity of substances with the same ability to combine with antibody and give flocculation. Purification of toxoid is accompanied by an increase in antigenic potency, perhaps due to elimination of inhibiting substances or of antigenically degraded toxoid which is still active in flocculation.[66]

c. Physical Status of Antigen. Insoluble and particulate antigens are much more potent than soluble antigens when given intravenously, while the opposite situation holds with subcutaneous injections. Furthermore, the addition of adsorbing agents to antigens will increase their strength to induce antibody formation, a property that has been used in preparation of toxoid. Freund and Bonanto[67] developed an adjuvant composed of an emulsion of antigen in lanolin with dead tubercle bacilli; unfortunately such adjuvant causes an intense local reaction which prevents its use in man.

d. Route of Administration. It has been mentioned that the route of administration of antigens is partly responsible for the intensity of the immune response. This difference seems to depend, at least with some antigens, on the presence of spleen, since Rowley has shown that it disappears after splenectomy.[68]

e. Interval between Several Doses. The same dose of antigen is more effective in stimulating antibody synthesis when it is fractionated in equal amounts and each is given on separate days than when it is injected all at once.[68] Furthermore, when the interval is prolonged the "anamnesic" response appears in which the appearance of circulating antibody is faster and higher than in the first response. This phenomenon has been used with antidiphtheria vaccine, typhoid vaccine and, recently, with poliomyelitis vaccine.[68]

f. Nutrition. Cannon et al.[69] showed that a protein-deficient diet and plasmapheresis inhibit antibody formation, and Lisker et al.[70] obtained similar results in malnourished patients with hypoproteinemia. The anamnesic response is also depressed by a decrease in nutritional factors,[71] the different vitamins play various roles in antibody production, but in general those favoring protein synthesis appear to be directly involved in the level of circulating antibody.[72] This is an open subject since other authors have published contradictory results.

g. Radiation. The extensive review by Taliaferro and Taliaferro[73] concludes that high doses of ionizing radiation decrease antibody synthesis but that small doses may stimulate it.

h. Hormones. Adrenalectomy increases precipitin to horse serum in rabbits,[74] as well as other antibodies.[75] There is an unsolved controversy on the effect of ACTH and cortisone on antibody formation. Some authors believe that these hormones increase the amount of circulating antibody[76] while others have failed to confirm such observations.[77] Germuth et al.[78] found complete suppression of antibody synthesis when ACTH and cortisone are given from the beginning of immunization, a result that has been repeatedly confirmed.[79] On the other hand, consistently negative results have been obtained in man. For instance, De Vries[80] was unable to modify circulating antibody levels with ACTH, and Larson and Tomlinson[81] could not inhibit precipitin formation in response to pneumococcus polysaccharide by the administration of cortisone and ACTH. No reduction was apparent in the formation of diphtheria antitoxin when toxoid was administered in addition to ACTH and cortisone[82] in patients with liver disease. Nilzen has shown that the effect of thyroid activity is opposed to that of the pituitary adrenal hormones,[83]

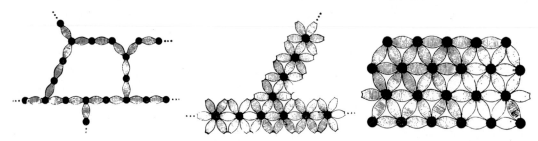

Fig. 8–4. Pauling's concept of antigen-antibody complex formation. *A*, Portion of anitgen-antibody complex with excess antigen. *B*, Antigen-antibody complex with excess antibody. *C*, Antigen-antibody complex with all active regions saturated. (Courtesy of Dr. L. Pauling and the Editor, Journal of the American Chemical Society.)

but so far there is no clear evidence that allergic manifestations of man are influenced by thyroid activity.[84]

C. ANTIGEN-ANTIBODY REACTION

Reactions between antigen and antibody are manifested in different ways which may be termed serologic and biologic. Serologic reactions are used to discover the immune response, to quantitate antibody, to study antigen-antibody combinations from a molecular viewpoint, to determine the presence and amount of antigen, and to study some genetic characteristics which induce antigenic specificity. Biologic reactions serve to determine the presence of serologically invisible antibodies, to study the immune response as a defense mechanism and as a pathogenetic mechanism of disease. Antigen-antibody reactions have been considered as protective in the discussion of defense mechanisms (p. 321), and their role in disease is reviewed in the next section of this chapter.

The structure of antigen-antibody complexes is explained by Pauling's theory of complementarity in the synthesis of antibody. This author[85] assumes that antibodies are divalent and antigens are multivalent, so after combination the result would be a network where the crossing points are antigen molecules and the threads antibodies, touching an antigen in each extreme.

Antigen-antibody complexes play an important role in the pathology of hypersensitivity. Germuth and McKinnon[86] induced anaphylactic shock in unsensitized guinea pigs by the administration of soluble antigen-antibody complexes, and the same phenomenon has been observed in white mice.[87] Such complexes will induce contraction of

isolated guinea pig smooth muscle[88] and inflammatory skin lesions[89] whose severity is proportional to the amount injected. The characteristic lesions of serum sickness were produced by McCluskey *et al.*[90] in only 36 hours in normal mice by means of intravenous injection of large amounts of soluble antigen-antibody complexes; the same authors have observed that the incidence of glomerulonephritis in experimental animals is greater than that of endocarditis or arteritis, and that it appears within 48 hours of the first injection. That the complexes are not dissociated was shown by failure to sensitize guinea pig skin to passive cutaneous anaphylaxis with injection of soluble complexes. Acute glomerulonephritis also has been produced passively in the rat by injection of antigen-antibody complexes.[91]

III. HYPERTENSIVITY

An important group of humoral defense mechanisms, dependent on antibody production, facilitate phagocytosis and block the toxic effects of parasitic poisons. But the combination of antigen with antibody is not always beneficial to the organism; sometimes it is responsible for pathologic changes as severe as, or more severe than, those caused by the antigen, and this may even occur in cases where the antigen is completely innocuous by itself. Antigen-antibody reactions detrimental for the organism are known as hypersensitivity reactions. The fundamental difference between protective and damaging immune mechanisms lies in what happens after the antigen-antibody re-

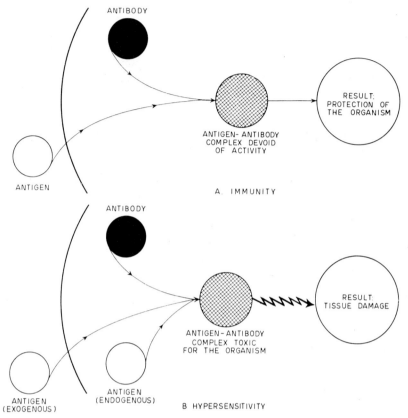

FIG. 8–5. The basic difference between immunity and hypersensitivity. Note that in hypersensitivity the antigen may be either exogenous or endogenous.

action has taken place, the ultimate fate of antigens being of no significance in hypersensitivity. These concepts are schematically represented in Figure 8–5.

Not all instances of hypersensitivity discussed in the following paragraphs enjoy identification of exciting antigen, mediating antibody and mechanism of tissue damage. Nevertheless, there are sufficient clinical and experimental similarities to classical humoral hypersensitivity to classify them as special types of immune responses.

A. TYPES OF HYPERSENSITIVITY

Experimental manifestations of hypersensitivity appear some time after sensitization of the animal. Portier and Richet's observations quoted above referred to 2 to 3 weeks, although 10 days suffice for most species. The first injection of antigen is known as preparatory; the time elapsing between this injection and the appearance of hypersensitivity is referred to as period of

induction; the administration of antigen to reveal the phenomenon is named eliciting injection. The induction period is the time necessary for synthesis of sufficient amounts of antibody to become demonstrable. If the preparatory dose of antigen is large enough it may still be circulating when antibody appears in the circulation and an antigen-antibody reaction may ensue, giving rise to clinical manifestations. Such appears to be the mechanism of serum sickness.[92]

The reaction occurring after the eliciting injection may appear in two different forms; either the animal responds immediately, within a few seconds or minutes, in a violent manner characterized by severe symptoms due to spasm of smooth muscle fibers which may cause rapid death, or the reaction may appear some hours later, be very localized, and suggest no specific tissue damage. These two types of response to the eliciting injection reveal some important differences in mechanism and are the basis for separating

Table 48. Some Differences between Immediate and Delayed Hypersensitivity

IMMEDIATE HYPERSENSITIVITY (URTICARIA)	DELAYED HYPERSENSITIVITY (BACTERIAL, TUBERCULIN)
Immediate onset	Delayed onset
Circulating antibody is demonstrable in most types	There is no demonstrable circulating antibody; cellular immunity
It affects smooth muscle, blood vessels and collagen	It is not limited to any type of tissue
Requires complete antigen	Antigen + tissues + microorganism
Uninfluenced by route of administration of antigen	Almost always through the skin
Passive transference by means of serum	Passive transference by means of cells or cell fractions
Histamine can be demonstrated in the circulation (except in Arthus phenomenon)	There is no histamine release
Types: Arthus phenomenon, anaphylactic shock, evanescent skin reactions, atopy	Types: bacterial, contact dermatitis, drug hypersensitivity

hypersensitivity in two general groups: immediate and delayed.[93] Table 48 summarizes some other important differences of these two types of reaction.

Perhaps the basic factor determining most or all variations between immediate and delayed hypersensitivity is in the nature of the antibody. In immediate hypersensitivity circulating antibody can be easily demonstrated by classic immunologic reactions, while in delayed hypersensitivity there is no measurable antibody (that is, not detectable within the limits of sensitivity of existing techniques) in the serum;[94] it is intimately associated with cells.[95] The term antibody is used here as defined (p. 321), namely, as a protein capable of reacting with the specific antigen, so even if in delayed hypersensitivity antibody cannot be separated from cells it is almost certain that it remains as a modification of intracellular proteins. Whether it lies on one or the other side of the cell membrane is of secondary importance in this context, since it still reacts with the antigen, but for the effects of the antigen-antibody complex on the host this topographic difference becomes of primary significance and appears to determine the special features of each type of hypersensitivity. Other differences in antibody will be pointed out below.

1. Immediate Hypersensitivity. As indicated by its name, this type of hypersensitivity appears a few seconds or minutes after the eliciting injection. Almost all forms show circulating antibody demonstrable by classic serologic techniques or, when serum titres of antibody are low, by means of passive transfer (Prausnitz-Küstner reac-

tion). Excepting the Arthus phenomenon, all other forms of immediate hypersensitivity appear to be caused by release of histamine, or a very similar substance[96] although the mechanism by which antigen-antibody complexes liberate histamine is not known. Histamine participation as mediator in immediate hypersensitivity has been much discussed, but today it is almost universally accepted for several reasons. Histamine injections reproduce the clinical manifestations of hypersensitivity;[97] antihistaminics decrease the intensity of anaphylactic shock and block other forms of immediate hypersensitivity[98] (although there are some controversial observations in this respect[99]); histamine has been isolated in large quantities in the venous blood of the liver in dogs[100] and of the lungs in guinea pigs[101] with anaphylactic shock, and such high levels decrease with disappearance of the symptoms; histamine is widely distributed in the organism, in amounts quite compatible with its role in hypersensitivity;[102] damage to mast cells as a result of anaphylaxis has been shown to occur in guinea pigs,[103] and mice.[104] The mechanism of histamine release in immediate hypersensitivity is believed to be proteolysis,[105] although it has not been demonstrated in rabbits (most histamine in these animals is contained in platelets and not in mast cells).[105]

The participation of histamine in immediate hypersensitivity does not eliminate other humoral factors which might explain some of the discrepancies. It has been shown that heparin, or a related sulphated mucopolysaccharide, is released to the blood during anaphylaxis.[107] Serotonin increases in rabbit's plasma during anaphylaxis,[108] but in amounts to which capillaries are completely insensitive,[109] so the significance of this finding is dubious. Perfusion of the isolated lungs of sensitized guinea pigs with antigen leads to the appearance in the perfusate of a substance causing delayed and slow contractions of the guinea pig ileum;[110] this activity is due to a substance called SRS-A.[111] A bradykinin-like substance has been found in blood taken from dogs during anaphylactic shock, which induces slower muscular contraction than histamine.[112] Some negative data should be mentioned regarding the role of histamine and other humoral substances in human immediate hypersensitivity. Rose et al.[113] failed to demonstrate histamine in arterial, pulmonary and femoral blood of patients studied during an attack of asthma, in spite of the fact that asthmatics are known to eliminate large amounts of histamine with the urine,[114] and such a substance is not found in normal subjects. It has been suggested that the proteolysis responsible for histamine release may also liberate other pharmacologically active compounds which would then be responsible for the production or modification of hypersensitivity.

Another interesting feature of immediate hypersensitivity is that it affects mainly smooth muscle, the wall of blood vessels and connective tissue fibers. Most or all manifestations of this type of hypersensitivity may be reduced to participation of such elements.[115] For instance, anaphylactic shock in the guinea pig is characterized by intense expiratory dyspnea which may cause death by asphyxia and which is associated histologically with forced contraction of bronchial muscles. By means of I[131]-labeled antigen, Dixon and Warren[116] showed that there is a higher concentration of antigen around bronchi and blood vessels than in the rest of the lung. Furthermore, the Arthus phenomenon does not occur in avascular areas such as the cornea[117] nor in explanted tissues,[118] where the cells preserve their motility in spite of the presence of both antigen and antibody in the medium.

The most important types of immediate hypersensitivity are anaphylaxis, the Arthus phenomenon, serum sickness and the group of diseases known as atopic which include bronchial asthma, hay fever, vasomotor rhinitis, gastrointestinal atopy, some forms of headache and dermatoses, conjunctivitis, purpura, etc. In the following paragraphs a brief reference is made to some of them, with special emphasis on mechanisms.

a. Anaphylactic Shock. "We call *anaphylaxis* (contrary to phylaxis) the property of a poison of decreasing, instead of reinforcing, immunity, when administered in nonfatal doses." Thus, Portier and Richet[1] defined the term used to designate this form of immediate hypersensitivity. The characteristics of anaphylaxis have been extensively studied in many animal species;[119] fortunately, its occurrence in man is rare, approximately 0.1 per cent of subjects receiving some form of serum.[120] The picture of anaphylaxis in man resembles that in guinea pigs, with anxiety, dyspnea, cyanosis and cough; all these manifestations reveal the intense contraction of bronchial muscle, and disappear with the injection of adrenaline.

b. Arthus Phenomenon. In 1903, Arthus[121] observed that when repeated subcutaneous injections of horse serum are given in the same area to rabbits the first two or three injections have no effect, but that starting with the fourth administration of horse serum the injected site shows some edema and following a few more injections the local reaction is each time more severe and lasts longer, until actual necrosis is produced. Later it was shown that the first changes occur in blood vessels and are always more intense in these structures;[122, 123] furthermore, passive transfer of this phenomenon was accomplished. The intensity of tissue damage depends on the amount of circulating antibody.[124] The first microscopic reaction is characterized by endothelial damage with stickiness of platelets and endothelium, and thrombi formation; in a few hours a homogeneous material precipitates in the vessel lumen, possibly derived from normal plasma proteins, and the blood vessel wall undergoes necrosis, followed by death of irritated tissues.[125] It is believed that antigen-antibody complexes are directly toxic to the blood vessels and that no mediators are released during most of the reaction.[126]

In his original paper, Arthus asked the

question, "Can man present, under the influence of repeated serum injections, an anaphylactic status, and local and systemic accidents similar to those described in rabbits?" With reference to human observations, Arthus goes on to answer his own question, ". . . after a certain number [variable according to the subject under study] of therapeutic injections given after intervals of several [8 to 15] days, a more or less extensive area of edematous infiltration is observed at the site injected." Arthus phenomenon has been described in man, especially after the application of a series of antirabies vaccine,[127] in which the nervous substance acts as antigen; furthermore, progressively severer reactions to typhoid vaccine and diphtheria toxoid, as well as some of the abscesses observed in diabetics treated with parenteral insulin, admit the same explanation. Arthus phenomena have been produced in many organs other than skin, such as the frog's mesentery, the eye, lungs, testes, peritoneum, joints, brain, etc.[123]

c. Serum Sickness. This disease appears 5 to 10 days after the therapeutic use of heterologous serum. The main clinical manifestations are fever, wheals, generalized lymphadenopathy and arthralgias. It lasts from a few hours to several days and only rarely has proved fatal.[128] Serum sickness differs from anaphylactic shock and Arthus phenomenon in that it can result from a single injection of a large amount of antigen, and this is also an important clue to its mechanism. In 1905, von Pirquet and Shick suggested that antigen is still present in the circulation when the antibody appears, and antigen-antibody reaction occurs and the resulting complex is the cause of the lesions.[129] A few years later, Longcope and Rackeman[130] showed that precipitins appear in the circulation during the latter part of the clinical course of serum sickness. Karelitz and Stempien[131] found that when horse serum is given to an individual and is followed a few hours later by the administration of serum from patients convalescing from serum sickness (and therefore containing precipitins for horse serum), then the entire clinical picture of serum sickness appears in a few hours to a few days, instead of the 5 to 10 days required when only horse serum is given.

Experimental serum sickness was produced by Rich using a single large injection of horse serum in rabbits.[132] Suppression of antibody production by means of nitrogen mustard inhibited the development of visceral lesions.[133] Visceral lesions were strikingly similar to polyarteritis nodosa; in addition, endocardial changes were interpreted as suggestive of rheumatic fever-like lesions, and renal changes were considered as resembling glomerulonephritis.[134] The relationship of antigen elimination, antibody synthesis and tissue damage was studied by several authors but has been clearly defined by Germuth.[135] During the phase of antigen elimination from the blood, when antibody is being synthesized in the presence of excess antigen, visceral lesions appear at their earliest stages of development, but once antibody can be demonstrated and antigen has disappeared from the circulation, the lesions enter a healing stage. The effect of antigen-antibody complexes prepared *in vitro* has been mentioned above. Dixon et al.[92] have beautifully shown that vascular and renal lesions of experimental serum sickness closely parallel the increase in rate of antibody synthesis, and that the onset of tissue damage is accompanied by an almost simultaneous localization of antigen and probably antibody in the sites of the lesions. Furthermore, they also showed that the regression of the lesions followed the disappearance of antigen from the circulation and from the areas of damage, and paralleled the decline in rate of antibody production. Hypersensitivity manifestations elicited by sulfonamides and penicillin may show similar tissue lesions[136] and appear to be mediated by the same mechanisms.

d. Atopy. This is the most frequent form of immediate hypersensitivity in man. The term "atopy" means displacement, or estrangement; it was introduced by Coca to refer to certain hypersensitivity states with two distinguishing features, namely that they were inherited and seemed to appear exclusively in man. The following features characterize atopic hypersensitivity. (1) It occurs spontaneously only in man (although there are some rare exceptions[137]); (2) antigens responsible reach the organism slowly and by inefficient routes, or they have little antigenic potency;[138] (3) early studies indicated the existence of a familial susceptibility to atopy, although at present it is believed that what is inherited is an unusual proneness to make antibody of the "reagin" type;[139] (4) it is difficult to reproduce atopy experimentally;[140] (5) a special feature of atopic antibody is that it can be demonstrated only by passive transfer (Prausnitz-Küstner reaction); (6) in contrast with other forms of immediate hypersensitivity, atopy seems to have a well defined shock organ and become apparent through congestion and edema of skin and/or mucosas.[141] Atopic hypersensitivity includes bronchial asthma, hay fever, vasomotor rhinitis, some gastrointestinal disturbances, etc.

There are two types of bronchial asthma, namely atopic and intrinsic. The atopic form is characterized by being inherited, by giving clinical manifestations usually before the subject is 20 years old, by the presence of other signs of hypersensitivity which may be detected by means of skin reactions, by the presence of the special "reagin" type of antibody and by a good response to treatment.[142] Reagins are not always demonstrable but when present they differ from antibodies formed in other types of immediate hypersensitivity by a series of features summarized in Table 49. The mechanism of atopic bronchial asthma is probably the same as in other forms of hypersensitivity; antigen comes in contact and combines with antibody, the resulting complex releasing histamine directly or indirectly, which then damages the cells.[138] Clinical manifestations of asthma are pulmonary rales, dyspnea, cyanosis and hypersonority of the lungs, which are explained by bronchiolar spasm, edema of surrounding tissues and mucus hypersecretion.[143] The inspired air is trapped within the lungs which become distended and, eventually, emphysematous. Possibly, antibody is present in the smooth muscle cells of bronchial walls. Intrinsic asthma appears in subjects 40 years of age or older, without a family history of similar ailments, may remain stationary throughout life or progress rapidly to status asthmaticus; in addition, it presents a therapeutic problem. A subsidiary type of asthma may be associated with bacterial infections of the bronchial tree, and is sometimes referred to as "bacterial" asthma. The role of chronic bron-

Table 49. Some Differences between Reagins and Other Antibodies

REAGINS	OTHER ANTIBODIES
Sensitize the skin	Do not sensitize the skin
Attached to cells	Freely circulating
Unable to sensitize guinea pigs	Will sensitize guinea pigs
Fail to precipitate	Precipitate
Fail to neutralize the antigen	Neutralize the antigen
Thermolabile	Thermostable

chitis in this type of bronchial spasm is difficult to assess, some authors believing that it is cause, and others effect, of the pathologic state; frequently, however, the symptoms decrease or disappear with control of infection.

Hay fever has a close relation with seasons, which determine the type and nature of air particles. It is characterized by seasonal paroxysmal attacks of nasal catarrh and conjunctivitis, which are revealing of the mucosal localization of reagins; this peculiar antibody is frequently demonstrated by skin tests or by passive transfer. Vasomotor rhinitis has the same pathologic meaning but here the antigen is more often some type of dust or food; sinusitis is a frequent complication and the symptoms may persist as long as bacteria are not eliminated.

2. Delayed Hypersensitivity. In this type of hypersensitivity the reaction appears several hours after the eliciting injection.[145] No antibody is demonstrated either by serologic tests or by passive serum transfer (with the exception of Cole and Favour's report).[146] Delayed hypersensitivity can be transferred only by means of cells,[147] either lymphocytes or leukocytes, or cellular fractions.[148, 149] The immune response is not limited to some special types of tissue, as in immediate hypersensitivity, but it may appear in almost any site in the organism. Antigen must be given through the percutaneous route in order to obtain this form of hypersensitivity. Neither histamine nor any other possible humoral mediator has been shown to play any role in this type of immune response. Both immediate and delayed hypersensitivity may be present in the same animal, and it is possible to eliminate the former type through desensitization without affecting the latter.[150]

Many different substances may elicit the delayed form of hypersensitivity, but in general they may be separated into two different categories: substances associated with biologic agents of disease, such as bacteria, fungi and viruses, and chemical compounds of simple structure. Pappenheimer and Freund suggest that all infections induce delayed sensitivity in the susceptible host to a greater or lesser degree;[151] substances associated with living organisms are mostly protein in nature, while simple chemicals are substances or chemical groups of low molecular weight, i.e., less than 1000, and more often less than 500.[152] The tuberculin reaction in animals or man infected with virulent tubercle bacilli or attenuated strains such as BCG has generally been considered the prototype of a delayed hypersensitivity reaction; consequently, this form of immune response is also known as tuberculin- or bacterial-type hypersensitivity.[153] The preparation of tuberculin involves prolonged heating of culture filtrates of tubercle bacilli to 100°C and old tuberculin contains a mixture of breakdown products of protein and polysaccharides. Therefore, they represent very complex and artificial antigens. Recently, Uhr, et al.[154] showed that when guinea pigs are infected intradermally with toxigenic *C. diphtheriae* and are protected a few hours later with antitoxin, they develop delayed sensitivity to diphtheria toxin; furthermore, the same type of sensitivity is obtained in both guinea pig and man by one intradermal injection of a small amount of antigen (1 Gm. or less) in the form of its complex with excess antibody.[155] The advantage of these techniques is that the antigen is a single and purified protein, which facilitates study of the phenomenon, and at the same time they may be revealing a closer relation between immediate and delayed hypersensitivities, since when such antigens are used intravenously in larger amounts they stimulate abundant formation of circulating antibody. Antigenic simple chemicals must react *in vivo* with tissue protein in order to form complete antigenic particles. They have the advantages of being easy to purify; isotopic labeling can be accomplished with specific in-

formation as to where in the molecule the label is situated, and specific competitive inhibitors can be found or synthesized with greater ease since the molecular composition is well known.[152]

The injection of antigen into an animal may result in the presence of two separate and distinct systems, that concerned with delayed hypersensitivity reactions and that concerned with the release of circulating antibody gamma globulin. That these two systems are under separate genetic control is indicated by studies in agammaglobulinemic patients;[156, 157] such work has shown that subjects suffering from agammaglobulinemia, while unable to form either antibody or gamma globulin in significant amount, readily develop delayed hypersensitivity.

If no antibody has been identified in delayed sensitivity, then what is the nature of the cellular change induced by these antigens? The answer to this question is not available, although it has been suggested that modifications occur at the cellular surface and are in the form of proteins of configuration complementary to antigen molecules.[150] Furthermore, Pappenheimer, *et al.* believe that such cell-surface change is the specific factor which accounts for the inflammatory reactions characteristic of the delayed hypersensitive state, and that antibody synthesis may be a two step process characterized by the cell-surface change and followed, upon additional antigenic stimulation, by antibody synthesis. Perhaps the antigen-induced modification of cells is also directly related to the transfer of delayed tuberculin sensitivity in animals and man. Landsteiner and Chase,[158] and Chase,[147] demonstrated that tuberculin sensitivity is conferred upon normal guinea pigs by the injection of leukocytes isolated from peritoneal exudates, blood, spleen or lymph nodes of sensitive guinea pigs. Lawrence[95] adapted this technique to man and was able to transfer tuberculin sensitivity by means of intact, viable leukocytes, and other authors have been able to transfer delayed sensitivity to other bacterial,[159] viral[160] and simple chemical antigens.[161] Furthermore, delayed hypersensitivity to streptococcal proteins (M substance) has been transferred by means of leukocytic extracts obtained by osmotic rupture,[149] and by the same material after treatment with desoxyribonuclease and ribonuclease, and trypsin.[162] Using DNAse-treated leukocyte extracts prepared from sensitized donors, Lawrence *et al.* have also been able to transfer delayed sensitivity to skin homografts in man.[163] The cellular component responsible for this phenomenon has been called "transfer factor," and it appears to be released from intact leukocytes when incubated in the presence of antigen (tuberculin) to which the donor is sensitive.[164] It seems that the main difference between the cellular transfer system in animals and man is the requirement of intact, viable cells for the experiment to be successful in animals.[165] Other differences may be that the dosage of leukocytes necessary to sensitize animals seems to be much greater,[166] and that the duration of delayed sensitivity in guinea pigs and rabbits is 3 to 5 days[167] while in man it may extend from months to 1 or 2 years.[168]

Lawrence[162] has summarized the following data against the interpretation of the "transfer factor" as antibody of the conventional type: (1) Transfer factor is not neutralized by adding antigen to leukocytes. (2) Antibody is not detectable in leukocyte extracts effective in passive transfer of delayed sensitivity. (3) Antibody is not detectable in the sera of recipients at the time of maximal delayed reactions resulting from transferred sensitivity. (4) Antibody is not detectable at the site of the transferred delayed inflammatory reaction. (5) Agammaglobulinemic patients accept and donate transfer factor in the absence of the capacity to synthesize gamma globulin or conventional serum antibody.

If the nature of the cellular change induced by antigen in delayed hypersensitivity is not well known, the mechanism of tissue damage in this type of immune response is even less understood. Waksman[138] suggests that the specific tuberculin response may be a primary reaction of antigen with cells, a point clearly demonstrated in tissue culture by Rich and Lewis several years ago,[169] and confirmed since by many others.[170] When tuberculin or tubercle bacilli are added to tissue cultures prepared from the tissues of sensitive animals the cells are usually killed;

the phenomenon has been demonstrated with cells derived from spleen, lymph nodes, bone marrow, buffy coat and testis, whereas cells from liver, kidney, skin and corneal epithelium are not affected. Whether the killed cells release other substances which are toxic for the tissues or act as mediators for liberation of some of the factors involved in inflammation (p. 82) must remain conjecture.

The most frequent types of delayed hypersensitivity are usually classified as bacterial, contact dermatitis and some forms of drug hypersensitivity.

a. Bacterial Hypersensitivity. Tuberculosis and many other infections, such as brucellosis, streptococcal and pneumococcal infections, glanders, typhoid, lymphogranuloma inguinale, smallpox vaccination and the various mycoses, induce delayed sensitivity of the bacterial type. Manifestations of this form of immune response are very variable and go from necrosis and destruction of all tissue elements to slight erythema and edema. In tuberculosis, delayed sensitivity probably contributes to the production of caseous necrosis and liquefaction, which are highly important events in the pathology of the disease.[171] Bacterial hypersensitivity is widely used for diagnostic tests, since subcutaneous administration of small amounts of antigen will result in a measurable reaction. Tuberculin and substances derived from fungi, such as histoplasmin, coccidioidin, etc., are some of the most widely used antigens.

b. Contact Dermatitis and Drug Sensitivity. Repeated contact of the skin with certain substances may be followed by a reaction characterized by erythema and blister formation. The nature of the irritating substances is very variable and they include cosmetics, plants, leather, nylon and other synthetic fibers, soap, formalin, etc. Contact dermatitis is a form of delayed sensitivity because the skin reaction is specific for the antigen, because it takes some time to develop and because it requires repeated contacts with the antigen; furthermore, erythema and blisters appear several hours after the last contact with the causing substance. A similar problem is drug sensitivity, which appears not only as contact dermatitis, but also after parenteral administration, and then the symptoms are similar to serum sickness, with fever, generalized lymphadenopathy, wheals, arthralgias, etc. Many drugs may produce the reaction, among them arsenic, sulfonamides, penicillin, thiouracil, etc. This form of hypersensitivity is characteristically delayed, without demonstrable antibody in the circulation.

HYPERSENSITIVITY AND IMMUNITY

It has been mentioned that immunity and hypersensitivity are different manifestations of the same basic phenomenon, i.e., combination of antigen with antibody. This is the reason some authors believe, and many doctors assume unconsciously, that hypersensitivity is an important defense mechanism. It is not rare to hear that a patient is in good immunologic condition because a skin reaction was positive and it is tacitly assumed that negativization of a previously positive skin test is a sign of poor prognosis in certain infectious diseases. Indeed, it is sometimes observed in tuberculous patients that during the last stages of the disease tuberculin skin tests become negative. According to Rich,[172] hypersensitivity may contribute to the defense of the organism in two possible ways: (1) Antibodies involved in immunity are the same as those determining hypersensitivity. In this case, the detrimental effect of antigen-antibody reactions becomes a collateral accident, a necessary evil acceptable only because of the protective and beneficial role of antibody. (2) Inflammation is exaggerated and accelerated by hypersensitivity, and since inflammation is such an effective local defense mechanism, hypersensitivity contributes indirectly to protect the individual.

A close examination of the first possibility suggests that hypersensitivity should be limited to the delayed type, since this is the form most frequently associated with infections. Nevertheless, it is convenient to point out that in pneumococcal infections the same antigen is responsible for both hypersensitivity and immunity, namely the capsular polysaccharide, and that in this case the immune response is immediate, of the Arthus type; delayed sensitivity produced by pneumococci is due to a nucleoprotein unrelated to virulence.[173] The main argument against the suggestion that sensi-

tivity and immunity are mediated through the same antibody is that experimental animals may be desensitized to tuberculin without changing their immunity,[174] and the same has been observed in infections other than tuberculosis. This, however, is indirect evidence only. A very clear experiment is that reported by Bailly[175] a few years ago. Rabbits were infected with streptococci Type 30 and shown to have delayed sensitivity to specific protein M and polysaccharide C. In this bacterial strain, specific protein M is related to virulence. Bailly proceeded to desensitize animals in two groups, one to protein M and the other to polysaccharide C, and once skin tests and precipitin reactions were negative all animals were reinoculated with streptococci Type 30. All animals desensitized to protein M, with full preservation of sensitivity to polysaccharide C, died in a few days, while the animals preserving hypersensitivity to protein M survived. This isolated experiment shows that the relation between immunity and hypersensitivity should not be judged in general, but only in those specific cases where there is demonstration that the same antibody is responsible for both phenomena.

The second possible role of hypersensitivity in defense is enhancement of inflammation, and this has been discussed in Chapter II (p. 80). Briefly, it can be recalled that the inflammatory process is supposed to limit bacterial spreading, so that an exaggerated inflammation would favor this mechanism even more. Experimental studies, however, have shown the opposite. The injection of bacteria into the inflammatory process of animals with delayed hypersensitivity is followed by a more rapid spread of the infection than in controls.[176]

AUTOIMMUNITY AND DISEASE

This is one of the most fascinating fields in medicine today, and during the last decade it has attracted the attention of many investigators. The following discussion will center around some instances of autoimmunity in disease and has no pretense of giving an adequate coverage of the literature; some recent reviews[177, 178] should be consulted for additional information.

If the organism is capable of synthesizing antibodies, and at the same time there are so many potentially antigenic substances in it, how is it that no antibodies are continuously formed against the organism itself? The question has received different answers, of which only four will be considered.

(1) Ehrlich's suggestion, although not actually an answer to the question, but the first clear recognition of the problem, states that by some mechanism the antibody-forming apparatus is capable of discriminating between the organism and everything that is foreign to it; this is the meaning of the concept of "horror autotoxicus," which is just another way of saying that as a rule no autoantibodies are formed in normal subjects.

(2) Burnet and Fenner[50] proposed that all cells of a given organism possess a unique, distinguishing characteristic called "self-marker" and that the antibody-forming apparatus is able to recognize it. When in the presence of "self-marker" the cells in charge of antibody synthesis will remain still, but as soon as a foreign substance or cell gains access to the organism the antibody-forming apparatus would recognize the absence of "self-marker" and would immediately react to it by producing antibody. Indeed, the "self-marker" is just the voicing of Ehrlich's discriminating mechanism.

(3) Felton[63] observed that when massive doses of antigen are given, antibody synthesis is blocked for a long time, a phenomenon usually referred to as "immunologic paralysis." It has been suggested that the same explanation is adequate for the lack of autoimmunity in most individuals, since the organism contains large amounts of most potentially antigenic substances and, therefore, would be in a constant state of "immunologic paralysis."[79]

(4) More recently, Burnet[60] has proposed the clonal selection theory of acquired immunity (p. 373), a vital part of which is the existence of a mechanism by which forbidden clones can be prevented from developing. The immune response is viewed in this theory as a homeostatic mechanism continuously eliminating clones of abnormal globulin producing cells, and disease would appear with failure of the eliminating mechanism. According to this theory, autoantibodies are produced by very few cells through somatic mutations, but are rapidly eliminated through secondary contacts with antigens. A more detailed discussion of this theory is given in the last section of this chapter.

Whatever the explanation, a growing body of evidence has accumulated in support of the concept of autoimmune disease. Briefly stated, it has been demonstrated that both in animals and in man the process of autoimmunization exists and is manifested either by circulating antibodies or cellular sensitivity capable of reacting with the host's own tissues. It must be understood, however, that this does not represent the burial of the concept of "horror autotoxicus," which holds for normal individuals; autoimmunity in disease is the exception to this rule. Furthermore, the presence of autoimmunization in a given pathologic state can represent a collateral, almost incidental phenomenon, and play no significant role in pathogenesis or in clinical manifestation.

Autosensitization may be theoretically explained in three different ways, not necessarily exclusive. First, some tissue component which is normally inaccessible to the antibody-forming apparatus may, as the result of pathologic changes, become accessible and act as an antigen; the result would be the formation of antibodies directed against such a tissue component and the combination of antigen and antibody wherever they happen to come in contact. Endophthalmitis phacoanaphylactica and Hashimoto's disease are apparently explained by this mechanism. The second theoretical alteration of the organism leading to autoimmunity would be a change in a body component, leading to development of antigenic determinants. This change might be caused by infection or by chemical action. Antibody formed against this changed body component is assumed to act also against the corresponding normal, unmodified component. The third theoretical alteration causing autoimmunity is a disturbance in the antibody-forming apparatus which may be produced by infection or somatic mutation, causing the cells to synthesize antibody against normal components of the organism; an instance of this mechanism might be the symptomatic hemolytic anemias of infectious mononucleosis and atypical pneumonia.

There are three categories of evidence implicating autoimmune mechanisms in experimental and human disease.[177] First, in some thyroid and hematologic disorders autoantibodies have been demonstrated beyond reasonable doubt, and very similar conditions have been reproduced in experimental animals. Second, experimental responses in animals to the injection of their own tissues adequately mixed with adjuvants show changes in the peripheral and central nervous systems, uvea, testes, articular tissues and skin, and circulating autoantibodies and/or cutaneous sensitivity to the injected antigens have been demonstrated; so-called allergic encephalomyelitis has been successfully transferred by means of cells in experimental animals. The clinicopathologic features of these experimental diseases are similar to certain human diseases. Third, in some human diseases such as disseminated lupus erythematosus, scleroderma, chronic hepatitis and macroglobulinemia, affinity of the host's gamma globulin for constituents of his own tissues has been demonstrated. Some instances of each one of these three levels of evidence are discussed in the following paragraphs.

1. Thyroid. In a series of papers, Witebsky et al.[180-183] showed that the thyroid has an antigen peculiar to it, not shown by other tissues of the body, but present in different species. Immunization against this antigen has been obtained in rabbits, dogs and guinea pigs, and antithyroid antibodies have been identified by complement fixation, precipitation and hemagglutination of tanned cells. The antigen is thyroglobulin, which normally exists only in thyroid colloid and, therefore, may be considered as foreign to the rest of the organism. In addition to forming detectable circulating autoantibodies, experimental animals injected with thyroid develop marked inflammatory and degenerative changes in their thyroids, bearing a strong resemblance to those of thyroiditis in man.[184, 185] For that reason, a search for thyroid autoantibodies in human cases of chronic thyroiditis, myxedema, subacute thyroiditis of viral origin and thyrotoxicosis was conducted by Roitt, et al. It was found that there were high levels of serum gamma globulin returning to normal within six months after removal of the thyroid;[186] in addition, precipitating antibodies to human thyroid extract and to thyroglobulin were also present in the blood.[187] Some patients with Hashimoto's disease do not show circulating antibody (and no correlation has been observed between the amount of circulating antibody and the extension of the lesions),[188] an observation valid also for dogs and guinea pigs. It has been suggested that the essential feature is the reaction of inflammatory and antibody-producing cells against thyroglobulin *in situ;* it is of only secondary significance whether circulating antibody is liberated. Nevertheless, the mechanism by which circulating antibodies damage the thyroid is not clear,[189] since experimental passive immunization of monkeys with large amounts of Hashimoto sera containing more than 5 mg. per ml. of precipitating antibody protein failed to produce any thyroid changes. The Hashimoto serum cross reacted strongly with monkey thyroid in the precipitin test; the concentration of precipitins in the injected monkey's blood was similar to that found in many Hashimoto patients, but no antibody was fixed in the thyroid according to Coons' fluorescent antibody technique.[190] Participation of delayed sensitivity in this condition has not been ruled out and should be considered.

2. Hematologic System. Autoimmune mechanisms have been described in disorders involving the red blood cells, leukocytes and platelets, both in isolation and in different combinations. Some cases of acquired hemolytic anemia were known to cause red cell agglutination,[191] but the meaning of this change was not clear until Coombs et al.[192] introduced their direct antiglobulin test, which shows the presence of antibodies attached to the patient's erythrocytes.[193] According to the temperature at which such antibodies are effective they are called "warm" and "cold." The former produce hemolysis at environmental temperatures and may be identified by means of antiglobulin during hemolytic crises and not during remissions, while the latter are effective only at lower temperatures and may be identified at all times, irrespective of the presence or absence of hemolysis.[194] Two forms of hemolytic anemia are usually distinguished, which are idiopathic or primary, and symptomatic or secondary; warm and cold antibodies have been identified in both types.[195] Primary hemolytic anemia is a chronic disease accompanied by jaundice and splenomegaly, whereas these manifestations are rare in the symptomatic or secondary forms of hemolytic anemia,[196] which appear after viral pneumonias or infectious mononucleosis, or are secondary to disseminated lupus erythematosus, malignant lymphomas, polyarteritis nodosa and many other diseases.[197] Two mechanisms have been suggested to explain the presence of antibodies: (a) Red cells are altered and acquire antigenic determinants capable of stimulating antibody synthesis.[198] (b) Gamma globulins are abnormal and function as antibodies against normal red blood cells.[199] In view of the frequent elevation of gamma globulins in the serum of these patients, as well as the association with lymphomas and other tumors of the lymphoid organs (lymphocytes are strongly implicated in the synthesis of antibodies), Dacie[194] believes that the second possibility is more plausible. Additional reasons would be that circulating antibodies react as readily with cells from other persons with the same blood type as with the patient's own cells,[200] and that thrombocytopenia is frequently associated with hemolytic anemia.[201] The mechanism by which autoantibodies produce hemolysis is triple:[202] (1) There is autoagglutination of red blood cells with formation of masses which are unable to circulate through the capillaries. They are thus detained in the spleen and in other tissues where they are destroyed by lytic substances. (2) Spherocytosis is also produced by autoantibodies which bring about the same effect as agglutination. (3) Phagocytosis is increased, perhaps through the two preceding mechanisms.

Autoimmunization to leukocytes has been implicated in many cases of leukopenia or agranulocytosis, usually combined with anemia and/or thrombocytopenia.[203, 204] Evans and Duane[205] suggested that destruction of red blood cells, leukocytes and platelets is due to different antibodies, and this has been confirmed on several occasions. Antigens are complex, but appropriate antisera may be obtained by injecting these cells into laboratory animals,[206] Tullis[207] believes that antigens are similar to blood groups A and B, but Rejholec, et al.[208] have identified two leukocytic antigens not correlated with red blood cell groups. Antileukocytic autoantibodies may develop in some forms of drug sensitivity, such as benzene and aminopyrine,[209] or without association with demonstrable exogenous agents. Agranulocytosis may be transferred in humans by means of serum[203, 209] and the same occurs in rabbits;[210] leukoagglutinins move with gamma globulins in electrophoresis and are stable at 56°C and destroyed at 65°C for 30 minutes;[209] leukoagglutinins may be removed from serum specifically by absorption in normal leukocytes and then later eluted from the leukocytes and still possess agglutinating activity for white blood cells.

Thrombocytopenic purpura caused by autoimmunization to the patient's own platelets has been found in two situations: first, in the course of hypersensitivity reactions to drugs in which the drug combines with platelets and makes up an antigenic compound, the condition being known as symptomatic thrombocytopenic purpura; second, without any exogenous influence, in idiopathic thrombocytopenic purpura.[211] The latter may occur alone or in the course of diseases such as leukemia or disseminated lupus erythematosus.[212] Drugs capable of inducing autosensitization to platelets are many, those most frequently encountered being allylisopropylacetylcarbamide (Sedormid),[213] quinine[214] and quinidine;[215] the mechanism of destruction of platelets requires three components, namely the patient's serum, the drug and platelets.[216] In idiopathic thrombocytopenic purpura the patient's platelets serve as complete antigens; according to Harrington, et al.[217] approximately two thirds of the patients show circulating autoantibodies to their platelets. Transfer of the patient's serum or blood to normal recipients will, in most instances, cause a prompt thrombocytopenia with or without associated purpura; this thrombocytopenia lasts 1 to 2 weeks, during which antiplatelet antibodies can be detected in the serum of the recipient and his platelets are coated with globulin.[218] The mechanism of destruction of platelets by autoantibodies seems to be combined. On one hand, platelets are agglutinated and lysed, as observed in *in vitro* tests; on the other hand, platelets are made more susceptible to elimination by phagocytic cells of the spleen and elsewhere. The role of the spleen in eliminating platelets is indicated by the postsplenectomy improvement of some patients in whom antiplatelet antibodies persist in the circulation.[219] In addition, autoantibodies in idiopathic thrombocytopenic purpura damage the megakaryocytes, as shown by transfer studies of a patient's serum to normal recipients and subsequent examination of the latter's bone marrow.[220, 221] Within 30 minutes megakaryocytes show redistribution in the cytoplasmic granules from the normal peripheral clumping to a uniform distribution throughout the entire cytoplasm, and platelets can no longer be identified in their immediate surroundings.

3. Central and Peripheral Nervous Systems. In 1933, Rivers *et al.*[222] reported that repeated injections of homologous or heterologous brain into monkeys were sometimes followed by destructive demyelinating and inflammatory lesions in the central nervous system. Later, this experimental allergic encephalomyelitis was also produced in dogs, cats, pigs, guinea pigs, pigeons, rats, rabbits and mice, by immunization with heterologous, homologous and even autologous brain, mixed with Freund's adjuvant, sometimes after a single or only a few injections.[223] The antigen seems related to myelin, since it is more concentrated in white matter,[224] is absent in the newborn[225] and appears simultaneously with the development of myelin.[226] These observations, plus the fact that the autoimmune response results in extensive destruction of myelin,[227, 228] strongly suggest that the antigen is related to myelin. In animals with experimental allergic encephalomyelitis there are destructive lesions in the brain which develop simultaneously with circulating antibrain antibodies and with delayed sensitivity to brain.[229] Although passive transfer cannot be accomplished by means of circulating antibodies, it has been effected by transfer of cells in rats[230] after some failures in other species.[231] Additional proof of the autoimmune nature of this form of en-

cephalomyelitis is that cortisone inhibits its development[232] and pretreatment with *H. pertussis* vaccine enhances the disease in mice.[233] Many of these studies were stimulated by the existence of rare cases of acute demyelinization following the administration of rabies vaccine, which is prepared with brain substance, and of acute and subacute necrotizing encephalomyelopathy following measles, mumps, influenza, smallpox and other viral diseases.[234] Attempts to explain other human diseases such as diffuse sclerosis, Schilder's disease, metachromatic encephalopathy, etc., have been analyzed by Hurst,[235] who believes that demyelinization is a nonspecific response of the white matter; on this account, suggestions based on morphologic similarities cannot be accepted as evidence in favor of an autoimmune mechanism. Perhaps some authors have gone beyond the evidence in their enthusiasm to find a possible pathogenesis for a group of diseases of unknown etiology; on the other hand, there is much indirect evidence in favor of the idea that autoimmunization may play a role in human demyelinating diseases.[236]

Waksman and Adams [237, 238] produced experimental allergic neuritis in rabbits, guinea pigs and mice by immunization with heterologous or homologous peripheral nerve emulsion with Freund's adjuvant. Complement-fixing antibody and delayed skin sensitivity to the injected antigen were present but were not correlated with the severity of the disease, which appeared mainly in the spinal ganglion, then the dorsal roots, ventral roots and finally the peripheral nerves. The lesions were focal perivascular demyelinization with destruction of axis cylinders and infiltration of histiocytes and lymphocytes with phagocytosis of the altered myelin. These changes resemble acute infectious polyneuritis, the Guillain-Barré syndrome and Landry's paralysis, which are held to be in a single category.[239] The relation between the experimental changes and human disease is still uncertain.

4. Testis. Following the observations of Joisin *et al.*[240] Freund *et al.*[241, 242] injected homologous or autologous testes or sperm in complete adjuvant into guinea pigs and rats and noted an autoimmune response characterized by complement-fixing, sperm-immobilizing and antihyaluronidase antibodies, delayed skin sensitivity and aspermatogenesis. The effective antigen was present only in homologous testes, in a mitochondrial fraction of testis, in washed sperm and in a polysaccharide-like extract of testis. Complement-fixing antibody and delayed skin sensitivity were roughly related to the degree of testicular damage, which could not be transferred by large amounts of serum from immunized guinea pigs. The lesions were complete loss of spermatogenic cells with preservation of Sertoli cells in the tubules; interstitial cells and other structures were not involved, including epididymis and prostate. A somewhat different histologic picture was described by Waksman[243] who found aspermatogenesis complete in young animals and focal in older ones, a predominantly mononuclear infiltration around veins and secondary arrest of spermatogenesis; the areas most severely involved were the epididymis and the rete. The relation of this mechanism for inducing aspermatogenesis to human male infertility is not known, but recently there have been reports of patients with sperm-immobilizing antibodies and infertility.[244, 245]

5. Uvea. Sympathetic ophthalmia is characterized by granulomatous inflammation of the uveal tract occurring some time after traumatic or other lesions of the uveal tract of the opposite eye.[246] For a long time this disease was thought to be the result of an autoimmune response to the antigens of the injured eye (a) because of the interval existing between injury to an eye and development of the lesion in the other, (b) because the uveal pigment serves as antigen and frequently gives positive skin tests in patients with the disease and (c) because of the granulomatous nature of the inflammatory lesion.[247] Experimentally, Collins[248, 249] was able to produce inflammation of the uveal tract in guinea pigs and monkeys by the injection of homologous uvea with complete Freund's adjuvant; in immunized animals trauma to the iris precipitated a reaction in the traumatized eye. Both circulating antibody and delayed hypersensitivity to uveal antigens have been observed in animals inoculated with homologous or heterologous tissue with Freund's adjuvant.[250]

6. Kidney. On the basis of clinical observations glomerulonephritis has long been considered an autoimmune disease. Some of the reasons are as follows: (1) Almost without exception, acute attacks of glomerulonephritis or exacerbations occur some 7 to 14 days after a streptococcal infection, usually in the upper respiratory tract. (2) Streptococci are not found in the kidneys. (3) There are some reports of antikidney antibodies in patients with glomerulonephritis and other renal diseases.[251, 252] (4) Using the fluorescent antibody technique in human cases of glomerulonephritis, Mellors and Ortega[253] showed that there is deposition of gamma globulin in the glomeruli, a finding confirmed and extended to other diseases such as diabetes mellitus, nephrotic syndrome, etc.[254] Experimental production of renal lesions by means of nephrotoxic serum, although resembling those of human glomerulonephritis,[255] may attest more to the limited variety of histologic responses of the kidney than to a similarity in pathogenesis of the two conditions. Cavelti's reports[256–258] that in rats injected with mixtures of homologous or autologous kidney and killed beta-hemolytic streptococci, morphologic and functional renal changes similar to glomerulonephritis are produced, has not been confirmed by many others.[259] Nevertheless, in view of the highly suggestive clinical characteristics of glomerulonephritis, it has been speculated that the pathogenesis may be as follows.[260] The foreign protein of bacteria would combine with a nonantigenic glycoprotein of the glomerulus and would form the antigen; antibodies formed against such antigen would appear and, following their combination, the lesions would be produced. The basement membrane glycoprotein would act as complete hapten, and tissue damage would obey a mechanism similar to the Arthus phenomenon.

7. Adrenal. Colover[261] described an inflammatory reaction in the adrenals of guinea pigs injected with whole guinea pig adrenal and mycobacterial adjuvant. The first lesions appeared in the cortical tissue 40 days after the first inoculation. In a more recent paper, Steiner *et al.*[262] found the same adrenal injury in guinea pigs given homologous or autologous adrenal tissue homogenates in Freund's adjuvant. Since the idiopathic form of Addison's disease has been conceived as an autoimmune process (because of the presence of lymphoid infiltrations in the involved adrenal and the finding of complement-fixing autoantibodies to adrenal extracts in two patients with Addison's disease[263]) these experimental models may serve to explore this possibility further.

8. Others. Affinity of the host's gamma globulin for his own or other tissue components has been reported recently by Gajdusek[264, 265] in patients with chronic liver disease of the type known as lupoid hepatitis, in disseminated lupus erythematosus and macroglobulinemia. Human liver may act as an antigen in a complement-fixation reaction with gamma globulins of these patients, but it is not the only nor the best antigen; these reactions are not tissue- or species-specific, rat tissues providing antigens of almost equivalent reactivity. Using the fluorescent antibody technique Cohen et al.[266] found that in hepatitis and postnecrotic cirrhosis there is deposition of gamma globulin in many reticuloendothelial cells of the hepatic sinusoids and of the fibrous tracts; other liver diseases were negative even in the presence of hypergammaglobulinemia. What role these globulins capable of reacting with tissues play in the pathogenesis of the various diseases remains to be seen. Reference has been made to the L.E. cell and the several instances of autoimmunization in collagen diseases (p. 294).

D. BIOLOGY OF THE IMMUNE RESPONSE

When considered against the background of the organism as a whole, the immune response is at first sight paradoxical. When first discovered, the immune response was held to be defensive in nature since it blocked the deleterious effects of toxins and favored the destruction of microorganisms. This narrow and finalistic interpretation was soon upset, however, by the discovery that the same mechanism was operative in some reactions which injured the host more than the causal agent, and that sometimes such reactions could be elicited by otherwise innocuous substances. Indeed, there is very little proof that delayed sensitivity, the type induced by most infections, plays any role

as a protective mechanism, and there is plenty of evidence that it can create damage and destruction in the host's tissues to a degree usually unwarranted by the hazard of the infection itself. Speculations about the biologic significance of the immune response have been stimulated by the growing body of evidence supporting the same general mechanism as the basis of graft rejection. The untenability of the concept of the immune response as a defense mechanism in view of recent studies on reactions to homologous or heterologous grafts is remarked upon by Thomas.[267] "Nature may have provided checks and balances for all conceivable kinds of untoward events, but I seriously doubt that she deliberately planned for this one. It is an artificial situation, created by meddlesome human begins and, in itself, not a regular circumstance in biology." But rejection of the immune response as a defense mechanism is no answer to the problem of the biologic significance, as neither is Haurowitz's[268] contention that antibody synthesis is an aberration of normal protein synthesis. What is needed is a general interpretation of the immune response which will fit all available facts and, without being unduly finalistic, will lend itself to experimental analysis. Perhaps it would be better to say that such an interpretation should indicate further areas of experimentation, since an heuristic concept has no other value.

Several authors have expressed almost simultaneously a general concept of the immune response which fulfills the requirements set up in the preceding paragraph. The clonal selection theory or acquired immunity of Burnet[60] is perhaps the most complete and coherent analysis of this concept, although Thomas,[267] and Lawrence,[269] have also contributed to it with both pertinent facts and thoughtful discussions. Perhaps the starting point is the recognition that the immune response appears when there is something within the organism that is foreign to it, be it bacteria, toxic protein, inert substance, or cells belonging to another individual; the property of "foreignness" may be acquired also by the host's own components and serve as a stimulus for the immune response. This last observation is the clue to the concept of the immune response as a homeostatic mechanism. Multicellular organisms require preservation of a constant *milieu interne,* which is represented not only by concentration of various substances in the different fluid compartments but by all those features that are recognized as "self." Therefore, uniformity of cell type is necessary for homeostasis, even in the face of wide differentiation of individual cells or tissues. Burnet's theory demands the existence of clones of mesenchymal cells, each carrying immunologically reactive sites corresponding in appropriate complementary fashion to one (or possibly a small number of) potential antigenic determinants. Such clones form part of a mobile population of mesenchymal cells constantly undergoing physiologic and mutational change; when a new clone is initiated through mutational change, it may not deviate from the accepted pattern of the organism and no modification of homeostasis is produced. But if the new clone were to present a marked difference from the rest of the cell population of the organism, it would immediately stimulate the corresponding clone of antibody-forming mesenchymal cells to produce in one way or another more globulin molecules of the cell's characteristic type. The obvious way of achieving this is to postulate that stimulation initiates proliferation of the antibody-forming element. The result would be the inhibition of development and the rapid disappearance of the "foreign" cells.

This theory places the immune response at the level of a homeostatic mechanism; therefore, disease can be understood as a failure, by defect or exaggeration, of this mechanism. A rapid review of those instances in which abnormalities result from the immune response should convince one that the theory fits well with the facts. But this homeostatic mechanism may also be at fault in other conditions which are usually not considered as disturbances of the immune response, the most prominent being cancer. In Chapter V, Green's immunologic theory of the mechanism of cancer was described, but here it is mentioned only to illustrate that preservation of uniformity of cell type is necessary for survival.

REFERENCES

1. Portier, P., and Richet, C.: Action anaphylactique des quelques venins, Compt. rend. Soc. biol. *54:*170, 1902.
2. Boyd, W. C.: Fundamentals of Immunology, ed. 3, New York, Interscience Publications, 1956.
3. Raffel, S.: Immunity. Hypersensitivity. Serology, New York, Appleton-Century-Crofts, 1953.
4. Cushing, J. E., and Campbell, D. H.: Principles of Immunology, New York, McGraw-Hill, 1957.
5. Landsteiner, K.: The Specificity of Serological Reactions, ed. 2, Cambridge, Harvard University Press, 1945.
6. Maurer, P. H.: Antigenicity of gelatin in rabbits and other species, J. Exper. Med. *100:*515, 1954.
7. Maurer, P. H.: The antigenicity of polyvinyl pyrolidone, J. Immunol. *77:*105, 1956.
8. Avery, O. T.: The role of specific carbohydrates in pneumococcus infection and immunity, Ann. Int. Med. *6:*1, 1932.
9. Oliver González, J.: Functional antigens in helminths, J. Infect. Dis. *78:*232, 1946.
10. Burger, M.: Bacterial Polysaccharides, Springfield, Charles C Thomas, 1950.
11. Kabat, E. A.: Blood Group Substances. Their Chemistry and Immunochemistry, New York, Academic Press, 1956.
12. Sussman, L. N.: Blood grouping tests in disputed paternity proceedings, J.A.M.A. *155:*1143, 1954.
13. Owen, R. D., Stormont, C., Wexler, I. B., and Wiener, A. S.: Committee on Medico Legal Problems. Medicolegal applications of blood grouping tests, J.A.M.A. *164:*2036, 1957.
14. Sussman, L. N.: Pitfalls of paternity blood grouping tests, Am. J. Clin. Path. *33:*406, 1960.
15. Race, R. R., and Sanger, R.: Blood Groups in Man, London, Oxford University Press, 1954.
16. Mourant, A. E.: The Distribution of Human Blood Groups, London, Oxford University Press, 1954.
17. Kauffman, F., Mørch, E., and Schmith, K.: On serology of pneumococcus-group, J. Immunol. *39:*397, 1940.
18. Lancefield, R. C.: Cellular Constituents of Group A Streptococci Concerned in Antigenicity and Virulence, in McCarthy, M. (ed.): Streptococcal Infections, New York, Columbia University Press, 1954.
19. Rothbard, S., and Watson, R. F.: Variations occurring in group A streptococci during human infection; progressive loss of M substance correlated with increasing susceptibility to bacteriostasis, J. Exper. Med. *87:*521, 1948.
20. Wertheim, A. R., Lyttle, J. D., Loeb, E. N., Earle, D. P., Seegal, B. C., and Seegal, D.: The association of type specific streptococci with acute glomerulonephritis, J. Clin. Invest. *32:*359, 1953.
21. Kuttner, A. G., and Krumwiede, E.: Observations on the effect of streptococcal upper respiratory infections in rheumatic children: a three year study, J. Clin. Invest. *20:*273, 1941.
22. Dubos, R. J.: The Bacterial Cell in Its Relation to Problems of Virulence, Immunity, and Chemotherapy, Cambridge, Harvard University Press, 1945.
23. Felix, A., and Pitt, R. M.: Virulence of *B. typhosus* and resistance to O antibody, J. Path. & Bact. *38:*409, 1934.
24. Burnet, F. M., and Stanley, W. M.: The Viruses. Biochemical, Biological and Biophysical Properties. Vol. III. Academic Press, Inc., New York, 1959.
25. Forssman, J.: Die Herstellung hochwertiger spezi-

fischer Schafhämolysine ohne Verwendung von Schafblut: Ein Beitrag zur Lehre von heterologen Antikörperbildung. Biochem. Ztschr. *37:* 78, 1911.

26. Zinsser, H.: On the essential identity of the antibodies, J. Immunol. *6:*289, 1921.

27. Askonas, B. A., Humphrey, J. H., and Porter, R. R.: On origin of multiple forms of rabbit γ-globulin, Biochem. J. *63:*412, 1956.

28. Kabat, E. A.: The Unity and Diversity of Antibodies, in Pappenheimer, A. M., Jr. (ed.): The Nature and Significance of the Antibody Response, New York, Columbia University Press, 1953.

29. Enders, J. F.: Chemical, clinical, and immunological studies on human plasma fractionation X. Concentrations of certain antibodies in globulin fractions derived from human blood plasma, J. Clin. Invest. *23:*510, 1944.

30. Faure, R., Fine, J. M., Saint-Paul, M., Eyquem, A., and Grabar, P.: Etude immunoélectrophorétique des hémagglutinines du sérum humaine, Bull. Soc. chim. biol. *37:*783, 1955.

31. Keckwick, R. A., and Record, B. R.: Some physical properties of diphtheria antitoxic horse serum, Brit. J. Exper. Path. *22:*29, 1941.

32. Smith, E. L., and Jager, B. V.: The characterization of antibodies, Ann. Rev. Microbiol. *6:*207, 1952.

33. Gitlin, D., Hitzig, W. H., and Janeway, C. A.: Multiple serum protein deficiencies in congenital and acquired agammaglobulinemia, J. Clin. Invest. *35:*1199, 1956.

34. Oncley, J. L.: Physical Characteristics of Gamma Globulins, in Tullis, J. L. (ed.): Blood Cells and Plasma Proteins: Their State in Nature, New York, Academic Press, 1953.

35. Pappenheimer, A. M., Jr.: Valence of Antibodies, in Pappenheimer, A. M., Jr. (Ed.): The Nature and Significance of the Antibody Response, New York, Columbia University Press, 1953.

36. McMaster, P. D.: Sites of Antibody Formation, in Pappenheimer, A. M., Jr. (Ed.): The Nature and Significance of the Antibody Response, New York, Columbia University Press, 1953.

37. Harris, T. N., and Harris, S.: The genesis of antibodies, Am. J. Med. *20:*114, 1956.

38. Roberts, K. B.: The failure of macrophages to produce antibodies, Brit. J. Exper. Path. *36:* 199, 1955.

39. Stevens, K. M., and McKenna, J. M.: Studies on antibody synthesis initiated *in vitro,* J. Exper. Med. *107:*537, 1958.

40. McKenna, J. M., and Stevens, K. M.: Studies on antibody formation by peritoneal exudate cells *in vitro,* J. Exper. Med. *111:*573, 1960.

41. Harris, T. N., and Harris, S.: Influenzal antibodies in lymphocytes of rabbits following the local injection of virus, J. Immunol. *61:*193, 1949.

42. Wesslén, T.: Studies on the role of lymphocytes in antibody production, Acta dermat.-venereol. *32:*265, 1952.

43. Roberts, J. C., and Dixon, F.: The transfer of lymph node cells in the study of the immune response to foreign proteins, J. Exper. Med. *102:*379, 1955.

44. Bjørneboe, M., Gormsem, H., and Lundquist, F.: Further experimental studies on the role of plasma cells as antibody producers, J. Immunol. *55:*121, 1947.

45. Fagraeus, A.: The plasma cellular reaction and its relation to the formation of antibodies in vitro, J. Immunol. *58:*1, 1948.

46. Coons, A. H., Leduc, E. H., and Connolly, J. M.: Studies on antibody production. I. A method for histochemical demonstration of specific antibody and its application to a study of the hyperimmune rabbit, J. Exper. Med. *102:*49, 1955.

47. Nossal, G. J. V.: Antibody production by single cells. IV. The histology of antibody production, Brit. J. Exper. Path. *40:*301, 1959.

48. Reiss, E., Mertens, E., and Ehrich, W E.: Agglutination of bacteria by lymphoid cells *in vitro,* Proc. Soc. Exper. Biol. & Med. *74:*732, 1950.

49. Craig, J. M., Gitlin, D., and Jewett, T. C.: Response of lymph node of normal and congenitally agammaglobulinemic children to antigenic stimulation, Am. J. Dis. Child. *88:*626, 1954.

50. Burnet, F. M., and Fenner, F.: The Production of Antibodies, ed. 2, Melbourne, Macmillan, 1949.

51. Roberts, J. C., Dixon, F. J., and Weigle, W. O.: Antibody-producing lymph node cells and peritoneal exudate cells, Arch. Path. *64:*324, 1957.

52. Roberts, J. C.: Role of the Lymphocyte in Antibody Production, in Rebuck, J. W. (Ed.): The Lymphocyte and Lymphocytic Tissue, New York, P. B. Hoeber, 1960.

53. Oakley, C. L.: The Localization of Antibody Production, in Collins, D. H. (Ed.): Modern Trends in Pathology, London, Butterworth, 1959.

54. Breinl, F., and Haurowitz, F.: Chemische Untersuchung des Präzipitates aus Hämoglobin und Anti-Hämoglobin-Serum und Bemerkung ueber die Natur der Antikörper, Ztschr. physiol. Chem. *192:*45, 1930.

55. Kaplan, M. H., Coons, A. H., and Deans, H. W.: Localization of antigens in tissue cells, J. Exper. Med. *91:*15, 1950.

56. Pauling, L.: A theory of the structure and process of formation of antibodies, J. Am. Chem. Soc. *62:*2643, 1940.

57. Smith, E. L., McFadden, M. L., Stockell, A., and Buettner-Janusch, V.: Amino acid composition of four rabbit antibodies, J. Biol. Chem. *214:* 197, 1955.

58. Stavitsky, A. B.: *In vitro* production of diphtheria antitoxin by tissues of immunized animals. III. Incorporation of amino acids into antibody; relationship to antibody synthesis and sensitivity relative to other methods, Brit. J. Exper. Path. *39:*661, 1958.

59. Jerne, N. K.: The natural selection theory of antibody formation, Proc. Nat. Acad. Sc. *41:*849, 1955.

60. Burnet, M.: The Clonal Selection Theory of Acquired Immunity, Cambridge, Cambridge University Press, 1959.

61. Edsall, G.: Factors Affecting the Antibody Response, in Pappenheimer, A. M., Jr. (Ed.): The Nature and Significance of the Antibody Response, New York, Columbia University Press, 1953.

62. Edsall, G., Banton, H. J., and Wheeler, R. E.: The antigenicity of single, graded doses of purified diphtheria toxoid in man, Am. J. Hyg. *53:*283, 1951.

63. Felton, L. R.: The significance of antigen in animal tissues, J. Immunol. *61:*107, 1949.

64. Dixon, F. J., and Maurer, P. H.: Immunologic unresponsiveness induced by protein antigens, J. Exper. Med. *101:*245, 1955.

65. Stark, O. K.: Studies on pneumococcal polysaccharide. II. Mechanism involved in production of "immunological paralysis" by type I pneumococcal polysaccharide, J. Immunol. *74:*130, 1955.

66. Levine, L., Wyman, L., and Edsall, G.: Chemical and immunological properties of diphtheria tox-

oid purified by ammonium sulfate fractionation, J. Immunol. *63:*219, 1949.

67. Freund, J., and Bonanto, M. V.: The effect of parafin oil, lanolin-like substances and killed tubercle bacilli on immunization with diphtheria toxoid and *Bact. typhosum,* J. Immunol. *48:* 325, 1944.

68. Rowley, D. A.: The effect of splenectomy on the formation of circulating antibody in the adult male albino rat, J. Immunol. *64:*289, 1950.

69. Cannon, P. R., Chase, W. E., and Wissler, R. W.: The relationship of protein reserves to antibody production. I. The effects of a low protein diet and of plasmapheresis on the formation of agglutinins, J. Immunol. *47:*133, 1943.

70. Lisker, R., Chagoya, V., and Laguna, J.: Respuesta immunológica en la desnutrición, Rev. Invest. Clin. *6:*473, 1954.

71. Axelrod, A. E.: The role of nutritional factors in the antibody responses of the anamnestic process, Am. J. Clin. Nutr. *6:*119, 1958.

72. Axelrod, A. E., and Pruzansky, J.: Role of the vitamins in antibody production, Vitamins and Hormones *13:*1, 1955.

73. Taliaferro, W. H., and Taliaferro, L. G.: The effect of x-rays on immunity: a review, J. Immunol. *66:*181, 1951.

74. Murphy, J. B., and Sturm, E.: The lymphoid tissue and antibody formation, Proc. Soc. Exper. Biol. & Med. *66:*303, 1947.

75. Dews, P. B., and Code, C. F.: Anaphylactic reactions and concentrations of antibody in rats and rabbits. Effect of adrenalectomy and of administration of cortisone, J. Immunol. *70:*199, 1953.

76. Hammond, C. W., and Novak, M.: Relation of adrenal cortical steroids to antibody release, Proc. Soc. Exper. Biol. & Med. *74:*155, 1950.

77. Germuth, F. G., Jr.: The role of adrenocortical steroids in infection, immunity, and hypersensitivity, Pharmacol. Rev. *8:*1, 1956.

78. Germuth, F. G., Jr., Ottinger, B., and Oyama, J.: Influence of cortisone on experimental hypersensitivity and circulating antibody in the guinea pig, Proc. Soc. Exper. Biol. & Med. *80:*188, 1952.

79. Kilbourne, E. D.: Influence of cortisone on experimental viral infection. II. Effects on antibody formation and acquired immunity, Proc. Soc. Exper. Biol. & Med. *90:*685, 1955.

80. De Vries, J. A.: The effect of adrenocorticotrophic hormone on circulating antibody levels, J. Immunol. *65:*1, 1950.

81. Larson, D. L., and Tomlinson, L. J.: Quantitative antibody studies in man. I. The effect of adrenal insufficiency and of cortisone on the level of circulating antibodies, J. Clin. Invest. *30:*1451, 1951.

82. Havens, W. P., Jr., Shaffer, J. M., and Hopke, C. J.: The capacity of patients with chronic hepatic disease to produce antibody and the effect of ACTH and cortisone on this function, J. Clin. Invest. *30:*647, 1951.

83. Nilzen, A.: The influence of the thyroid gland on the histamine and anaphylactic reactions in animals. III. The influence of thyroidectomy on the precipitin reaction, the Arthus phenomenon and the Schulz-Dale reaction in guinea pigs, Acta allergol. *8:*103, 1955.

84. Rose, B.: Hormones and allergic responses, in Shaffer, J. H., *et al.* (Eds.): Mechanisms of Hypersensitivity, Boston, Little, Brown, 1959.

85. Pauling, L.: Antibodies and specific biological forces. Endeavour *7:*43, 1948.

86. Germuth, F. G., Jr., and McKinnon, G. E.: Studies on the biological properties of antigen-antibody complexes. I. Anaphylactic shock induced by soluble antigen-antibody complexes in unsensitized normal guinea pigs, Bull. Johns Hopkins Hosp. *101:*13, 1957.

87. Tokuda, S., and Weiser, R. S.: Production of anaphylaxis in the white mouse with soluble antigen-antibody complexes, Science *127:*1327, 1958.

88. Trapani, I. L., Garvey, J. S., and Campbell, D. H.: Stimulating action of soluble antigen-antibody complexes in normal guinea pig smooth muscle, Science *127:*700, 1958.

89. Ishizaka, K., and Campbell, D. H.: Biological activity of soluble antigen-antibody complexes. I. Skin reactive properties, Proc. Soc. Exper. Biol. & Med. *97:*635, 1958.

90. McCluskey, R. T., Benacerraf, B., Potter, J. L., and Miller, F.: The pathologic effects of intravenously administered soluble antigen-antibody complexes. I. Passive serum sickness in mice, J. Exper. Med. *111:*181, 1960.

91. Benacerraf, B., Potter, J. L., McCluskey, R. T., and Miller, F.: The pathologic effects of intravenously administered soluble antigen-antibody complexes. II. Acute glomerulonephritis in rats, J. Exper. Med. *111:*195, 1960.

92. Dixon, F. J., Vázquez, J. J., Weigle, W. O., and Cochrane, C. G.: Pathogenesis of serum sickness, Arch. Path. *65:*18, 1958.

93. Lawrence, H. S.: The delayed type of allergic inflammatory response, Am. J. Med. 428, 1956.

94. Angevine, D. M.: A comparison of cutaneous sensitization and antibody formation in rabbits immunized by intravenous or intradermal injections of indifferent or hemolytic streptococci, J. Exper. Med. *73:*57, 1941.

95. Lawrence, H. S.: The cellular transfer of cutaneous hypersensitivity to tuberculin in man, Proc. Soc. Exper. Biol. & Med. *71:*516, 1949.

96. Rose, B.: Role of histamine in anaphylaxis and allergy, Am. J. Med. *3:*545, 1947.

97. Gaddum, J. H.: Histamine, Brit. M. J. *1:*867, 1948.

98. Rosenthal, S. R., and Brown, M. L.: Thymoxyethyldiethylamine as antagonist of histamine and of anaphylactic reactions, J. Immunol. *38:*259, 1940.

99. Brocklehurst, W. E., Humphrey, J. H., and Perry, W. L. M.: The role of histamine in cutaneous antigen-antibody reactions in the rat, J. Physiol. *129:*305, 1955.

100. Dragstedt, C. A., and Gebauer-Fuelnegg, E.: Studies in anaphylactic shock, Am. J. Physiol. *102:*512, 1932.

101. Code, C. F.: The histamine content of the blood of guinea pigs and dogs during anaphylactic shock, Am. J. Physiol. *127:*78, 1939.

102. Feldberg, W.: Distribution of Histamine in the Body, in Woltensholme, G. E. W., and O'Connor, C. M. (Eds.): Histamine, Ciba Symposium, London, J. & A. Churchill, 1956.

103. Fulton, G. P., Maynard, F. L., Riley, J. F., and West, G. B.: Humoral aspects of tissue mast cells, Physiol. Rev. *37:*221, 1957.

104. Carter, P. B., Higginbotham, R. D., and Dougherty, T. F.: The local response of tissue mast cells to antigen in sensitized mice, J. Immunol. *79:* 259, 1957.

105. Ungar, G.: Biochemical mechanism of the allergic reaction, Internat. Arch. Allergy *4:*258, 1953.

106. Humphrey, J. H., and Jacques, R.: The histamine and 5-hydroxytryptamine content of platelets and leucocytes in various species, J. Physiol. *124:*305, 1954.

107. Jaques, L. B., and Waters, E. T.: The isolation of crystalline heparin from the blood of dogs in

anaphylactic shock, Am. J. Physiol. *129:*389, 1940.

108. Waalkes, T. P., Weissbach, H., Bozicevich, J., and Undefriend, S.: Serotonin and histamine release during anaphylaxis in the rabbit, J. Clin. Invest. *36:*1115, 1957.

109. Sparrow, E. M., and Wilhelm, D. L.: Species differences in susceptibility to capillary permeability factors. Histamine, 5-hydroxytryptamine and compound 48/80, J. Physiol. *137:*51, 1957.

110. Kellaway, C. H., and Trethewie, E. R.: The liberation of a slow-reacting smooth muscle stimulating substance in anaphylaxis, Quart. J. Exper. Physiol. *30:*121, 1940.

111. Brocklehurst, W. E.: A Slow Reacting Substance in Anaphylaxis "SRS-A," in Woltensholme, G. E. W., and O'Connor, C. M. (Eds.): Histamine, Ciba Symposium, London, J. & A. Churchill, 1956.

112. Beraldo, W. T.: Formation of bradykinin in anaphylactic and peptone shock. Am. J. Physiol. *163:*283, 1950.

113. Rose, B., Rusted, I., and Fownes, J. A.: Intravascular catheterization studies of bronchial asthma. I. Histamine levels in arterial and mixed venous blood of asthmatic patients before and during attacks, J. Clin. Invest. *29:*1113, 1950.

114. Adam, H. M.: Excretion of histamine in human urine, Quart. J. Exper. Physiol. *35:*281, 1950.

115. Seegal, B. C.: Anaphylaxis, in Gay, F. P. (Ed.): Agents of Disease and Host Resistance, Springfield, Charles C Thomas, 1935.

116. Dixon, F. J., and Warren, S.: Antigen tracer studies and histologic observations in anaphylactic shock in the guinea pig, Am. J. Med. Sc. *219:*414, 1950.

117. Rich, A. R., and Follis, R. H., Jr.: Studies on the site of sensitivity in the Arthus phenomenon, Bull. Johns Hopkins Hosp. *66:*106, 1940.

118. Raffel, S.: Immunity, Hypersensitivity, Serology, New York, Appleton-Century-Crofts, 1953.

119. Dragstedt, L. A.: Anaphylaxis, Physiol. Rev. *21:*563, 1941.

120. Kojis, F. G.: Serum sickness and anaphylaxis, Am. J. Dis. Child. *64:*93, 313, 1942.

121. Arthus, M.: Injections répétées de serum de cheval chez le lapin, Comp. rend. Soc. biol. *55:*817, 1903.

122. Goddard, J. W.: Vascular changes in the Arthus phenomenon, Arch. Path. *66:*384, 1958.

123. McMaster, P. D.: General and Local Vascular Reactions in Certain States of Hypersensitivity, in Lawrence, H. S. (Ed.): Cellular and Humoral Aspects of Hypersensitive States, New York, Hoeber-Harper, 1959.

124. Benacerraff, B., and Kabat, E. A.: A quantitative study of the Arthus phenomenon induced passively in the guinea pig, J. Immunol. *64:*1, 1950.

125. Stetson, C. A.: Similarities in the mechanisms determining the Arthus and Schwartzman phenomena, J. Exper. Med. *94:*347, 1951.

126. Culbertson, J. T.: The relationship of circulating antibody to the local inflammatory reaction to antigen (the Arthus phenomenon), J. Immunol. *29:*29, 1935.

127. Tumpeer, I. H., and Cope, E. J.: The Arthus phenomenon, Am. J. Dis. Child. *45:*342, 1933.

128. Dammin, G. J.: Serum Sickness and Related States, in Lawrence, H. S. (Ed.): Cellular and Humoral Aspect of Hypersensitive States, New York, Hoeber-Harper, 1959.

129. von Pirquet, C. F., and Schick, B.: Serum sickness, ed. 2, Baltimore, Williams and Wilkins, 1951.

130. Longcope, W. T., and Rackemann, F. M.: The relation of circulating antibodies to serum disease, J. Exper. Med. *26:*341, 1918.

131. Karelitz, S., and Stempien, S. S.: Studies on the specific mechanism of serum sickness, passive serum sickness, J. Immunol. *44:*271, 1942.

132. Rich, A. R.: The experimental demonstration that periarteritis nodosa is a manifestation of hypersensitivity, Bull. Johns Hopkins Hosp. *72:*65, 1943.

133. Dammin, G. J., Bukantz, S. C., and Alexander, H. A.: Modification of biologic response in experimental hypersensitivity, J.A.M.A. *139:*358, 1949.

134. Rich, A. R.: Hypersensitivity in disease, with special reference to periarteritis nodosa, rheumatic fever, disseminated lupus erythematosus, and rheumatoid arthritis, Harvey Lect. *42:*106, 1947.

135. Germuth, F. G., Jr.: A comparative histologic and immunologic study in rabbits of induced hypersensitivity of the serum sickness type, J. Exper. Med. *97:*257, 1953.

136. Waugh, D.: Myocarditis, arteritis, and focal hepatic, splenic and renal granulomas apparently due to penicillin sensitivity, Am. J. Path. *28:*437, 1952.

137. Wittich, F. W.: Allergic diseases in animals, Progr. Allergy *2:*58, 1949.

138. Waksman, B. H.: The Toxic Effects of the Antigen-Antibody Reaction on the Cells of Hypersensitive Reactors, in Lawrence, H. S. (Ed.): Cellular and Humoral Aspects of the Hypersensitive States, New York, Hoeber-Harper, 1959.

139. Kuhns, W. J., and Pappenheimer, A. M., Jr.: Immunochemical studies of antitoxin produced in normal and allergic individuals hyperimmunized with diphtheria toxoid, J. Exper. Med. *95:*363, 375, 1952.

140. Reddin, L., Jr.: A classification of allergic diseases and their specific manifestations in animals, Ann. New York Acad. Sc. *50:*692, 1949.

141. Halpern, B. N., Biozzi, G., and Benacerraf, B.: Mise en évidence du role des facteurs irritatifs et des traumatismes dans la localisation élective des anticorps dan les organes de choc, Acta allergol. *8:*181, 1955.

142. Lowell, F. C.: Bronchial asthma, Am. J. Med. *20:*778, 1956.

143. Schiller, I. W., and Lowell, F. C.: Pulmonary function in bronchial asthma, J. Allergy *25:*364, 1954.

144. Kountz, W. B., and Alexander, H. L.: Emphysema, Medicine *13:*251, 1934.

145. Lawrence, H. S.: The delayed type of allergic inflammatory response, Am. J. Med. *20:*428, 1956.

146. Cole, L. R., and Favour, C. B.: Correlations between plasma protein fractions, antibody titers, and the passive transfer of delayed and immediate cutaneous reactivity to tuberculin PPD and tuberculopolysaccharides, J. Exper. Med. *101:*391, 1955.

147. Chase, M. W.: The cellular transfer of cutaneous hypersensitivity to tuberculin, Proc. Soc. Exper. Biol. & Med. *59:*134, 1945.

148. Jeter, W. S., Tremaine, M. M., and Seebohm, P. M.: Passive transfer of delayed hypersensitivity to 2,4-Dinitrochlorobenzene in guinea pigs with leucocytic extracts, Proc. Soc. Exper. Biol. & Med. *86:*251, 1954.

149. Lawrence, H. S.: The transfer in humans of delayed skin sensitivity to streptococcal M-substance and to tuberculin with disrupted leucocytes, J. Clin. Invest. *34:*219, 1955.

150. Pappenheimer, A. M., Jr., Scharff, M., and Uhr, J. W.: Delayed Hypersensitivity and Its Possible Relation to Antibody Formation, in Shaffer, J. H., LoGrippo, G. A., and Chase, M. W. (Eds.): Mechanisms of Hypersensitivity, Boston, Little, Brown, 1959.

151. Pappenheimer, A. M., Jr., and Freund, J.: Induction of Delayed Hypersensitivity to Protein Antigens, in Lawrence, H. S. (Ed.): Cellular and Humoral Aspects of Hypersensitive States, New York, Hoeber-Harper, 1959.

152. Eisen, H. N.: Hypersensitivity to Simple Chemicals, in Lawrence, H. S. (Ed.): Cellular and Humoral Aspects of Hypersensitive States, New York, Hoeber-Harper, 1959.

153. Pappenheimer, A. M., Jr.: Hypersensitivity of the delayed type, Harvey Lect., *52*:100, 1956.

154. Uhr, J. W., Pappenheimer, A. M., Jr., and Yoneda, M.: Induction of delayed hypersensitivity to diphtheria toxin in guinea pigs by infection with *C. diphtheriae,* J. Exper. Med. *105*:1, 1957.

155. Uhr, J. W., Salvin, S. B., and Pappenheimer, A. M., Jr.: Induction of delayed hypersensitivity in guinea pigs by means of antigen-antibody complexes, J. Exper. Med. *105*:11, 1957.

156. Good, R. A., Zak, S. J., Jensen, D. R., and Pappenheimer, A. M., Jr.: Delayed allergy and agammaglobulinemia, J. Clin. Invest. *36*:908, 1957.

157. Porter, H. M.: Demonstration of delayed type reactivity in congenital agammaglobulinemia, Ann. New York Acad. Sc. *64*:932, 1957.

158. Landsteiner, K., and Chase, M. W.: Studies on the sensitization of animals with simple chemical compounds. VII. Skin sensitization by intraperitoneal injection, J. Exper. Med. *71*:237, 1940.

159. Good, R. A., and Zak, S. J.: Disturbances in gamma globulin synthesis as "experiments of nature," Pediatrics *18*:109, 1956.

160. Warwick, W. J., Page, A., and Good, R. A.: Passive transfer with circulating leucocytes of delayed hypersensitivity to cat scratch antigen, Proc. Soc. Exper. Biol. & Med. *93*:253, 1956.

161. Ebstein, W. L., and Kligman, A. M.: Transfer of allergic contact-type delayed sensitivity in man, J. Invest. Dermat. *28*:291, 1957.

162. Lawrence, H. S.: The Transfer of Hypersensitivity of the Delayed Type in Man, in Lawrence, H. S. (Ed.): Cellular and Humoral Aspects of Hypersensitive States, New York, Hoeber-Harper, 1959.

163. Lawrence, H. S., Rapaport, F. T., Converse, J. M., and Tillet, W. S.: Transfer of delayed hypersensitivity to skin homografts with leukocyte extracts in man, J. Clin. Invest. *39*:185, 1960.

164. Lawrence, H. S., and Pappenheimer, A. M., Jr.: Effect of specific antigen on release from human leucocytes of the factor concerned in transfer of delayed hypersensitivity, J. Clin. Invest. *36:*908, 1957.

165. Stavitsky, A. B.: Passive cellular transfer of the tuberculin type of hypersensitivity, Proc. Soc. Exper. Biol. & Med. *67*:225, 1948.

166. Lawrence, H. S., and Pappenheimer, A. M., Jr.: Transfer of delayed hypersensitivity to diphtheria toxin in man, J. Exper. Med. *104*:321, 1956.

167. Metaxas, M. N., and Metaxas-Bühler, M.: Studies on the cellular transfer of tuberculin sensitivity in the guinea pig, J. Immunol. *75*:333, 1955.

168. Good, R. A., Bridges, R. A., Zak, S. J., and Pappenheimer, A. M., Jr.: Delayed Hypersensitivity, in Shaffer, J. H., LoGrippo, G. A., and Chase, M. W. (Eds.): Mechanisms of Hypersensitivity, Boston, Little, Brown, 1959.

169. Rich, A. R., and Lewis, M. R.: The nature of allergy in tuberculosis as revealed by tissue culture studies, Bull. Johns Hopkins Hosp. *50*:115, 1932.

170. Favour, C. B.: *In vitro* studies on cell injury in the tuberculin-type reaction: implications in homotransplantation, Ann. New York Acad. Sc. *64:* 842, 1957.

171. Rich, A. R.: The Pathogenesis of Tuberculosis, ed. 2, Springfield, Charles C Thomas, 1951.

172. Rich, A. R.: The significance of hypersensitivity in infections, Physiol. Rev. *21*:70, 1941.

173. MacLeod, C. M.: The Pneumococci, in Dubos, R. J. (Ed.): Bacterial and Mycotic Infections of Man, ed. 2, Philadelphia, J. B. Lippincott, 1952.

174. Rothschild, H., Friedenwald, J. S., and Bernstein, C.: The relation of allergy to immunity in tuberculosis, Bull. Johns Hopkins Hosp. *54.*232, 1934.

175. Bailly, M. D.: quoted in Seegal, B. C.: Allergy in infection: relation to immunity, Ann. New York Acad. Sc. *50*:758, 1949.

176. Cannon, P. R.: The functional significance of specific agglutinins and precipitins, Physiol. Rev. *20*:89, 1940.

177. Dixon, F. J.: Autoimmunity in disease, Ann. Rev. Med. *9*:257, 1958.

178. Clough, P. W.: Auto-immunization and auto-antibodies, Ann. Int. Med. *52*:930, 1960.

179. Wiener, A. S.: Solution of certain fundamental immunological problems by studies on Rh sensitization, Ann. Allergy *10*:535, 1952.

180. Witebsky, E., Rose, N. R., and Shulman, S.: Studies on organ specificity. I. Serological specificity of thyroid extracts, J. Immunol. *75*:269, 1955.

181. Rose, N. R., and Witebsky, E.: Studies on organ specificity. II. Serological interrelationships among thyroid extracts of various species, J. Immunol. *75*:282, 1955.

182. Shulman, S., Rose, N. R., and Witebsky, E.: Studies on organ specificity. III. Ultracentrifugal and electrophoretic examinations of thyroid extracts, J. Immunol. *75*:291, 1955.

183. Witebsky, E., and Rose, N. R.: Studies on organ specificity. IV. Production of rabbit thyroid antibodies in the rabbit, J. Immunol. *76*:408, 1956.

184. Rose, N. R., and Witebsky, E.: Studies in organ specificity. V. Changes in thyroid glands of rabbits following active immunization with rabbit thyroid extracts, J. Immunol. *76*:417, 1956.

185. Terplan, K. L., Witebsky, E., Rose, N. R., Paine, J. R., and Egan, R. W.: Experimental thyroiditis in rabbits, guinea pigs and dogs, following immunization with thyroid extracts of their own and of heterologous species, Am. J. Path. *36:* 213, 1960.

186. Roitt, I. M., Doniach, D., and Campbell, P. N.: The nature of the gamma globulins in lymphadenoid goitre, Biochem. J. *64*:54, 1956.

187. Doniach, D., and Roitt, I. M.: Auto-immunity in Hashimoto's disease and its implications, J. Clin. Endocrinol. *17*:1293, 1957.

188. Roitt, I. M., and Doniach, D.: Thyroid auto-immunity, Brit. M. Bull. *16*:152, 1960.

189. Roitt, I. M., Doniach, D., Campbell, P. N., and Hudson, R. V.: Auto-antibodies in Hashimoto's disease (lymphadenoid goitre), Lancet *2*:820, 1956.

190. Roitt, I. M., and Doniach, D.: The Incidence, Nature, and Significance of Auto-antibodies in Thyroid Disease, in Shaffer, J. H., LoGrippo, G. A.,

and Chase, M. W. (Eds.): Mechanisms of Hypersensitivity, Boston, Little, Brown, 1959.

191. Dameshek, W., and Schwartz, S. O.: Hemolysins as the cause of clinical and experimental hemolytic anemias with particular reference to the nature of spherocytosis and increased fragility, Am. J. Med. Sc. *196:*759, 1938.

192. Coombs, R. R. A., Mourant, A. E., and Race, R. R.: A new test for the detection of weak and incomplete Rh agglutinins, Brit. J. Exper. Path. *26:*255, 1945.

193. Loutit, J. F., and Mollison, P. L.: Haemolytic icterus (acholuric jaundice) congenital and acquired, J. Path. & Bact. *58:*711, 1946.

194. Dacie, J. V.: The auto-immune hemolytic anemias, Am. J. Med. *18:*810, 1955.

195. Wiener, A. S., Samwick, A. A., Morrison, M., and Loewe, L.: Acquired hemolytic anemia, Am. J. Clin. Path. *22:*301, 1952.

196. Dacie, J. V.: The Hemolytic Anemias: Congenital and Acquired, London, J. & A. Churchill, 1954.

197. Marshall, J., Zoutendyk, A., and Gear, J.: Serum auto-antibodies in diseases of skin, South African M. J. *25:*764, 1951.

198. Stats, D., and Wasserman, L. R.: A critique of our knowledge of the etiology of hemolytic anemia, Tr. New York Acad. Sc. *14:*238, 1952.

199. Rosenthal, M. C., Komninos, Z. D., and Dameshek, W.: Multiple antibody formation in autoimmune hemolytic anemia; report of case, New Eng. J. Med. *248:*537, 1953.

200. Dacie, J. V., and Cutbush, M.: Specificity of autoantibodies in acquired hemolytic anemias, J. Clin. Path. *7:*18, 1954.

201. Evans, R. S., Takahashi, K., Duane, R. T., Layne, R., and Liu, C. K.: Primary thrombocytopenic purpura and acquired hemolytic anemia. Evidence for a common etiology, Arch. Int. Med. *87:*48, 1951.

202. Wasastjerna, C.: Immunohemolytic mechanisms in vivo: mode of destruction of sensitized red cells in living organism, Blood *8:*1042, 1953.

203. Moeschlin, S., Siegenthaler, W., Gasser, C., and Hasseg, A.: Immunopancytopenia associated with incomplete cold hemagglutinins in a case of primary atypical pneumonia, Blood *9:*214, 1954.

204. Matoth, Y., Elian, E., Nelken, D., and Nevo, A.: Specificity of lytic factors for erythrocytes, leukocytes and platelets in a case of pancytopenia, Blood *11:*735, 1956.

205. Evans, R. S., and Duane, R. T.: Acquired hemolytic anemia. Relation of erythrocyte antibody production to activity of disease; significance of thrombocytopenia and leukopenia, Blood *4:*1196, 1949.

206. Finch, S. C., Ross, J. F., and Ebaugh, F. F.: Immunologic mechanisms of leukocyte abnormalities, J. Lab. & Clin. Med. *42:*555, 1953.

207. Tullis, J. L.: Blood Cells and Plasma Proteins, New York, Academic Press, 1953.

208. Rejholec, V., Donner, L., Wagner, V., and Mandlikova, Z.: Certain antigenic properties of the leucocytes, Casop. lék. česk. *93:*242, 1954.

209. Dausset, J., Nenna, A., and Brecy, H.: Leukoagglutinins. V. Leukoagglutinins in chronic idiopathic or symptomatic pancytopenia and in paroxysmal nocturnal hemoglobinuria, Blood 9: 696, 1954.

210. Miescher, P.: Nucléophagocytose et phénomene L. E., J. suisse méd. *83:*1042, 1953.

211. Lozner, E. L.: The thrombocytopenic purpuras, Bull. New York Acad. Med. *30:*184, 1954.

212. Robson, H. N.: Idiopathic thrombocytopenic purpura, Brit. M. J. *2:*971, 1950.

213. Ackroyd, J. E.: Allergic purpura including purpura due to foods, drugs and infections, Am. J. Med. *14:*605, 1953.

214. Steinkamp, R., Moore, C. V., and Doubek, W.: Thrombocytopenic purpura caused by hypersensitivity to quinidine, J. Lab. Clin. Med. *14:*605, 1953.

215. Barkham, P., and Tocantins, L.: Observations on the thrombocytopenia due to hypersensitivity to quinidine, Blood *9:*134, 1954.

216. Bolton, F. G.: Thrombocytopenic purpura due to quinidine: serologic mechanisms, Blood *11:*547, 1956.

217. Harrington, W. J., Sprague, C. C., Minnich, V., Moore, C. V., Ahlvin, R. C., and Dubach, R.: Immunologic mechanisms in idiopathic and neonatal thrombocytopenic purpura, Ann. Int. Med. *38:*433, 1953.

218. Harrington, W. J., Minnich, V., Hollingsworth, J. W., and Moore, C. V.: Demonstration of a thrombocytopenic factor in the blood of patients with thrombocytopenic purpura, J. Lab. & Clin. Med. *38:*1, 1951.

219. Harrington, W. J.: The clinical significance of antibodies for platelets, Sang *25:*712, 1954.

220. Dameshek, W., and Miller, E. B.: The megakaryocytes in idiopathic thrombocytopenic purpura, a form of hypersplenism, Blood *1:*27, 1946.

221. Stefanini, M., Dameshek, W., Chatterjea, J. B., Adelson, E., and Mednicoff, I. B.: Studies on platelets. IX. Observations on the properties and mechanism of action of a potent platelet agglutinin detected in the serum of a patient with idiopathic thrombocytopenic purpura (with a note on the pathogenesis of the disease). Blood *8:*26, 1953.

222. Rivers, T. M., Sprunt, D. H., and Berry, G. P.: Observations on attempts to produce acute disseminated encephalomyelitis in monkeys, J. Exper. Med. *58:*49, 1933.

223. Waksman, B. H.: Experimental allergic encephalomyelitis and the "auto-allergic" diseases, Internat. Arch. Allergy *14* (Suppl.), 1959.

224. Alvord, E. C., Jr.: Studies on the etiology and pathogenesis of experimental meningoencephalomyelitis in the guinea pig, J. Immunol. *61:*355, 1949.

225. Kabat, E. A., Wolf, A., and Bezer, A. E.: Studies in acute disseminated encephalomyelitis produced experimentally in rhesus monkeys. III, J. Exper. Med. *88:*417, 1948.

226. Kabat, E. A., Wolf, A., and Bezer, A. E.: Experimental studies on acute disseminated encephalomyelitis in the rhesus monkey, Ann. Allergy *6:*109, 1948.

227. Ferraro, A., and Roizin, L.: Neuropathologic variations in experimental allergic encephalomyelitis. Hemorrhagic encephalomyelitis, perivenous encephalomyelitis, diffuse encephalomyelitis, patchy gliosis, J. Neuropath. & Exper. Neurol. *12:*373, 1953.

228. Wolf, A., Kabat, E. A., and Bezer, A. E.: The pathology of acute disseminated encephalomyelitis produced experimentally in the rhesus monkey and its resemblance to human demyelinating diseases, J. Neuropath. & Exper. Neurol. *6:*333, 1947.

229. Hill, K. R.: An investigation into the presence of antibodies and hypersensitivity in the encephalitis produced experimentally by the injection of homologous brain suspensions, Bull. Johns Hopkins Hosp. *84:*302, 1949.

230. Paterson, P. Y.: Transfer of allergic encephalomyelitis in rats by means of lymph node cells, J. Exper. Med. *111:*119, 1960.

231. Chase, M. W.: A Critique of Attempts at Passive Transfer of Sensitivity to Nervous Tissue, in Kies, M. W., and Alvord, E. C., Jr. (Eds.): "Allergic" Encephalomyelitis, Springfield, Charles C Thomas, 1959.

232. Ferraro, A., and Roizin, L.: Experimental allergic encephalomyelitis during and following cortone acetate treatment, J. Neuropath. & Exper. Neurol. *12:*373, 1953.

233. Lee, J. M., and Olitzky, P. K.: Simple method of enhancing development of acute disseminated encephalomyelitis in mice, Proc. Soc. Exper. Biol. & Med. *89:*263, 1955.

234. Adams, R. D., and Kubik, C. S.: Morbid anatomy of demyelinating diseases, Am. J. Med. *12:* 510, 1952.

235. Hurst, E. W.: Experimental demyelination in relation to human and animal disease, Am. J. Med. *12:*547, 1952.

236. Paterson, P. Y.: Organ-specific Tissue Damage Induced by Mammalian Tissue-Adjuvant Emulsions, in Lawrence, H. S. (Ed.): Cellular and Humoral Aspects of Hypersensitive States, New York, Hoeber-Harper, 1959.

237. Waksman, B. H., and Adams, R. D.: Allergic neuritis: an experimental disease of rabbits induced by the injection of peripheral nervous tissue and adjuvants, J. Exper. Med. *102:*213, 1955.

238. Waksman, B. H., and Adams, R. D.: A comparative study of experimental allergic neuritis in the rabbit, guinea pig, and mouse, J. Neuropath. & Exper. Neurol. *15:*293, 1956.

239. Haymaker, W., and Kernohan, J. W.: Landry-Guillain-Barré syndrome; clinico-pathologic report of 50 fatal cases and critique of the literature, Medicine *28:*59, 1949.

240. Voisin, G., Delaunay, A., and Barber, M.: Sur des lesions testiculaires provoquées chez le cobaye par iso- et auto-sensibilization, Ann. Inst. Pasteur *81:*48, 1951.

241. Freund, J., Lipton, M. M., and Thompson, G. E.: Aspermatogenesis in the guinea pig induced by testicular tissue and adjuvants, J. Exper. Med. *97:*711, 1953.

242. Freund, J., Thompson, G. E., and Lipton, M. M.: Aspermatogenesis, anaphylaxis, and cutaneous sensitization induced in the guinea pig by homologous testicular extract, J. Exper. Med. *101:* 591, 1955.

243. Waksman, B. H.: A histologic study of the auto-allergic testis lesion in the guinea pig, J. Exper. Med. *109:*311, 1959.

244. Wilson, L.: Sperm agglutinin in human semen and blood, Proc. Soc. Exper. Biol. & Med. *85:* 652, 1954.

245. Rümke, P., and Hellinga, G.: Autoantibodies against spermatozoa in sterile men, Am. J. Clin. Path. *32:*357, 1959.

246. Joy, H. H.: Sympathetic ophthalmia. The history of its pathogenic studies, Am. J. Ophth. *36:*1100, 1953.

247. Woods, A. C.: Endogenous Uveitis, Baltimore, Williams and Wilkins, 1956.

248. Collins, R. C.: Experimental studies on sympathetic ophthalmia, Am. J. Ophth. *32:*1687, 1949.

249. Collins, R. C.: Further experimental studies on sympathetic ophthalmia, Am. J. Ophth. *36:*150, 1953.

250. Suie, T.: An immunologic study of rabbits sensitized with homologous uveal tissue, Am. J. Ophth. *39:*377, 1955.

251. Lange, K., Gold, M. M. A., Wiener, D., and Simon, V.: Autoantibodies in human glomerulonephritis, J. Clin. Invest. *28:*50, 1949.

252. Liu, C. T., and McCrory, W. W.: Autoantibodies in human glomerulonephritis and nephrotic syndrome, J. Immunol. *81:*492, 1948.

253. Mellors, R. C., and Ortega, L. G.: Analytical pathology. III. New observations on the pathogenesis of glomerulonephritis, lipoid nephrosis, polyarteritis nodosa and secondary amyloidosis in man, Am. J. Path. *32:*455, 1956.

254. Freedman, P., Peters, J. H., and Kark, R. M.: Localization of gamma-globulin in the kidney, Arch. Int. Med. *105:*524, 1960.

255. Smadel, J.: Experimental nephritis in rats induced by injection of antikidney serum: preparation and immunological studies of nephrotoxin, J. Exper. Med. *64:*921, 1936.

256. Cavelti, P. A., and Cavelti, E. S.: Studies on the pathogenesis of glomerulonephritis. I. Production of autoantibodies to kidney in experimental animals, Arch. Path. *39:*148, 1945.

257. Cavelti, P. A., and Cavelti, E. S.: Studies on the pathogenesis of glomerulonephritis. II. Production of glomerulonephritis in rats by means of autoantibodies to the kidney, Arch. Path. *40:* 158, 1945.

258. Cavelti, P. A., and Cavelti, E. S.: Studies on the pathogenesis of glomerulonephritis. III. Clinical and pathologic aspects of the experimental glomerulonephritis produced in rats by means of autoantibodies to the kidney, Arch. Path. *40:* 163, 1945.

259. Middleton, E., Jr., Middleton, E. B., and Seegal, B. C.: Effect of injecting rats with homologous renal tissue mixed with adjuvants or streptococci, Arch. Path. *56:*125, 1953.

260. Jones, D. B.: The Kidney, Inflammatory and Vascular Diseases of the Glomerulus, in Mellors, R. C. (Ed.): Analytical Pathology, New York, Blakiston, 1957.

261. Colover, J., and Glynn, L. E.: Experimental isoimmune adrenalitis, J. Immunol. *1:*172, 1958.

262. Steiner, J. W., Langer, B., Schatz, D. L., and Volpe, R.: Experimental immunologic adrenal injury. A response to injections of autologous and homologous adrenal antigens in adjuvant, J. Exper. Med. *112:*187, 1960.

263. Anderson, J. R., Goudie, R. B., Gray, K. G., and Timbury, G. C.: Auto antibodies in Addison's disease, Lancet *1:*1123, 1957.

264. Gajdusek, D. C.: An "autoimmune" reaction against human tissue antigens in certain acute and chronic diseases. I. Serological investigations, Arch. Int. Med. *101:*9, 1958.

265. Mackay, I. R., and Gajdusek, D. C.: An "autoimmune" reaction against human tissue antigens in certain acute and chronic diseases. II. Clinical correlations, Arch. Int. Med. *101:*30, 1958.

266. Cohen, S., Ohta, G., Singer, E. J., and Popper, H.: Immunocytochemical study of gamma globulin in liver in hepatitis and postnecrotic cirrhosis, J. Exper. Med. *111:*285, 1960.

267. Thomas, L.: in discussion of Medawar, P. B.: Reactions to Homologous Tissue Antigens in Relation to Hypersensitivity, in Lawrence, H. S. (Ed.): Cellular and Humoral Aspects of the Hypersensitive States, New York, Hoeber-Harper, 1959.

268. Haurowitz, F.: The mechanism of the immunological response, Biol. Rev. *27:*247, 1952.

269. Lawrence, H. S.: Homograft sensitivity, Physiol. Rev. *39:*811, 1959.

CHAPTER IX

GENERAL PATHOLOGY OF

BODY FLUIDS AND ELECTROLYTES

I. INTRODUCTION

Perhaps in no other field of physiology and pathology is Claude Bernard's concept of the constancy of the internal environment better exemplified than in the body fluids and electrolytes. Many physiologic mechanisms contribute to maintain volume, distribution and concentration of water and solutes constant within very narrow limits; pathologic processes resulting in deviations from the normal are many and very important, but the variety of compensating mechanisms and the inability of the organism to withstand more than minor variations in pH, potassium and sodium concentrations, etc., make abnormal changes quantitatively small. The constancy of the internal environment becomes a major issue in independent life with the appearance of the structure isolating a group of self-replicating chemical compounds from the world at large, i.e., the membrane. According to Szent-Györgyi,[1] the membrane is the fundamental scheme of the biological universe.

"If I look on this world from the point of view of the cell, every individual, you and me, and every cell, is the center of his own universe, which is divided into two parts: the inside and the outside. The plane which separates these two worlds is what we call 'the membrane' . . . It is something like God used to be: nobody has seen him, but he did everything. So does the membrane which divides the whole world into two parts. The intracellular atmosphere depends on what the membrane lets through, and what the intracellular machinery will do depends on this intracellular atmosphere. Moreover, any messages arriving from the outside will reach the cell at the membrane, which will be the first to receive any message and to give the very answer, and trigger off the function of the internal machinery . . . Last, but not least, the membrane is always the seat of energy, there being a potential jump. This energy can be spent in action for triggering off the internal mechanism as a response to outside stimuli. So the membrane is really the most important part of the cell, which, schematically, consists of a membrane and the inside machinery. This is the basic blueprint."

But for multicellular organisms the internal environment is not within the cellular membrane. It occupies an extracellular compartment, which may be further divided into intra- and extravascular areas. Interstitial fluids bathing the cellular surfaces, serving as passageway and transporting mechanisms of substances required by, and eliminated from, the cells represent the true *milieu interne*. In a recent editorial, Robin and Bromberg[2] speak of intracellular contents as the real internal environment, but here one is tempted to ask, internal "environment" to what? Should the cell itself be considered as surrounding medium of subcellular particles, which accordingly acquire the category of organisms? It can be expected that further refinements will eventually bring the organism into striking similarity with the Cheshire cat, of which the last visible manifestation, before completely vanishing, was the grin.

This chapter is devoted to a review of the general pathology of body fluids and electrolytes, important components of the internal environment. It is characteristic of the spirit of this book that a discussion of such problems is included, in spite of the few and relatively unimportant tissue changes accompanying most pathologic conditions of water and electrolytes. Hypokalemia is as pathologic a process as atrophy of the brain, despite the fact that appreciation of the former rests on chemical and electrocardiographic findings, while a study of the latter requires specialized morphologic techniques. A brief physiological introduction precedes the discussion of abnormal changes in volume, composition and concentration in body fluids and electrolytes, as well as the different mechanisms at play in each of these conditions. Detailed description of specific clinical situations is not attempted

since it goes beyond the scope of this book and may be found in specialized texts.[3, 4, 5] Hernández Peón's[6] excellent chapter on the physiology of body fluids in Fulton's textbook has been freely used to prepare this section.

II. DISTRIBUTION, COMPOSITION AND EXCHANGE OF BODY FLUIDS

Water is the most abundant compound in the organism. At birth it amounts to 82 per cent of body weight, and in the adult it is nearly 72 per cent;[7] these figures are averages obtained from many determinations in different individuals, which show wide variations not only from one subject to another but also from one type of tissue to another.[8] Such variations are partly due to the low water content of fat[9] and to the wide differences in the amount of fatty tissue present in different subjects. This is the main reason why it is not convenient to use body weight to estimate total water content, but only lean body weight. When calculations are made using lean body weight it is found that the relation to water content is quite constant.[10] Body water content tends to decrease progressively with age; a significant difference in mean body water content exists between males and females which appears at puberty and persists throughout the life span.[11] Water is the solvent of many substances in the organism, electrolytes of which play a very important role in its distribution in different compartments.

A. DISTRIBUTION OF WATER IN THE ORGANISM

Theoretically, it is possible to consider two large compartments in the organism separated by the cell membrane: the intracellular and the extracellular compartments; the former is characterized by a rather definite electrolyte pattern consisting predominantly of potassium, magnesium, phosphate and protein[12] (*vide infra*). Further studies will probably demonstrate subdivisions of intracellular water and electrolytes but at present the concept of a single intracellular phase is useful in describing the organization of the organism as a whole. On

Table 50. Body Water Distribution in an "Average" Normal Young Adult Male

SOURCE	ML./KG. OF BODY WEIGHT	% OF TOTAL BODY WATER
Plasma	45	7.5
Interstitial-lymph	120	20.0
Dense connective tissue and cartilage	45	7.5
Inaccessible bone water	45	7.5
Transcellular	15	2.5
Total extracellular	270	45.0
Total body water (D_2O)	600	100.0
Total intracellular	330	55.0

(From Edelman and Liebman[8])

the other hand, the extracellular compartment may be subdivided into two more parts, separated by the vascular membrane, which are the intravascular and the extravascular (or interstitial) compartments. Such separation is valid for total body water, but a topographic distribution is also feasible and useful, as in lymph, cerebrospinal fluid, joint fluid, urine, aqueous humor, gastrointestinal secretions, interstitial fluid, etc. In many of these compartments water is, strictly speaking, outside the organism, but it is still part of total body water. The topographic analysis of water compartments is not only of anatomic interest, but also is significant as an index of specialized cellular activity in each of these different areas of the organism. Extracellular water has been divided by Edelman and Leibman[8] into the following four categories: (1) plasma; (2) interstitial and lymph fluid, (3) dense connective tissue, cartilage and bone, and (4) transcellular fluids. The last category was introduced to designate a variety of extracellular fluids which have the common property of being formed by the transport activity of cells,[13] such as saliva, tears, bile, urine, etc. The actual figures obtained in an average man appear in Table 50.

Intracellular water volume is more than twice the extracellular volume of water, although part of the cellular water is considered as "fixed" or combined; i.e., it does not participate freely in exchange with the extracellular compartment. This concept, however, is not applicable to individual water molecules, which are in continuous ionic exchange, but to a certain amount of water held continuously within the cell membrane.

B. COMPOSITION OF BODY FLUIDS

Tradition has consecrated Gamble's simple and useful diagrams to represent the composition of the different fluid compartments of the body.[14] Such compartments are formed by water, as solvent, and two different types of solutes, separated according to the direction of their displacement in an electric field, into anions (negatively charged ions which move towards the anode) and cations (positively charged ions which move towards the cathode). Whatever the total amount of solutes, electrostatic equilibrium is reached when equivalent amounts of anions and cations are present; the sum of anions and cations tends to remain constant and equals the total concentration of solutes in water. The concept of equivalence must be clearly separated from that of weight, since amounts in grams are not the same as ionizing capacity of different substances, nor do all ions have the same number of valences. An equivalent is the number of ions necessary to neutralize the electrical charge of a molecular gram in solution. For instance, NaOH has a molecular weight of 40 (Na, 23; O, 16; H, 1), while HCl has a molecular weight of 36.5 (H, 1; Cl, 35.5); 40 Gm. of NaOH and 36.5 Gm. of HCl deposited in one liter of water will be completely ionized and will induce no change in pH, since H^+ ions neutralize all OH^- ions, which are present in the same amounts, although the initial weight deposited for each substance is not the same. For the same reason, 23 Gm. of Na^+ and 35.5 Gm. of Cl^- are equivalents. In this case both ions are monovalents but in the case of Ca^{++}, with atomic weight of 40, an equivalent amount in grams would be half the atomic weight, or 20, since the combining power is double. The equivalence of a given compound is related not only to ionic valence, but also to degree of ionization reached in solution; plasma proteins are only weakly dissociated in solution, and for this reason they play a secondary role in pH determination. Since the actual amounts of solutes in the organism are very small, instead of using equivalents as units the custom is to speak of milliequivalents, which are one thousandth of an equivalent; thus, one milliequivalent of Na^+ in weight is 23 mg., one milliequivalent of Cl^+ is 35.5 mg., and one milliequivalent of Ca^{++} is 20 mg.

Plasma pH is slightly alkaline (7.4) and varies within very narrow limits. Neutrality indicates that cations are balanced by anions; it may be of interest to compare the concentration of solutes in plasma, both in milligrams and in milliequivalents, in order to demonstrate the difference between these two types of units. This is important because the functions of different electrolytes (maintenance of pH, osmotic pressure, etc.) are the result of their ionization and electrical charge, and not of their amount in weight. Figure 9–1 is a comparison of anion and cation concentration in plasma according to Gamble. Table 51 gives the concentrations of anions and cations in normal human plasma.

The composition of interstitial fluid is more variable and is mainly determined by differences in protein concentration. All other electrolytes diffuse freely through capillary endothelium, so that differences in the total amount of cations will be compensated by opposite changes in the amount of anions. It has been mentioned that proteins are weak anions because of their limited dissociation in solution, so that differences are not clinically significant as far as concentrations go; on the other hand, the fact that capillary membranes are impervious to proteins is fundamental in the exchange of fluids between the different body compartments.[15]

By the same token, the composition of

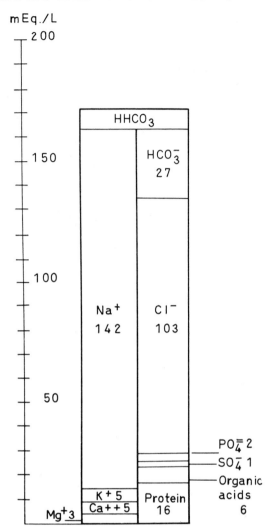

FIG. 9–1. Concentration of anions and cations in extracellular fluids (plasma).

intracellular fluid is variable according to the functions of different tissues; the most abundant protoplasm in the organism corresponds to striated muscle, the composition of which appears in Fig. 9–2, with data given by Muntwyler.[16]

Finally, the composition of special fluids such as bile, cerebrospinal fluid, urine, gastrointestinal secretions, etc., is even more variable since it depends on the functions of different organs and systems. Furthermore, some of these fluids (saliva, sweat, urine) vary in composition as a result of a series of mechanisms tending to maintain constancy of the interstitial fluid, so that for practical purposes the most important

Table 51. Electrolyte Composition of Human Plasma

CATIONS	mEq./1	ANIONS	mEq./1
Na^+	142	Cl^-	103
K^+	5	HCO_3^-	27
Ca^{++}	5	$PO_4^{\equiv}$	2
Mg^{++}	3	$SO_4^=$	1
		Proteins	
		Organic acids	
	155		155

mEq./L

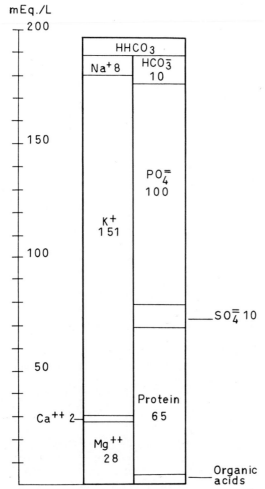

FIG. 9–2.   Concentration of anions and cations in intracellular fluids (muscle).

fluid is the plasma, which reflects the composition of the fluid in direct contact with cells and tissues.

C. THE EXCHANGE OF FLUIDS IN THE BODY

The fluids of the body are in continuous movement.[17] Plasma circulates within the vascular system, passes through the capillary walls and moves in the interstitial spaces, where it comes in contact with cellular membranes; through these membranes cells obtain a series of compounds necessary for their metabolism and eliminate others, the result of metabolic processes. In specialized tissues, such as the choroid plexus or the renal glomerulus, plasma undergoes filtration and clearance of different substances. Nevertheless, in the end the plasma returns to the circulatory system via veins or lymphatics, and the entire cycle is initiated again. Cellular products carried by the circulation are not only waste metabolites, but also a series of substances acting in various areas of the organism and that must reach these areas by the blood. This exchange of fluids between the different compartments of the organism is in a steady state of equilibrium, ruled by a series of physicochemical principles which were first established by Starling,[18] in 1896. At that time, vitalism and mechanicism were fighting one of their most bitter, and probably their last, fights. Vitalists believed that capillaries actively absorbed fluids from the interstitial spaces, especially when hydrostatic intracapillary pressure was very low. In his memorable paper, Starling asks:

". . . Are the capillary walls so constituted as to react to a lowering of the capillary pressure with an active absorption of extravascular fluid, *i.e.* is the absorption due to vital activity of the cells? or can we find mechanical conditions that will account for this absorption?"

Some paragraphs below, he states:

"I believe the explanation is to be found in a property on which much stress was laid by the older physiologists, and which they termed the high endosmotic equivalent of albumen. . . . The application of semi-permeable membranes by Pfeffer to the measurement of osmotic pressures, showed that the osmotic pressures of salts and other crystalloids are enormously higher than those of such substances as albumen, and it has therefore been supposed that the osmotic pressure of the proteids in serum being so insignificant must be of no account in physiological processes. The reverse is however the case. Whereas the enormous pressures of the salts and crystalloids in the various fluids of the body are of very little importance for the function of absorption by the blood vessels, the comparatively insignificant osmotic pressure of the albumens is I believe of great importance, ...

. . . In the limbs and connective tissues generally of the peripheral parts of the body, we have capillaries which are more or less impervious to proteids. As the blood passes under pressure through these capillaries, a certain amount of lymph is filtered through their walls, but in the process it loses the greater part of its proteids. We have therefore on one side of the capillary wall blood-plasma with 8% proteids, on the other side lymph containing 2 to 3% proteids. In this separation of proteid a certain amount of work must have been done, and if the proteids of serum . . . possess an osmotic pressure, there must be a difference of osmotic pressure between intra- and extravascular fluids tending to a reabsorption of the latter."

Table 52. Factors in Fluid Filtration from Capillaries in Starling's Equilibrium

FAVORING FILTRATION	OPPOSING FILTRATION
Hydrostatic blood pressure	Intracapillary osmotic pressure
Extracapillary osmotic pressure	Interstitial tissue tension
Increased capillary permeability	Decreased capillary permeability

By means of an osmometer consisting

"of a small glass bell provided near the top with two vertical tubulures. Over the mouth of the bell is tied a peritoneal membrane . . . . . . rendered absolutely watertight by soaking it for some minutes, after it had been tied on, in a 10% solution of gelatin,"

Starling measured the osmotic pressure of serum proteins and found figures ranging from 30 to 40 mm. Hg. Therefore, he concluded that this pressure

"is of an order of magnitude comparable to that of the capillary pressures; and whereas capillary pressure determines transudation, the osmotic pressure of the proteids of the serum determines absorption."

Exchange occurs between two different pairs of systems, one formed by intravascular and extravascular spaces, separated by the capillary membrane, the other consisting of the interstitial and intracellular compartments, separated by the cellular membrane. According to Elkinton and Danowski,[3] the complex formed by the intravascular, interstitial and intracellular spaces is "open" in both extremes, since blood plasma is continuously subject to volume and concentration regulating mechanisms, while the cell itself is capable of changing the composition and volume of circulating fluids by means of metabolic adjustments. But in a system composed of a semipermeable membrane separating two compartments with solutions possessed of hydrostatic and osmotic pressures, the exchange is ruled by purely physicochemical mechanisms.

Exchange between the two divisions of the extracellular compartment (intravascular and interstitial) clearly follows Starling's rules.[19] Table 52 gives the forces favoring filtration towards the interstitial space and opposing absorption into the vascular lumen, as well as the forces acting in an opposite sense in the interstitial space.

Even in pathologic situations, in which there are other factors at play such as blockage of lymphatic circulation, decrease in oncotic pressure, changes in the permeability of membranes, etc., the net result in filtration will be the algebraic sum of hydrodynamic forces as proposed by Starling.

A superficial examination of fluid exchange between the interstitial, extracellular space and the intracellular compartment would seem to negate Starling's principle. Especially in organs with high metabolic activity such as the kidney or liver, osmotic pressure is much higher within the cells than outside, in the extracellular compartment, and even here hydrostatic pressure is lower than within capillary vessels. The explanation lies in "active" transport of solutes through the cellular membrane and passive diffusion of others in the opposite direction, plus the formation of certain compounds of high molecular weight (phosphates and proteins) which are unable to traverse the cell membrane. The difference between "active" and "vital" is simply the word, since both indicate energy expenditure necessary to move a given ion against a concentration gradient.[20]

The passage of fluids and electrolytes through membranes obeys four different mechanisms: (1) Diffusion by concentration gradient, in which solutes exert no osmotic pressure since they can pass freely through the membrane. Movement occurs from the compartment with a higher solute concentration to that with less solute, while water moves in the opposite direction until an equilibrium is reached. (2) Diffusion by osmosis, in which one of the compartments has a higher concentration of a solute which cannot pass through the separating membrane, in which case water will move from the compartment of less solute concentration into the other compartment until an equilibrium is reached (considering the system without hydrostatic pressure). (3) "Active" transport, in which solute concentration increases in one compartment as the result of energy expenditure, the result being a diffusion by concentration gradient of solutes in opposite direction, if the membrane is permeable to them, and/or water passage in the same direction as the "ac-

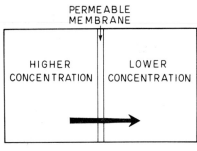

EXCHANGE DUE TO CONCENTRATION
GRADIENT

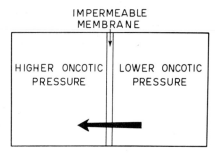

EXCHANGE DUE TO OSMOTIC PRESSURE
GRADIENT

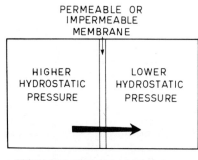

EXCHANGE DUE TO HYDROSTATIC
PRESSURE GRADIENT

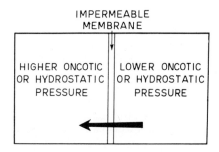

EXCHANGE DUE TO "ACTIVE TRANSPORT"

FIG. 9–3. The four mechanisms of fluid and electrolyte exchange in the body.

tive" transport until the increase in osmotic pressure produced by the greater concentration of the solute is equilibrated. (4) Diffusion by hydrostatic pressure gradient, in which both water and solute pass from the compartment with higher pressure into the other compartment, until pressures are in equilibrium. These different mechanisms are illustrated in Fig. 9–3.

Pappenheimer[21] suggested that diffusion of lipid-soluble substances (oxygen and carbon dioxide) occurs throughout the entire capillary surface, but that water and solutes which are not soluble in lipids (sodium chloride, urea and glucose) are filtered only through an area not greater than 0.2 per cent of the total capillary surface; the smallness of the filtration area suggests the intercellular cement as the actual site of passage. Furthermore, the speed of filtration through the capillary wall is against free diffusion, but would seem to depend on molecular size; this is the basis of the pore theory of molecular sieving, which was mentioned in Chapter II.

The amount of intracellular water is partly regulated by hormones. The absence of adrenocortical hormones will produce an increase in the intracellular compartment and a decrease in the extracellular compartment before any changes are observed in Na^+ plasma concentration. Cortisone and ACTH determine an increase in extracellular volume accompanied by increased Na^+ and Cl^-, although plasma Na^+ is not modified.[22]

III. CONTROL OF VOLUME AND CONCENTRATION OF BODY FLUIDS

The organism maintains the volume and concentration of body fluids within very narrow limits, which is not surprising in view of the many and important functions of water and electrolytes. Water is so ubiquitous that it is difficult to conceive some physiologic process in which it does not participate. Electrolytes play important roles in many functions which may be separated in three groups: (1) the maintenance of neutrality in pH, (2) the osmotic pressure responsible for exchange and distribution of fluids and (3) their role in energy metabolism. It has been mentioned that the body pH is in equilibrium near neutrality, i.e., 7.4, and that this is due to the existence of equivalent amounts of anions and cations. Nevertheless, there are some differences in electrostatic potential in several more or less localized areas of the organism, which are necessary for "active" transport through membranes, nerve and muscle excitability, etc. Anyhow, these differences in potential are small and do not affect the pH of the body fluids as a whole. It has also been mentioned that osmotic pressure is one of the most important factors in fluid exchange and distribution, both in the extracellular and in the intracellular compartments, although the latter may be more difficult to define. Finally, the concentration of electrolytes is very important for energy metabolism. For instance, K^+ and Mg^{++} activate, and Na^+ inhibits, some reactions involved in the enzymatic breakdown of large molecules and the production of high energy bonds. Cannon et al.[23] showed that lack of K^+ inhibits protein synthesis, and Gardner et al.[24] observed that the same situation blocks the use of carbohydrates by the cell. Besides influencing the energy metabolism electrolytes have many other functions, such as the participation of Ca^{++} in nerve excitability and blood coagulation, of Cl^- in gastric secretions, etc.

Since solutes are ionized and in electrostatic equilibrium, there are three types of constants to be considered in the body fluids, which are volume, concentration (also known as osmolarity or tonicity) and composition. The difference between the last two is apparent when considering that concentration is the total amount of solutes in a given solvent, while composition refers to the partial amounts of each one of the solutes considered individually. For instance, the concentration of plasma is 310 mEq./l. separated in equivalent amounts of anions and cations, but when the amount of anions decreases and that of cations increases (as observed in certain instances of acidosis),

concentration is maintained at 310 mEq./l. but composition has changed.[4] Modifications in composition of body fluids are usually accompanied by changes in volume and concentration, but the controlling mechanisms are somewhat different and therefore will be considered in a later section, when discussing the equilibrium of H^+. In this section reference is made to the regulation of volume and concentration of body fluids.

A. VOLUME

The mechanisms of regulation of volume of body fluids belong to two general categories: those operated through modifications in concentration, and those sensible to changes in volume itself. The former are better understood than the latter.

A normal adult will gain water as drinking fluid, in food ingested and from his own cellular metabolism (so-called "oxidation water"); on the other hand, the same subject loses water as urine, with the feces and as insensible loss, a term reserved for tears, sweat, saliva, cutaneous evaporation, etc.[25] The normal amounts of water entering and leaving the organism every 24 hours appear in Table 53, where it can be seen that they are in equilibrium. Mechanisms regulating the volume of body fluids operate mainly through thirst, which favors ingestion, and through the excretion of urine. Water absorption in the intestine is indiscriminate and ingestion of fluids is quite variable, since they are taken even in the absence of thirst; furthermore, insensible loss varies with temperature, exercise, etc. All these variations are not part of volume regulation, but rather provide stimuli for the participation of mechanisms involved in maintenance of constant fluid volume in the organism.

Table 53. Intake and Output of Water in 24 Hours in Normal Man

INTAKE		OUTPUT	
Water ingested as fluid	1200 ml.	Urine	1500 ml.
Water in solid foods	1000 ml.	Feces	100 ml.
"Oxidation" water	300 ml.	Insensible loss (sweat, tears, etc.)	1000 ml.
	2500 ml.		2500 ml.

Fluid ingestion is controlled by the sensation of thirst.[26] According to Cannon,[27] a homeostatic mechanism should stimulate the search not only of the effector organ, but also of the stimulus, the receptor and, possibly, integrative mechanisms. In the case of thirst the stimulus seems to be a decrease in water and an excess of solutes, which is the same as an increase in concentration or tonicity of plasma.[28] Whether this state of extracellular fluids is accompanied by a similar hypertonicity of intracellular fluids is still a matter of conjecture.[29] It is important that Na^+, which fails to penetrate within cells, is more effective in inducing thirst than urea and other substances which pass freely through the cellular membrane.[30] This would suggest that the cells are losing water by osmotic diffusion,[31] but if this loss refers to the intracellular compartment as a whole or only to certain specialized areas is not known at present. Adolph et al.[32] believe that a water deficit in excess of solutes is the cause of thirst, but they suggest additional factors involved in this response and which might tend to modify it, such as gastric distention, administration of water by routes other than mouth, large doses of Pitressin, cocainization of the mouth, hyperosmotic or hypotonic water, etc. It is possible that the hypothalamus may participate in the thirst mechanism as a receptor or regulator.[33]

Fluid loss is regulated by a mechanism stimulated by changes in concentration; the receptor is in the hypothalamus and the pars nervosa of the pituitary gland; the integration is of hormonal nature; the effector organ is the kidney, and more specifically the distal convoluted tubule. Other stimuli may start the homeostatic mechanism since the receptor is sensible to pain, emotions, nicotine, morphine, alcohol, etc.[28]; furthermore, it has been suggested that the receptor is also sensible to isotonic modifications in extracellular fluid volume.[34]

Verney[35] showed that intracarotideal injections of hypertonic NaCl solutions resulted in antidiuresis (inhibition of urine elimination), and that this effect was absent in hypophysectomized animals. Furthermore, a hypertonic urea solution fails to induce the same result, so the conclusion was that there were "osmoreceptors" since urea will pass freely through cell membranes and fail to create differences in osmotic pressure. Such osmoreceptors are probably located in the supraoptic and paraventricular nuclei, which are extraordinarily rich in blood vessels.[36] Both nuclei are joined to the posterior pituitary by two different mechanisms: one is a nervous tract, the supraoptic-hypophyseal tract, and the other is a vascular connection, through the portal venous system leading from the median eminence to the pituitary gland. The antidiuretic hormone is formed by neurosecretory cells within the hypothalamus and transported along their axons to be stored in dilated nerve endings closely applied to the capillaries of the neurohypophysis.[37] The chemical structure of antidiuretic hormone varies in different animal species,[38] but in man it has been identified as arginine vasopressin.[39] Antidiuretic hormone is partially eliminated with the urine and the rest is inactivated by the liver, under the influence of the adrenals. This hormone acts directly on the cells of the distal convoluted tubule, modifying the "facultative" reabsorption of water, [40, 41] which amounts to approximately 15 per cent of the volume filtered through the glomerulus. This phase of water reabsorption is known as "facultative" because it is not determined by osmotic forces; on the contrary, it is carried out against the plasmatic osmotic gradient and, therefore, is a form of "active" transport of water.[42] Lack of antidiuretic hormone, as in diabetes insipidus, may increase the urinary output up to 50 liters a day.

The mechanisms mentioned above regulate volume of body fluids through changes in concentration, but there are many data (recently analyzed by Epstein,[43] Smith,[44] Grossman[45] and others[46, 47]) strongly suggesting the presence of mechanisms sensible to modifications in volume itself. Receptors for these mechanisms are not adequately localized yet, but suggested sites are in the peripheral veins,[48] in the cephalic portion of the body,[49] in the left atrium,[50] etc. Whatever their location, the effective stimulus is an isotonic change in fluid volume and the response is increased or decreased secretion of antidiuretic hormone in the pituitary, with a consequent stimulation or inhibition of water reabsorption in the distal convoluted tubule of the kidney.[51] But in this case there is a double response, since modifications in the volume of urine are not accompanied by changes in concentration, especially of sodium;[45] therefore, an isotonic fluid will be eliminated or retained as long as there is enough solute to maintain such concentration, but when the limit is approached water will no longer be freely handled by the organism. Regulation of tonicity has precedence over regulation of volume.

Both thirst and antidiuretic hormone show several common features revealing of their effectiveness in homeostasis: (1) Both may be started by small changes in fluid tonicity, as long as they are rapidly induced, in which case the response will be adequate. (2) Both mechanisms respond better to loss of water than to an increase, since water loss will result in thirst and increased secretion of antidiuretic hormone. Water excess, on the other hand, will cause absence of thirst, which is no effective inhibitor of fluid ingestion, and the inhibition of antidiuretic hormone secretion may also be obtained by morphine, emotions and alcohol. (3) Both mechanisms are relatively insensible to volume changes, which should be pronounced before the posterior pituitary will respond. In view of these reasons it is clear that the most important role of thirst and antidiuretic hormone is the preservation of fluid tonicity, and that volume regulation comes in second place.[52]

B. CONCENTRATION

In the same manner as with volume regulation, mechanisms involved in maintaining the concentration of body fluids constant refer especially to the extracellular compartment. Little is known of intracellular concentration, which is probably changing according to cell metabolism and type of tissue. For practical purposes the tonicity of body fluids depends on the most abundant anions and cations, which are Na^+, Cl^-, and HCO_3^-. Changes in K^+, Ca^{++}, Mg^{++}, HPO_4^-, proteins and other cations bring about no important modifications in concentration, but are very significant in ionic equilibrium (composition, acid-base balance, H^+ equilibrium), so they will be discussed later. Again, care must be exercised in distinguishing between physiologic variations in the concentration of plasma solutes and their regulating mechanisms; while the former result from many different factors, such as the amount ingested with various foods, the amount lost by sweating, in vomiting, etc., the regulating mechanisms are centered in the kidney, which is the single most important organ in the regulation of concentration of body fluids. Knowledge in this area is less complete than that relating to water and certain organic substances, because renal function is both excretory and regulatory at the same time, and also because changes in a given electrolyte may be very small and yet of great physiologic significance. For instance, lack of reabsorption of one per cent of filtered glucose may be entirely unimportant, but lack of reabsorption of one per cent of filtered Na^+ represents a daily loss of approximately 15 Gm. of salt, which may bring about disastrous consequences to the organism.[53]

Na^+ is filtered by the glomerulus at a rate of 15 to 20 mEq./min., but in the urine there appear only 30 to 300 mEq./day; i.e., in 24 hours the renal tubules have reabsorbed 1200 Gm. of NaCl, although daily ingestion is not greater than 5 Gm. and the normal balance of Na may be maintained with 0.5 Gm. per day.[54] This reabsorption is one of the most extraordinary operations of the organism, and one of the best regulated. Water reabsorption is dependent on it and is probably carried out throughout the length of the renal tubule. Most of the filtered Na^+ is reabsorbed in the proximal convoluted tubule against a very slight pressure gradient, the amount reabsorbed depends mostly on the amount filtered and, at least under physiologic conditions, it does not seem to be limited by an upper degree of saturation.[55] The thin portion of the tubule, or Henle's loop, may be considered as an "osmotic" dialyzer, where the tubular contents achieve osmotic equilibrium and reach the distal tubule in isosmotic form.[56] Here the rest of the filtered Na^+ is reabsorbed against a high pressure gradient and with a well defined upper limit. Finally, a small portion may be reabsorbed in the collector tubules.[57] Therefore, sodium reabsorption depends on the amount reaching the tubules (filtered fraction) and on tubular activity, and the results of any experiment on sodium elimination should take into account at least these two variables.

Decrease in glomerular filtration may result from low cardiac output or general decrease in total circulating volume, although some experimental data seem to oppose such a conclusion.[58] The problem is that regulation of tubular activity suggests a homeostatic mechanism, and this mechanism requires a stimulus. It has been postulated that the stimulus is the sodium concentration in the extracellular fluid and that the receptor is the adrenal cortex, responding to low sodium concentrations with a greater secretion of mineralocorticoids, especially aldosterone,[59] and that this hormone would act on the effector organ, which is the renal tubule. Patients with edema on salt-free diets show an increased secretion of aldosterone;[60] chronic suppression of Na+ results in hypertrophy of the adrenals;[61] in primary hyperaldosteronism there is retention of large amounts of Na+, etc.[62] The relation between aldosterone and Na+ reabsorption in renal tubules seems established but the stimulus for hormonal secretion is still under discussion. Low Na+ in extracellular fluids,[63] increased K+[64] decreased total extracellular volume,[65] decreased extracellular volume in a critical area of the organism,[66] etc., have been suggested as possible stimuli for aldosterone secretion. Farrell believes that in the basal ganglia (perhaps the pineal gland) a substance is secreted that stimulates aldosterone secretion;[67] such substance has been baptized "glomerulotrophin" or "adrenoglomerulotrophin"[68] since it has been shown that aldosterone is secreted in the glomerulosa of the adrenal cortex.[69] Recently, evidence is accumulating favoring some influence of ACTH on aldosterone secretion.[70, 71] Many aspects of the physiology of aldosterone are covered in recent reviews.[72, 73, 74] Aldosterone is not the only hormone capable of causing Na+ retention; this property is shared by other corticoids such as cortisone, halogenated corticosteroids, the synthetic product desoxycorticosterone (DOCA), methyltestosterone, estrogens, etc.[54] The exact site of action of these hormones on the renal tubule remains to be determined. A role has been suggested for the central nervous system in renal tubular activity, but it is not clear if it is played through hemodynamic changes, hormone secretions, or directly on Na+ reabsorption by renal tubules. Cl− homeostasis parallels that of Na+, and this parallelism is so great that it has been suggested that Na+ is passively carried and that all mechanisms act directly on Cl−; nevertheless, in different pathologic processes such parallelism is lost and these ions may vary independently in concentration.

Potassium regulation is still more complicated than that of Na+, partly because most K+ is intracellular and, therefore, is away from the excretory routes of the organism, partly because the renal tubule reabsorbs and excretes K+ simultaneously, and partly because K+ competes with Na+ for H+ in the renal tubule, as part of the mechanisms regulating H+ equilibrium.[75] The accepted opinion is that filtered K+ is reabsorbed in the proximal convoluted tubule, while that appearing in the urine is secreted by the cells of distal convoluted tubules, in competition with Na+ for H+ ions.[76] In general, extracellular fluid K+ decreases when there is less ingestion of K+ and increases in the opposite situation, although almost all K+ may be accommodated within cells.[77] On the other hand, administration of large amounts of Na+ provokes intracellular K+ to leave the cells, a movement which would tend to increase the K+ plasma concentration were it not for the renal elimination of excess K+ and the simultaneous expansion of extracellular fluid volume, which tend to decrease the concentration of plasmatic K+.[78] Therefore, the outcome will be the algebraic addition of those two processes and the usual result is that in the presence of excess Na+ the plasma K+ concentrations are normal or even low. On the other hand, with low extracellular Na+ there are higher concentrations of K+, despite the amounts eliminated with the urine. For these reasons it seems that the predominating factor is a change in extracellular volume, and not the replacement of Na+ for K+ within the cells.

Since K+ is closely linked with intracellular metabolism, disturbances in metabolic processes will be reflected in K+ concentrations in plasma. The best known example is the sudden decrease in plasma and urinary K^+ with intracellular penetration of glucose, which in diabetics recovering from hyperglycemia may produce disturbances in muscular contraction.[79] In the metabolic response to trauma, where there is rapid catabolism of intracellular proteins the plasma K^+ rises, which is explained not only as secondary to K^+ release with protein breakdown, but also to intracellular water loss and inefficiency of the energetic metabolism that keeps K^+ within the cells.[80] Plasma K^+ decreases under the influence of insulin and adrenal corticoids, especially aldosterone, which causes a marked elevation of urinary K^+.[81] Attacks of weakness in familial periodic paralysis are usually associated with a shift of K^+ from the extracellular to the intracellular space, thus resulting in hypopotassemia.[82] All these factors suggest a homeostatic mechanism in the regulation of potassium, but it is not possible as yet to assign a stimulus, a receptor, an effector and integrative mechanisms among them.

C. INTEGRATION OF MECHANISMS REGULATING VOLUME AND CONCENTRATION OF BODY FLUIDS

From the preceding paragraphs it should be clear that mechanisms regulating volume and concentration of body fluids, although independent, are intimately related. Changes in concentration (hypo- or hypertonicity) stimulate reactions which result in modifications of water and solute reabsorption in different proportions and, therefore, affect volume. On the other hand, changes in volume precipitate readjustments in renal tubular work which end by restoring the corresponding proportions of water and solute to the organism.[83] In both situations the mechanisms involve independent changes in the elimination of water and solutes; nevertheless, modifications in the amount of Na^+ are followed by others in water volume as to maintain osmotic pressure constant within very narrow limits. The apparent contradiction can be solved by reference to the time element. It seems that mechanisms related to the elimination of Na^+ are slower than those involved in water excretion; furthermore, even when Na^+ reabsorption or elimination carries with it a certain amount of "obligatory" water, 15 per cent of the glomerular filtrate is free from Na^+ and may be reabsorbed or eliminated through the influence of antidiuretic hormone. An illustration will clarify these differences, which become quite apparent with the ingestion of water, as compared with that of saline. Water will result in diuresis in a short period, since after being absorbed from the intestine it dilutes the plasma, and this hypotonicity inhibits the secretion of antidiuretic hormone. On the other hand, ingestion of saline is not followed by diuresis; on the contrary, it may be retained in the organism for hours or days, since there has been no modification in plasma concentration.[52]

IV. PATHOLOGIC CHANGES IN VOLUME AND CONCENTRATION OF BODY FLUIDS

From a general standpoint the body fluids may undergo pathologic changes in three different parameters, namely volume, concentration and composition. This separation is artificial, since isolated types may be encountered only under experimental conditions and very early in rare human cases. Nevertheless, it may be useful to consider the mechanism at play in each one of the three separate types before considering them together. Again, changes in body fluid composition, which are intimately linked to volume and concentration, will not be treated here but in the section on H^+ ion equilibrium. The different forms of edema are combined alterations with variable changes in fluid volume, concentration, composition and distribution; they are included here as instances of complex pathologic states.

A. CHANGES IN VOLUME OF BODY FLUIDS

The total amount of body fluid may be lower than normal, a state known as dehydration, or may be greater than normal, which is referred to as "water intoxication." In practice there are no isolated changes in volume of body fluids; they are always accompanied by secondary modifications in concentration, which may result from the same cause as the disturbance in volume or represent the expression of mechanisms regulating the tonicity of plasma.

1. Dehydration. Decrease in total body fluids may appear in subjects who are not receiving, or cannot retain, the normal amount of water; i.e., comatose or unconscious patients, small children, subjects with obstructive lesions in the digestive tract or with intense diarrhea, etc.[84] In addition to the restriction on fluid intake, the organism continues to eliminate water in the form of urine, feces and by insensible loss. Although urinary volume may decrease considerably, there is an irreducible minimum of 250 to 350 ml. per 24 hours.[85] The effects of dehydration are frequently complicated by those of malnutrition, since most of the subjects unable to drink water are also incapable of feeding themselves.

Clinical manifestations of pure dehydration are oliguria, increased plasma concentration which appears as hypernatremia and intracellular dehydration, which appears as apathy, muscular weakness, impaired mental faculties, etc.;[86] such manifestations are rarely observed since patients are usually unconscious, so the only and most useful sign is increased Na+ concentration in the plasma. Although water loss is greater in the extra- than in the intracellular compartment, the relative increase in interstitial oncotic pressure results in passage of water from within the cells to the extracellular space until the difference in oncotic pressure is equilibrated, and this reaction in itself tends to improve the state of extracellular dehydration, but not that of the organism as a whole. Advanced cases may show the so-called "dehydration reaction," in which the kidney eliminates K+ in exchange for Na+; intracellular osmotic pressure decreases while that of the interstitial space increases, and water passes from within the cells into the extracellular space.[46]

2. "Water Intoxication." It is impossible to induce more than a transient increase in the total amount of water in a normal subject, since after a short interval the kidney will eliminate all fluids ingested to the upper limit of gastric capacity. In fact, the kidney may eliminate 10 or more liters of fluid in 24 hours, which correspond to "facultative" absorption in the distal convoluted tubule and is regulated by antidiuretic hormone. But water intoxication may appear in subjects unable to eliminate excess fluids, usually dehydrated and unconscious patients in the hands of enthusiastic physicians.[87] Clinical manifestations, which again are only apparent in those rare conscious subjects, are confusion, mental fatigue, headache and nausea; experimental animals may also show convulsions, coma and death.[88] The plasma is hypotonic because of hyponatremia, hypoproteinemia and low hematocrit value, although the last may be normal, indicating that part of the water remaining in the blood is equally distributed between plasma and red cells.[89] There is also polyuria with diluted urine and increased elimination of Cl−, which Wrong attributes to decreased aldosterone secretion as a response to a volume receptor somewhere in the organism.[90] Fluid excess is also intracellular, as a result of decreased osmotic pressure in the interstitial space, which favors passage of fluid inside the cells.

B. CHANGES IN CONCENTRATION OF BODY FLUIDS

Reference will be made only to changes in Na+ and K+ concentrations, since those of Cl− are similar to Na+, and changes in HCO$_3$− are discussed in the section of equilibrium of H+ ion.

1. Sodium. *a. Hyponatremia.* Decrease in plasma Na+ has been observed in many clinical conditions having as common denominator the loss of this ion with digestive tract secretions, sweat and urine.[91] Pure undernutrition or a low-salt diet will not produce hyponatremia because of the immediate reaction of the kidney with complete reabsorbtion of all filtered Na+;[92] in the patient with adrenal insufficiency, however, no aldosterone is secreted and there is loss of Na+ with the urine.[93] Fluid losses through the digestive tract are caused by repeated vomiting, diarrhea, fistulas and continuous aspirations, and are usually complicated by either acidosis or alkalosis; in severe diarrhea, as occurs in cholera or pseudomembranous enterocolitis, sodium loss may be massive and fatal. Excessive sweating will not produce hyponatremia because sweat is hypotonic, but with a decrease in fluid volume and ingestion of large amounts of water the loss of sodium becomes apparent, as is the case in the heat exhaustion syndrome.[94] Polyuria is not necessarily followed by hyponatremia; rather, this is the result of tubular insufficiency as in Addison's disease,[95] in osmotic diuresis caused by either glucose or urea,[96] in the polyuric phase of acute tubular necrosis,[97] in excessive loss of Cl^- caused by administration of mercurial diuretics,[98] etc.

Whatever the cause of hyponatremia, severe cases are usually accompanied by important hemodynamic modifications. Sodium loss decreases the tonicity of interstitial fluid, which can pass inside the cell and aggravate dehydration while causing hemoconcentration and increased viscosity of the blood. This is reflected in decreased cardiac output, venous return and arterial pressure, while at the same time there is an increase in circulating time. The final result is vascular collapse which includes renal failure with oliguria and azotemia, commonly observed in advanced cases of Na^+ depletion.[99] This extrarenal uremia may be mistaken for a primary renal condition, but in the latter Na^+ elimination with the urine is normal or high, while in the former there are only traces. The clinical picture of hyponatremia is very varied, and depends in part on the main disease producing it and on its severity. Sodium concentration in plasma may be high, normal or low, but the results of chemical determinations should not be judged in isolation from the clinical picture; indeed, a high sodium concentration is no contraindication for the use of saline solutions, nor does a low sodium level demand immediate replacement therapy.[100] The type of solution to be used in treatment varies with the H^+ ion equilibrium.

b. Hypernatremia. The most common manifestation of sodium excess in the organism is edema, but this requires retention of other anions and water. Hypernatremia without water retention cannot be induced by dietary means in normal subjects, since the renal tubules stop reabsorption of Na^+ and eliminate all excess. On the other hand, hypernatremia may be present when there is a defect in renal function, which might be caused by an intrinsic disease of the tubules, a circulatory disturbance decreasing the amount of Na^+ presented for reabsorption to the tubules, an excess of aldosterone, etc.[101] In acute nephritis or acute tubular necrosis, renal tubules show morphologic changes which can be correlated with their inability to reabsorb sodium.[102] In shock, in massive hemorrhage, and in other forms of acute hypotension, the amount of blood reaching the kidney is much less than normal and, therefore, the amount of Na^+ reabsorbed by the tubules decreases.[103] This is a transitory situation, but some data seem to favor this mechanism for Na^+ retention in patients with heart failure, especially of acute onset, as in myocardial infarction.[104]

Excessive aldosterone secretion may be primary or secondary;[105] primary aldosteronism is caused by a tumor or hyperplasia of the adrenal cortex which secretes large amounts of the hormone, and the patients show severe loss of K^+ by the kidney, arterial hypertension and sodium retention.[106] Most of these patients show no edema, but in some cases it has been present and may even be massive in character.[107] Of greater significance because of its frequency is secondary hyperaldosteronism, which appears in patients with generalized edemas of cardiac, renal, hepatic and other origins, and with increased concentration of Na^+ in plasma. This aspect of hypernatremia is further discussed under Edema.

2. Potassium. *a. Hypokalemia.* According to Black,[52] the term hypokalemia is preferred to its popular rival hypopotassemia because "Not only is it less offensive to the ear, but it does not beguile the fancy with thoughts of a bizarre zoological infestation of the blood." Anyhow, "hypokalemia" is not entirely correct since it literally means a low concentration of K^+ in blood, although the term actually refers to plasma.

Decrease of K^+ in plasma may be due to renal or extrarenal losses, especially through the digestive tract. Increased renal elimination of K^+ may occur when the concentration of this ion in the interstitial space is increased as the result of being displaced from inside the cells because of hypernatremia, acidosis, dehydration, or exaggerated protein catabolism, as in the metabolic response to trauma.[108] Furthermore, increased renal elimination of K+ is characteristic of primary or secondary hyperaldosteronism, of chronic salicylate administration and of some renal diseases such as pyelonephritis, renal tubular acidosis and the polyuric phase of acute renal necrosis.[109] Vomiting is not accompanied by important losses of K+ but in cases of chronic pyloric obstruction gastric aspiration of fluids associated with malnutrition and increased protein catabolism may produce hypokalemia. In the lower intestinal tract K+ is eliminated through ionic exchange with Na+[110] so that severe fluid and solid losses, as in chronic ulcerative colitis, steatorrhea, ureterosigmoidostomy[111] and even repeated enemas,[112] may lead to hypokalemia.

Potassium is lost not only from the extracellular compartment to the environment, but also to the intracellular compartment.[113] In glucose administration or in recovery from diabetic coma,[79] K+ is necessary for the passage of glucose through the cellular membrane, and if this process is much increased there may be hypokalemia. Chronic administration of testosterone is usually accompanied by slight hypokalemia. In familial periodic paralysis, immediately before or during a convulsive attack, there is a rapid penetration of K+ inside the cells with marked hypokalemia.[82]

Recently, attention has been called to a peculiar form of tubular dilation and vacuolation in the kidneys of patients with hypokalemia;[114] Kulka, et al.[115] called this condition "vacuolar nephropathy," and other names, such as hypokalemic or kaliopenic nephropathy, have been used.[116] It is characterized by the presence of dilated convoluted tubules, usually proximal, with large, empty vacuoles in the cytoplasm which displace the nucleus towards the base of the cell.[117] The condition seems to be reversible;[118] similar, but not identical, lesions are produced in experimental animals with hypokalemia.[119, 120] The main differences in the experimental, as against human, renal lesions of potassium deficiency appear to be that, at least in rats, a short episode of K+ depletion followed by prolonged periods of normal K+ concentrations leads to a progression of pathologic changes in the kidney[121] which has been compared to those occurring spontaneously in old age.[122] Furthermore, histochemical studies reveal abnormalities in the distal portions of the nephron, namely the thin limbs of Henle's loops and collecting ducts,[123] whereas microdissection studies in man have shown that the most severely involved portion of the nephron is the proximal convoluted tubule.[124] The most conspicuous effect of potassium deficiency on renal function is impairment of the urinary concentrating mechanism[125] which has been attributed to decreased water diffusion through damaged collecting ducts;[119] nevertheless, this explanation is adequate only for the experimental model since in man these structures have not been shown to be damaged.[126]

Focal areas of myocardial degeneration or necrosis and interstitial infiltration with mononuclear cells have been described in one fatal case of potassium depletion due to chronic diarrhea.[127]

b. Hyperkalemia. No condition is known in which the total amount of potassium in the organism is increased, although the hyperkalemias of Addison's disease and renal failure have been interpreted as such.[128] On the other hand, intracellular K+ increases in familial periodic paralysis, passing from the interstitial space into the cells during the convulsive attacks.[82] The most frequent forms of intracellular hyperkalemia occur during treatment of diabetes with insulin and glucose, or during administration of potassium salts in cases of renal failure, especially during the oliguric phase, when care must be exercised to eliminate all K+ from the diet. Extracellular K+ is increased during the metabolic response to trauma, in acidosis, in diabetic coma, in severe hemolytic crises and in agonal states with severe anoxia.[124] In all these cases hyperkalemia is transitory, but if it becomes persistent then it is indicative of a renal defect. The most important effects of hyperkalemia appear in striated muscle, both skeletal and cardiac. In the heart, hyperkalemia produces changes of progressively increasing severity as the concentration of potassium rises, which begin by slow idioventricular rhythm, ventricular fibrillation and diastolic standstill; levels at which cardiac stop occur vary between 7 and 13 mEq./1.[130] Skeletal muscles show paralysis, which may involve the intercostal muscles and produce asphyxia, but this is very rare and usually the heart stops before any changes are observed in skeletal muscles.

C. EDEMA

"Edema is a simple little word of humble Greek origin; and that is as far as edema walks with humility and simplicity. Its pathogenesis now presents one of the most complex problems in pathophysiology and many theories have already foundered in the uncharted sea of edema fluid."[131] The most important change in edema is an increase in interstitial fluid; in many forms of edema there is also an expansion in circulating volume, which would suggest that not only interstitial but all extracellular fluid is increased although this is not true of all cases, as it is not true also that all types of edema show an increased retention of Na^+ and water by the kidney. Generalizations from one, or a few, types of edema usually ignore two fundamental facts: (a) Edema is not a disease, but a symptom, a manifestation of another pathologic process, which occurs in the course of many different diseases. (b) Factors determining volume and concentration of body fluids are many and varied, thus suggesting the possibility that in different types of edema there may be different factors involved. The last decade has witnessed important advances in renal physiology, hormonal factors, fluid and electrolyte balance, etc., which make untenable many of the classical concepts of edema, although they cannot be replaced as yet by a completely satisfactory scheme. A survey of some general concepts of edema is presented in the following paragraphs.

There are two general types of edema, localized and systemic, which differ not only in their topographic distribution but also in their physiopathology. As suggested by its name, localized edema is that increase in extracellular (interstitial) fluid which is limited to a more or less well defined area of the organism. The most important aspects of the pathogenesis of localized edema are that it represents a derangement of Starling's mechanisms determining fluid exchange in the intimacy of tissues, and that it rarely involves an increase in circulatory volume; rather, it is due to a redistribution of existing fluids. On the other hand, systemic edema is a generalized increase in fluid volume in the extracellular space, which in addition to representing a disturbance in the mechanisms of fluid exchange in tissues is accompanied by endocrine, circulatory and renal modifications. Each one of these two types of edema is separately analyzed.

1. Localized Edema. There are several instances of this type of edema, which at the same time serve to illustrate some of the factors involved in Starling's equilibrium. It is convenient to emphasize that in no form of localized edema is there an absolute increase in body fluids; the basic disturbance is a redistribution of fluids existing in normal volume. Table 54 is a list of some types of localized edema. Starling's equilibrium has been summarized (p. 390) so here it should suffice to say that forces determining fluid exchange through a semipermeable membrane need not involve energy expenditure, and that in fact they may be considered as purely physicochemical in nature without any violence to observation.[21] Nevertheless, disturbances in one of those forces is immediately followed by changes in the others, so that no single factor can be incriminated as the cause of any type of edema; at most, it may be pointed out which factor seems to play the initiating, or most prominent, role.

Allergic edema, occurring in wheals, evanescent cutaneous responses and "angioneurotic" or Quincke's edema, appears after contact with an antigen and awakes a sudden and violent reaction.[132] Such a reaction is characterized by capillary dilation and marked increase in capillary permeability, comparable to that occurring after an injection of histamine. Vasodilation is accompanied by increased hydrostatic pressure which, together with the increased capillary permeability, favors the passage of fluid and proteins to the interstitial space, faster than they can be reabsorbed by the lymphatic system.[133] At the same time tissue pressure increases, which not only contributes to increased hydrostatic pressure in the arterial side of circulation by inducing partial collapse of veins, as shown by Starling in 1896, but also tends to oppose filtration from the capillary bed into the interstitial space.

Table 54.   Some Forms of Localized Edema

TYPE	BASIC CHANGE	RESULT	CLINICAL INSTANCE
Allergic edema	Increase in capillary permeability	Passage of proteins to interstitial space, increasing extravascular oncotic pressure and decreasing intravascular oncotic pressure	Angioneurotic edema; urticaria
Lymphedema	Blockage of lymphatic drainage	Accumulation of proteins and lymph in interstitial space increasing extravascular oncotic pressure	Elephantiasis caused by *W. bancrofti;* Milroy's disease
Inflammatory edema	Increase in capillary permeability and hydrostatic pressure	Passage of fluid and proteins to interstitial space; blockage of lymphatics by fibrin; local acidosis with increased retention of sodium and water by connective tissue	Infections such as pneumonia, scarlet fever, carbuncle
Venous insufficiency	Increase in intracapillary hydrostatic pressure	Filtration of fluid to interstitial space, with failure to reabsorb at the venular portion of capillaries	Varicose veins of the lower extremities
Acute pulmonary edema	Increase in hydrostatic pressure? Increase in capillary permeability?	Passage of fluid to alveolar sacs with blockage of gas exchange, anoxia and further increase in capillary permeability	Paroxysmal dyspnea in mitral stenosis

Plasma proteins are also present outside the capillary wall (after having left the circulation) and add their oncotic pressure to tissue pressure to oppose filtration pressure within the capillaries. In the end, the equilibrium is reached when all these hydrodynamic factors cancel each other; the effect of the antigen-antibody reaction vanishes; hydrostatic pressure in the capillaries is lowered to normal, and interstitial fluid is absorbed, especially by lymphatic vessels. The lymphatics are not collapsed because of the existence of firm anchorages to surrounding collagen fibers which, on becoming separated by edema fluid, keep the lymphatic vessels open.[134]

Lymphedema is perhaps the simplest form of disturbance in Starling's principle, since it is caused by inability of the lymph vessels to reabsorb interstitial fluid and proteins, the result being an increase in extracapillary oncotic pressure which favors greater filtration.[135] A frequent form of lymphedema is seen after radical mastectomy for the treatment of carcinoma of the breast, which includes removal of all lymph nodes in the homolateral axilla; lymphedema appears in the arm, which is left without lymphatic drainage.[136] It has been shown in a group of cases that cicatricial scarring in the axilla with compression of veins plays no role in this type of edema.[137] Some cases are on record of malignant transformation of lymphatics in arms affected by postmastectomy lymphedema.[138]

A similar form of edema, caused by pure obstruction of lymphatic drainage, is that produced by *Wuchereria bancrofti,* which is transmitted as the microfilaria by mosquitoes; microfilarias then migrate to the draining lymph nodes and in 12 to 18 months produce adult worms which may measure 5 to 8 cm. in length and which block lymph vessels and lymph nodes.[139] In addition to the mechanical blockade produced by the parasite there is also a connective tissue proliferation, especially after the worm dies, which contributes effectively to obstruct lymphatic, and sometimes even venous, channels. Interstitial fluid is then accumulated in large amounts in the areas peripheral to the blockage, usually lower extremities and scrotum. The resulting edema has at first a high protein content (1.9 to 4 Gm./100 ml.); later, a fibrous proliferation appears in the interstitial tissues which advances slow but relentlessly until grotesque enlargement of the involved areas is produced.[140] Not only because of the size, but also because of the skin which appears thickened, hard and dark, the phenomenon is known as elephantiasis.

A similar picture is caused by a congenital, inherited malformation known as Milroy's disease appearing in puberty or youth and characterized by the presence of many malformed lymph vessels in the interstitial tissue.[141] Lymphatic vessels may be so numerous that it has been thought to represent a true tumor, but such an interpretation is probably incorrect. In summary, lymphatic obstruction causes edema because of the drainage difficulty thus created and because of elevation of oncotic pressure in interstitial fluid, secondary to protein accumulation.

Venous insufficiency, especially that of the lower extremities, is known as varices and may occasionally lead to edema, especially in patients that must remain in the standing position for prolonged periods. In these cases, venous valves are unable to retain the blood and the result is venous hypertension,[142] which is transmitted to capillaries hindering the reabsorption of filtered fluid. Lymphatic capillaries drain at their maximal capacity, but beyond that there is accumulation of interstitial fluid. In this case edema is secondary to increased hydrostatic pressure, and later on, to increased interstitial oncotic pressure because of accumulation of proteins.

Inflammatory edema has many points of contact with the allergic type, since it is only a less exaggerated form of the same process of increased hydrostatic pressure and capillary permeability, as can be supposed from the important role played by chemical mediators in the pathogenesis of inflammation (*see* Chapter II). But soon other factors appear on the scene, as the blockage of lymphatic capillaries by fibrin clots, and biochemical changes in the area of injury which lower the pH and favor hydration of intercellular substances, perhaps under the influence of modified affinities for Na^+. There are still many unknown aspects in inflammatory edema.

Acute pulmonary edema is a special problem of great complexity; the mechanisms involved are not completely clarified. It should be remembered that in this form of edema, as in all other localized types, accumulation of fluid in the interstitial spaces is not due to an increase in total volume, but rather to a redistribution of existing fluids. Therefore, there seem to be two main problems connected with acute pulmonary edema: one, the mechanisms leading to an extra load of fluid in the pulmonary circulation, and the other, the manner by which this extra load disrupts Starling's equilibrium and produces edema. The complexity of the situation is reflected in

Experimental Methods of Producing Acute Pulmonary Edema

Acute ventricular overload:
  Ligature of aortic arch
  Multiple pulmonary embolism
Acute ventricular damage:
  Reduction of the left ventricle
  Necrosis of the left ventricle
  Necrosis of the right ventricle
Acute obstruction of pulmonary veins
Adrenalin administration
Trauma of the thorax
Localized pulmonary embolism
Massive intravenous injection of fluid
Rapid intracarotid injection of plasma or hypertonic
  solution
Bronchial irritation with gases
Toxic substances:
  Methyl salicylate
  Muscarine
  Alloxan
  Thiourea derivatives
  Ammonium chloride
Cerebral damage:
  Occlusion of carotid arteries
  Cerebral trauma
  Destruction of hypothalamus
  Cisternal injection of veratrine or fibrinogen +
    fibrin
Combined methods:
  Aortic insufficiency + adrenalin
  Aortic insufficiency + unilateral nephrectomy

the list of conditions in which pulmonary edema may occur: left ventricular failure, cranioencephalic traumatisms, pulmonary embolism and infarction, shock, infections, etc. In a series of 100 consecutive autopsies in which the patients had had acute pulmonary edema, Cameron[143] found advanced coronary disease, heart failure, malignant tumors of different origins, moderate or severe malnutrition, bronchopneumonia and arterial hypertension, among the most frequent causes. Furthermore, the number of experimental situations producing acute pulmonary edema is impressive, as can be seen in the outline above, constructed with data from Luisada.[144] It appears unlikely that a process developing in so many different conditions should have a single, simple mechanism.

There are many theories to explain acute pulmonary edema,[145] of which only three will be mentioned, namely the left ventricular failure theory, the neurogenic theory and the more recent neurohemodynamic theory. In 1878, Welch[146] produced acute pulmonary edema by obstructing the aorta before the emergence of the left subclavian artery, and showed that arterial pressure is elevated in both carotid arteries and pulmonary veins, but that it remains normal or low in the pulmonary artery. Acute pulmonary edema was also obtained by destroying the left ventricle without injuring the right ventricle. It was postulated that a dissociation between the output of both ventricles, with decreased output in the left and increased output in the right, would produce increased hydrostatic pressure in the pulmonary capillaries and edema. For 80 years this theory has been held, with minor modifications, by many physiologists and cardiologists, despite the unphysiologic experiments on which it is based (complete obstruction of the aorta, open chest, crushing of left ventricle) and the obvious impossibility of the main postulate, a dissociation of output between the two ventricles. According to Katz,[147] "a moment's reflection will show that if the left heart were to pump 5 cc. more per stroke than the right, and if the right pumped 60 cc. per stroke, and the heart beat 80 times per minute, and if the circulating blood volume is of the order of 5 liters, then in about 10 minutes all of the blood would have been pumped into the systemic circuit and none would remain in the lungs." Reversing the instance will give the same results for the right side of the heart. In addition, increased pulmonary vein pressure is not always accompanied by pulmonary edema, and direct measurement of pulmonary capillary pressure in patients with mitral stenosis sometimes reveals figures surpassing the normal capillary oncotic pressure[148] (oncotic pressure: 25 to 30 mm. Hg; hydrostatic pressure: 35 to 42 mm. Hg) although the situation need not be the same in pathologic lungs, where anatomic changes in the alveolar walls might impose additional obstacles to the free diffusion of fluid.[149] Furthermore, in many cases of pulmonary edema the left ventricle is normal and the main disease involves either the brain or other part of the organism. It is possible, however, that some agonal forms of acute pulmonary edema, or that developing in extensive and rapidly fatal myocardial infarction, are caused by a mechanism involving some degree of dissociation between the output of both ventricles.[150]

The neurogenic theory of pulmonary edema is based on the frequency with which cerebral diseases are accompanied by it. It has received experimental support from Cameron and De,[151] who were able to induce acute pulmonary edema in cats by the intracysternal injection of fibrinogen and thrombin, and from McKay, who observed[152] that encephalic traumatisms in rats are accompanied by pulmonary edema, and furthermore, that section of vagal nerves inhibits the development of this type of edema. Removal of stellate ganglia will prevent edema produced by adrenaline; anesthetics and sympathicolytic drugs inhibit pulmonary edema more than vasodilators.[153]

The neurohemodynamic theory of the mechanism of pulmonary edema is based on several experimental findings. First, the rapid injection of large amounts of serum into the carotid arteries in a cephalic direction will result in pulmonary edema; second, denervation of the carotid sinus inhibits the development of this type of experimental edema; third, the same amounts of fluid injected at the same speed into the femoral artery will produce edema with less frequency; fourth, section of vagal nerves has no influence on this form of edema, but the use of morphine and barbiturates will block its development.[154] Sarnoff[155] has suggested that the mechanism is as follows: Pressoreceptors of carotid sinus and other areas are stimulated by the rapid increase in volume and produce a generalized vasoconstriction which decreases cardiac output, increases peripheral resistance and displaces the blood from capillaries, venules and reservoirs, increasing the venous return and the right cardiac output, while emptying of the left ventricle is made difficult. This rapid redistribution of circulating volume would result in acute pulmonary edema.

Pulmonary edema produced by breathing toxic substances is easier to understand, since in this case the toxicant will damage the capillary wall directly, increasing its permeability and initiating the passage of fluid and protein into the alveolar space, in amounts beyond the draining ability of the lymphatic system.[156] In many cases of acute pulmonary edema the concentration of protein in the edema fluid is greater than could be expected from a simple increase in hydrostatic pressure, and this points out the participation of capillary permeability, as demonstrated experimentally by Cheng.[157] It is believed that increased protein content of edema fluid is caused by anoxia, since the presence of fluid within the alveoli interferes with adequate oxygenation of alveolar cells, the result being an increase in capillary permeability. Furthermore, anoxia brings about a contraction of pulmonary vessels and an increase in cardiac output,[158, 159] which are manifested by hypertension in the pulmonary circuit, and this tends to favor the passage of fluid from the capillaries into the alveolar cavities. A vicious circle is thus established, in which the greater outpouring of fluid from the capillaries increases anoxia, and this results in greater permeability and higher hydrostatic pressure in the capillaries. Nevertheless, even in the case of toxic substances, drugs with an inhibiting effect on the sympathetic nervous system and, in general, all depressants of the cerebral cortex, such as anesthetics, alcohol, morphine, etc., decrease mortality in acute experimental pulmonary edema.[160]

In view of the preceding data, it may be convenient to conclude that hemodynamic factors redistributing the circulatory volume and overloading the pulmonary circulation, together with all of Starling's factors regulating fluid exchange in the intimacy of tissues,[161] and with some mysterious influence of the nervous system, act in a combined and variable manner in the different types of acute pulmonary edema.

2. Systemic Edema. Systemic or generalized edema requires the presence of two different types of factors: (a) disturbances in the mechanisms regulating the exchange of fluids in tissues, which result in the accumulation of fluid in the interstitial space as a consequence of overwhelming the draining capacity of the lymphatic system; (b) disturbances in the mechanisms regulating the total volume and concentration of body fluids, especially water and Na^+ reabsorption in the renal tubule, which result in a positive balance of water and Na^+. The first type point to disturbances in fluid distribution, and are similar to those encountered in localized edema, while the second type of factors refer to volume and occur only in

systemic edema. Therefore, a satisfactory explanation of any type of systemic edema should involve mechanisms for the increase in total fluid volume, as well as for its extravascular localization. There is a limit to the accumulation of fluids in the organism, which is set at different levels for different individuals, i.e., the patient does not go on swelling indefinitely; unfortunately, the mechanisms operating to set such a limit are not known.

Changes in Starling's factors have been discussed with localized edema, but some of them have been supposed to occur in a systemic form in some types of generalized edema. The clearest instance is hypoproteinemia, which would lower the oncotic pressure of the plasma, leaving the hydrostatic pressure to predominate throughout the capillary length and resulting in increased passage of fluid into the interstitial spaces.

Experimentally it was shown by Weech et al.[162] that plasmapheresis in dogs results in edema, and clinically this form of edema has been postulated in the nephrotic syndrome,[163] in cirrhosis of the liver,[164] and in starvation,[165] since in all these instances there is hypoproteinemia, especially hypoalbuminemia. The significance of this factor is made less certain, however, by consideration of the following facts. Kylin[166] induced plasmapheresis in rabbits and failed to observe edema despite the fact that plasma proteins were near zero; no reason is apparent as to why the experiment in dogs should be preferred to that in rabbits, other than the personal animal preferences of the different authors. Furthermore, there are cases of nephrotic syndrome with generalized edema and normal figures of plasma proteins, others with very low hypoalbuminemia and no edema, and still others in which there is coincidence of hypoproteinemia and edema, but during a remission there will be polyuria with elimination of much interstitial fluid without any coincident modification in plasma proteins.[167]

Similar observations are available for starvation edema. In many cases there is coincidence of edema and hypoalbuminemia, but there are others in which edema will not appear until sodium is ingested, and then what edema there is bears no relation to plasma protein levels.[168] Keys *et al.*[169] kept a series of young men in a state of starvation for approximately 6 months, and although many of them developed edema the actual average decrease in plasma protein was only 0.7 Gm. In cirrhosis of the liver it has been observed that there is a critical level of 3.1 Gm. per cent of albumin below which edema and ascites will accumulate.[170] This seems to be true, however, only in patients with the postnecrotic type of cirrhosis since another study of a group of patients mostly with Laennec's cirrhosis failed to show such correlation.[171]

Armstrong, *et al.*[172] published what may be the explanation for all these contradictory observations. They made careful measurements of the oncotic pressure actually present at different levels of albumin in plasma of nephrosis and cirrhosis and found that there is no linear correlation between protein concentration and osmotic pressure, probably because of differences in the spatial configuration of the molecule in various diseases. This suggests that correlations would have to be established between the actual value of plasma oncotic pressure and edema, and not between plasma proteins and edema. Nevertheless, that hypoalbuminemia by itself is unlikely to be the only, or even the most important, factor in any form of edema is strongly supported by the striking finding of two cases with congenital analbuminemia by Bennhold *et al.*[173] One of them, a 31 year old woman, complained of fatigability and slight edema of the joints; the other subject was her brother, who was able to do heavy farm work and had never suffered from edema.

Another factor involved in Starling's equilibrium is capillary permeability, and this too has been postulated to be altered in a systemic way in some forms of generalized edema, such as the edema of acute nephritis and even that of the nephrotic syndrome. Peters[174, 175] has summarized the arguments against this hypothesis, which are as follows: (a) Systemic alteration in capillary permeability would result in hypoproteinemia and increased protein concentration in the edema fluid. Measurement of these two parameters has shown them to be incompatible with such a theory. (b) Direct measurement of capillary permeability by means of radioactive isotopes has revealed normal values in several types of systemic edema. (c) Extensive histologic study of peripheral capillaries in some forms of generalized edema has failed to show any abnormality. (d) The existence of other factors adequately demonstrated makes increased capillary permeability unnecessary as an explanation of generalized edema.

Schade[176] suggested that edema might be explained by a change in colloid hydrophilia. This author considered that interstitial connective tissue (the site of edema accumulation) became acid, and through this lowered pH its affinity for water was increased. Although in principle this hypothesis is correct, in practice the change in pH necessary for an increase in hydrophilia is entirely incompatible with life, especially at a systemic level. On the other hand, Blumberg, *et al.*[177] have shown *in vitro* that different electrolyte concentrations, especially Na^+, can modify the spatial structure of acid mucopolysaccharides such as hyaluronic acid, which is abundant in the interstitial space. This change in structure is parallel to an increase in affinity for Na^+, and therefore for water, which may be fixed to the interstitial space in larger amounts than normal. The spatial structure of hyaluronic acid is similar to that of an ionic exchange resin, and this would probably explain, at least in part, why water is retained in the interstitial space, which is another unsolved problem in generalized edema.[178] In this case, Starling's equilibrium would be modified by an increase in extravascular osmotic pressure, which would promote both the outpouring of fluid from the capillaries and the retention of excess fluid in the interstitial space.

Finally, a generalized increase in hydrostatic pressure has also been invoked as responsible for a special type of systemic edema, that of heart failure. This hypothesis is common to both "forward"[104] and "backward"[179] theories of heart failure; whatever the mechanism for increased circulating volume, in the end it is increased hydrostatic pressure in veins that will cause edema.

The preceding considerations deal only with factors involved in redistribution of fluids. Those determining the total volume of body fluids operate at the level of renal tubules through reabsorption of water and sodium. It has been mentioned that the total amount of fluids in the organism is the result of glomerular filtration and tubular reabsorption, so that an increase in fluid volume may result from: (a) decrease in filtration with normal reabsorption; (b) normal filtration and increased reabsorption; and (c) decrease in filtration and increase in reabsorption. In most cases what has been found to occur is that filtration remains normal while reabsorption is increased; some factors involved in this process are hormonal and some are of another nature.[180]

It has been mentioned that several hormones participate in tubular reabsorption of water and Na$^+$, and that the two most important are aldosterone and antidiuretic hormone. An early observation was the presence in the urine of normal subjects of a factor capable of inducing Na$^+$ retention in the kidney, which was considered to be antidiuretic hormone. Nevertheless, quantitative studies in patients with heart failure and cirrhosis of the liver showed that antidiuretic hormone was present in normal amounts[181] and that the diseased liver was perfectly capable of inactivating it.[182] Furthermore, White et al.[183] observed that the administration of antidiuretic hormone to patients with edema produced the same reactions as in normal subjects, so the possibility of increased sensitivity to this hormone was eliminated. On the other hand, in a long series of papers Luetscher[184] has shown that aldosterone is elevated in patients with various types of edema, and that with disappearance of edema the amount of aldosterone returns to normal. It appears to be definitely established that aldosterone is one of the most important factors in Na$^+$ and water retention in edematous patients;[185] a moot point is whether this increased level of aldosterone is a primary disturbance or an adaptation of the organism to higher levels of Na$^+$ and water.

The sensitivity of different subjects to equal amounts of hormones is very variable, as appears in patients with Addison's disease or arterial hypertension, who are very sensitive to desoxycorticosterone, or in patients with chronic glomerulonephritis and diabetes insipidus, who are resistant to antidiuretic hormone.

Nonhormonal factors are represented by decreased glomerular filtration, which is present in some cases of advanced heart failure and in any other cause of venous hypertension, and with increased intrarenal pressure. However, most patients with heart failure have normal glomerular filtration rates[187] and venous hypertension increases tubular reabsorption of Na$^+$.[188] Sodium and water retention may also occur as a part of the metabolic response to trauma,[189] probably because of K$^+$ loss with increased protein catabolism and intracellular sequestration of Na$^+$ (p. 456).

In summary, in generalized edema there are two types of factors operating to determine distribution and total volume of body fluids: the former are those in Starling's equilibrium of fluid exchange in the intimacy of tissues, the latter are related to Na$^+$ and water retention in the organism. No explanations are available for the maximum limit set to Na$^+$ and fluid volume in many types of edema, nor for the mechanism of fluid retention in the interstitial space.

V. REGULATION OF H$^+$ION EQUILIBRIUM

The preceding paragraphs contained a discussion of volume and concentration of body fluids under both normal and abnormal conditions. In this section the physiologic and pathologic aspects of the composition of body fluids are presented. This field can also be characterized as H$^+$ ion equilibrium or "acid-base" balance. Relman[190] has pointed out the reasons why the terms "acid" and "base" are easily confusing and should be abandoned: From a physicochemical standpoint, reactions occurring between acids and bases are only exchange of protons (H$^+$ ions), in which acids act as proton donors and bases serve as proton receptors. Both may be either anions or cations or even nonionized compounds. Following this idea, Cl$^-$ and SO$_4^=$ (anions or "acids" in the clinical sense) are not acids but very weak bases, while Na^+ and K^+ (cations or "bases") are neither acids nor bases. The application of this, the Brönsted nomenclature, to acid-base disorders in surgery is discussed by Kaufman and Rosen.[191]

Biologic reactions frequently release groups of H^+ donor compounds and others of H^+ receptors; in addition, some substances are easily ionized and liberate protons. Enzymatic reactions are exquisitely sensitive to the pH of the medium, a property shared by the spatial structure of macromolecules, especially proteins. The continuous production of H^+ ions in the organism demands the existence of adaptation mechanisms that will maintain a constant pH at a level where enzymatic reactions are optimal. The existence of such mechanisms is witnessed by the fact that the concentration of H^+ is jealously guarded despite there being almost infinitesimal quantities of this ion in the organism ($10^{-7.4}$ Eq./l. of extracellular fluid).

The basic principles ruling the characteristics of H^+ ion equilibrium are very simple and require only a small effort to grasp them. That, however, seems to be the main difficulty, since as all things easy to learn, they are also easy to forget.

A. BASIC PRINCIPLES

Most of the knowledge necessary to understand the H^+ ion equilibrium can be reduced to two general principles: electrolytic dissociation and the Henderson-Hasselbalch equation. They explain the way in which buffer systems work.[192]

1. Electrolytic Dissociation. A simple acid substance in solution separates into its components according to the following reversible reaction:

$$HA \rightleftharpoons H^+ + A^- \qquad (1)$$

In order to transform this qualitative expression into a quantitative equation, one must take into account that the dissociation of HA is proportional to its concentration, which is represented as [HA], and to its intrinsic instability, which is a constant k for each acid. Therefore, the speed at which the reaction moves from left to right may be represented as follows:

$$[HA] \, k_1 = [H^+] + [A^-] \qquad (2)$$

On the other hand, the speed with which the reaction moves from right to left depends on the concentrations of H^+ and of A^-, since the greater the concentration of dissociated particles the higher the probability that they will come in contact; furthermore, the affinity of H^+ for A^- depends on another constant, which is different for each ion and may be represented as k_2. In equilibrium, the dissociation of HA may then be represented as follows:

$$[HA] \, k_1 = [H^+] \, [A^-] \, k_2 \qquad (3)$$

Since k_1 and k_2 are constants, the reaction may be simplified by writing

$$k_1 \, / \, k_2 = Ka \qquad (4)$$

so the representation of equilibrium in the dissociation of HA would be

$$[HA] \, Ka = [H^+] \, [A^-] \qquad (5)$$

and solving Ka in order to know the dissociation constant of the acid

$$Ka = \frac{[H^+] \, [A^-]}{[HA]} \qquad (6)$$

which is an expression following the mass action law.

In order to learn the concentration of H^+ ions in a given solution of a simple acid, equation (6) is rearranged as follows:

$$[H^+] = Ka \frac{[HA]}{[A^-]} \qquad (7)$$

The dissociation of salts is similar in most respects, but the resulting ions are not playing all their electrostatic activity because they are in equilibrium with other anions and cations in solution. Therefore, the activity of a given salt in solution refers to the total composition of electrolytes, which is a constant g called "activity coefficient." The effective concentrations of cations and anions derived from a salt are proportional to the product of the salt concentration and its activity coefficient, which may be expressed as follows:

$$g \, [BA] = [B^+] \, [A^-] \qquad (8)$$

2. The Henderson-Hasselbalch Equation. This famous equation expresses the relations existing between weak acids and their salts, when in solution in plasma, and pH.

It is extremely useful to understand the mechanism of action of buffers, and the actual situation in certain pathologic conditions such as acidosis and alkalosis.

When HA and BA are placed in solution, and it is assumed that all H$^+$ ions in equation (7) are derived from HA, and that all [A$^-$] in the same equation arise from BA, since α [BA] = [A$^-$] it may be written

$$[H^+] = Ka \frac{[HA]}{\alpha [BA]} \qquad (9)$$

but since Ka and g are constants, it may be considered that

$$Ka / g = k \qquad (10)$$

and the equation may now be written as follows:

$$[H^+] = k \frac{[HA]}{[BA]} \qquad (11)$$

which is Henderson's equation, stating that the concentration of H$^+$ ions is equal to the product of a constant multiplied by the result of dividing the concentration of undissociated acid by the concentration of undissociated base.

Hasselbalch simplified this equation in order to handle the figures of H$^+$ ions naturally occurring in the organism, which vary between 0.0000001 and 0.00000016 Gm./l., which would make all operations rather cumbersome. Writing the reciprocal of all terms in equation (11)

$$\frac{1}{[H^+]} = \frac{1}{k} + \frac{[BA]}{[HA]} \qquad (12)$$

and then using logarithms for the same expression

$$\log \frac{1}{[H^+]} = \log \frac{1}{k} + \log \frac{[BA]}{[HA]} \qquad (13)$$

By using Sorensen's nomenclature, where

$$pH = \log \frac{1}{H^+} \qquad (14)$$

and expressing pK as follows

$$pK = \log \frac{1}{k} \qquad (15)$$

the final equation may now be written

$$pH = pK + \log \frac{[BA]}{[HA]} \qquad (16)$$

which is known as the Henderson-Hasselbalch equation. Its usefulness becomes apparent when the values actually occurring in man are replaced in it, using NaHCO$_3$ as the base and H$_2$CO$_3$ as the acid. Thus:

$$pH = pK + \log \frac{[NaHCO_3]}{[H_2CO_3]} \qquad (17)$$

Constant pKHCO$_3^-$ is 6.1; the normal amount of NaHCO$_3$ is 27 mEq./l., and that of H$_2$CO$_3$ is 1.35 mEq./l.; i.e., the relation of sodium carbonate to carbonic acid is 20 to 1. Substituting these values in equation (17)

$$pH = 6.1 + \log \frac{20}{1} \qquad (18)$$

The logarithm of 20 is 1.3, so the numeric expression may be written as follows:

$$pH = 6.1 + 1.3 \qquad (19)$$

and by solving it is shown that the normal pH of the plasma is 7.4.

When the normal ratio of $\frac{20}{1}$ is modified there will be a change in pH, but if both members of the equation are proportionally changed the equilibrium will be maintained and the pH will remain constant.

3. Buffers. A buffer system is formed by a weak acid in solution and its salt. It functions by opposing radical changes in pH which would otherwise occur upon addition of a strong acid. The most important buffer system in the organism is formed by H$_2$CO$_3$ and the sodium salt NaHCO$_3$. When HCl is added to this system the reaction is as follows:

$$HCl + NaHCO_3 = NaCl + H_2CO_3$$

The result is a decrease in the amount of NaHCO$_3$ and an increase in H$_2$CO$_3$, but the deviation in pH is much smaller than if HCl had become dissociated in the absence of a buffer system, since H$_2$CO$_3$ is a weak acid and a large part of its H$^+$ ions remain undissociated. Furthermore, the organism has efficient mechanisms to eliminate excess

H_2CO_3 and regain $NaHCO_3$; otherwise, buffer systems would be soon exhausted, since they follow the mass action law.

B. PHYSICOCHEMICAL REGULATION

There are two great systems of regulation of H^+ ion equilibrium in the organism: one is of physicochemical nature and resides in plasma and red blood cells, while the other is physiologic and depends on the functioning of lungs and kidneys. Another distinction is possible between these two systems: the physicochemical regulation is immediate, its effects begin as soon as there is any deviation in the pH of the plasma, while physiologic mechanisms are slower in action and their net effect is to maintain the ratio of base to weak acids in the normal proportion of 20 to 1.

Physicochemical regulation is carried out by means of buffer systems distributed throughout the different fluid compartments of the body.[193] These whole body buffers take care of most of the acid or alkaline load in acute respiratory acidosis or alkalosis, the renal mechanism accounting for only 4 to 6 per cent of the total disposal.[194] In the plasma and interstitial compartments, body buffers are represented by the carbonate-carbonic acid, phosphate-phosphoric acid and proteinate-protein systems, while in red cells the oxyhemoglobin-hemoglobin system predominates. Quantitatively, the most important system is that formed by carbonate-carbonic acid; according to Swan and Pitts,[193] in nephrectomized dogs 40 per cent of the total buffering is done extracellularly, 10 per cent is done by the erythrocyte, and 50 per cent by cellular buffers. This is fortunate, since the organism is continuously forming CO_2 as part of the metabolism, and this gas is easily removed by the respiration. Furthermore, the usual clinical determinations are made of the total concentration of CO_2 in plasma, which in view of the preponderance of $NaHCO_3$ over H_2CO_3 $\left(\dfrac{20}{1}\right)$ may be taken as representative of modifications in $NaHCO_3$ and are known as "alkaline reserve." The term is a misnomer since it measures not only "alkaline" but also "acid" reserve, and it also fails to include proteins, phosphates, hemoglobin, and other buffer systems which are quantita-

tively less important. It may be pertinent to point out at this moment that changes in H_2CO_3 usually result from CO_2 retention in the lungs (respiratory acidosis) or excessive elimination with the respiration (respiratory alkalosis), while deviations in the buffer system as a whole are usually of a metabolic nature, regardless of whether they increase or decrease their concentration.

C. PHYSIOLOGIC REGULATION

Physiologic regulation of the H^+ ion equilibrium is carried out in the organs which are related to the environment, the lungs and the kidneys.

1. Respiratory Regulation. The main outlet of CO_2 is the respiratory tract. The pCO_2 in breathed air is in equilibrium with the plasma concentration of H_2CO_3. When the pCO_2 decreases in the breathed air, as is the case in hyperventilation, there is an increased elimination of H_2CO_3 as H_2O and CO_2; the plasma concentration of H_2CO_3 falls, and there is alkalosis with elevation in pH. The opposite process, observed in pulmonary emphysema, tends to produce acidosis.[195] The pCO_2 of breathed air is a function of the volume per minute, and as the respiratory center is sensitive to pO_2, pCO_2, and to plasma pH, the number of respirations will be adjusted to the physicochemical constants of plasma.[196] The respiratory regulation of H^+ ion equilibrium is a homeostatic mechanism admirably adapted to carry out its function by changing the concentration of one of the components of the carbonate-carbonic acid buffer system in plasma.[197]

2. Renal Regulation.[198] The kidney is the most important physiologic regulator of plasma pH, since the lung can only eliminate volatile anions and cations, and for practical purposes its activities are limited to CO_2. All "fixed" acids and bases must be eliminated by the kidney, which in addition is capable of subtracting small amounts of free H^+ ion from the organism through the synthesis of NH_3. The mechanisms used by the kidney in the maintenance of pH are of three types: (1) the conservation of base as bicarbonate ($NaHCO_3$, $KHCO_3$, etc.); (2) the elimination of H^+ ions through ionic exchange with Na^+ and K^+, (3) the removal of H^+ ions by the synthesis of

NH$_3$.[199] These three mechanisms function simultaneously and are intimately related, although the contribution of each one in the maintenance of plasma pH is quantitatively different. The first one, or conservation of base as bicarbonate, seems to be the most important.[200]

Every 24 hours the renal glomeruli filter 5000 to 5400 mEq. of HCO$_3^-$, or close to 4 kg. if expressed as NaHCO$_3$, which represents five times the total amount of bicarbonate in the normal individual. Nevertheless, the urine contains only 1 to 2 mEq. every day, which should give an idea of the effectiveness of the reabsorbing mechanisms in the renal tubules.[201, 202] Furthermore, if excess bicarbonate is administered it will appear in the urine in the amount given and no more. The significance of HCO$_3^-$ reabsorption may be estimated when considering that the most abundant buffer system in the body is that formed by carbonate-carbonic acid; failure in the mechanism for conservation of bicarbonate by the kidney results in disastrous changes in plasma pH.

A small fraction of the base preserved by the kidney contributes to the elimination of H$^+$ ions produced by the cells during their metabolism in the form of "fixed" acids such as sulphuric and phosphoric acids. These acids are neutralized by the carbonate-carbonic acid system, thus decreasing the amount of HCO$_3^-$ in the fluids of the body. The entire HCO$_3^-$ of plasma might be exhausted in less than a week were it not for the renal tubule, which retains a large fraction of the filtered anion and returns it to the circulation. The mechanism appears to be as follows: neutral salts of weak acids reaching the tubules after being filtered in the glomerulus become acid salts or free acids and the base is retained as bicarbonate. For instance:

$$\text{Na}_2\text{HPO}_4 + \text{H}_2\text{CO}_3 \rightarrow \text{NaH}_2\text{PO}_4 \text{ (excreted)}$$
$$+ \text{ NaHCO}_3 \text{ (reabsorbed)}$$

Disodium phosphate reacts with carbonic acid and forms monosodium phosphate, which is eliminated with two H$^+$ ions, and monosodium carbonate, which is reabsorbed, thus preserving half of the base. The origin of carbonic acid is in plasma CO$_2$ which may combine slowly with H$_2$O, but in the presence of an enzyme, carbonic anhydrase, the combination is instantaneous. Therefore, the complete mechanism

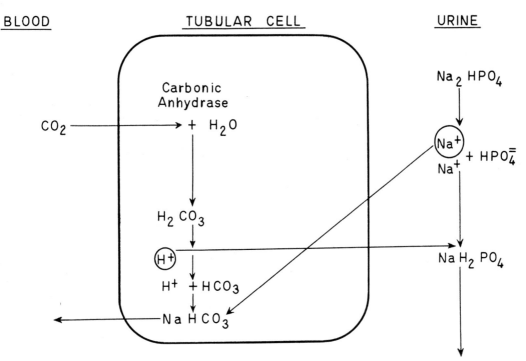

FIG. 9–4. Mechanism of Na retention by the kidney in exchange for H$^+$ ions.

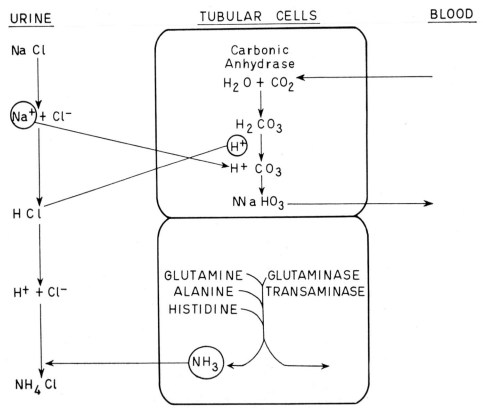

FIG. 9–5. Mechanism of NH_3 synthesis in renal tubular cells.

may be represented as in Figure 9–4 and is usually known as ionic exchange, since one H^+ is exchanged for one Na^+ ion, which is preserved. It has been suggested that energy for this process is derived from cellular metabolism, probably as a transformation of electric into electrochemical energy.[203]

In 1921, Nash and Benedict[204] showed that the kidney was capable of synthesizing ammonia which appears in large quantities in the urine. The compounds used by the kidney for this synthesis are glutamine, asparagin, alanine, histidine and other amino acids,[205] and the transformation is catalyzed by the enzymes glutaminase, L-amino acid oxidase, glycine oxidase and transaminases.[206] Once it has been formed, ammonia combines with Cl^- or other anions and with H^+ to form an ammonium salt, which is the way in which it appears in the urine. The process is depicted in Figure 9–5. The process is carried out in the distal tubule and is influenced by two separate factors, which are rate of production of ammonia in the tubule cells and rate

of diffusion from the cells into the intra-tubular fluid.[207]

The three mechanisms described function at the same time, but the way they react when there is a sudden increase in the amount of H^+ ions is as follows: first, there is an increased base elimination, beginning only a few minutes after acidosis; then, there is an increased formation of ammonia, and finally, large amounts of acid salts appear in the urine.

VI. DISTURBANCES IN THE EQUILIBRIUM OF THE H+ ION

Acidosis and alkalosis are not absolute, but relative terms; "acidosis" does not mean that plasma pH is lower than 7, but lower than 7.4, and it has been mentioned that life is possible only within very narrow deviations from this figure. By the same token, alkalosis is only a very slight increase

Table 55. Types of Acidosis

TYPE	MECHANISM	CAUSES
Respiratory	Increase in pCO$_2$ in alveolar air caused by interference with normal ventilation.	Pulmonary emphysema Bronchial asthma Pulmonary fibrosis Bronchial obstruction Poliomyelitis with respiratory paralysis Heart failure
Metabolic		
(a) Increase in H$^+$ ions	1. Greater production of "fixed" acids such as lactic, pyruvic, etc.	Diabetes mellitus
	2. Administration of acid substances such as HCl, NH$_4$Cl, etc.	Iatrogenic
(b) Decrease in base	1. Loss of carbonate	Diarrhea, biliary fistula, vomiting of intestinal contents
(c) Renal failure	1. Accumulation of H$^+$ ions produced in normal amounts caused by renal elimination defect	Acute or chronic renal failure

in pH above 7.4. Furthermore, acidosis and alkalosis are not static changes but very dynamic processes, so that determinations carried out within a few hours may show wide variations, sometimes caused by the main disease, sometimes as a response to medical treatment. Finally, acidosis and alkalosis are very frequently complications of certain diseases, and not entities in themselves. Diagnosis, and therefore treatment, should rest in a complete appreciation of the entire clinical situation and not only on one electrolyte determination.

A. ACIDOSIS

By definition, acidosis is an increase in plasma concentration of H$^+$ ions, or a decrease in pH below 7.4. Such an elevation in H$^+$ ions may be caused by the following mechanisms or several combinations of them: (1) metabolic production of "fixed" acids such as pyruvic, lactic, diacetic, etc., in amounts greater than can be compensated by, or eliminated through, plasmatic and renal mechanisms; (2) exaggerated ingestion or administration of acid substances; (3) retention of "fixed" acids (produced in normal amounts) by defective compensating mechanisms; (4) abnormal retention of CO$_2$ with increased dissociated H$_2$CO$_3$ in the circulation; (5) excessive loss of base. The different types of acidosis, according to the mechanisms just described, appear in Table 55.

The homeostatic compensation of aci-

dosis takes place in the lung and kidneys; in the latter, the mechanism is always retention of larger amounts of bicarbonate and the removal of H$^+$ ions in the form of acid urine, due to both a high concentration of acid phosphates and increased excretion of ammonia. Respiratory compensation differs according to the type of metabolic acidosis.

1. Respiratory Acidosis. This form of acidosis is caused by respiratory retention of plasma CO$_2$. The result is an increase in the denominator of the carbonate-carbonic acid buffer system, and a concomitant decrease in the normal 20:1 ratio, with the consequent decrease in plasma pH. The most frequent causes are those interfering with normal ventilation and increasing the partial tension of CO$_2$ in breathed air, as chronic pulmonary emphysema,[208] asthma, pulmonary fibrosis and in general all diffuse pulmonary diseases, bronchial obstruction, infections, poliomyelitis with paralysis of respiratory muscles, heart failure, etc.[209]

Compensatory mechanisms are mainly renal, with considerable retention of bicarbonate and increased elimination of acid phosphates and ammonia.[210, 211] The result may be a discrete hypernatremia, secondary to increased Na$^+$ reabsorption as bicarbonate and a heightened ionic exchange of Na$^+$ for H$^+$ ions, while excessive elimination of chloride as NH$_4$Cl partly drains the Cl$^-$ reserves and there may be a slight hypochloremia.[212]

2. Metabolic Acidosis. Metabolic acidosis results from the excessive (absolute or relative) retention of acid substances which cannot be eliminated through the lungs. There are three general types, caused: (1) by an increase in H^+ ions; (2) by a decrease in base; (3) by renal insufficiency.[213]

Metabolic acidosis caused by an absolute increase in H^+ ions occurs in decompensated diabetes mellitus, where there is an overproduction of ketogenic acids as the result of the disturbance in the normal lipid metabolism,[214] in the excessive administration of HCl or NH_4Cl,[215] and in the exaggerated metabolic response to trauma with massive protein catabolism.[216] In these cases compensation is mainly renal, with bicarbonate conservation and, therefore, Na^+, and increased elimination of H^+ ions as acid phosphates and NH_3.[217] There is also hyperventilation with removal of part of the plasma CO_2, which tends to compensate acidosis. In diabetic patients it is of great importance to know the status of the kidneys, since they represent the most significant compensating mechanism;[218] unfortunately, there is frequently atherosclerotic nephrosclerosis, intercapillary glomerulosclerosis, pyelonephritis, or a combination of all these changes which greatly limit the compensating renal mechanisms.

Metabolic acidosis caused by loss of base is usually secondary to chronic diarrhea, to repeated vomiting of intestinal contents, to biliary or pancreatic fistulas, to intestinal occlusion, etc., and in general to all important causes of loss of base from the organism. Probably, bicarbonate is secreted in the intestine where there is dissociation of H_2CO_3, release of H^+ ions which are reabsorbed and of HCO_3^- ions which are lost. Therefore, in diarrhea there is loss of base accompanied by a loss of Na^+. This type of acidosis must be compensated by the kidney, by retaining bicarbonate and eliminating H^+ ions in the form described.

Finally, renal failure is accompanied by inability of the kidney to carry out its normal functions in maintaining the equilibrium of H^+ ions, which accumulate in the organism.[219] Compensation is respiratory, but not very efficient since the nature of the acids retained makes the elimination of CO_2 of limited value for the organism.[220]

B. ALKALOSIS

1. Respiratory Alkalosis. In respiratory alkalosis there is hyperventilation with excessive loss of CO_2,[221] thus decreasing the denominator of the carbonate-carbonic acid relation; the 20:1 index increases and the plasma pH tends to be more alkaline. This is the less frequent type of disturbance of the H^+ ion equilibrium.[222] It is usually the result of a strong central stimulation, as occurs in emotional disturbances, anoxia, fever, encephalitis, brain tumors and intracranial surgery.[223] The compensation is at the level of the kidney with increased elimination of bicarbonate and retention of chloride, and there may be salt depletion of the plasma.[224]

2. Metabolic Alkalosis. Metabolic alkalosis may be caused by an excessive loss of H^+ ions in the form of fixed anions, as HCl in repeated vomiting or gastric suction,[225] by retention of fixed Na^+, as in cases of administration of large doses of antiacids;[226] finally, it may also be the result of increased elimination of Cl^- under the influence of diuretics.[227] In these cases the relation of carbonate-carbonic acid is disturbed by an increase in the numerator and the 20:1 ratio becomes higher, with a displacement of plasma pH towards alkalinity.

The immediate result is hypoventilation, which results in CO_2 retention and an increase in the denominator in the Henderson-Hasselbalch equation. In addition, renal elimination of Na_2CO_3 is increased, rendering the urine alkaline. In the serum there is elevated CO_2, hypernatremia and hyperchloremia; slight hypokalemia may also be present.[228]

REFERENCES

1. Szent-Györgyi, A.: Ions, Function and Permeability, in Jasmin, G., and Robert, A. (Eds.): The Mechanism of Inflammation, An International Symposium, Montreal, Acta, 1953.
2. Robin, E. D., and Bromberg, P. A.: Claude Bernard's milieu interieur extended: intracellular acid-base relationships (editorial), Am. J. Med. 27:689, 1959.
3. Elkinton, J. R., and Danowski, T. S.: Body Fluids, Baltimore, Williams and Wilkins, 1955.
4. Welt, L. G.: Clinical Disorders of Hydration and Acid-Base Equilibrium, Boston, Little, Brown, 1955.
5. Strauss, M. B.: Body Water in Man: The Acquisition and Maintenance of the Body Fluids, Boston, Little, Brown, 1957.

6. Hernández Peón, R.: Physiology of Body Fluids, in Fulton, J. F. (Ed.): A Textbook of Physiology, ed. 17, Philadelphia, W. B. Saunders, 1955.

7. Edelman, I. S., Haley, H. B., Schloerb, P. R., Sheldon, D. B., Friis-Hansen, B. J., Stoll, G., and Moore, F. D.: Further observations on total body water. I. Normal values throughout the life span, Surg. Gynec. & Obst. 95:1, 1952.

8. Edelman, I. S., and Leibman, J.: Anatomy of body water and electrolytes, Am. J. Med. 27:256, 1959.

9. Osserman, E. F., Pitts, G. C., Welham, W. C., and Behnke, A. R.: In vivo measurement of body fat and body water in a group of normal men, J. Appl. Physiol. 2:633, 1950.

10. Keys, A., and Brozek, J.: Body fat in adult man, Physiol. Rev. 33:245, 1953.

11. Friis-Hansen, B.: Changes in body water compartment during growth, Acta paediat. 46: (Suppl. 110) 1, 1957.

12. Wallace, W. M.: Some aspects of the chemical composition, physiology, and pathology of intracellular fluid, Pediatrics 9:141, 1952.

13. Edelman, I. S., Olney, J. M., James, A. H., Brooks, L., and Moore, F. D.: Body composition: studies in the human being by the dilution principle, Science 115:447, 1952.

14. Gamble, J. L.: Anatomy, Physiology and Chemical Pathology of Extracellular Fluids, Cambridge, Harvard University Press, 1947.

15. Manery, J. F.: Water and electrolyte metabolism, Physiol. Rev. 34:334, 1954.

16. Muntwyler, E.: Electrolyte and Water Equilibria, in Glasser, O. (Ed.): Medical Physics, Chicago, Year Book Publishers, 1950.

17. Peters, J. P.: Body Water. The Exchange of Fluids in Man, Springfield, Charles C Thomas, 1935.

18. Starling, E. H.: On the absorption of fluids from the connective tissue spaces, J. Physiol. 19:312, 1896.

19. Tobian, L.: The Influence of Hydrostatic Pressure and Colloid Osmotic Pressure on Fluid Transfer Across the Capillary Membranes, in Moyer, J. H., and Fuchs, M. (Eds.): Edema. Mechanisms and Management, Philadelphia, W. B. Saunders, 1960.

20. Rosenberg, T.: The Concept and Definition of Active Transport, in Active Transport and Secretion, New York, Academic Press, 1954.

21. Pappenheimer, J. R.: Passage of molecules through capillary walls, Physiol. Rev. 33:387, 1953.

22. Gaunt, R., Birnie, J. H., and Eversole, W. J.: Adrenal cortex and water metabolism, Physiol. Rev. 29:281, 1949.

23. Cannon, P. R., Frazier, L. E., and Hughes, R. H.: Influence of potassium on tissue protein synthesis, Metabolism 1:49, 1952.

24. Gardner, L. I., Talbot, N. B., Cook, C. D., Berman, H., and Uribe, C.: The effect of potassium deficiency on carbohydrate metabolism. J. Lab. Clin. Med. 35:592, 1950.

25. Elkinton, J. R.: Water metabolism, Ann. Rev. Physiol. 12:145, 1950.

26. Wolf, A. V.: Thirst: Physiology of the Urge to Drink and Problems of Water Lack, Springfield, Charles C Thomas, 1958.

27. Cannon, W. B.: Organization for physiological homeostasis, Physiol. Rev. 9:399, 1929.

28. Strauss, M. B.: Body Water in Man: The Acquisition and Maintenance of the Body Fluids, Boston, Little, Brown, 1957.

29. Strauss, M. B.: Thirst: The acquisition of water, Arch. Int. Med. 101:216, 1958.

30. Gilman, A.: The relation between blood osmotic pressure, fluid distribution and voluntary water intake, Am. J. Physiol. 120:323, 1937.

31. Holmes, J. H., and Gregersen, M. I.: Relation of the salivary flow to the thirst produced in man by intravenous injection of hypertonic salt solution, Am. J. Physiol. 151:252, 1947.

32. Adolph, E. F., Barker, J. P., and Hoy, P. A.: Multiple factors in thirst, Am. J. Physiol. 178:539, 1954.

33. Andersson, B., and McCann, S. M.: A further study of polydipsia evoked by hypothalamic stimulation in the goat, Acta physiol. scandinav. 33:333, 1955.

34. Leaf, A., and Mamby, A. R.: An antidiuretic mechanism not regulated by extracellular fluid tonicity, J. Clin. Invest. 31:60, 1952.

35. Verney, E. B.: Antidiuretic hormone and the factors which determine its release, Proc. Roy. Soc. London s.B 135:25, 1947.

36. Van Dyke, H. B.: The regulation of water excretion by the neurohypophysis, Bull. New York Acad. Med. 29:24, 1953.

37. Scharrer, E., and Scharrer, B.: Hormones produced by neurosecretory cells, Rec. Progr. Hormone Res. 10:183, 1954.

38. Sawyer, W. H., Munsick, R. A., and Van Dyke, H. B.: Antidiuretic hormones, Circulation 21: 1027, 1960.

39. Light, A., and Du Vigneaud, V.: On the nature of oxytocin and vasopressin from human pituitary, Proc. Soc. Exper. Biol. & Med. 98:692, 1958.

40. Berliner, R. W., Levinsky, N. G., Davidson, D. G., and Eden, M.: Dilution and concentration of urine and action of antidiuretic hormone, Am. J. Med. 24:730, 1958.

41. Smith, H. W.: The fate of sodium and water in the renal tubules, Bull. New York Acad. Med. 35:293, 1959.

42. Robinson, J. R.: The active transport of water in living systems, Biol. Rev. 28:158, 1953.

43. Epstein, F. H.: Renal excretion of sodium and the concept of a volume receptor, Yale J. Biol. & Med. 29:282, 1956.

44. Grossman, J.: Volume factors in modern medicine, Arch. Int. Med. 99:93, 1957.

45. Smith, H. W.: Salt and water volume receptors, Am. J. Med. 23:623, 1957.

46. Wrong, O.: The volume control of body fluids, Brit. M. Bull. 13:10, 1957.

47. Welt, L. G.: Volume receptors, Circulation 21: 1002, 1960.

48. Aviado, D. M., Jr., and Schmidt, C. F.: Reflexes from stretch receptors in blood vessels, heart and lungs, Physiol. Rev. 35:247, 1955.

49. Viar, W. N., Oliver, B. B., Eisenberg, S., Lombardo, T. A., Willis, K., and Harrison, T. R.: Effect of posture and of compression of the neck on excretion of electrolytes and glomerular filtration: further studies, Circulation 3:105, 1951.

50. Henry, J. P., Gauer, O. H., and Reeves, J. L.: Evidence of the atrial location of receptors influencing urine flow, Circulation Res. 4:85, 1956.

51. Sieker, H. O., Gauer, O. H., and Henry, J. P.: The effect of continuous negative pressure breathing on water and electrolyte excretion by the human kidney, J. Clin. Invest. 33:572, 1954.

52. Black, D. A. K.: Essentials of Fluid Balance, Oxford, Blackwell Scientific Publications, 1957.

53. Smith, H. W.: Principles of Renal Physiology, New York, Oxford University Press, 1957.

54. Selkurt, E. E.: Sodium excretion by the mammalian kidney, Physiol. Rev. 34:287, 1954.

55. Berliner, R. W.: Renal excretion of water, sodium,

chloride, potassium, calcium, and magnesium, Am. J. Med. *9:*541, 1950.

56. Gottschalk, C. W., and Mylle, E.: Micropuncture study of the mammalian urinary concentrating mechanism: evidence for the countercurrent hypothesis, Am. J. Physiol. *196:*927, 1959.

57. Ullrich, K. J.: Function of the collecting ducts, Circulation *21:*869, 1960.

58. Wesson, L. G., Jr.: Glomerular and tubular factors in the renal excretion of sodium chloride, Medicine *36:*281, 1957.

59. Luetscher, J. A., Jr., and Axelrad, B. J.: Increased aldosterone output during sodium deprivation in normal men, Proc. Soc. Exper. Biol. & Med. *87:*650, 1954.

60. Gaunt, R., Renzi, A. A., and Chart, J. J.: Aldosterone—a review, J. Clin. Endocrinol. *15:*621, 1955.

61. Hartroft, P. M., and Eisenstein, A. B.: Alterations in adrenal cortex of rat induced by sodium deficiency: correlations of histologic changes with steroid hormone secretion, Endocrinology *60:*641, 1957.

62. Crane, M. G., Short, G., and Peterson, J. E.: Observations on a case of primary aldosteronism, Am. J. Med. *24:*313, 1958.

63. Rosnagle, R. S., and Farrel, G. L.: Alterations in electrolyte intake and adrenal steroid secretion, Am. J. Physiol. *187:*7, 1956.

64. Laragh, J. H., and Stoerk, H. C.: Study of mechanism of secretion of sodium retaining hormone (aldosterone), J. Clin. Invest. *36:*383, 1957.

65. Bartter, F. C., Liddle, G. W., Duncan, L. E., Jr., Barber, J. K., and Delea, C.: Regulation of aldosterone secretion in man: role of fluid volume, J. Clin. Invest. *35:*1306, 1956.

66. Bartter, F. C., and Gann, D. S.: On the hemodynamic regulation of the secretion of aldosterone, Circulation *21:*1016, 1960.

67. Farrel, G.: Regulation of aldosterone secretion, Physiol. Rev. *38:*709, 1958.

68. Farrell, G.: Adrenoglomerulotrophin, Circulation *21:*1009, 1960.

69. Stachenko, J., and Giroud, C. J. P.: Functional zonation of the adrenal cortex: Pathways of corticosteroid biogenesis, Endocrinology *64:*730, 1959.

70. Davis, J. O., Yankopoulos, N. A., Lieberman, F., Holman, J., and Bahn, R. C.: The role of anterior pituitary in the control of aldosterone secretion in experimental secondary hyperaldosteronism, J. Clin. Invest. *39:*765, 1960.

71. Ross, E. J., Van'T Hoff, W., Grabbé, J., and Thorn, G. W.: Aldosterone excretion in hypopituitarism and after hypophysectomy in man, Am. J. Med. *28:*229, 1960.

72. Luetscher, J. A., Jr., and Lieberman, A. H.: Aldosterone, Arch. Int. Med. *102:*314, 1958.

73. Zimmerman, B., and Moran, W. H.: Aldosterone, Am. J. Surg. *99:*503, 1960.

74. August, J. T., Nelson, D. H., and Thorn, G. W.: Aldosterone, New Eng. J. Med. *259:*917, 967, 1958.

75. Black, D. A. K.: Current concepts of potassium metabolism, J. Pediatrics *56:*814, 1960.

76. Black, D. A. K., and Emery, E. W.: Tubular secretion of potassium, Brit. M. Bull. *7,* 1957.

77. Danowski, T. S.: Fundamental features of metabolism of sodium and potassium, Am. J. Clin. Path. *23:*1095, 1953.

78. Danowski, T. S., and Elkinton, J. R.: Exchanges of potassium related to organs and systems, Pharmacol. Rev. *3:*42, 1951.

79. Holler, J. W.: Potassium deficiency occurring dur-

ing the treatment of diabetic acidosis, J.A.M.A. *131:*1186, 1946.

80. Moore, F. D.: Bodily changes in surgical convalescence. The normal sequence—observations and interpretations, Ann. Surg. *137:*289, 1953.

81. Cortes, F., Shuman, C. R., and Channick, B. J.: Primary aldosteronism, observations on two cases, Am. J. Med. Sc. *239:*324, 1960.

82. Grob, D., Johns, R. J., and Liljestrand, A.: Potassium movement in patients with familial periodic paralysis, Am. J. Med. *23:*356, 1957.

83. Elkinton, J. R.: Regulation of water and electrolytes, Circulation *21:*1184, 1960.

84. Black, D. A. K.: Body fluid depletion, Lancet *1:* 305, 353, 1953.

85. Marriot, H. L.: Water and Salt Depletion, Oxford, Blackwell Scientific Publications, 1950.

86. Black, D. A. K.: Symptoms and signs in disorders of body fluids, J. Chron. Dis. *11:*340, 1960.

87. Zimmerman, B., and Wangensteen, O. H.: Observations on water intoxication in surgical patients, Surgery *31:*654, 1952.

88. Wynn, V., and Robb, C. G.: Water Intoxication, Lancet *1:*587, 1954.

89. Wynn, V.: Water intoxication and serum hypotonicity, Metabolism *5:*490, 1956.

90. Wrhong, O.: The relationship between water retention and electrolyte excretion following administration of anti-diuretic hormone, Clin. Sc. *15:*401, 1956.

91. Elkinton, J. R.: Hyponatremia: clinical state or biochemical sign? Circulation *14:*1027, 1956.

92. Elkinton, J. R., and Widdowson, E. M.: The effect of severe chronic undernutrition on body composition of the rat, Metabolism *8:*404, 1959.

93. Holmes, J. H.: Mechanisms Producing the Hyponatremic Syndrome, in Moyer, J. H., and Fuchs, M. (Eds.): Edema. Mechanisms and Management, Philadelphia, W. B. Saunders, 1960.

94. Edelman, I. S.: The pathogenesis of hyponatremia; physiologic and therapeutic implications, Metabolism *5:*500, 1956.

95. Hills, A. G., Chalmers, T. M., Webster, G. D., Jr., and Rosenthal, O.: Adrenal cortical regulation of distribution of water and electrolytes in human body, J. Clin. Invest. *32:*1236, 1953.

96. Brodsky, W. A., and West, C. D.: Mechanism of glycosuric diuresis in diabetic man, J. Clin. Invest. *29:*1021, 1950.

97. Swan, R. C., and Merrill, J. P.: Clinical course of acute renal failure, Medicine *32:*215, 1953.

98. Pitts, R. F., and Sartorius, O. W.: Mechanism of action and therapeutic use of diuretics, J. Pharmacol. & Exper. Therap. *98:*161, 1950.

99. Elinton, J. R., Danowski, T. S., and Winkler, A. W.: Hemodynamic changes in salt depletion and in dehydration, J. Clin. Invest. *25:*120, 1946.

100. Black, D. A. K.: Sodium Metabolism in Health and Disease, Springfield, Charles C Thomas, 1952.

101. Knowles, H. C.: Hypernatremia, Metabolism *5:*508, 1956.

102. Oliver, J.: Correlations of structure and function and mechanisms of recovery in acute tubular necrosis, Am. J. Med. *15:*535, 1953.

103. Zierler, K. L.: Hyperosmolarity in adults: a critical review, J. Chron. Dis. *7:*1, 1958.

104. Merrill, A. J.: Mechanism of water and salt retention in heart failure, Am. J. Med. *6:*357, 1949.

105. Streeten, D. H. P.: Primary and Secondary Aldosteronism: Definition and Diagnosis, in Moyer, J. H., and Fuchs, M. (Eds.): Edema. Mechanisms and Management, Philadelphia, W. B. Saunders, 1960.

106. Baulieu, E. E., Robel, P., Siguier, F., and Jayle,

M. F.: Metabolic observations in a case of pure primary hyperaldosteronism, J. Clin. Endocrinol. *19:*1081, 1959.

107. Ross, E. J., Crabbé, J., Renold, A. E., Emerson, K., and Thorn, G. W.: A case of massive edema in association with an aldosterone-secreting adrenocortical adenoma, Am. J. Med. *25:*278, 1958.

108. Overman, R. R.: Sodium, potassium, and chloride alteration in disease, Physiol. Rev. *31:*285, 1951.

109. Scribner, B. H., and Burnell, J. M.: Interpretation of the serum and potassium concentration, Metabolism *5:*468, 1956.

110. Field, H., Dailey, R. E., Boyd, R. S., and Swell, L.: Effect of restriction of dietary sodium on electrolyte composition of the contents of the terminal ileum, Am. J. Physiol. *179:*477, 1954.

111. Stamey, T. A.: The pathogenesis and implications of the electrolyte imbalance in ureterosigmoidostomy, Surg., Gynec. & Obst. *103:*736, 1956.

112. Schwartz, W. B., and Relman, A. S.: Metabolic and renal studies in chronic potassium depletion resulting from overuse of laxatives, J. Clin. Invest. *32:*258, 1953.

113. Darrow, D. C.: Body fluid physiology: The role of potassium in clinical disturbances of body water and electrolytes, New Eng. J. Med. *242:*978, 1950.

114. Relman, A. S., and Schwartz, W. B.: The kidney in potassium depletion, Am. J. Med. *24:*764, 1958.

115. Kulka, J. P., Pearson, C. M., and Robbins, S. L.: A distinctive vacuolar nephropathy associated with intestinal disease, Am. J. Path. *26:*349, 1950.

116. Conn, J. W., and Johnson, R. D.: Kaliopenic nephropathy, Am. J. Clin. Nutr. *4:*523, 1956.

117. Williams, R. H., and MacMahon, H. E.: Gastroenterocolitis; carcinoma of the pancreas; "clearcell" nephrosis, Bull. New Eng. Med. Center *9:*274, 1947.

118. Relman, A. S., and Schwartz, W. B.: The nephropathy of potassium depletion, New Eng. J. Med. *255:*195, 1956.

119. Oliver, J., MacDowell, M., Welt, L. G., Holliday, M. A., Hollander, W., Jr., Winters, R. W., Williams, T. F., and Segar, W. E.: The renal lesions of electrolyte imbalance. I. The structural alterations in potassium-depleted rats, J. Exper. Med. *106:*503, 1957.

120. Tauxe, W. N., Wakim, K. G., and Baggenstoss, A. H.: The renal lesion in experimental deficiency of potassium, Am. J. Clin. Path. *28:*221, 1957.

121. Fourman, P., McCance, R. A., and Parker, R. A.: Chronic renal disease in rats following a temporary deficiency of potassium, Brit. J. Exper. Path. *37:*40, 1956.

122. Kennedy, G. C., Flear, C. T. G., and Parker, R. A.: Renal disease and secondary potassium depletion in aging rats, Quart. J. Exper. Physiol. *45:*82, 1960.

123. Wachstein, M., and Meisel, E.: Enzymatic staining reactions in the kidneys of potassium depleted rats, Am. J. Path. *35:*1189, 1959.

124. Darmady, E. M., and Stranack, F.: Microdissection of the nephron in disease, Brit. M. Bull. *13:*21, 1957.

125. Hollander, W., Jr.: The Effects of Potassium Deficiency on Renal Function, in Moyer, J. H., and Fuchs, M. (Eds.): Edema. Mechanisms and Management, Philadelphia, W. B. Saunders, 1960.

126. Chalmers, T. M., Fitzgerald, M. G., James, A. H., and Scarborough, H.: Conn's syndrome with severe hypertension, Lancet *1:*127, 1956.

127. Perkins, J. G., Petersen, A. B., and Riley, J. A.: Renal and cardiac lesions in potassium deficiency due to chronic diarrhea, Am. J. Med. *8:*115, 1950.

128. Mudge, G. H.: Potassium imbalance, Bull. New York Acad. Med. *29:*846, 1953.

129. Moore, F. D., Edelman, I. S., Olney, J. M., James, A. H., Brooks, L., and Wilson, G. M.: Body sodium and potassium. III. Interrelated trends in alimentary, renal and cardiovascular disease. Lack of correlation between body stores and plasma concentration, Metabolism *3:*334, 1954.

130. Villarreal, H.: El metabolismo del potasio y su importancia en la clínica, Principia Cardiol. *1:*242, 1954.

131. Marriot, H. J. L.: Some observations on the pathogenesis of cardiac edema, Ann. Int. Med. *41:*377, 1954.

132. Milton, S.: Urticaria and angioedema, Ann. Allergy *12:*659, 1954.

133. Landis, E. M.: Capillary pressure and capillary permeability, Physiol. Rev. *14:*404, 1934.

134. Pullinger, B. D., and Florey, H. W.: Some observations on structure and functions of lymphatics: their behaviour in local edema, Brit. J. Exper. Path. *16:*49, 1935.

135. Drinker, C. K., Field, M. E., and Homans, J.: The experimental production of edema and elephantiasis as a result of lymphatic obstruction, Am. J. Physiol. *108:*509, 1934.

136. Villasor, R. P., and Levison, E. F.: Postmastectomy lymphedema, Surg. Gynec. & Obst. *100:*743, 1955.

137. West, J. P., and Ellison, J. B.: A study of the causes and prevention of edema of the arm following radical mastectomy, Surg. Gynec. & Obst. *109:*359, 1959.

138. Nelson, W. R., and Morfit, H. M.: Lymphangiosarcoma in the lymphedematous arm after radical mastectomy, Cancer *9:*1189, 1956.

139. Jordan, P.: Notes on elephantiasis and hydrocele due to *W. bancrofti*, J. Trop. Med. *58:*113, 1955.

140. Lichtenberg, F., and Medina, R.: Bancroftian filariasis in the etiology of funiculoepididymitis, periorchitis and hydrocele in Puerto Rico, Am. J. Trop. Med. *6:*739, 1957.

141. Milroy, W. F.: Chronic hereditary edema: Milroy's disease, J.A.M.A. *91:*1172, 1928.

142. Edwards, J. E., and Edwards, E. A.: The saphenous valves in various veins, Am. Heart. J. *19:*338, 1940.

143. Cameron, G. R.: Pulmonary edema, Brit. M. J. *1:*965, 1948.

144. Luisada, A. A., and Cardi, L.: Acute pulmonary edema; pathology, physiology, and clinical management, Circulation *13:*113, 1956.

145. Altschule, M. D.: Acute Pulmonary Edema, New York, Grune and Stratton, 1954.

146. Welch, W. H.: Zur Pathologie des Lungenödems, Arch. path. Anat. *72:*375, 1878.

147. Katz, L. N.: The mechanism of cardiac failure, Circulation *10:*663, 1954.

148. Richards, D. W., Jr., Cournand, A., Darling, R. C., Gillespie, W. H., and Baldwin, E. D.: Pressure of blood in the right auricle in animals and in man: under normal conditions and in heart failure, Am. J. Physiol. *136:*115, 1942.

149. Hayward, G. W.: Pulmonary edema, Brit. Med. J. *1:*1361, 1955.

150. Drinker, C. K.: The Clinical Physiology of the Lungs, Springfield, Charles C Thomas, 1954.

151. Cameron, G. R., and De, S. N.: Experimental pulmonary edema of nervous origin, J. Path. & Bact. *61:*375, 1949.

152. McKay, E. M.: Experimental pulmonary edema. IV. Pulmonary edema accompanying trauma to the brain, Proc. Soc. Exper. Biol. & Med. *74:* 695, 1950.

153. Luisada, A. A.: The pathogenesis of paroxysmal pulmonary edema, Medicine *19:*475, 1940.

154. Sarnoff, S. J., and Berglund, E.: Neurohemodynamics of pulmonary edema. IV. Effect of systemic vasoconstriction and subsequent vasodilatation of flow and pressures in systemic and pulmonary vascular beds, Am. J. Physiol. *170:* 588, 1952.

155. Sarnoff, S. J.: Some Physiologic Considerations in the Genesis of Acute Pulmonary Edema, in Adams, W., and Weith, I. (Eds.): Pulmonary Circulation, New York, Grune and Stratton, 1959.

156. Maurer, F. W.: Effects of decreased blood oxygen and increased blood carbon dioxide on flow and composition of cervical and cardiac lymph, Am. J. Physiol. *131:*331, 1940.

157. Cheng, K. T.: quoted in Cameron, G. R.: Pulmonary edema, Brit. M. J. *1:*965, 1948.

158. Liljestrand, G.: Regulation of pulmonary arterial pressure, Arch. Int. Med. *81:*162, 1948.

159. Motley, H. L., Cournand, A., Werkö, L., Himmelstein, A., and Dresdale, D.: The influence of short periods of induced acute anoxia upon pulmonary artery pressures in man, Am. J. Physiol. *150:*315, 1947.

160. Luisada, A. A., and Sarnoff, S. J.: Paroxysmal pulmonary edema consequent to stimulation of cardiovascular receptors. III. Pharmacologic experiments. Am. Heart. J. *31:*293, 1946.

161. Goldberg, H., Bentivoglio, L., and Sgarminaga, X.: Mechanisms of Pulmonary Edema, in Moyer, J. H., and Fuchs, M. (Eds.): Edema. Mechanisms and Management, Philadelphia, W. B. Saunders, 1960.

162. Weech, A. A., Goettsch, E., and Reeves, E. B.: Nutritional edema in the dog. I. Development of hypoproteinemia on a diet deficient in protein, J. Exper. Med. *61:*266, 1935.

163. Adams, D. A.: The pathophysiology of the nephrotic syndrome, Arch. Int. Med. *106:*117, 1960.

164. Björneboe, M., Bruun, C., and Raaschou, F.: Colloid osmotic pressure in chronic hepatitis, Arch. Int. Med. *83:*539, 1949.

165. Denz, F. A.: Hunger oedema, Quart. J. Med. *16:* 1, 1947.

166. Kylin, E.: Studien ueber den kolloidosmotischen (onkotischen) Druck. XXVIII Mitteilung Tierexperimentelle Untersuchungen ueber die Bedeutung der Senkung des kolloidosmotischen Druck für die Oedempathogenese, Arch. exper. Path. u. Pharmakol. *170:*407, 1933.

167. Derow, H. A.: The nephrotic syndrome, New Eng. J. Med. *258:*77, 1958.

168. Sodeman, W. A., and Mekheiji, K. L.: Observations on malnourished patients with edema, Am. J. Med. *16:*610, 1954.

169. Keys, A., Taylor, H. L., Mickelsen, O., and Henschel, S.: Famine edema and the mechanism of its formation, Science *103:*669, 1946.

170. Post, J., and Patek, A. J., Jr.: Serum proteins in cirrhosis of the liver. I. Relation to prognosis and to formation of ascites, Arch. Int. Med. *69:* 67, 1942.

171. Giges, B., and Kunkel, H. G.: Osmotic pressure measurements of serum and ascitic fluid in patients with cirrhosis of the liver, J. Clin. Invest. *33:*257, 1954.

172. Armstrong, S. H., Jr., Kark, R. M., Schoenberger, J. A., Shatkin, J., and Sights, R.: Colloid osmotic pressures of serum proteins in nephrosis and cirrhosis: relation to electrophoretic distributions and average molecular weights, J. Clin. Invest. *33:*297, 1954.

173. Bennhold, H., Peters, H., and Roth, E.: Ueber einen Fall von kompletter Analbuminaemie ohne wesentiche klinische Krankheitszeichen, Verhand. deutsch. Gesellsch. inn. Med. *60:*630, 1954.

174. Peters, J. P.: Sodium, water, and edema, J. M. Sinai Hosp. *17:*159, 1950.

175. Peters, J. P.: Edema of acute nephritis, Am. J. Med. *14:*448, 1953.

176. Schade, H.: Die Molekulärpathologie in ihren verhaltnis zur Zellulärpathologie und zum klinischen Krankheitbild am Beispiel der Entzündung, München. med. Wchnschr. *71:*1, 1924.

177. Blumberg, B. S., Oster, G., and Meyer, K.: Changes in the physical characteristics of the hyaluronate of ground substance with alterations in sodium chloride concentration, J. Clin. Invest. *34:*1454, 1955.

178. Farber, S. J.: Mucopolysaccharides and sodium metabolism, Circulation *21:*241, 1960.

179. McMichael, J.: Cardiac venous congestion. Its causes and consequences, Am. J. Med. *6:*651, 1949.

180. Thorn, G. W., Renold, A. E., Froesch, E. R., and Crabbé, J.: Pathophysiology of edema, Helvet. med. acta *23:*334, 1956.

181. Stein, M., Schwartz, R., and Mirsky, I. A.: The antidiuretic activity of plasma of patients with hepatic cirrhosis, congestive heart failure, hypertension, and other clinical disorders, J. Clin. Invest. *33:*77, 1954.

182. Miller, G. E., Townsend, C. E., and Jones, M. C.: The *in vitro* inactivation of Pitressin by normal and cirrhotic human liver, J. Clin. Invest. *33:* 549, 1954.

183. White, A. G., Rubin, G., and Leiter, L.: Studies in edema. III. The effect of Pitressin on the renal excretion of water and electrolytes in patients with and without liver disease. J. Clin. Invest. *30:*1287, 1951.

184. Luetscher, J. A., Jr., and Johnson, B. B.: Observations on the sodium-retaining corticoid (aldosterone) in the urine of children and adults in relation to sodium balance and edema, J. Clin. Invest. *33:*1441, 1954.

185. Bartter, F. C.: The role of aldosterone in normal homeostasis and in certain disease states, Metabolism *5:*369, 1956.

186. Merrill, A. J.: Edema and decreased renal blood flow in patients with chronic congestive heart failure. Evidence of "forward failure" as the primary cause of edema, J. Clin. Invest. *25:*389, 1946.

187. Barger, A. C., Muldowney, F. P., and Liebowitz, M. R.: Role of the kidney in the pathogenesis of congestive heart failure, Circulation *20:*273, 1959.

188. Frieden, J.: Effects of chronic peripheral venous congestion on renal sodium excretion, Am. J. Physiol. *168:*650, 1952.

189. Moore, F. D.: Common patterns of water and electrolyte changes consequent to injury, surgery, and disease, New Eng. J. Med. *258:*277, 325, 377, 428, 1958.

190. Relman, A. S.: What are "acids" and "bases"? Am. J. Med. *17:*435, 1954.

191. Kaufman, H. E., and Rosen, S. W.: Clinical acid-base regulation—the Brönsted schema, Surg. Gynec. & Obst. *103:*101, 1956.

192. Clark, W. M.: Topics in Physical Chemistry, Baltimore, Williams and Wilkins, 1952.

193. Swan, R. C., and Pitts, R. F.: Neutralization of infused acid by nephrectomized dogs, J. Clin. Invest. 34:205, 1955.

194. Elkinton, J. R.: Whole body buffers in the regulation of acid-base equilibrium, Yale J. Biol. & Med. 29:191, 1956.

195. Grodins, F. S.: Respiration and the regulation of acid-base balance, Arch. Int. Med. 99:569, 1957.

196. Liljestrand, A.: Neural control of respiration, Physiol. Rev. 38:691, 1958.

197. Pitts, R. F.: The organization of the respiratory center, Physiol. Rev. 26:609, 1946.

198. Pitts, R. F.: Acid-base regulation by the kidneys, Am. J. Med. 9:356, 1950.

199. Gilman, H., and Brazzeau, P.: The role of the kidney in the regulation of acid-base metabolism, Am. J. Med. 15:765, 1953.

200. Orloff, J.: The role of the kidney in the regulation of acid-base balance, Yale J. Biol. & Med. 29:211, 1956.

201. Pitts, R. F., Ayer, J. L., and Schiess, W. A.: The renal regulation of acid-base balance in man. III. The reabsorption and excretion of bicarbonate, J. Clin. Invest. 28:35, 1949.

202. Roberts, K. E., Randall, H. T., Vanamee, P., and Popell, J. W.: Renal mechanisms involved in bicarbonate absorption, Metabolism 5:404, 1956.

203. Pitts, R. F.: Some reflections on mechanisms of action of diuretics, Am. J. Med. 24:745, 1958.

204. Nash, T. P., and Benedict, S. R.: The ammonia content of the blood and its bearing on the mechanism of acid neutralization in the animal organism, J. Biol. Chem. 48:463, 1921.

205. Kamin, H., and Handler, P.: The metabolism of parenterally administered aminoacids. III. Ammonia formation, J. Biol. Chem. 193:873, 1951.

206. Davies, B. M. A., and Yudkin, J.: Studies on biochemical adaptation. The origin of urinary ammonia as indicated by the effect of chronic acidosis and alkalosis on some renal enzymes in the rat, Biochem. J. 52:407, 1952.

207. Milne, M. D., Scribner, B. H., and Crawford, M. A.: Non-ionic diffusion and the excretion of weak acids and bases, Am. J. Med. 24:709, 1958.

208. Cohn, J. E., Carroll, D. G., and Riley, R. L.: Respiratory acidosis in patients with emphysema, Am. J. Med. 17:447, 1943.

209. Stanbury, W. W., and Thomson, W. E.: The renal response to respiratory alkalosis, Clin. Sc. 11:357, 1952.

210. Schwartz, W. B., Falbriard, A., and Lemieux, G.: The kinetics of bicarbonate reabsorption during acute respiratory acidosis, J. Clin. Invest. 38:939, 1959.

211. Sullivan, W. J., and Dorman, P. J.: The renal response to chronic respiratory acidosis, J. Clin. Invest. 34:268, 1954.

212. Epstein, F. H., Branscome, W., and Levitin, H.: The mechanism of hypochloremia in chronic respiratory acidosis, Clin. Res. Proc. 5:17, 1957.

213. Frazer, S. C., and Stewart, C. P.: Acidosis and alkalosis: a modern view, J. Clin. Path. 12:195, 1959.

214. Dole, V. P.: Fat metabolism in diabetes, Bull. New York Acad. Med. 34:21, 1958.

215. Sleisenger, M. H., and Freedberg, A. S.: Ammonium chloride acidosis. Report of six cases, Circulation 3:837, 1951.

216. Cuthbertson, D. P.: Protein metabolism in relation to energy needs, Metabolism 8:787, 1959.

217. Sprague, R. G., and Power, M. H.: Electrolyte metabolism in diabetic acidosis, J.A.M.A. 151:970, 1953.

218. Trever, R. W., and Cluff, L. E.: The problem of increasing azotemia during management of diabetic acidosis, Am. J. Med. 24:368, 1958.

219. Elkinton, J. R.: Renal acidosis, Am. J. Med. 28:165, 1960.

220. Schwartz, W. B., Hall, P. W., Hays, R. M., and Relman, A. S.: On the mechanism of acidosis in chronic renal disease, J. Clin. Invest. 38:39, 1959.

221. Brown, E. B., Jr.: Physiological effects of hyperventilation, Physiol. Rev. 33:445, 1953.

222. Sattler, T. H., Marquardt, G. H., and Cummins, G. M., Jr.: Alkalosis due to hyperventilation. Report of three cases, J.A.M.A. 146:1125, 1951.

223. Rice, R. L.: Symptom patterns of hyperventilation syndrome, Am. J. Med. 8:691, 1950.

224. Schwartz, W. B., Lemieux, G., and Falbriard, A.: Renal reabsorption of bicarbonate during acute respiratory alkalosis, J. Clin. Invest. 38:2197, 1959.

225. Davies, H. E. F., Jepson, R. P., and Black, D. A. K.: Some metabolic sequels of gastric surgery in patients with and without pyloric stenosis, Clin. Sc. 15:61, 1956.

226. Kirsner, J. B., and Palmer, W. L.: Alkalosis complicating the Sippy treatment of peptic ulcer, Arch. Int. Med. 69:789, 1942.

227. Grossman, J.: Electrolyte Abnormalities Associated with Mercurial, Thiazide, and Carbonic Anhydrase-inhibiting Diuretics, in Moyer, J. H., and Fuchs, M. (Eds.): Edema. Mechanisms and Management, Philadelphia, W. B. Saunders, 1960.

228. Elkinton, J. R., Squires, R. D., and Crosley, A. P., Jr.: Intracellular cation exchanges in metabolic alkalosis, 30:369, 1951.

Chapter X

GENERAL PATHOLOGY OF

METABOLISM AND NUTRITION

I. INTRODUCTION

No single thing abides; but all things flow.
Fragment to fragment clings—the things
     thus grow
  Until we know and name them. By
     degrees
They melt, and are no more the things we
     know.
Globed from the atoms falling slow or swift
I see the suns, I see the systems lift
  Their forms; and even the systems and
     the suns
Shall go back slowly to the eternal drift.
Thou too, oh earth—thine empires, lands,
     and seas—
Least, with thy stars, of all the galaxies,
  Globed from the drift like these, like
     these thou too
Shalt go. Thou art going, hour by hour, like
     these.
Nothing abides. Thy seas in delicate haze

Go off; those mooned sands forsake their
    place;
  And where they are, shall other seas in
    turn
Mow with their scythes of whiteness other
    bays.
Observe this dew-drenched rose of Tyrian
    grain—
A rose today. But you will ask in vain
  Tomorrow what it is; and yesterday
It was the dust, the sunshine and the rain.

    (fragment from *De Rerum Natura,* by
    Lucretius, translated by Mallock)

II. NORMAL METABOLISM

The living protoplasm is characterized by its ability for self preservation and self replication. Mechanisms responsible for these two fundamental properties may be analyzed at various levels of organization, which at one end of the scale go beyond the individual to the structure and functions of societies, and at the other end are now reaching the submolecular realm. Between these two extremes lie the isolated organism, the different organs and systems, the separate tissues and cells, and the subcellular particles. The nature of the problems appearing for study at each level of organization determines to a great extent the techniques to be used.[1] These have been developed in different epochs and in accordance with the interests of each generation and its methodologic ingenuity. Almost one hundred years ago Rudolf Virchow began the systematic use of the microscope in the study of diseased tissues and cells, with magnificent results; today, morphologists are busy probing with the electron microscope a new world in pathology, the limits of which are unknown. Similarly, the use of chemical and physicochemical methods in the study of metabolism has produced an enormous mass of data important for the physician, not only for the diagnosis and treatment of disease but, what is even more significant, for the better understanding of pathology.[2]

It would be unfair to conclude that methods other than chemical and physicochemical have contributed little or nothing in the realm of metabolism. The admirable work of Oliver and his group on the kidney[3] and the growing literature in histochemistry are two clear examples of what can be done in the field by combining morphology with biochemical understanding. But it is in the nature of things that many important questions arising in the analysis of metabolism are more adequately answered in chemical terms.

Metabolism means all physical and chemical processes occurring in living beings, but usage has limited the application of the term to the changes in different foods within the organism, where they are used for building up cellular structure and as energy carriers. These two aspects of metabolism are known respectively as intermediary and energetic. Two other terms in use are anabolism and catabolism. The first indicates the process of synthesis or the building of high molecular weight compounds starting from others of lower molecular weight, while the second term designates the breakdown of substances within the organism. These two concepts are useful for descriptive purposes but the processes cannot be separate; indeed, they are so intimately coupled that energy released in catabolism is used for synthesis, as in the degradation of carbohydrates and their transformation into fats. For these reasons the separation of metabolism into intermediary metabolism and energy metabolism is preferred. A brief review of those aspects more closely related to pathology is given in the next paragraphs.

A. ENERGY METABOLISM

The living protoplasm is formed by the same elements found in the inert environment; the only difference is that of organization.[4] The maintenance of this organization requires the expenditure of energy, so death might be defined as the absence of energy exchange, which is the same as a static equilibrium between organism and surrounding medium. This is in sharp contrast with the frequent description of living beings in "equilibrium," which indicates their tendency to maintain a constant composition; it might be wise, therefore, to clarify what is meant by "equilibrium."[5]

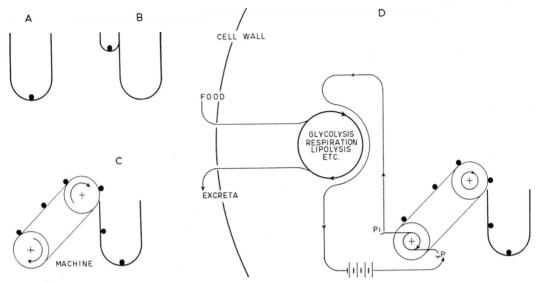

FIG. 10–1. Different types of equilibrium which are encountered in the organism. *A,* Static equilibrium. *B,* Kinetic stability. *C,* Metabolic machine which is being charged while it works. *D,* Dynamic maintenance of steady equilibrium or steady state, where energy derived from food serves to charge the metabolic machine. (Courtesy of Dr. D. Stetten and the Editor, American Journal of Medicine.)

A physicochemist understands by equilibrium that state in which there is a minimum of free energy; such a state can only be modified by investing energy from another source, i.e., with work within the system.[6] The situation may be represented as a sphere lying in the bottom of a concave receptacle (Fig. 10–1, *A*). It is obvious that the sphere will remain there as long as it is not moved by an external influence. The organism shows very few instances of this type of equilibrium, but one might be the situation existing between the solid and fluid phases of bone mineral.[7] Another form of equilibrium is the so-called "kinetic stability" which may be represented by the small sphere placed in a small compartment next to the concave recipient and separated from it by an edge (Fig. 10–1, *B*). In order to roll down into the recipient the sphere must get to the top of the edge; the energy necessary for this jump is known as activation energy. There are many instances of this type of equilibrium in the organism, since it can be accepted that enzymes act by decreasing activation energy. Nevertheless, collagen fibers lying in the interstitial spaces represent a good example, since their metabolic activity is so slow that they probably have a longer half-life than the organism of which they are a

part.[8] This metabolic inertia is probably due to their extracellular position, where enzymes cannot reach them; therefore, it might be considered that the constancy of this special protein is a result of its kinetic stability.

The vast majority of the body components, however, are undergoing continuous modification, breakdown and resynthesis, catalyzed by numerous enzymes and with a very active energetic metabolism. It is therefore necessary to conceive a machine continuously moved by the energy derived from the difference in potential between inorganic and high-energy phosphates, which function as electric piles and discharge (Fig. 10–1, *C*). In this machine respiration, glycolysis, fat breakdown, etc., consume inorganic phosphate and recharge the pile, so the entire cycle is self-supported and requires the introduction of external sources of energy in the form of different food substances (Fig. 10–1, *D*). This state is far from what the physicochemist knows as "equilibrium," and it is perhaps better characterized as the "dynamic maintenance of steady equilibrium" or "steady state," for lack of more adequate terminology.[9]

Perhaps the most important form of equilibrium in the organism is that existing between the synthesis and breakdown of cellular components; growth is partly the predominance of synthesis, as the result of which the amount of cytoplasm increases although breakdown never ceases. The adult subject is characterized by a balance between formation and destruction of cytoplasmic building stones, and although no external change is apparent, almost every single piece is in a state of continuous activity.[10] The entire process may become apparent with specific studies of metabolic turnover of different cytoplasmic components in health, or with the dynamic study of disease.

1. Energy Exchange. The study of mechanisms of release, storage and utilization of energy by the organism shows that they follow the same thermodynamic principles ruling inert systems. There are four important types of energy in the body, namely mechanical, chemical, electric and caloric. Nevertheless, since energy is the capacity to perform work, cells use only chemical energy to carry out their metabolic processes, and caloric energy to maintain a constant temperature. Work is manifested by mechanical, electric, chemical and osmotic changes, of which the three former are synthetic or anabolic, while the latter participates in the exchange of fluids and solutes among the various body compartments. Caloric energy is not used in work; therefore, the greater the amount of heat produced in a chemical reaction the lesser will be the energy released in a useful form to perform any type of work, which is the same as saying that the efficiency of the reaction is inversely proportional to the amount of heat released. Still another expression of the same principle is that the organism is not a heat machine, since caloric energy cannot be transformed into the other three (mechanical, chemical, electric) which can perform work.[11]

The source of all energy is the sun. The organism acquires part of this energy with food, which a moment of reflection will show is all reducible to vegetables. Plants are capable of synthesizing large compounds with high molecular weight starting from very simple fragments through their mechanism for capturing solar energy (photosynthesis).[12] On the other hand, humans, for instance, cannot use all energy-rich compounds but need, among other things, substances with a structure somewhat similar to those making up the cytoplasm; the result is that foods are limited to carbohydrates, lipids and proteins. After entering the organism, most foods are broken down and mixed with similar fragments constituting a general deposit known as the metabolic pool, where they can be reached indiscriminately when needed. Furthermore, when chemical bonds are broken not all released energy is used immediately; part of it is stored in special phosphate compounds until it is needed again.[13, 14]

A bioenergetic system[15] is formed by the following four stages: (1) a source of energy, represented by the different foods; (2) a mechanism capable of releasing that energy, which is composed of several enzymes; (3) some form of economic storage of energy released and which is not being used immediately, formed by high-energy phosphates; (4) the transformation of energy in work, which may be mechanical, as in muscle contraction, or chemical, as in anabolic reactions.

2. Basal Metabolism. Most of the energy released during metabolism appears as heat, and when the organism is not carrying out any work it is possible to measure the energy liberated in combustion (oxidation) of foods by determining the temperature. This is important because from a thermodynamic viewpoint the intermediate stages may be disregarded; the point at issue is the energy content of reacting compounds and that of their results. Therefore, it is possible to classify foods according to the amount of caloric energy released during their combustion. It has been determined that this energy is the same both within the organism and *in vitro*. The unit used is the calorie, which is defined as the amount of heat necessary for raising the temperature of 1 Gm. of H_2O from $14.5°C$ to $15.5°C$; a kilocalorie is equal to 1000 calories. Each type of food has a characteristic heat of combustion, which for carbohydrates and fats is 4.1 Kcal./Gm. and for proteins is 9.3 Kcal./Gm.

Energy released in the organism from the various foods is used in three different ways, which are work, storage and heat; the first two are useful in metabolism, the third serves to maintain a constant temperature. Therefore, the following equation may be established:

Caloric value of foods =
work + stored energy + heat

based on the first law of thermodynamics, which may be expressed by saying that the total amount of energy within a given system is constant. In basal metabolic conditions (absolute rest and fast) all the energy released may be expressed as heat minus stored energy:

energy released = heat − stored energy

where the energy stored has a negative sign because without ingestion of food the organism will use it in its metabolism.

The relative amounts of carbohydrates, fats and proteins used by a given subject in basal metabolic conditions may be calculated from the respiratory quotient, i.e., the ratio between the volumes of inspired O_2 and expired CO_2:

Respiratory quotient =
$$\frac{\text{Volume of expired } CO_2}{\text{Volume of inspired } O_2}$$

Oxidation of carbohydrates requires minimal oxygen consumption, so the respiratory quotient will be equal to 1; in the case of fats it is necessary to use oxygen in greater proportion, so the respiratory quotient will be less than unit, i.e., 0.71. For proteins the situation is similar, and the respiratory quotient is 0.80. It has been calculated that each gram of nonprotein nitrogen eliminated with the urine (usually as urea) represents 6.25 Gm. of oxidized protein. When the total respiratory quotient of a subject, and the amount of urea eliminated, are known, that part of the respiratory quotient corresponding to proteins may be calculated, and the proportion corresponding to carbohydrates and fats may be established in special tables prepared *ex profeso*.[16]

The basal metabolic rate is modified by many physiologic conditions, such as age, exercise, emotions, pregnancy, height, etc., which should be taken into account when interpreting results.[17] Furthermore, although at one time the study of basal metabolic rates was very popular, at present it is being replaced by other determinations of greater

Table 56. Alterations in Basal Metabolism in Disease

INCREASED B.M.R.	DECREASED B.M.R.
Hyperthyroidism	Myxedema
Toxic adenomas of thyroid gland	Cretinism
Malignancy of thyroid gland	Thyroiditis (Riedel's struma)
Polycythemia	Nephrosis
Severe anemia	Hypopituitarism
Leukemia	Simmonds' disease
Diabetes insipidus	Addison's disease
Advanced cardiac decompensation	Undernutrition (starvation, anorexia nervosa)
Drug poisoning (a) thyroid (b) dinitrophenol	Shock
Diabetic pseudodwarfism	
Febrile disorders	

value and simpler performance; conditions modifying the basal metabolic rate appear in Table 56.

Normally the organism produces 1 Kcal. per Kg. of body weight per hour, or 38 to 40 Kcal. per square meter of body surface per hour, or 1500 to 2000 Kcal. per day; under the influence of intense exercise, 5000 to 7000 Kcal. may be produced, which should be replaced in the diet. Nevertheless, when the amounts of carbohydrates, lipids and proteins in the diet are calculated it is necessary to make room for the so-called "specific dynamic action" of foods, which consists of an elevation of metabolism and, therefore, of heat production.[18] Proteins have a more marked effect, approximately 30 per cent, so in order to provide 2000 calories in proteins, 2600 should be given. The specific dynamic action of fats is 6 per cent and that of carbohydrates is 4 per cent.

3. Regulation of Energy Exchange. The fact that most healthy subjects preserve a relatively constant weight suggests the existence of mechanisms regulating the amount of food ingested and of energy expended as heat and work. It seems certain that it is precisely the expenditure of energy that determines the amount of food ingested.[19] Some avenues for energy expenditure such as glandular secretion, absorption against a gradient, the transmission of the nerve impulse, etc., are difficult to measure and to study for practical purposes.[20] Therefore, it is convenient to study that part of energy which is applied to muscular movement. Factors influencing movement in locomotion have been analyzed by means of "activity" cages, which maintain experimental animals in continuous exercise; it has been observed that fasting exaggerates, and the postprandial state slows down, locomotion in different animal species. Estrus in rats increases their motor activity 8 to 10 times, but during pregnancy and lactation they tend to move less; ovariectomy erases differences in activity between sexes, darkness stimulates locomotion and light slows it. Cold temperatures increased the activity of blind rats, while warm temperatures had the opposite effect. It is of interest that when food ingestion is limited to the amount required by inactive animals to gain weight, rats in "activity" cages keep moving and lose weight, sometimes in considerable amounts.[21] Although it is not possible to give a common interpretation to all these observations, the general impression is that they do not appear aimed at providing an energetic balance, in the sense that the energy spent was similar in amount to that ingested with foods. Many other factors seem to operate in man: genetic, psychologic, emotional, social, the degree and duration of adaptation, etc. Nevertheless, there are several studies in obese and non-obese boys and girls showing that the degree of physical activity can be correlated with the amount of food intake when caloric expenditures reach a certain level characteristic of the individual.[22, 23]

Motor activity is regulated by the central nervous system, especially the hypothalamus and the frontal lobes; lethargic encephalitis shows degenerative lesions in the neurones of the posterior portion of the hypothalamus. Hetherington and Ranson[24] produced experimentally a syndrome characterized by hypomotility and hypersomnia by puncturing the posterior hypothalamus, and suggested the existence of a "wake center" in this area; on the other hand, it has been observed in rats, cats, dogs and monkeys, that lesions in the frontal lobes can induce continuous locomotion, and that in monkeys this increased activity is associated with ingestion of more food, so they tend to lose very little weight.[25] In man, motor activity is regulated by even higher centers, probably by the cortex, and variations in this activity agree with homeostatic modifications of food ingestion.[19]

Energy storage is also a dynamic process and may be defined as the state in which deposition is larger than utilization, since both mechanisms are occurring simultaneously and in a continuous manner. Energy storage is made especially as lipid, and much less as carbohydrate; energy reserves are easily accessible and may be used wherever external sources are not available. The normal adult organism has approximately 300 Gm. of reserve glycogen, providing some 400 to 600 Kcal., one tenth of which is in the liver and the rest in skeletal muscles. The transformation of glycogen into glucose, and vice versa, depends on their relative concentrations; furthermore, there is an upper limit beyond which all carbohydrates turn into fat instead of increasing the glycogen reserve.[26] Energy storage as fat is also in dynamic equilibrium with circulating lipids and those in tissue depots; it is characterized by being practically unlimited. Fat represents a very compact form of energy storage because of its high caloric value and its low water content.

Regulation of food ingestion is closely associated with the sensation of "appetite," which is difficult to analyze objectively in laboratory animals; nevertheless, conditions modifying the amount of food ingested may be enumerated as follows. After fasting, animals increase their ingestion of food, and the same occurs if they are submitted to increased exercise; during the period of growth, young animals eat more than adults, while hypophysectomy will depress growth and food ingestion; the administration of insulin in fasting increases even more the amount of food ingested, and the same effect is observed after pancreatectomy with hyperglycemia and glycosuria; estrus decreases, and lactation increases, food ingestion; low temperatures increase, and fever and high temperatures decrease, the amount of food eaten.[11] In general, all conditions, except fever, show a response of a homeostatic nature. It has been shown that the regulating center is in the hypothalamus, since lesions in this area frequently produce hyperphagia and obesity, and when symmetrical and on both sides of the medial eminence, the experimental animal dies of starvation, despite the presence of adequate amounts of food in its cage.[27] Furthermore, the feeding mechanism can be selectively activated by adrenergic stimulation of one area in the lateral hypothalamus.[28]

B. INTERMEDIARY METABOLISM

While studies of energy metabolism are aimed at understanding energy production and consumption during chemical reactions in the body, experiments in intermediary metabolism are designed to analyze the chemical transformations of different foods within the organism and the metabolic pathways of the different individual compounds.[29, 30] This aspect of biochemistry has received great impulse with the introduction of isotopic techniques, with which it is feasible to follow whole molecules or their fragments throughout their intricate exchanges and combinations, and to measure the speed with which all these changes occur in different compounds. Schoenheimer's fundamental contribution to knowledge of "the dynamic state of body constituents,"[10] although made with nonradioactive isotopes (deuterium), followed the same principle of marking molecules by means of recognizable labels which would not change their behavior.

Each one of the three main groups of foods (carbohydrates, lipids and proteins) undergoes a series of transformations leading to a two-carbon fragment, and in this form they penetrate a common final pathway known as the citric acid cycle, the tricarboxylic acid cycle, Krebs' cycle or the common metabolic cycle. Some of the most salient aspects of the intermediary metabolism of each of the three main groups of foods are presented in the next paragraphs, together with a brief note on the common metabolic cycle.

1. Carbohydrates. Absorption of carbohydrates is carried out in the small intestine, especially in the upper portion, after they have been hydrolyzed to form monosaccharides; the rate of absorption is variable for the different types; from higher to lower these are galactose, glucose, fructose and the pentoses.[31] Glucose is elim-

inated with the urine and ruled by a special Tm imposing a maximum limit to reabsorption of 250 to 400 mg. per minute.[32] Glucose can diffuse freely through the wall of peripheral capillaries and serous membranes,[33] as well as glomerular capillaries; for some time it was believed that phosphorylation was a necessary step for glucose to pass through the cell membrane,[34] but recent studies have shown that glucose can diffuse freely through the cell membrane and that immediately after doing so it is transformed into glucose-6-phosphate by hexokinase in the presence of ATP.[35] It seems certain that glucose transport through the cell membrane is a rate-limiting step for glucose utilization[36] and that the mechanism involves a specialized "carrier system,"[37] although the nature of this system still remains unknown. Glucose-6-phosphate may be converted into glycogen, or else it may continue its metabolic pathway to reach pyruvic acid and enter Krebs' cycle. In becoming glycogen, glucose-6-phosphate is transformed into glucose-1-phosphate by a phosphoglucomutase, and hence is polymerized while phosphorus is being released by a phosphorylase, until large molecules are formed.[38] When glucose is required glycogen is hydrolyzed going in reverse through the same stages as during polymerization until glucose-6-phosphate is again formed, when a phosphatase is necessary for it to become glucose and leave the cell. This enzyme is present in the liver, which therefore contributes to maintain the level of blood glucose, but the muscle lacks such phosphatase, a deficiency which appears as protective in cases of hypoglycemia since otherwise the muscle would lose most or all glycogen.[39]

There are three possible pathways for glucose-6-phosphate to reach pyruvic acid: first, through the formation of pentoses by means of phosphogluconic acid, which is one mechanism of synthesis of ribose and ribulose and, therefore, of nucleic acids ("hexose monophosphate shunt");[40] second, through fructose-1-2-diphosphate, then breaking into two 3-carbon fragments which may form glycerol, and further transformation into fats and phospholipids;[41] third, through phosphoric compounds and glyceric acid to pyruvic acid (Embden-Meyerhof cycle)[42] (Fig. 10–2). These three pathways lead to the same common end, pyruvic acid and acetyl-coenzyme A, which represent the "entry" to Krebs' tricarboxylic acid cycle.[43] Within the red blood cell there is a pure glycolytic system which produces lactic acid from pyruvic acid, and the same thing occurs throughout the rest of the organism when there is lack of oxygen. Formation of lactic acid from glucose results in only one fourth of the energy obtained from complete oxidation of sugar to CO_2 and H_2O. During violent exercise the skeletal muscles form lactic acid which passes to the blood, lowers the pH and stimulates respiration, which increases the oxygenation of blood; furthermore, the liver uses lactic acid to synthesize glucose which again passes to the circulation and is utilized by the skeletal muscle (Cori's cycle).[44]

The intermediary metabolism of carbohydrates is regulated by the endocrine and nervous systems; the influence exerted is one of coordination, since chemical reactions continue in their absence. Hormones with a definite influence on carbohydrate metabolism are insulin, glucagon, adrenal steroids, epinephrine, pituitary secretions and, probably, the thyroid hormone.[45] The most spectacular action is that of insulin, which seems to have two fundamental effects:[46] (1) It facilitates the utilization of glucose by accelerating its passage through muscular, and other, cell membranes[47] (but not all, since intestinal absorption and renal tubular reabsorption are not modified), its phosphorylation, its conversion into glycogen, etc. (2) It accelerates the synthesis of fat from carbohydrates.[48] This second effect is of great significance in understanding some of the most important physiopathologic disturbances in diabetes mellitus. Other effects, such as decrease in protein catabolism with low plasma amino acid concentration, appear secondary to the main actions of insulin in glucose metabolism and lipogenesis.[49] Glucagon is secreted by alpha cells in the islands of Langerhans and it causes hyperglycemia by increasing hepatic glycogenolysis;[50] it does not seem to play any role in diabetes mellitus.[51] Adrenal cortical hormones decrease the capacity of peripheral utilization of glucose and, at the same time, increase hepatic glycogenolysis;

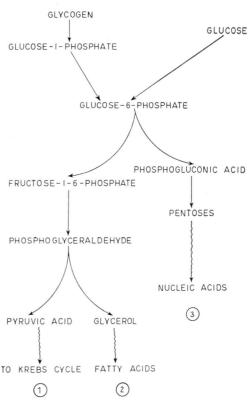

FIG. 10–2. The three pathways of glucose-6-phosphate metabolism. *1*, Through pyruvic acid to the Krebs cycle. *2*, Through glycerol to fatty acids. *3*, Through phosphogluconic acid to nucleic acids.

the activity of different compounds is quite variable; i.e., it is much higher in those with a hydroxyl or oxygen molecule in carbon 11, which accelerates protein catabolism and increases the formation of glycogen in the liver while decreasing the same compound in skeletal muscle. Prolonged administration of these steroids induces hyperglycemia and glucosuria; in adrenalectomized animals the liver glycogen is decreased and the consumption of carbohydrates is increased, while protein gluconeogenesis is decreased.[52] If these animals (or patients with adrenal insufficiency) are deprived of dietary carbohydrates they develop hypoglycemia very easily. Epinephrine causes a rise in blood glucose, glucosuria, increased concentration of lactic acid and ketone bodies in blood and ketonuria; these effects have been attributed to mobilization of liver glycogen, although a blockage of aerobic metabolism with deviation towards anaerobic type may also be responsible. Of pitui-

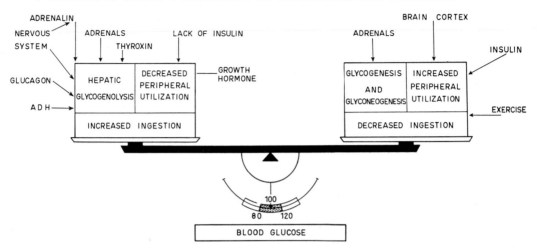

FIG. 10–3. Schematic representation of different factors regulating blood glucose levels.

tary secretions, growth and antidiuretic hormones seem to have direct influence on the intermediary metabolism of carbohydrates, since ACTH and thyrotropin act respectively through adrenals and thyroid. Growth hormone inhibits protein catabolism and carbohydrate oxidation in tissues, the result being hyperglycemia and glycosuria when foods contain sugar; prolonged administration of growth hormone to dogs and cats may end in permanent diabetes with atrophy of the islands of Langerhans. Antidiuretic hormone has an effect similar to epinephrine, i.e., it elevates blood sugar levels through increased hepatic glycogenolysis, and it is therefore capable of counteracting insulin hypoglycemia when the liver has an adequate amount of glycogen.

Since Claude Bernard's celebrated experiment of the "piqûre" of the fourth ventricle, ending in glycosuria, it is accepted that the central nervous system exerts a definite influence on carbohydrate metabolism.[54] Lesions in the basal ganglia and/or in the hypothalamus are frequently accompanied by hyperglycemia and, less often, by hypoglycemia; in certain emotional reactions there may be marked hyperglycemia. An interesting observation is the possibility of producing marked hypoglycemia in dogs by conditioning; Alvarez Bullya[55] has shown that this effect is mediated by the pituitary gland, since it disappears with hypophysectomy. Different factors regulating the blood glucose level appear in Figure 10–3.

Other sugars such as lactose, fructose, galactose and certain pentoses such as xylocetoses and ribose are absorbed in the intestine and transformed before utilization by the organism, although a small fraction may persist in the original structure.[56] Fructose can be utilized by the organism in the absence of insulin and this feature has been used in the past for the treatment of mild cases of diabetes mellitus,[57] although continuous or very frequent administration is necessary and limits its usefulness.[58]

2. Lipids. The intermediary metabolism of lipids is less well known than that of carbohydrates, partly because individualization of the different chemical types of lipids is not easy.[59] Table 57, taken from Peters,[30] is an incomplete list of some of the best known lipids; the following discussion refers to fatty acids in general, phospholipids (phosphatids) and cholesterol, which have been studied somewhat better.

Lipids are almost entirely insoluble in water, and to be absorbed require the presence of bile, which acts by decreasing surface tension and favoring a more intimate mixing of intestinal fluids and fats.[60] Nevertheless, it is possible that this effect is not purely on surface tension since the replacement of bile by other detergents such as Tween 80 is not as favorable for absorption and although labeled fatty acids appear to be adequately absorbed by rats with bile fistulas, only one fourth of free fatty acids appeared in the intestinal lymphatics.[61] Thus, bile might regulate the path by which lipids are absorbed

Table 57.   Classification of Lipids

I. True fats and oils, triglycerides of fatty acids
II. Nitrogen-containing lipids
    A. Phospholipids, nitrogenous lipids containing phosphoric acid
        1. Phosphatides, triglycerides in which one fatty acid is replaced by a phosphoric acid ester
        2. Sphingomyelins, nitrogenous lipids with only one molecule of fatty acid to each molecule of phosphoric
           acids
    B. Cerebrosides, compounds containing fatty acids, nitrogen and galactose, but no phosphoric acid
III. Unsaponifiable materials
    A. Sterols and steroids, compounds having a perhydrocyclopentanophenanthrene nucleus
        1. Cholesterol, free
           cholesterol esters, with a fatty acid attached to C_4
        2. Steroid hormones
        3. Bile acids
        4. Steroid vitamins and provitamins

(From Peters[30])

rather than the quantity assimilated.[62] Lack of bile will result in poor or no absorption of fats and liposoluble vitamins A, C, D and K. Pancreatic lipase is also necessary for absorption of fats, since many triglycerides pass the intestinal wall after they have been hydrolyzed to di- or monoglycerides; neutral fats are again formed in the intestinal cells and pass to the lymphatic capillaries and the portal circulation.[63] Neutral fats with chains longer than 12 carbons are usually absorbed by the lymphatics, while those with shorter carbon chains go into the blood directly. Phospholipids may be absorbed without any change or after partial hydrolysis; cholesterol absorption requires at least partial sterification, which occurs in the distal portion of the small intestine.[64]

Fecal fat is formed by unabsorbed fat and, especially, by fat of intestinal bacteria; under certain conditions the intestinal mucosa may also be one source of fat. There are also sterols with rings that cannot be oxidized, and cholesterol eliminated with the bile that has failed to be reabsorbed and is eliminated in different forms with the feces.[65]

Triglycerides are found in the fat depots of the organism, such as subcutaneous adipose tissue, mesentery, omentum and retroperitoneal space.[66] Phosphatides are widely distributed in the organism since they are part of the cell membrane and have been identified in the mitochondria. There is free and esterified cholesterol in serum. The free form occurs in many cells while esters are found only in ovaries, adrenals, liver and intestinal mucosa; in the last structure they are probably derived from absorption,

while in the former organs they represent precursors of steroid hormones.[65]

The organism can synthesize glycerol and most fatty acids. Those beyond the synthetic ability of the body are polyunsaturated acids such as linoleic, linolenic and arachidonic acids. Synthesis begins with the condensation of two molecules of acetyl-coenzyme A to form one of aceto-acetyl-coenzyme. A, and another of reduced coenzyme A.[67] This reaction requires energy expenditure, since the amount of glucose produced by a fatty acid will provide only 75 per cent of its caloric value, and this energy is probably derived from the oxidation of pyruvic acid to acetyl.[68]

Fatty acids may be synthesized in the liver,[69] but most of them are formed in adipose cells in fatty depots;[70] on the other hand, plasma phospholipids are produced in the liver, while those in each tissue are locally synthesized.[71] Cholesterol is easily formed throughout the organism starting with two-carbon units (acetate)[72, 73] while esterification is performed primarily by the liver, intestine and some endocrine glands as adrenals and testes. The interrelations of lipid synthesis appear in Figure 10–4.

Oxidation of fatty acids and phospholipids is carried out by two different pathways, which are "direct utilization" and ketone body formation.[74] In both cases the breakdown mechanism is the same, and is usually referred to as β-oxidation;[75] it consists of oxidation of the two terminal carbons with production of a fatty acid with two carbons less and a fragment with acetic acid structure. The discovery of acetyl coenzyme A clarified the mechanism of β-oxi-

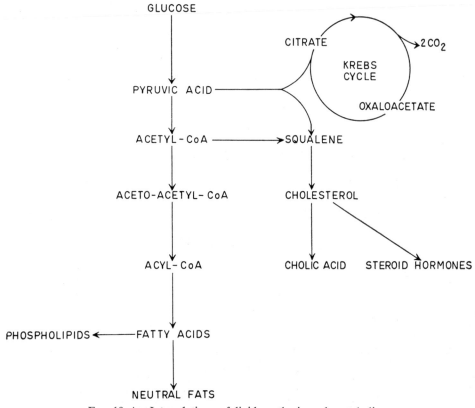

FIG. 10–4. Interrelations of lipid synthesis and metabolism.

dation and led Lynen[76] to propose the "fatty acid cycle," in which breakdown occurs by the combination of a molecule of acetate derived from fatty acid with another molecule of reduced coenzyme A, producing acetyl-coenzyme A and a molecule of fatty acid with two carbons less. Release of H_2O from carboxyl and sulfhydryl liberates a large amount of energy (during fatty acid synthesis combination of H_2O with carboxyl and sulfhydryl consumes two high energy bonds of ATP, which is transformed into AMP). In "direct utilization," acetyl-coenzyme A combines with oxalacetic acid to form citric acid and reduced coenzyme A, and enters the Krebs cycle. Indeed, coenzyme A serves as a link in the intermediary metabolism of carbohydrates, fats and proteins, supplying the two-carbon fragment (acetate) for the transformation of the four-carbon oxalacetic acid into the six-carbon citric acid.

When fatty acid oxidation results in ketone body formation, two molecules of

acetyl-coenzyme A are condensed to form aceto-acetyl-coenzyme A, which through catalysis by a diacetylase is irreversibly hydrolyzed to form acetoacetic acid and other ketone bodies.[77] This transformation occurs only in the liver, from which ketone bodies pass to the blood and are used by the cells, where they complete their metabolism to CO_2 and H_2O. Formation of β-hydroxy-butyric acid, aceto-acetic acid and acetone depends, at least in part, on the presence of carbohydrates or, better still, of pyruvic acid.[78] A diet poor in carbohydrates, or inability to utilize those present in a well balanced diet, will considerably decrease the amount of pyruvic acid produced, and also, therefore, the amount of oxalacetic acid, and this makes possible the condensation of two acetyl molecules in the peripheral tissues.[79]

Of the two methods of oxidation, direct and ketone body formation, the most important is the former, since even when the entire energy of the organism is derived from fat, as is the case in severe diabetes

Table 58.   Concentrations and Proportions of Lipids in Blood Plasma of Normal Adults

SUBSTANCE	MAXIMUM	MINIMUM	MEAN	STANDARD DEVIATION
Total lipid, mg. per 100 ml.	820	360	570	
Total fatty acid, mEq. per liter	36.9	7.3	12.3	± 3.37
Neutral fatty acids, mEq. per liter	17.8	0	3.1	± 1.49
Lipid phosphorus, mg. per cent	14.5	6.1	9.2	± 1.41
Total cholesterol, mg. per cent	320	107	194	±35.6
Ratio of free cholesterol to total cholesterol	0.32	0.24	0.28	
Ratio of cholesterol to lipid phosphorus at mean normal cholesterol concentration	31.7	14.9	21.4	± 2.48

(From Peters[30])

with ketosis, ketone body formation provides no more than 30 per cent of metabolized fat.[80]

Serum lipids show variable concentration (Table 58); all lipids are insoluble in water, but when combined with proteins they become soluble, which explains the transparency of serum in fasting subjects.[81] The nature of the combination of lipids and proteins is unknown, but by ultracentrifugation it has been found that most lipids are combined with the alpha$_2$ and beta fractions of globulins, and that the former contain more phospholipid than cholesterol, while the latter have equal amounts of both fats.[82] The total amount of fatty acids in serum is very small, but after a fat-rich meal it increases and the serum becomes opalescent. If these fatty acids are separated by centrifugation and the amount of protein is determined it is found to be very small whereas a few hours later, when the serum is again clear, most of the lipid is associated with protein and there are almost no emulsified fatty acids left.[83] The transition of emulsified fatty acid to lipoprotein obeys many unknown factors but at least two have been found, namely heparin and the clearing factor, a lipase of lipoprotein.

In 1943, Hahn[84] found that heparin abolished alimentary lipemia *in vivo,* an observation extended a few years later by showing that postheparin plasma cleared lipemia *in vitro.*[85] It has been established that this result is due to disappearance of triglyceride, appearance of unesterized fatty acids in combination with plasma albumin and, because the triglyceride was in a turbid lipid system and the unesterized fatty acids are in a water-soluble state, a clearing of

the lipid emulsion.[86] There is no change in the total fatty acid content of such a system.[87] Changes occurring *in vivo* during the absorption of a fatty meal with the administration of heparin are adequately explained by assuming that the same lipolytic system active *in vitro* is active in the whole animal. In addition to the decrease in chylomicrons and the increase in unesterized fatty acids and lipoproteins, the products of lipolytic action disappear very rapidly from the circulation;[88] this effect has been interpreted as indicating a certain influence on the transport of fatty acids out of the blood.[89] An enzyme, lipoprotein lipase, has been isolated from plasma, adipose tissue and myocardium.[90] It has been estimated that only a small percentage of the clearing of ingested fat entering the blood during fat absorption can be explained by lipoprotein lipase activity.[91] Other lipases may be present, especially in adipose tissue.[92]

Plasma lipids are being transported, and since there is no direct correlation between the plasma levels and the relative or absolute concentration of fatty acids, phospholipids and cholesterol in other parts of the organism, no inferences can be made from such a determination.[93] Furthermore, plasma lipids represent the outcome of two different processes, namely ingestion and consumption of fats, which occur simultaneously. Theoretically it is possible to find the same plasma concentration of lipids with high ingestion and consumption, or with both processes decreased to a minimum; furthermore, low ingestion and active oxidation will produce the same effect as decreased lipogenesis from carbohydrates.[94] The fate of plasma lipids may be storage in

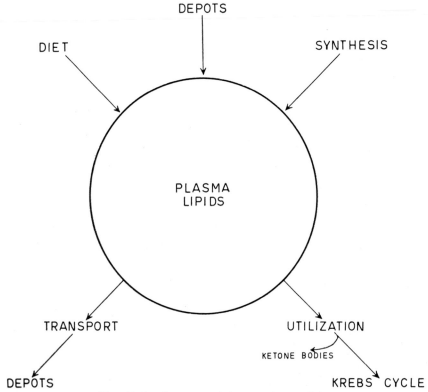

FIG. 10–5. Sources and fate of plasma lipids.

body depots or utilization; some interrelations of plasma lipids appear in Figure 10–5.

The role of the liver in the intermediary metabolism of lipids is of great significance: (a) The same as adipose cells and other tissues, the liver synthesizes fatty acids from acetyl groups, and with these fatty acids and glycerol derived from carbohydrates, forms triglycerides.[95] (b) Although phospholipids are formed in the intestinal mucosa during absorption of fats, the main organ involved in the synthesis of serum phospholipids is the liver, which uses fatty acids from serum triglycerides for it.[96] (c) Serum cholesterol is also synthesized by the liver, although this is not its only origin.[97, 98] From the liver cholesterol passes to the blood and/or to the bile; furthermore, the liver esterizes cholesterol and forms bile acids, which favor cholesterol absorption in the intestine.[99]

The normal amount of fat in the liver derives from three main sources: (a) food ingestion, (b) body depots and (c) local synthesis. On the other hand, fat may leave the liver in two different ways, which are transport or oxidation. Therefore, liver fat content is a manifestation of the equilibrium existing between processes favoring deposit, and those stimulating mobilization or breakdown.[95] Deposit is favored by fat-rich diets, by the activity of the pituitary gland, which secretes a hormone capable of mobilizing fat from the body depots (adipokinin) and deposits it in the liver for oxidation[100] (see below) and by an adequate supply of cystine and thiamine, among other factors, which favor synthesis.[101] On the other hand, fat mobilization from the liver depends on the presence of phospholipids, especially lecithin, cholesterol esters and fatty acids; transport requires lipotropic factors such as choline, inositol and others, which participate in phospholipid synthesis. Fat oxidation demands normal carbohydrate metabolism with combination of pyruvic acid and coenzyme A to form acetyl-coenzyme A and the two-carbon fragment that will transform oxalacetic acid into citric acid in Krebs' cycle. Lipotropic factors may also accelerate oxidation of fatty acids in the liver.[102] Participation of all these factors determines the amount of fat in the liver, and is depicted in Figure 10–6.

Endocrine glands participate in the regulation of intermediary metabolism of lipids, some directly, some through their influence in carbohydrate metabolism.[103] The effects of insulin and epinephrine have been mentioned as secondary to their role in glucose metabolism. Thyroid hormone is apparently related to the speed of utilization of plasma lipids, since in hypothyroidism there is hyperlipemia, mainly due to increased cholesterol and phospholipid, while in hyperthyroidism these substances tend to be low.[104] Adrenalectomy suppresses the effect of pancreatectomy on the liver, which is the lack of synthesis of long chain fatty acids;[105] this effect is even more pronounced after hypophysectomy.[103] These changes, however, are secondary to modifications in carbohydrate metabolism. Although there is general agreement on the proposition that the pituitary gland secretes a fat-mobilizing factor, its identity has not been established as yet. It has been claimed to be a separate hormone,[106] thyrotropin,[107] or somatotrophin.[108]

3. Proteins. The intermediary metabolism of proteins is less well known than that of carbohydrates and fats. This is probably because of the complexity of these substances, which in addition to carbon, hydrogen and oxygen (as sugars and fats) contain nitrogen, sulphur, phosphorus, iron and other metals, and whose molecular weight may be many millions. The number of possible combinations among the 22 or more known amino acids forming compounds of such high molecular weights defies imagination; furthermore, structure may be varied in spatial as well as in chemical composition, which modifies the properties of the molecule and, almost certainly, its handling by the cell.[109]

The vast majority of proteins ingested with food are digested by gastric pepsin, trypsin and other intestinal proteolytic enzymes which induce almost complete hydrolysis;[31] nevertheless, the use of oral vaccines and the existence of hypersensitivity acquired through the gastrointestinal tract

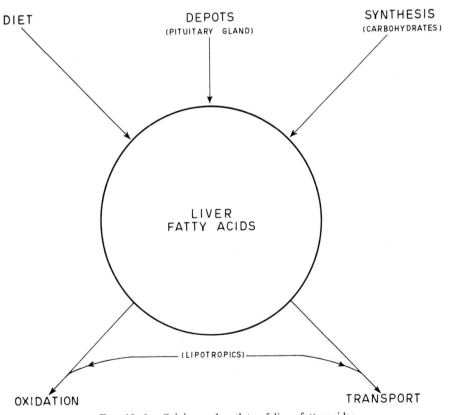

Fig. 10–6.   Origins and outlets of liver fatty acids.

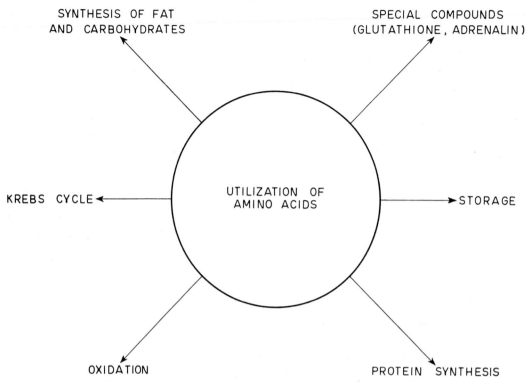

FIG. 10–7. Some pathways of utilization of plasma amino acids.

suggests that at least some of the ingested proteins are absorbed partially, or completely, unhydrolyzed.[110] A large amount of absorbed amino acids reaches the liver through the portal circulation, while the rest is found in the intestinal lymphatics; from there it passes to the venous circulation and is taken in part by the liver and in part by other organs such as skeletal muscle. Amino acids may be utilized in several ways, but in all the liver plays a very important role: (a) some are stored in cells, both hepatic and of other tissues; (b) they are used for protein synthesis; (c) they are oxidized and form NH_3, H_2O and CO_2; (4) they may be transformed into glucose and/or fats; (5) they may be used by the tissues to synthesize other special compounds such as glutathione, epinephrine, melanin, creatine, etc.[111] (Fig. 10–7).

Protein breakdown results in smaller fragments every time until α-amino acids are formed, which are deaminated to give NH_3; the latter may be reutilized in the synthesis of new amino acids, or combined with ornithine to form arginine, which through the action of arginase is separated

into urea and ornithine.[112] Finally, NH_3 may combine with glutamic acid to form glutamine, which in the kidney is again separated by glutaminase with elimination of NH_3 as one of the mechanisms of acidification of urine.[113] Ammonia is very toxic[114] and it may appear in high concentrations in the blood in cases of hepatic disease[115] or when amino acids fail to reach the liver, as is the case in certain shunting operations creating a short-circuit between the portal vein and the inferior vena cava.[116]

Proteins are the most important structural elements of cells, but at the same time their turnover is very active in most tissues.[10] Liver protein has a half life of 7 days, which means that half the amino acids of the liver are replaced every week. In man it has been calculated that the average half life of proteins is approximately 80 days, and that exchange is faster in the liver and slower in skeletal muscle.[30]

Some amino acids are not synthesized in the organism, at least in the amounts necessary to maintain normal growth, and for this reason they are considered "essential;"[117] a list of such amino acids is given in Table 59, together with daily requirements for man. When essential amino acids are given, the rest of the protein calories may be supplied in any combination of amino acids, or even as urea, glutamine or glycine. The content of essential amino acids and their proportions determine the nutritive value of a given protein.

One of the most fascinating problems in biochemistry is the synthesis of proteins, which is based on the combination of amino acids through peptide linkages.[118] Protein synthesis occurs throughout the cell but is faster in mitochondria;[119] it is believed that nucleic acids, and especially ribonucleic acid, participate in some way in the formation of proteins.[120] Synthesis depends on the requirements of the organism and occurs whenever amino acids are present in amounts greater than those necessary for energetic metabolism.[121] The incorporation of one amino acid to a protein molecule probably demands the complete breakdown and resynthesis of the protein, together with the amino acid.[122] The energy required for protein synthesis is probably derived from acetyl-coenzyme A, since rats deprived of pantothenic acid (a component of acetyl-coenzyme A) are almost completely unable to form antibodies.[123] Transference of a group amino from an amino acid to a ketonic acid is known as "transamination" and occurs in the presence of the enzyme transaminase and pyridoxine, which acts as coenzyme.[124] In spite of many efforts, it has not been possible to obtain protein synthesis in a cell-free system; many combinations of amino acids and different enzymes *in vitro* have failed to provide an adequate instance of protein formation.

The functions of proteins in the body are many and very varied; the following are some instances: most enzymes are proteins; genes are formed by proteins and determine inherited characteristics of organisms; fibrous proteins are abundant and provide support to the body; plasma proteins play a fundamental role in the exchange of fluids in tissues; antibodies are gamma globulins, etc. The relation between proteins and the synthesis of carbohydrates and fats is also significant, since it has been shown that in the absence of carbohydrates every 6.25 Gm. of protein can produce 3.65 Gm. of

Table 59. Essential Amino Acids

AMINO ACID	REQUIREMENTS (GM./DAY)
Isoleucine	0.70
Leucine	1.10
Lysine	0.80
Methionine	1.10
Phenylalanine	1.10
Treonine	0.60
Tryptophan	0.25
Valine	0.80

glucose, i.e., approximately 58 per cent of the protein will become carbohydrate.[125] Furthermore, deamination of amino acids results in compounds identical to those found in the intermediary metabolism of carbohydrates, and through them lipids may be formed; for instance, through pyruvic and acetic acids the synthesis of fats is possible, and with them, the storage of energy.

Amino groups released by oxidation of amino acids to H_2O and CO_2 are transformed into urea by the liver and eliminated by the kidney. The classic observations of Bollman, *et al.*[126] showed that in hepatectomized dogs urea formation ceases completely and that if no glucose is given the animal dies in hypoglycemia. Such a result is due not only to lack of hepatic glycogenolysis, but also to inability to change proteins into carbohydrates. Urea synthesis requires energy expenditure, and this energy is derived from the oxidation of foods, a possible explanation of the "specific dynamic action" of such substances mentioned above.[18] The liver forms urea through the "ornithine cycle."

The endocrine system influences protein metabolism but direct effects are difficult to separate from those exerted through carbohydates and fats.[127] Insulin inhibits carbohydrate formation from protein, while lack of this hormone accelerates protein catabolism and a similar effect is obtained with carbohydrate-poor diets. Thyroid hormone increases the metabolism of peripheral tissues and, therefore, of proteins, but this effect is purely energetic and it is possible to maintain an adequate protein balance by increasing carbohydrate and calorie supplies without giving more protein. The opposite effect

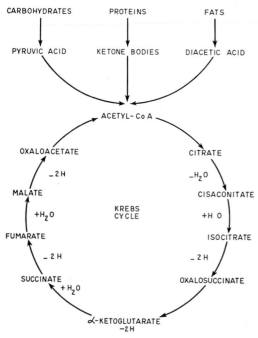

FIG. 10–8. The Krebs cycle.

can be seen in hypothyroidism. Adrenocorticoid hormones accelerate protein breakdown and increase glycogen deposits in the liver, while growth hormone inhibits protein catabolism and accelerates protein synthesis.[128]

C. THE COMMON METABOLIC CYCLE

The common metabolic cycle, tricarboxylic acid cycle, citric acid cycle or Krebs cycle, represents the most important mechanism for energy production as a result of oxidation of foods.[129, 130] All substances metabolized may enter the cycle as two-carbon fragments, since the terminal product of the cycle is oxalacetic acid, with 4 carbons, and the next step is represented by citric acid, which is a six-carbon compound. Carbohydrates provide the two-carbon fragment as pyruvic acid, fats as acetate, proteins as ketone bodies (Fig. 10–8). Nevertheless, several compounds formed during the cycle are also present in the organism as the result of other reactions, especially of proteins, and may enter the cycle at the corresponding level and continue in it. On the other hand, some of the substances appearing in the cycle play other roles in the organism, such as citric acid, which is im-

portant in the formation of bone mineral, and α-ketoglutaric acid, which participates in the synthesis of glutamic acid. The net result of the common metabolic cycle is the formation of high-energy phosphate bonds, such as ATP. This energy is utilized in many metabolic processes in the organism, including Krebs' cycle, where 4 high-energy bonds are invested and 14 are recovered in each turn, a net benefit of 10.

III. DISTURBANCES OF METABOLISM

If metabolism is the sum total of chemical changes occurring in the living organism, and disease is "life under abnormal conditions," then all diseases may be interpreted as disturbances in metabolism. This concept has great biologic value, but it encloses too many different phenomena to be of practical use in medicine. Indeed, practice has limited the use of the term "diseases of metabolism" to those in which the main disturbance is in some phase of metabolism and the cause remains obscure.[17] The field has been the domain of internists and endocrinologists for some time, but in recent years it has become more and more extensive involving other specialties such as pediatrics, surgery, psychiatry, etc. Today it would be as unthinkable for the psychiatrist to overlook the metabolic consequences of severe emotional upsets, or for the surgeon to ignore the metabolic response to trauma, as for the internist to ignore the profound metabolic disturbances of his diabetic patient.

Following the artificial division in the preceding section, metabolic disturbances may be separately discussed considering those involving intermediary, and those affecting energy, metabolism. Since pathologic changes in energy metabolism are closely linked to malnutrition and obesity, they are presented in the next section of this chapter, while in the following paragraphs some instances of disturbed intermediary metabolism are presented, together with a brief review of inborn errors of metabolism and the metabolic response to trauma.

A. DISTURBANCES IN INTERMEDIARY METABOLISM

1. Carbohydrates. Changes in carbohydrate metabolism are usually reflected in modifications in the blood concentration of glucose; when there is hyperglycemia the most common cause is diabetes mellitus, and when there is hypoglycemia there is frequently a tumor formed by islands of Langerhans.

a. *Diabetes Mellitus*.[131] Diabetes mellitus is a chronic disturbance of carbohydrate metabolism caused by a relative or absolute deficiency of insulin. There are enough data supporting the view that this disease, characterized by hyperglycemia, glycosuria and changes in fat and protein metabolism, may be due to different causes and, therefore, may be considered a syndrome.[132] Indeed, pancreatic destruction caused by acute or chronic pancreatitis,[133] carcinoma of the pancreas[134] and hemochromatosis[135] are three instances of diseases producing the same syndrome, and there may still be others.

Lawrence[136] has called attention to the existence of three different types of diabetes, called "lipoplethoric," "lipoatrophic" and "insulin deficiency." Although very few cases of these varieties have been reported, they serve to emphasize that diabetes is really not a specific disease but may result from many causes. Lipoatrophic diabetes has been interpreted as a primary defect in the mechanism for subcutaneous storage of fat leading to disordered carbohydrate metabolism.[137] Absolute or relative deficiency of insulin may be secondary to a lesion of the islands of Langerhans, and this idea has been widely accepted since Opie described hyalinization in this tissue.[138] Nevertheless, hyalinization of the islands of Langerhans is present in no more than half the patients with diabetes, namely those suffering from the disease for long periods.[139] So at present it is agreed to consider such change as a result of the metabolic disturbance and not as its cause; obviously, once the islands are hyalinized insulin secretion becomes impossible.

Mirsky[140] has described an insulinase in plasma which is capable of degrading insulin proteolytically and, therefore, could be the cause of some cases of diabetes. Mirsky has suggested that in some cases of human diabetes excessive activity of insulinase or deficiency of a normally occurring insulinase-inhibitor might be of etiologic significance.[141] However, tracer experiments with I^{131}-labeled insulin have failed to show an abnormally rapid rate of insulin degradation in untreated human diabetic subjects.[142] Other forms of insulin antagonists have been studied, especially in relation to insulin-resistant diabetes, but their role in the etiology and pathogenesis of the syndrome remains to be elucidated.[143] Additional studies of these interesting observations have been summarized recently.[143]

In other cases it would appear that the insulin requirements of the organism increase and the pancreas is unable to respond with secretion of adequate amounts, so diabetes supervenes.[144] Experimentally, diabetes is usually produced by destruction of the islands of Langerhans,[145] but the large number of patients with normal islands of Langerhans suggests the existence of other factors important in the development of the disease; those that have encountered more support are obesity, a certain hereditary tendency and other endocrine disturbances.

Diabetes is more frequent in obese people, but whether this is a cause and effect relation or the result of metabolic disturbances at a preclinical stage is not known. It has been clearly shown that the tendency to develop diabetes is inherited as a mendelian recessive character, although the subject may die before showing any signs of the disease or diabetes may become apparent after the age of 50. Houssay observed that hypophysectomy in dogs made diabetic by pancreatectomy was followed by a spectacular reduction in the clinical and chemical manifestations of the disease,[146] and this phenomenon has been documented in several human cases;[147] a similar observation is on record for the effect of adrenalectomy. The explanation of this phenomenon is to be found in the opposite influences of pituitary and adrenal secretions on insulin; the latter favors peripheral glucose utilization and accelerates lipogenesis, while the former inhibits utilization of glucose and favors gluconeogenesis. Therefore, the lack of insulin in pancreatectomized dogs or in diabetic patients will result in a predominance of pituitary and adrenal secretions with hyperglycemia, while elimination of these glands will bring about a fall in blood glucose and considerable improvement in diabetes.

The mechanism of action of insulin has been much discussed,[46, 47] but at present it is believed that it accelerates glucose transport through the cell membrane; the idea that it blocked the inhibiting effect of the pituitary on hexokinase and thus promoted the transformation of glucose into glucose-6-phosphate has been abandoned,[148] among other reasons because the passage through the cell membrane seems to be simultaneous with, but independent of, phosphorylation.[149] The controversy on the origin of hyperglycemia in diabetics (overproduction versus lack of utilization[150]) seems to have been solved in favor of both ideas,[151] since in the absence of insulin glucose will not pass through cell membranes and will not be utilized,[152] but at the same time it has been shown by means of C^{14}-labeled glucose and diabetic dogs that there is an increased production of glucose by the liver.[153] The studies of Shreeve, et al.[154] suggest that the relative importance of overproduction and underutilization of glucose might vary with the clinical type of diabetic patient. It has been postulated that insulin affects the formation of ATP, thus influencing phosphorylation by hexokinase, but decrease in ATP in alloxan-diabetic animals does not parallel the metabolic disturbance.[155] In anaerobiosis, liver ATP decreases to very low figures, while the organ preserves its ability to metabolize glucose in the presence of insulin.[156] The intracellular transfer of glucose is accompanied by extracellular potassium and a concomitant outflow of intracellular sodium; there is no adequate explanation for this phenomenon, but it should be kept in mind because without insulin potassium will not gain the inside of the cells and may be lost through the kidney in diabetic coma, which is then complicated by hypokalemia.[157] On the other hand, the simultaneous administration of potassium and glucose facilitates the peripheral utilization of glucose and prevents the consequences of sudden hypokalemia following injection of insulin, which would otherwise cause a sudden fall in plasma potassium.

One of the main difficulties in determining the mechanism of action of insulin is that its effects are difficult to reproduce in cell-free systems, or with cell particles such as microsomes or mitochondria. These facts suggested to Stadie that whole cells are required for the hormone to be active. By means of ingenious experiments, this author and his colleagues have shown that insulin is concentrated in tissues, with which it is firmly bound since it cannot be removed by careful and prolonged washings.[158] Finally, it has been mentioned that insulin acts on the intermediary metabolism of glucose, not only favoring transport through cell membranes, but also the transformation of glucose into pyruvic acid and the utilization of this acid in Krebs' cycle. This oxidative action of insulin is blocked with addition of acetate or β-hydroxybutyric acid, which suggests a less intense effect than the facilitation of glucose transfer through membranes. Acceleration of lipogenesis from pyruvic acid is of great significance and seems to be a primary effect,[159] while the increase in protein synthesis through glycine and phenylalanine is apparently secondary to insulin's action on glucose transfer.[160]

In view of the preceding observations on the mechanism of action of insulin, metabolic disturbances in diabetes will result from inadequate utilization of glucose, while hyperglycemia will be secondary both to this effect and to overproduction of glucose by the liver.[151] Changes in intermediary metabolism may be summarized as follows:[49] (1) lack of transport (decreased utilization) of glucose through cell membranes, with resulting hyperglycemia and glycosuria; (2) lack of glycolytic degradation caused by absence of substrate, with consequent decrease in pyruvic acid and material available for Krebs' cycle; (3) decrease in fat synthesis and increase in gluconeogenesis, which also contributes to hyperglycemia and glycosuria; (4) disturbance of fat metabolism, with acceleration of oxidation, cholesterol synthesis and ketone body formation, with a consequent decrease in fat depots in the organism and accumulation of ketone bodies in the blood;[161] (5) possible metabolic acidosis caused by loss of water

Table 60. Mechanism of Some Metabolic Disturbances in Diabetes Mellitus

METABOLIC DISTURBANCE	MECHANISM
Hyperglycemia and glycosuria	1. Increased glyconeogenesis from fats and proteins 2. Increased glycolysis in the liver 3. Peripheral inability to utilize glucose, because of insulin lack
Hypercholesterolemia and hyperlipidemia	1. Increased synthesis of cholesterol and fatty acids
Hyperaminoacidemia	1. Inhibition of protein synthesis 2. Increase in protein catabolism
Hyperketonemia and ketonuria	1. Increased formation of ketone bodies from fats
Acidosis and dehydration	1. Accumulation of ketone bodies in blood, loss of bicarbonate and water through the kidney

and bicarbonate resulting from overloading of the kidneys by ketone bodies which are "fixed" acids and must be eliminated through them; (6) decreased protein synthesis and increased protein catabolism, resulting in negative nitrogen balance with mobilization of tissue proteins and increase of plasma amino acids, succinic dehydrogenase and liver transaminase (which may be considered as an index of decreased synthesis and increased catabolism of these compounds). The mechanism of each one of those metabolic disturbances is summarized in Table 60, which refers to decompensated diabetes with acidosis and dehydration.

The consequences of such severe disturbances of intermediary metabolism are of two types, immediate and late. Immediate consequences are represented by coma and infection. Diabetic coma is usually the result of inadequate insulin treatment, of infection, or of some gastrointestinal complication producing fluid loss with vomiting or diarrhea. Diabetic coma develops slowly and there is marked hyperglycemia, hyperketonemia and ketonuria, hypokalemia, metabolic acidosis and dehydration.[162] Acidosis results in hyperventilation with Kussmaul's respiration and the patient exhales a peculiar acetone odor. Focal infections are very common in diabetics, especially in the lower extremities, and seem to be caused by a decrease in the phagocytic ability of leukocytes and by the presence of hyperglycemia, which favors the production of an acid environment in any infection (*see* Chapter II).

Late consequences of diabetes are vascular, renal, retinal and nervous, and with adequate treatment of immediate complications they have increased a great deal in recent years; in fact, the pathology of diabetes has been modified because patients live longer and give opportunity for metabolic disturbances to produce degenerative changes.[163] The mechanism of these changes is obscure, but it is probably related to modifications in the intermediary metabolism of fats and proteins.

The frequency and severity of atherosclerosis in diabetics is unsurpassed. Considering only 50 year old or older subjects, mortality from vascular disease is 80 times greater in diabetics than in nondiabetics;[164] gangrene of lower extremities is 50 to 70 times more frequent;[165] myocardial infarction is 1.3 times more frequent in males and 14 times in females. Curiously enough, it has been pointed out that atherosclerosis is more intense in all vessels except the aorta.[166] The relation of vascular changes to modifications in plasma lipids has been suspected for a long time, but so far it is still in the nature of a statistical correlation;[167] diabetics show high cholesterol in plasma[168] as well as elevated lipoproteins of class Sf 12-20, and the latter change is more pronounced in women with atherosclerosis and hypertension.[169]

There are four main renal complications in diabetes (Fig. 10–9): acute and chronic pyelonephritis, which has a much higher frequency in diabetics than in nondiabetics;[170] necrotizing papillitis, which is nothing other than a very acute and severe pyelonephritis with necrosis of the renal papillae probably caused by vascular obstruction;[171] atherosclerotic nephrosclerosis, more intense in diabetes on account of the

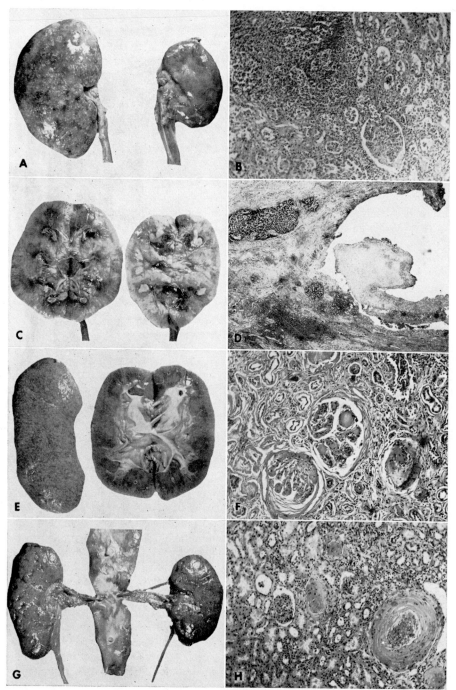

FIG. 10–9.   Some renal complications of diabetes mellitus. *A,* Gross aspect of acute and chronic pyelo-nephritis with abscess formation. *B,* Microscopic picture of an abscess in the kidney. *C,* Necrotizing papil-litis in a case of diabetes, with bilateral and extensive lesions. *D,* Sequestrum of a renal papilla with mul-tiple abscess formation in the vicinity. *E,* Kimmelstiel-Wilson disease. The kidneys are finely granular and pink in color. *F,* Microscopic aspect of the previous case. *G,* Advanced atherosclerosis and arterial nephro-sclerosis in diabetes. *H,* Hyalinized glomeruli, atrophic tubules and thickened arteries in arterial nephro-sclerosis.

increased severity of atherosclerosis;[172] and the Kimmelstiel-Wilson syndrome or intercapillary glomerulosclerosis.[173-175] This lesion is characterized by glomerular deposits of hyaline material with high fat content, which may take three different anatomic forms: globular, diffuse or exudative (*see* Chapter I). According to Gellman, *et al.,*[176] the diffuse form is more frequently associated with clinical manifestations than the other two; clinically there may be proteinuria, hyperlipiduria, hypoproteinemia, generalized edema and hypertension. Glomerular lesions are never present without extensive hyaline arteriolosclerosis in the kidney, and it has been proposed that they represent the same type of lesion.[177] Retinal arterioles are also involved, giving rise to diabetic retinopathy.[198] Both complications (renal and retinal) are more frequent in older subjects with long histories of diabetes, usually poorly controlled;[179] it has been suggested that in rigorously controlled cases vascular and renal complications never occur.[180] The retina may show punctate hemorrhages, brilliant or waxy exudates, vascular changes which occasionally may be very severe and then the condition is known as "retinitis proliferans."

Neurologic changes referred to under the collective term of diabetic neuropathy may be quite diverse and appear as a decrease or abolition of reflexes, pupillary inequality, dullness of extremities, etc.[181] The anatomic substrate may be represented by degeneration of peripheral nerves secondary to vascular changes.[182] Occasionally there may be involvement of the spinal cord with pain in hips and muscles, fecal and urinary incontinence and sexual impotency.[183] Sensory disturbances may be severe and produce joint changes of the Charcot type.

The study of large groups of diabetics has revealed some patients with a marked tendency to develop complications, and this has been attributed to adrenal hyperactivity. Furthermore, it has been shown that vitamin B_{12} is not normally retained in these subjects who after the administration of 50 micrograms eliminate at least twice as much as normal controls, and the same thing happens in animals treated with cortisone.[184] The effect of adrenocortical hormones is an increase in gluconeogenesis from both fats

Table 61. Etiologic Classification of Spontaneous Hypoglycemia

I. Organic hypoglycemia (with anatomic lesions)

  A. Hyperinsulinism
    1. Adenoma of islands of Langerhans
    2. Carcinoma of islands of Langerhans
    3. Generalized hyperplasia of islands of Langerhans
  B. Hepatic disturbances
    1. Chronic diseases (cirrhosis, von Gierke's disease)
    2. Acute diseases (hepatitis, alcoholism)
  C. Hypopituitarism
    1. Neoplasias (craniopharyngioma, adenoma)
    2. Atrophy (Simmonds' disease)
    3. Surgical
  D. Hypoadrenalism
    1. Tuberculosis
    2. Cytotoxic atrophy
  E. Tumors: fibromas and sarcomas
  F. Cerebral lesions: hypothalamus

II. Functional hypoglycemia (without apparent anatomic lesions)

  A. Hyperinsulinism (idiopathic, neurogenic, etc.)
  B. Alimentary hyperinsulinism
  C. Hyperinsulinism of childhood
  D. Other types (renal glycosuria, lactation, etc.)

(Modified from Conn[186])

and proteins, and in addition there is inhibition of synthesis of proteins.[185] From a general standpoint it is convenient to ascribe most complications of diabetes to changes in intermediary metabolism, but the exact mechanisms are not known and will remain so until more is learned of normal metabolic interrelations and of the pathogenesis of atherosclerosis.

b. Hypoglycemia. As in hyperglycemia and glycosuria, there are many causes of hypoglycemia and it reveals the presence of factors capable of decreasing the passage of glucose to the blood and/or increasing the rate of removal. Therefore, hypoglycemia is not a disease but a syndrome which may be associated with different entities (Table 61).[186] Hypoglycemia might also be considered as exogenous or endogenous in origin, which is of some importance since excessive administration of insulin may induce severe falls in glycemia, accompanied by the same manifestations appearing in other forms of hypoglycemia. A clinical classification of some usefulness in differential diagnosis considers three main types of hypoglycemia: "fasting," "stimulative" and combined. Fasting hypoglycemia shows the lowest blood levels of glucose after the longest fasting period, i.e., immediately before breakfast. The most common causes are related to liver disease, adrenal and pituitary insufficiency and lesions in the central nervous system. Stimulative hypoglycemia is characterized by normal glucose blood levels during fasting but 2 to 4 hours after intestinal absorption of carbohydrates has been started there is hypoglycemia; furthermore, if the usual postprandial elevation of blood glucose is inhibited there is also no consequent hypoglycemia. The most common cause is functional hyperinsulinism. Finally, the combined forms of hypoglycemia are caused by the presence of adenoma of the islands of Langerhans, hyperplasia of the same tissue or surreptitious administration of insulin.

Hypoglycemia of hepatic origin appears in cases of lesions both severe and diffuse,[187] although not necessarily irreversible,[188] and may resemble coma in cirrhosis of the liver or cerebral anoxia in chronic heart failure.[189] The cause seems to be a substantial decrease in glycogenolysis and gluconeogenesis, although it has been shown that the liver preserves these functions much longer than others susceptible of clinical measurement. Functional adenomas of islands of Langerhans are rare, usually small and well encapsulated neoplasms, with pink to brownish color and abundant vascularization, which are found both in the head and the tail of the pancreas.[190] Approximately 10 per cent of the cases are multiple; most tumors occur between 30 and 40 years of age. Some 20 to 25 per cent of the cases show histologic signs of malignancy but metastases are less frequent; when there is dissemination it usually occurs in neighboring lymph nodes and the liver.[191] On the other hand, only 10 per cent of all adenomas of the islands of Langerhans are functional;[192] diffuse hyperplasia of insular tissue is very rare. Some fibrogenic tumors may cause hypoglycemia, and the mechanism seems to be the secretion of large amounts of insulin-like material.[193]

c. Other Diseases. The efficiency of mechanisms maintaining blood glucose levels is demonstrated by the rarity and slight significance of changes in this parameter other than those already mentioned. Hyperglycemia and glycosuria, occasionally observed after intense trauma, especially of the central nervous system, are partly the result of certain intolerance to carbohydrates and also lack of food ingestion, leading to glycogenolysis; severe infections may also be accompanied by slight hyperglycemia. In chronic renal failure, and especially in chronic glomerulonephritis, there is a certain degree of alimentary hyperglycemia which may reach levels of glycosuria, although the latter is usually small. Some hepatic and bile duct abnormalities may also produce alimentary hyperglycemia. In general, all disturbances in carbohydrate metabolism other than diabetes and hyperinsulinism are of more physiologic than clinical interest. Meliturias are mentioned with inborn errors of metabolism.

2. Lipids. Disturbances in intermediary metabolism of lipids are more complicated and difficult to study than those of carbohydrates. This is because of the participation of more compounds and the wide variations of their normal plasma concentrations,[194, 195] frequently falling within levels observed in several diseases. Furthermore, it should be remembered that abnormal changes in fat metabolism are closely linked to others in carbohydrate and protein metabolism. Among many that might be mentioned, in the following paragraphs steatorrhea, fatty deposition in the liver and atherosclerosis are described as instances of disturbances in fat metabolism.

a. Steatorrhea. Fatty diarrhea or steatorrhea is a symptom of several diseases in which there is defective intestinal absorption of fat.[196] Normally, feces contain little lipid, most of which originates not in the diet, but in intestinal secretions and bacteria. Steatorrhea occurs when fecal fat is higher than 10 per cent of fat ingested with foods; this loss of fat will be reflected in inability to absorb many other substances, especially fat-soluble vitamins, and the result will be weight loss and malnutrition.[197] Although the loss of calories may be very important, vitamin deficiencies predominate, especially vitamin D and folic acid. Lack of vitamin D will be accompanied by inability to absorb calcium and the results are hypocalcemia, osteoporosis, tetany and cataract formation.[198] Deficiency in folic acid results in macrocytic anemia.[199] Advanced steatorrhea is usually only part of a more complex defect in intestinal absorption, the so-called malabsorption syndrome, in which many substances other than fat fail to be absorbed.[200] Rarely deficient absorption may involve a single substance, as vitamin B_{12} in pernicious anemia or vitamin D in resistant osteomalacia. The malabsorption syndrome has been variously classified; Volwiler's division appears complete enough[201] (Table 62), although there are many instances where causes are multiple. In general, defective absorption may occur whenever food is not adequately prepared, or it remains too short a period in contact with the intestinal mucosa, or the latter is abnormal. Clinical manifestations of the intestinal malabsorption syndrome are extremely variable and depend on the severity of nutritional deficiency, the quality of preferential food loss and the time of duration; furthermore, in all secondary forms there are also data corresponding to the primary disease. The complete picture is characterized by diarrhea, osteomalacia and/or osteoporosis, weight loss, signs of multiple avitaminoses, hemorrhagic phenomena, edema, megaloblastic anemia, etc. (Fig. 10–10).

b. Fatty Deposition in the Liver. Some aspects of fatty deposition in the liver were presented in Chapter I, so here only a brief discussion of those features related to metabolic disturbances is included. According to Figure 10–6 the amount of fat in the liver depends on two main factors: those determining fat supply from diet and depots, and those regulating removal of lipids through oxidation and transport to depots. In the first group, a fat-rich diet will produce fatty deposition in the liver, but it is doubtful that this is an isolated factor. It is usually associated with defects in oxidation caused by deficiency in carbohydrates, or by insufficient supply of dietary lipotropic factors which inhibit lipid transport and oxidation. On the other hand, a fat-poor diet is also followed by fatty deposition in the liver, but in this case lack of lipotropic factors is more apparent, with accumulation of both cholesterol and phospholipids in the liver and a consequent decrease of the same compounds in plasma. An exaggerated mobilization of depot fat may also cause fatty deposition in the liver, and this has been postulated to occur as the result of hormonal stimuli (adipokinin from the pituitary gland, adrenocortical secretions) which would induce increased oxidation of fat.[95, 101]

Increased fatty synthesis occurs when the organism has a rich supply of calories and no outlet for them; carbohydrate and protein deposits have a maximum limit, whereas fat may be deposited almost *ad infinitum* in the omentum, the subcutaneous tissue, the retroperitoneal space, etc. Fat is a very economic form of energy storage because of its high caloric value and low water content. One storing place is the liver, and

Table 62. Classification of Malabsorption Syndrome

I. Inadequate mixing of food with bile salts, lipase

  A. Pyloroplasty
  B. Subtotal gastrectomy
  C. Total gastrectomy

II. Inadequate lipolysis—lack of lipase
  A. Pancreatic insufficiency
    1. Congenital cystic fibrosis of pancreas
    2. Chronic pancreatitis
    3. Cancer of pancreas or ampulla
    4. Pancreatic fistula
    5. Protein deficiency

III. Inadequate emulsification of fat   lack of bile salts

  A. Obstructive jaundice
  B. Severe liver disease

IV. Primary absorptive defect of small bowel

  A. Inadequate length of normal surface
    1. Surgical resection
    2. Internal fistula
  B. Obstruction of mesenteric lymphatics
    1. Lymphoma
    2. Carcinoma
    3. Whipple's disease
  C. Inadequate absorbing surface because of extensive mucosal disease
    1. Inflammatory—tuberculosis, regional enteritis
    2. Neoplastic
    3. Amyloid infiltration
    4. Scleroderma
  D. Biochemical dysfunction of mucosal cells
    1. Celiac disease
    2. Sprue
    3. Severe starvation
    4. Transient dysfunction associated with intestinal infections
    2. Malabsorption associated with blind loops, diverticula, strictures

(Volwiler[201])

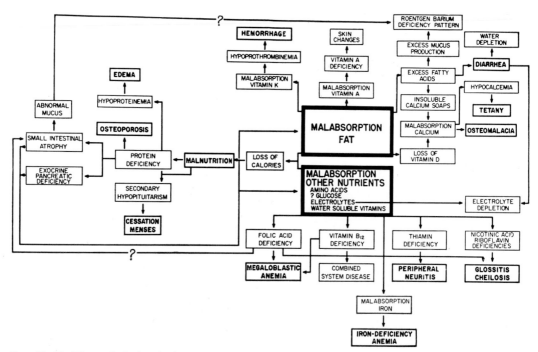

Fig. 10–10. The pathologic physiology of the malabsorption syndrome. (Courtesy of Dr. W. Volwiler and the Editors, American Journal of Medicine.)

this form of fatty deposition is not accompanied by metabolic disturbance. On the other hand, decreased synthesis caused by cellular damage, usually secondary to anoxia, is followed by accumulation of fat which cannot be oxidized.[202] One of the mechanisms is the deviation from aerobic to anaerobic metabolism of carbohydrates, which turn to lactic acid and provide little if any pyruvic acid for Krebs' cycle, decreasing energy release and hindering oxidation of fat. When the liver lesion is secondary to choline deficiency there is an additional difficulty in fat oxidation and transport to body depots. Finally King, *et al.*[203] have shown that cells in tissue cultures given colchicine or other toxic substances will rapidly increase their cholesterol content (*see* Chapter I). Therefore, there seem to be three factors affecting fatty deposition in the liver: disturbance in carbohydrate metabolism, defective oxidation and accelerated cholesterol synthesis.[204]

c. Atherosclerosis. The relation between plasma lipids and atherosclerosis has been suspected for a long time, among other reasons because in uncontrolled diabetes, hypothyroidism and xanthomatosis, where

there is intense hyperlipemia, the intensity of atherosclerosis is extreme.[205] Furthermore, atherosclerosis may be produced in animals by means of fat-rich diets;[206] many of the experimental and human vascular lesions contain large amounts of fat;[207] groups of population with various food habits differing in the amount and type of fat ingested also show variations in the extent and severity of atherosclerosis.[208, 209] In a recent study it has been shown that peptic ulcer patients treated with Sippy's diet (very rich in milk and other sources of fat) show a much higher incidence of myocardial infarction than control groups formed by nonulcer patients and ulcer patients treated by other means.[210] Many abnormalities in fat metabolism have been suggested as responsible for, or associated with, increased frequency and severity of atherosclerosis:[211] hypercholesterolemia, increase in β-lipoproteins, increase in cholesterol/phospholipid ratio in plasma, presence of abnormal lipoproteins and chylomicronemia. It should be recalled that whatever the metabolic disturbance associated with atherosclerosis, the present state of knowledge refers only to a statistically significant correlation between both phenomena, which is far from being a cause and effect relation.

Atherosclerosis may be produced experimentally by feeding rabbits a cholesterol-rich diet, but in addition to genetic differences between this animal species and man, the pathologic changes in this form of experimental atherosclerosis show marked differences from those of the human disease.[212] In addition, blood cholesterol rises 20 to 50 times; the cholesterol/phospholipid ratio increases from 0.5 to 2.0; atherosclerosis is also present in the pulmonary artery, and there is fatty deposition in the liver and xanthomatosis in the reticuloendothelial system. Furthermore, in addition to the increase in plasma cholesterol, phospholipids are elevated up to 7 times their normal level and triglycerides are at least 5 times more concentrated.[213] It has been demonstrated that in alloxan-diabetic animals the administration of cholesterol results in even higher concentrations of this lipid, but phospholipids are only slightly raised, the cholesterol/phospholipid ratio is altered little or not at all, and the intensity of atherosclerosis is much lower.[214] These observations suggest that the important change is not the absolute cholesterol figure but the ratio between the two types of lipids in plasma.[215] Furthermore, cholesterol is associated with α-lipoproteins but in rabbits on cholesterol-rich diets it appears in increasing amounts associated with β-lipoproteins, and especially with those with flotation density of Sf 12-30.[216] Therefore, experiments in rabbits successfully approximate conditions of plasma lipids to those normally existing in man, who shows a high proportion of blood cholesterol, an elevated cholesterol/phospholipid ratio and most of the cholesterol associated with β-lipoproteins.[217] Table 63 summarizes some data on the changes of plasma lipid concentration in rabbits in comparison with man.

In view of the association between high levels of plasma lipids and atherosclerosis, it may be convenient to examine the factors involved in causing such an increase. Figure 10–5 illustrates the different mechanisms determining whatever plasma lipid concentration is found at a given moment. The factors known to influence plasma lipid levels are mainly two, diet and hormones. It is possible that synthesis of lipids by the arterial wall *in situ* may contribute to fat deposition in arteries,[218] but no reasons exist to admit a simultaneous increase in plasma lipids. Diets rich in cholesterol and phospholipids tend to produce higher levels of these substances in plasma than diets with other types of fat,[219, 220] especially unsaturated fatty acids such as linoleic acid.[221, 222] Saturation of vegetable and fish fatty acids results in elevation of blood cholesterol.[223]

Other factors related to elevation of the level of plasma lipids (change in cholesterol/phospholipid ratio, increase in low density β-lipoproteins) include the endocrine glands, especially the gonads.[224, 225] Throughout active sex life the characteristics of plasma lipids in men are more similar to those of atherosclerotic rabbits than to those in women, who show lower cholesterol/phospholipid ratio, less total cholesterol associated with lipoproteins and less lipoproteins in class Sf 10-20. Nevertheless, after the menopause such differences tend to disappear, and this observation suggested that estrogens have a certain influence on plasma lipids; confirmation was obtained by giving estrogens to men.[226] Androgens have an opposite effect, and the mechanism of both groups of hormones is completely unknown, although it is suggestive of a partial explanation for the sex differences in frequency and severity of atherosclerosis.[227]

It is possible that lipoproteins may serve in lipid transport, so the central problem of

Table 63. Comparison of Plasma Lipids in Man, Rabbit and Atherosclerotic Rabbit

LIPID	MAN	RABBIT	ATHEROSCLEROTIC RABBIT
Total cholesterol, mg./100 ml.	200	51	1000–2500
Phospholipids, mg./100 ml.	250	88	400–616
Cholesterol /phospholipid ratio	0.8	0.58	2.1–4.2
Per cent of total cholesterol in β-lipoproteins	70	47	

the relation of plasma lipids to atherosclerosis may be connected with a disturbance in lipid transport.[228] It is noteworthy that in spite of the total insolubility of lipids in water, serum is transparent, and the only time there is some turbidity is immediately after meals, when fat concentration is very high. It has been reasoned that the combination of lipid and protein is a mechanism favoring solubility and, therefore, lipid transport.[229] Albrink, *et al.*[230] found that in order to observe serum turbidity it is necessary to have more than 590 mg. of neutral fat per 100 ml. of serum. On the other hand, hypercholesterolemia may be induced by infusion of triglycerides or phosphatides in rats, and the effect may be observed even in absence of the liver. Friedman and Byers[231] suggested that since hypercholesterolemia is secondary to changes in other lipids, this would explain other instances of hyperlipemia, as for instance the hypercholesterolemia of nephrosis, which might be secondary to hypoproteinemia; a similar explanation has been offered for the hyperlipemia of hypothyroidism.[232] Of equal significance is the mechanism of reduction of hyperlipemia, or at least of decrease in serum lactescence after meals or after lipid infusion. The original observation, that heparin accelerates disappearance of serum turbidity, led to the discovery of the "clearing" factor in serum, a lipase of lipoprotein which hydrolyzes triglycerides of soluble lipoproteins and makes them available to cells for metabolism (p. 431). It might be speculated that in the presence of hyperlipemia the "clearing" factor in serum is not present or its effect is being blocked,[89] but this or any other hypothesis linking disturbances in lipid transport with atherosclerosis is still awaiting experimental support.

Most hypotheses on the role of hyperlipemia in atherosclerosis assume that plasma lipids penetrate blood vessels, but other suggestions might explain the findings as well. It has been repeatedly shown that fatty acids, phospholipids and cholesterol accelerate blood coagulation,[233, 234] and Duguid[235] has suggested that growth of atherosclerotic plaques is caused by repeated deposit of thrombi in the intima of blood vessels. Therefore, hyperlipemia might act in atherosclerosis through an indirect mechanism, by accelerating blood clotting and thrombosis.[236] In close relation with these data is Swank's suggestion[237] that chylomicronemia increases blood viscosity and, therefore, decreases the speed of circulation and favors thrombosis. This hypothesis attempts to explain the growth of atherosclerotic plaques and not their presence.[238]

d. Other Diseases. Modifications in fat storage are discussed with obesity, and changes in diabetes and xanthomatosis have been mentioned. Hypothyroidism is also accompanied by hypercholesterolemia, and it is of interest that in order to induce the same change in plasma lipids in dogs they must be made hypothyroid.[239] Poisons such as guanidine and phloridzin produce hyperlipemia, although here the effect is not direct but through blockage of carbohydrate metabolism. In acute hepatitis there is increase in plasma lipids and normal levels are recovered in convalescence; a similar phenomenon is observed in biliary obstruction, while the opposite is the rule in cirrhosis of the liver.

3. Proteins. Most disturbances in intermediary protein metabolism result from malnutrition[240] or "inborn errors."[241] Some authors consider amyloidosis the result of abnormal protein metabolism, but there is not enough available information to accept this hypothesis; existing data are rather suggestive of deposition of an antigen-antibody complex (p. 35). Nevertheless, there is one disease in which the basic abnormality seems to be a disturbance in intermediary protein metabolism, namely, gout, and in association with some tumors there may be abnormal proteins in serum.

a. Gout. This disease is a disturbance in the intermediary metabolism of proteins characterized by hyperuricemia, recurring attacks of acute joint pains, deposit of urate crystals in cartilage, joint spaces, tendons and kidneys, tophus formation and renal failure.[242] The disease is caused by a single autosomal gene; it is inherited following a recessive mendelian line, and predominates in men.[243] The relative significance of an increase in endogenous production of uric acid, or of a decrease in its destruction and/or elimination, is difficult to decide.[244] In advanced stages the kidney is unable to

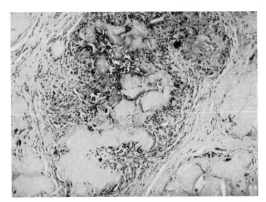

Fig. 10–11. Tophus, with urate crystals and foreign body reaction.

excrete uric acid, but before this happens there seems to be some overproduction.[245] In animals uric acid does not accumulate because of the presence of uricase, a hydrolytic enzyme which transforms uric acid into allantoin, but in man this enzyme is nonexistent and the acid must be eliminated without modification; a small amount appears in the feces and the rest leaves the organism with the urine. Purines arise from two different sources: nucleoproteins ingested with food, and endogenous synthesis from glycine, ammonia, formate and CO_2.[246] Purines may then be used in the synthesis of nucleic acids or of uric acid, and for this reason diets fail to reduce hyperuricemia in patients with gout. The relation between hyperuricemia and painful attacks is not clear, but they have been supposed to be caused by a precursor of uric acid, which would also be responsible for vascular and soft tissue lesions.[247] In chronic cases uric acid crystals are deposited in tissues and produce a histologic picture characterized by bland necrosis with some crystals and granulomatous inflammation, fibrosis and giant cells (Fig. 10–11); joints are deformed and function is lost, but renal sclerosis is the final cause of death in these patients.[248]

b. Abnormal Serum Proteins. The most clear instance of this disturbance in protein metabolism is the so-called Bence Jones protein, which appears in plasma and urine of patients with multiple myeloma. In truth, it is not a protein but several protein compounds which vary in composition and concentration from case to case, sharing only their enormous molecular weight and the fact that they precipitate with temperature changes.[249] Their concentration may be so high that plasma may precipitate spontaneously and have a viscous aspect. Of course, proteins appearing in the urine have a lower molecular weight, approximately 43,000. Osserman and Lawlor[250] suggested that abnormal serum proteins are combined with a glycoprotein and that this would explain their large size, whereas those filtered by the renal glomerulus are not combined with carbohydrate. Bence Jones proteins are not associated with any known serum protein and are precipitated in renal tubules producing tubular cell damage and basophilic casts surrounded by giant cells (Fig. 10–12). The increased frequency of amyloid in multiple myeloma has been associated with abnormal plasma proteins, probably formed by neoplastic plasma cells.[251]

c. Disturbances in Serum Proteins. Albumins and globulins may be altered in many diseases. Hypoalbuminemia is characteristic of the nephrotic syndrome, in which albumin escapes through the kidney in large amounts. It is also present in cirrhosis of the liver, where apparently albumin is not formed in adequate amounts by diseased hepatic cells; in advanced malnutrition, where the pathogenesis may be multiple; in the metabolic response to trauma, etc. On the other hand, hyperalbuminemia is almost always transitory and due to hemoconcentration. Globulins are altered in almost all cases with albumin modifications, and the most frequent change is hyperglobulinemia, probably because it accompanies the decrease in albumin.[252] β-lipoproteins are in-

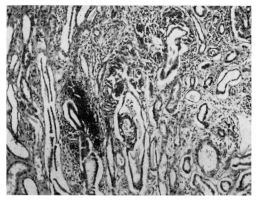

Fig. 10–12. Myeloma kidney, with dark cast formation and tubular degeneration.

creased in almost all cases of hyperlipemia, while gamma globulins show high values in many chronic infections. In other diseases, such as cirrhosis of the liver, the so-called "collagen diseases," sarcoidosis, schistosomiasis, kala-azar and granuloma inguinale, there is elevation of gamma globulins.[253] Their decrease is less frequent but it may be observed in agammaglobulinemia, a rare but extremely interesting "experiment of nature," which may occur after some viral infections or may appear as a congenital disturbance in protein metabolism.[254, 255]

B. INBORN ERRORS OF METABOLISM

Many disturbances in the intermediary metabolism of carbohydrates, lipids and proteins are congenital in nature. The doyen of this rare but extremely interesting aspect of medicine, Garrod,[256] called a group of four entities "inborn errors of metabolism" (albinism, alkaptonuria, cystinuria and pentosuria) but the field has been expanding and at present the number of diseases falling within this category is well over 80.[257] They are interesting not only because of their rarity, but also because of their mechanisms, which usually are reduced to the absence of enzymes necessary to complete a given metabolic cycle. Dent[258] defines an inborn error of metabolism as "a permanent and inherited condition, due to a primary enzymatic abnormality. The result is that one or more chemical compounds may follow an abnormal metabolic pathway or may be encountered in some of the body fluids in very elevated or very low concentrations." These diseases are all inherited and genetically transmitted, and viewed simply their main biochemical manifestations are: (a) absence of the enzyme responsible for a given metabolic step; (b) accumulation in the organism of the compound that fails to be metabolized; (c) decrease or absence of substances resulting from metabolism of the accumulated compound.[259] These biochemical manifestations may be complicated by the existence of several metabolic pathways for a single substance, so when one of them is closed because of enzymatic lack, other or others may be followed and the substance will not accumulate but the result will be the presence of abnormal compounds or of high concentrations of normal metabolites. At the same time, the intermediary metabolism of many compounds depends on the integrity of other metabolic steps, so the possibility of "chain reactions" should always be kept in mind. A simpler possibility is that the kidney may be eliminating a given substance in an abnormal way, a disturbance which Dent calls "deviation" instead of error. If these are genetic diseases it follows that all cells in the organism show the same disturbance, and the different clinical pictures may be due to the operation of two main factors: (a) functional specialization of organs and (b) environmental conditions. Inborn errors of metabolism may also be discussed according to the classification of foods into carbohydrates, lipids and proteins, although a few other additional points of interest have been added at the end of this section. Additional details may be obtained in some recent publications.[260, 261, 262]

1. Carbohydrates. *a. Von Gierke's Disease.* This disease was described by von Gierke in 1929[263] and is characterized by the inability of tissues to metabolize glycogen. Further studies showed that the disease described by von Gierke is only one of several defects in hereditary disturbances in glycogen metabolism which are known as glycogen storage diseases.[264] Recant[39] recognized four main types, which are: (1) the one described by von Gierke, or hepatorenal glycogenosis; (2) myocardial glycogenosis; (3) diffuse glycogenosis with cirrhosis of the liver, and (4) hepatic and muscular glycogenosis. The main clinical and chemical features of each one of these four types are summarized in Table 64.

From a metabolic standpoint the defect in most cases of von Gierke's disease is a decrease or absence of glucose-6-phosphatase, which limits glucose utilization by preventing glycogen degradation to glucose.[264] Nevertheless, the enzyme is normal in other cases, which suggests the existence of additional factors. Glycogen from liver, although greatly increased in quantity, has normal structural characteristics.[266] Patients show severe hypoglycemia, hyperlipemia and ketosis, and fail to respond to Adrenalin injection with hyperglycemia since hepatic glycogenolysis is low or absent.[267]

Table 64. Summary of Glycogen Storage Diseases

TYPE	ORGANS AFFECTED	AGE		HYPOGLYCEMIA KETOSIS HYPERLIPEMIA	EPINEPHRINE RESPONSE	GLYCOGEN STRUCTURE	ENZYMATIC ALTERATIONS
		ONSET	DEATH				
I	Liver, Kidney	Neonatal, infancy	Varies with severity	+ + + +	0– + +	Normal	Decreased to absent glucose-6-phosphate
II	Heart muscle, tongue, brain	Neonatal, infancy	Early	0	Normal	Normal	None found
III	Liver (cirrhosis), reticulo-endothelial system	Late infancy	1–10 yrs.	0	+ +	Abnormal: excessively long outer branches	Probably decreased brancher activity
IV	Liver, muscle	Late infancy	?	+ +	+	Abnormal: very short outer branches	Probably decreased de-brancher activity

(Recant[39])

Autopsy reveals considerable hepatomegaly and nephromegaly with extensive accumulation of glycogen in liver cells (Fig. 10–13) and renal tubular cells; in addition, hepatic cells contain abundant fat. Myocardial glycogenosis has no adequate biochemical explanation since the few cases so far studied have shown normal glycogen structure and glucose-6-phosphatase activity.[268] Myocardial cells are greatly enlarged and completely filled with glycogen, and the same aspect appears in the tongue, diaphragm and other muscles.[269] The two other types are much rarer. Knowledge of these diseases has been greatly advanced by biochemical studies, but they are fortunately very rare and sufficient cases are yet to be analyzed in order to have a more complete picture; possibly, enzymatic defects vary from one case to another while all maintain the inability to use glycogen as their common feature.[38]

b. Galactosemia. Galactosemia is characized by the inability to transform galactose into glucose and use it normally in metabolism.[270] The results are a high blood level of galactose, generalized anatomic changes and delay of growth.[271] Normally, galactose is transformed into glucose in three steps, each catalyzed by a different enzyme; the fundamental metabolic defect is an absence of P-gal-transferase in liver and red blood cells, so that galactose-1-phosphate cannot be changed into galactose-uridin-phos-

phate.[272] The main clinical manifestations are vomiting, jaundice, weight loss, hepatomegaly, ascites, cataracts, proteinuria and aminoaciduria.[273] They appear after ingestion of galactose, thus forcing the conclusion that they are caused by the "toxic" effect of galactose or a derived metabolite. Anatomic changes were described in one autopsied case by Edmonds *et al.*[274] who found advanced malnutrition, hepatomegaly and splenomegaly. The liver showed portal fibrosis and nodular regeneration, suggesting incipient biliary cirrhosis in some areas, and some groups of large liver cells contained abundant glycogen and fat. Chemical determinations in the liver showed less glycogen and more fat than normal.

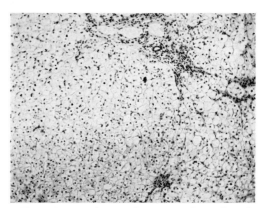

Fig. 10–13. Microscopic aspect of the liver in von Gierke's disease. (Courtesy of Dr. Edmundo Rojas.)

Table 65. Summary of Some Lipoidoses

DISEASE	STORED LIPID	INVOLVED ORGANS	AGE	SEX	CAUSE OF DEATH
Gaucher's disease	Kerasin (with glucose instead of galactose)	Spleen, liver, lymph nodes, bones, lungs	Children and adults	Even	Respiratory infections
Niemann-Pick disease	Sphingomyelin and lecithin	Liver, spleen, lungs, adrenals, brain, bone marrow	Children (6 mo.)	Even	Intercurrent infections
Tay-Sachs disease	Neuraminic acid	Brain and retina, spleen, myocardium, liver, lymph nodes.	Children (6 mo.)	Even	Intercurrent infections
Hand-Schüller Christian disease	Cholesterol	Cranial bones, spleen, lymph nodes, liver, skin	Children (2–5 yrs.)	Male	Intercurrent infections
Lipogranulomatosis	Sphingomyelin and other phosphatides	Pleura, pericardium, synovium, liver, spleen, brain, spinal cord	Children (1 yr.)	Even	?

c. Nondiabetic Meliturias. Nondiabetic meliturias are defined as the presence of excessive sugars in the urine in the absence of diabetes mellitus; they may be conveniently separated into glycosuric and nonglycosuric types. Those that can be considered as inborn errors of metabolism are renal glycosuria and nonglycosuric melituria; their significance lies in the possibility of confusion with diabetes mellitus.

Renal glycosuria is permanent, appears with blood sugar levels below 100 mg. per 100 ml. and curves of glucose tolerance are normal.[275] Nonglycosuric meliturias of interest here are galactosuria, which is a part of galactosemia, and pentosuria,[276] fructosuria and maltosuria which give no clinical manifestations of any type.

2. Lipids. The group of inborn errors of lipid metabolism is of little interest here since almost nothing is known of their intimate mechanism.[277] The most important are Gaucher's disease, Hand-Schüller-Christian disease, Niemann-Pick disease, xanthomatosis of several types and Farber's disseminated lipogranulomatosis,[278] redescribed by the same author under the name of glycolipoproteinosis. They are all congenital and hereditary, appear early in childhood, have a poor prognosis and entirely unknown etiology, and accumulate various lipids of a more or less specific type for each disease in the reticuloendothelial system. Table 65 summarizes some of the main features of these diseases. Hand-Schüller-Christian disease is included despite many data favoring the concept that in this form of lipid-storage disease the primary disturbance is proliferation of reticuloendothelial cells, while lipid accumulation is only secondary. Indeed, Lichtenstein[279] suggested that the other diseases apparently associated with Hand-Schüller-Christian disease, which are eosinophilic granuloma of bone and Letterer-Siwe disease, should be classified together as "Histiocytosis X," which emphasizes histiocytic proliferation and ignorance of etiology, and places no significance on lipid storage.

Hypercholesterolemia has been investigated recently and has appeared as a rather frequent inherited disturbance in lipid metabolism, since 4 to 5 per cent of a hospital population will show it.[280] It is inherited as an incomplete recessive mendelian character and is synonymous with xanthomatosis, although the term hypercholesterolemia is more distinctive of this type of lipoidosis. Its close association with atherosclerosis has been mentioned and is of interest because if a group of young people with atherosclerosis is studied, most if not all of them show familial hypercholesterolemia.[281]

3. Amino Acids. Three instances have been selected of the several that might be included, because they illustrate rather well the variety of metabolic disturbances that may occur as inherited errors; they are phenylpyruvic oligophrenia, cystinuria and Fanconi's syndrome.

a. Phenylpyruvic Oligophrenia. Phenylpyruvic oligophrenia, or phenylketonuria, is a fascinating example of correlation between a single gene, an enzyme and a bizarre clinical picture; indeed, it represents the most perfect instance of Garrod's classic concept of "inborn error of metabolism."[282] Phenylketonuria is transmitted by a single autosomic recessive gene; it affects both sexes with equal frequency since the gene is not located in sex chromosomes, and it appears only when the subject receives an abnormal gene from each of his parents. Since it is a recessive character, a heterozygotic couple with the abnormal gene will produce one normal child, two heterozygous and one with phenylketonuria.[283] The gene involved determines the presence of an enzyme catalyzing the transformation of phenylalanine into tyrosine, and is called phenylalanine hydroxylase.[284] In the disease, the enzyme may be entirely absent or perhaps the molecular structure is abnormal and cannot act on phenylalanine.[285] Should the second possibility be true, this would be the second instance of a "molecular disease," the first being the abnormal hemoglobin of sickle cell anemia.[286] The absence of normal activity of phenylalanine hydroxylase is manifested by an increase in concentration of phenylalanine, the lack of an elevation in tyrosine after the administration of the precursor amino acid[285] and the very limited transformation of radioactive phenylalanine into tyrosine.[287] This transformation seldom is more than 10 per cent of normal and has been interpreted as a sign of molecular alteration in the enzyme, although it could also represent the total yield of a different metabolic pathway.

Chemical and clinical disturbances may be correlated with this basic metabolic defect: (a) presence in serum and urine of large amounts of phenylalanine and other compounds derived from this amino acid;[288] (b) disturbances in pigmentation, since phenylalanine and tyrosine are precursors of melanin, with a tendency of the patients to be white, fair and have blue eyes;[285] (c) skin changes revealing a greater susceptibility to different agents such as light, antigens, bacteria, etc.;[282] (d) decreased tolerance to Adrenalin, which gives rise to severe hypertensive reaction,[289] and low levels of epinephrine in plasma;[290] (e) different neurologic disturbances such as reflex hyperactivity, muscular hypertonicity, ataxia, athetosis, etc., which are signs of changes in the extrapyramidal system.[285] In addition, there is epilepsy and in most patients there is a variable degree of mental deficiency ranging from decreased intelligence to complete imbecility, which unfortunately is more frequent. There is also decreased cerebral oxygen consumption[291] and electroencephalographic anomalies. Treatment consists of eliminating phenylalanine from the diet and giving tyrosine, and the result may be gratifying[292] although the degree of recovery of intelligence is not adequately established.

b. Cystinuria. Cystinuria is an inherited disease showing two different genetic types, one purely recessive, and the other incompletely recessive. Patients eliminate exaggerated amounts of cystine, lysine, arginine and ornithine in the urine, and form renal calculi composed almost exclusively of cystine.[293] Cystine crystals have been identified in bone marrow biopsy specimens and in the peripheral blood in one patient.[294] Cystinuria is then an aminoaciduria limited to the four amino acids mentioned and should be distinguished from other aminoacidurias, such as those occurring in Fanconi's syndrome and Wilson's disease, where many amino acids are involved and there is no calculi formation.[295] Dent, *et al.*[296] question the idea that cystine and other sulphur amino acids are eliminated through the kidney as part of an inborn error of metabolism, and suggest that the disturbance is in renal reabsorption. Intermediary metabolism would be normal since the four amino acids are not found in increased amounts in the organism;[297] their renal clearance is similar to that of inulin,[298] and the artificial increase in one of them stimulates the exaggerated elimination of the four.[299] This last observation suggests that the renal tubule is endowed with a single mechanism for reabsorption of cystine, lysine, arginine and ornithine. It has been proposed that it depends on the presence of two amino groups separated by a chain of 4 to 6 carbons, which is a structure common to the four amino acids.[300]

c. Fanconi's Syndrome. This is an inborn error of metabolism characterized by the elimination of excessive amounts of amino acids, glucose and phosphorus, inherited as a recessive character.[301] Anatomically there are deposits of cystine crystals in the reticuloendothelial system and a peculiar lesion of the proximal convoluted tubule in the kidney, consisting of an extraordinary elongation of the "neck" or first portion ("swan-neck" lesion).[302] The disturbance is very complex and, in addition to deposition of cystine crystals, there is marked aminoacidemia.[303] The renal lesion is associated with absence of alkaline phosphatase in the tubules, which fail to reabsorb glucose, amino acids and phosphorus; the same enzyme is missing in the liver and bone marrow.[304] Bickel, et al.[305] found that the kidney is unable to preserve base or bicarbonate in response to acidosis, which is probably due to decrease in carbonic anhydrase. The result of these metabolic disturbances is extensive demineralization of the skeleton with pathologic fractures, loss of glucose with tendency to ketosis and acidosis (which also favors osteoporosis) and a somatic development indistinguishable from rickets in children or osteomalacia in the adult.[306]

4. Other Congenital Disturbances of Intermediary Metabolism. A clear instance of enzyme deficiency is hypophosphatasia, in which there is absence or marked decrease in alkaline phosphatase, abnormal calcification of the skeleton and elimination of large amounts of phosphorylethanolamine. Fraser[307] reviewed 35 cases from the literature and found a slight predominance in males. Alkaline phosphatase is decreased in bones, kidney, intestinal mucosa and liver. Usually, there is hypercalcemia, especially in very young patients; blood phosphate is normal; most patients eliminate abundant phosphorylethanolamine with the urine and show extensive lesions in the skeleton and kidneys.[308] Bone changes are indistinguishable from rickets and appear as disturbances in calcification with deposit of abundant osteoid tissue, considered by some as abnormal. The kidneys reveal nephrocalcinosis with calcium deposition in the interstitial tissues and fibrosis. Parathyroid glands and adrenals are normal.[309]

Another disturbance of great interest is Wilson's disease, but here the inborn error is very complex and has not been adequately identified.[310] The disease is inherited as a recessive character and heterozygotes are normal, thus revealing that a double dose of abnormal genes is necessary for its appearance.[311] The fundamental disturbance seems to be related to copper, and is characterized by a defective synthesis of ceruloplasmin,[312] a protein with a molecular weight of 151,000 and eight copper atoms in the molecule. The functions of this protein are not known but is suspected that they are enzymatic in nature. In addition to low ceruloplasmin there is also a decreased amount of serum copper and an increased deposition of copper in tissues, especially liver and brain. Urinary copper is increased. Studies with Cu^{64} in subjects with Wilson's disease show that it is not coupled to protein and form the basis for suggesting a decreased synthesis of ceruloplasmin.[313] In addition, many patients show increased aminoacidemia, especially of threonine and cystine, although other amino acids such as serine, glycine, asparagin, valine, etc., are also found in large quantities. Proline and citrulline, which are not present in the urine of normal subjects, may also be found in these patients. Glycosuria, proteinuria and increased amounts of urates are also found.[314] Nevertheless, the most important changes are cirrhosis of the liver[315] and degenerative lesions in the basal ganglia, especially the lenticular and striated nuclei, where in addition to severe neuronal changes there may be cyst formation and bizarre, atypical glial cells.[316] These lesions in the central nervous system were considered rather characteristic at one time, but they have been described since in other forms of cirrhosis.[317] They are now believed to be secondary to the liver changes. The pathogenesis of this disease is obscure, and there are two main theories to explain it. One postulates a primary defect in the synthesis of ceruloplasmin, the other a disturbance in copper metabolism.[318]

C. THE METABOLIC RESPONSE TO TRAUMA

In the last decades knowledge of the metabolic response to trauma has shown an extraordinary and healthy increase.[319] Local reaction to a pathogenic agent producing cell injury or death is inflammation; hemorrhage or shock results in a series of homeostatic adjustments between circulating volume and vascular bed. But in addition to

Table 66.   Bodily Changes in First Phase of Metabolic Response to Injury

CIRCULATORY	METABOLIC	BLOOD
Tachycardia	Hepatic glycogenolysis	Increase in platelets and fibrinogen
Increase in cardiac output	Hyperglycemia	Decrease in prothrombin time
Generalized vasoconstriction	Increase in O₂ consumption	Accelerated coagulation
Splenic contraction	Decrease in adrenal cholesterol and vitamin C	Leukocytosis
Hypertension	Increase in urinary corticoids	Accelerated sedimentation rate and rouleaux formation
		Hypoferremia
		Fibrinolysis
		Eosinopenia

these localized and systemic changes, trauma is followed by a group of metabolic disturbances which are relatively independent from the nature and seat of injury and in which the endocrine and nervous system play a very important role.[320, 321] Such metabolic alterations may be separated into three more or less well defined stages, which are the emergency stage (Selye's "alarm" reaction),[322] the shock stage and the recovery stage. It is convenient to point out that this division is artificial, that many of the metabolic changes extend through two or three phases, that the response to trauma may be limited to the first stage when the intensity of injury is not great, or else the experimental animal or the patient may die early after severe trauma without revealing any tendency to an organized response. Nevertheless, the division is useful for descriptive purposes, and in the following paragraphs the metabolic changes in each one of the three stages are summarized, together with some influencing factors and the different mechanisms proposed to explain them.

1. First Phase or Emergency Stage. Immediately after the organism has been exposed to an intense stimulus, which may be trauma, burns, surgery, bone fractures, poisoning, hemorrhages, etc., a series of reactions occurs which are summarized in Table 66. These and other changes were described by Cannon[323] and others and represent a rather uniform response although occasionally some components may be masked or even be inverted by the peculiarities of the injurious agent, as occurs with intense total body radiation (500 r) in rats, when instead of thrombocytophilia there is thrombocyto-penia.[324] All parts of the first phase of the metabolic response to trauma may be reproduced by the injection of epinephrine, and many are absent in the adrenalectomized animal. It has been shown that epinephrine increases adrenal cortical secretions, and this represents the most satisfactory explanation for several metabolic changes.[325] Furthermore, for epinephrine to stimulate the adrenals the integrity of the hypothalamus and pituitary gland is necessary.[326] Therefore, it is accepted that the pathway followed by epinephrine to increase adrenal cortical hormone secretion is via the hypothalamus and pituitary, which releases ACTH.

Some components of the first phase of the metabolic response to trauma are directly produced by epinephrine, and others are caused by adrenal cortical hormones. Studies in stimulated rats with demedullated adrenals have shown that cholesterol and vitamin C decrease in the adrenal cortex.[327] The effects produced by increased secretion of adrenal steroids are eosinopenia, decrease in capillary permeability, increased elimination of corticoids in urine, decreased cholesterol and vitamin C in adrenals;[328] the other components of the emergency state are caused by norepinephrine. The duration of these changes also shows that they obey different hormonal stimuli, since those caused by epinephrine disappear rapidly while the remainder persist for variable periods and may be found even after 24 hours.[329]

2. Second Phase or Shock State. Circulatory reactions during shock are homeostatic in nature or result from decreased circulatory volume;[330] thus, hypotension,

Table 67. Bodily Changes in Second Phase of the Metabolic Response to Injury

CIRCULATORY	METABOLIC		WATER AND ELECTROLYTES
Tachycardia	Hypothermia	Hypoglycemia	Water retention
Decreased cardiac output	Anoxia	Hyperaminoacidemia	Na and Cl retention
Generalized vasoconstriction	Metabolic acidosis		Renal loss of K
Hypotension	Decrease in O_2 consumption		Oliguria
Low right atrium pressure	Decrease in energy production		Hemodilution
Hypovolemia			

decreased cardiac output and decreased right auricular pressure are manifestations of decreased circulatory volume, while tachycardia is a compensatory mechanism. Interesting as they are, however, circulatory disturbances are not metabolic in nature and will not be mentioned further. Exception should be made of the depression in cardiac output reported during major surgical procedures by Clowers and del Guercio,[331] which these authors compare to acute heart failure with metabolic acidosis. The cause is not known, but it has been attributed to depression of the myocardium[332] since no significant changes occurred in blood volume. Disturbances in body fluids and electrolytes, a prominent part of this second phase of the metabolic response to trauma, are more important in the third phase and will be discussed there (Table 67).

It is apparent that the most important metabolic consequence of trauma is a decrease in the amount of energy released by the organism, which is manifested as hypothermia, low utilization of oxygen and metabolic acidosis with accumulation of lactic acid in the peripheral blood.[333] These data can be explained by anoxia, which is sure to be present when there is copious hemorrhage and blood is not sufficient to transport all oxygen required by tissues for their metabolism (vide infra). But shock may be produced by agents other than hemorrhage, and in these cases anoxemic anoxia is not the cause of depressed metabolism. If the amount of oxygen reaching the peripheral tissues is normal, but the energy produced by them is decreased, as can be shown by the presence of hypothermia and increased venous oxygen, the defect must be in the tissues themselves, which have a decreased ability to maintain energetic metabolism at

a normal level. Green and Stoner[334] have summarized three possible mechanisms of decreased energy production by cells in shock, which are: (a) decrease in energy-storing compounds, such as ATP and phosphocreatine; (b) "uncoupling" of high-energy phosphate compounds with the Krebs cycle; (c) blockage of carbohydrate metabolism.

(a) Some authors observed that in shock there is a decrease in energy-storing compounds and a simultaneous increase in the amount of inorganic phosphate in plasma and red blood cells, which would explain the depression in energy-releasing processes.[335, 336] But this decrease in ATP is found only in certain types of shock, is more marked in the area experimentally damaged, and both phosphocreatine and ATP are found in normal concentration in the rest of the organism.[337] During the terminal phases of shock there may be some generalized decrease in high energy phosphates, but this is not the prevailing situation in the second phase of the metabolic response to trauma.

(b) If there is no decrease in energy-storing compounds, then another possibility to explain decreased energetic tissue metabolism would be "uncoupling" of high-energy phosphates with the tricarboxylic acid cycle. Glucose oxidation of glucose-6-phosphate to lactic acid is anaerobic; the enzymatic systems in charge of this transformation are also synthesizing ATP from ADP and inorganic phosphate. Both systems are intimately "coupled," and in the synthesis of ATP there is energy storage, which is released with the transformation of ATP into ADP and inorganic phosphate. "Uncoupling" would be expected to be accompanied by decreased ATP, increased

ADP and inorganic phosphate, but actual determinations have failed to show such a state of affairs in shock.[338]

(c) Engel[339] and others[340] have postulated an inhibition of carbohydrate metabolism as the explanation for decreased energetic metabolism in shock, in view of their findings in hemorrhagic shock. It has been observed that after hemorrhage there is a marked elevation of plasma lactic acid, with loss of the normal lactic acid/pyruvic acid ratio and acidosis. Since "entry" to Krebs' cycle is represented by pyruvic acid, a deviation in carbohydrate metabolism from aerobic to anaerobic would result in decreased supply of material available for oxidation to O_2 and H_2O and, therefore, of energy released. This attractive hypothesis has not been confirmed in other forms of shock, as those produced by intense trauma or nucleotide injection,[338] and it leaves without explanation the reason for the deviation towards anaerobiosis of carbohydrate metabolism.

Since the three possible mechanisms for explaining depressed energy metabolism in shock are unsatisfactory, Green and Stoner[334] have suggested another hypothesis: "A teleological view of these findings is that injury creates an excessive demand for carbohydrate in the injured area which, if unopposed by conservation elsewhere, would denude the body of the substrates required for energy production during recovery. Such a conservation is promoted first by the secretion of adrenaline, leading to the conversion of the carbohydrate stores to an inert form (glucose) which remains in the extracellular space, and second by the secretion of adrenocortical hormones which promote gluconeogenesis and inhibit glucose utilization." In other words, these authors believe that the cause of decreased energy metabolism is the inhibiting action of adrenocortical hormones on hexokinase, which catalyzes transformation of glucose to glucose-6-phosphate and, therefore, initiates oxidation of glucose; lack of oxidative degradation of glucose would decrease the amount of pyruvic acid, blocking the tricarboxylic cycle. Nevertheless, injection of products derived from glucose-6-phosphate such as hexose diphosphate or pyruvic acid, instead of improving experi-

mental animals in shock, makes them worse.[341] Green and Stoner remark: ". . . Anyone who builds hypotheses about shock does it at his peril and must be fully prepared to see them swept away by the advancing tide of biochemical knowledge!"

Since disturbances in carbohydrate metabolism have not been identified as the cause of decreased energetic metabolism in shock, some authors have examined the conditions of the energy "machine" itself, i.e., the tricarboxylic acid cycle. This is not a simple procedure, and results in general have been negative. Nevertheless, Threlfall, et al.[342] have found that citric acid is increased in the rat kidney in shock, which would indicate a blockage in the step from citric to cisaconitic acid, in Krebs' cycle. These experiments, however, were performed in shock produced by nucleotide (ATP) injections, and have not been observed in ischemic shock.

In summary, then, during the second or shock stage of the metabolic response to trauma there is depression of energy production by the organism, and although the mechanism of this disturbance is sure to involve carbohydrate metabolism and the tricarboxylic acid cycle, it has not been localized with certainty. Probably all circulatory, metabolic, and body fluid and electrolyte disturbances in this phase of shock are linked through homeostatic mechanisms, but this is no more than conjecture.

3. Third Phase or Recovery Stage. The third phase of the metabolic response to trauma has been called by Cuthbertson[343] the period of "traumatic inflammation," an unfortunate term since inflammation is classically known as the local response to injury and may be provoked by trauma. Nevertheless, this author was the first to observe the disturbance in protein metabolism characteristic of the third phase, which consists of a loss in protein nitrogen in the urine for periods varying from 2 to 8 days but reaching its maximum in 5 to 6 days.

Circulatory changes in the stage of recovery of the metabolic response to trauma are a return to normality probably due to adequate circulatory volume, which results from passage of interstitial fluid into the intravascular compartment, water retention in the kidney and bone marrow activity.

Table 68. Bodily Changes in Third Phase of Metabolic Response to Injury

CIRCULATORY	METABOLIC	WATER AND ELECTROLYTES	BLOOD
Tachycardia Normotension Normal cardiac output	Fever Increased consumption of O_2 Negative nitrogen balance Weight loss Hyperglycemia Increased urinary corticoids Retention of ascorbic acid Creatinuria Riboflavinuria	Water retention Na and Cl retention Renal loss of K, sulfur, phosphate Oliguria	Eosinopenia Leukocytosis Hypoalbuminemia Hyperglobulinemia Increased fibrinogen

Central problems in this phase are in body fluids and electrolytes, and in protein metabolism (Table 68). In his excellent review, Moore[345] points out a series of fundamental propositions in reference to water and electrolyte retention in trauma; those directly related to the metabolic problem are as follows: (a) Water and sodium chloride retention is one of the primary responses of the organism to disease, the usual result being hypotonicity of body fluids because water retention is in excess of sodium chloride. (b) Endogenous water is not under osmotic obligation to sodium and its retention is, therefore, another cause of hypotonicity. Endogenous water derives from cell water (approximately 750 ml./Kg. of lean tissue), from oxidation of proteins (approximately 150 ml./Kg. of lean tissue) and from fat oxidation (approximately 1080 ml./Kg. of fat). It is usual for a surgical patient to catabolize 500 Gm. of lean tissue and 500 Gm. of fat every day, which represent a daily production of 1000 ml. of water added to body fluids and contributing to their hypotonicity. (c) After an acute hemorrhage the reaction of the organism is to maintain volume at the expense of tonicity, and this mechanism is greatly altered or almost nonexistent in hypophysectomized or adrenalectomized animals or patients. (d) The total content of ions in the body and their concentration in plasma frequently change in opposite directions. (e) Trauma or surgery imposes difficulties on the compensating mechanisms for disturbances in the equilibrium of the H^+ ion. Another important modification is the loss of K^+ by the urine, which is associated with catabolic destruction of proteins and increase in extracellular Na^+, which passes inside the cells releasing K^+ to the interstitial space and facilitating its excessive elimination.

In 1929, Cuthbertson[346] found that after trauma (bone fracture) requiring immobilization there is urinary loss of nitrogen, phosphorus and sulphur, beginning shortly after 24 hours of injury and continuing for 8 to 10 days, with its maximum at 5 or 6 days. The proportion of nitrogen to phosphorus and sulphur suggested that protein catabolyzed was of muscular origin, but other tissues have similar proportions of these substances and in experimental animals it has been determined that nitrogen loss is not limited to the damaged extremity. The intensity of nitrogen loss is variable. Moore[347] finds an average of 350 Gm. per day; Paquin[348] found figures of 2 to 6 Gm./Kg. per day. In a case studied by Cuthbertson the total nitrogen loss in 10 days reached 137 Gm., which is equivalent to a reduction of 7.7 per cent of the total content of the organism and to an amount of nitrogen greater than that contained in the liver. Body weight losses estimated on the basis of the patient's body weight may be misleading since at the same time there is water retention. The diet is important in the amount of protein lost after trauma; in experimental animals maintained for some time with nonprotein diets the urinary loss of nitrogen is much less after trauma than in well-fed animals.[349] Furthermore, if some time before trauma there is an increase in the amount of protein in the diet, the urinary loss of nitrogen is proportional to the increment in protein ingestion, whereas such an effect is not observed when the animal is fed more proteins immediately after injury.[350]

Results obtained with different diets in experimentally traumatized animals reflect the behavior of protein metabolism in normal subjects since the amount of protein nitrogen eliminated with the urine depends on the ingestion of protein with foods. When a subject in protein balance is suddenly given a protein-free diet the amount of urinary nitrogen will decrease until a new level is reached; the opposite experiment gives inverse results. On this basis, Borsook[351] postulated that the protein lost is "labile" and is not represented by that recently ingested, the fate of which is apparently to become part of the cell structure; a similar conclusion was reached by Munro and Chalmers.[350] This observation is closely related to the origin of urinary nitrogen. The amounts lost suggest that it is not derived from plasma proteins or lymphoid tissue, or at least not exclusively from these origins, but that liver and skeletal muscles are also important contributors.[352] Although this phenomenon is commonly referred to as protein "catabolism," there are data indicating that the metabolic disturbance is more complicated. First, not all proteins are equally affected, since some, like fibrinogen, may increase instead of decrease; second, Yuile, et al.[353] have shown by means of C^{14}-labeled proteins that plasma albumin has an increased rate of both synthesis and breakdown, since half-life in dogs with turpentine abscesses was 2 days against 9 in controls, but the plasma levels remained unmodified; third, hemoglobin shows a decreased rate of synthesis without there being a change in catabolism.

4. Factors Influencing the Metabolic Response to Trauma. It has been mentioned that the type of injurious agent responsible for the metabolic response to trauma may influence some of the features of this reaction. Other factors of some interest are the severity of the lesion, which when very intense may end with the life of experimental animal or patient, and when very slight may produce only the first and/or second phases. Moore has proposed a "scale of ten" to indicate the approximate magnitude of injury. At one end of the scale, scale 1, are minor injuries such as a sprained ankle. At midscale lie the major abdominal operations, whereas at scale 7, 8 or 9 are the major multivisceral operations usually performed in cancer. Scale 10 is represented by serious and extensive tissue loss with trauma, penetration, infection and shock. Obviously this classification is quite subjective, but Moore himself remarks,[354] "This scale, like that used by mariners to express the force of a blow, may depend on the experience of the skipper, which way he is looking and how hard it blew yesterday. But still a hurricane looks different from a good stiff racing breeze, a zephyr from a flat calm." Whatever classification of the magnitude of tissue injury is employed, it is important to remember that the metabolic response to trauma depends in great part on the severity of injury.

Clinically, the nutritional status of the patient to be operated on is very important. An undernourished subject may present the so-called "depletion response," characterized by greater lability of the postoperative period, hypotension even in the presence of normal circulatory volume, oliguria with sodium loss and hypotonic expansion of plasma, increased eosinophils and low excretion of corticoids in the urine. All these features indicate that the adrenals failed to respond to trauma in an adequate manner.[355] Another interesting aspect is blood loss, which makes the second phase of the metabolic response to trauma more severe and prolonged. Multiple causes of injury, such as burns and radiation, or infection plus prolonged cold exposure will result in a more intense metabolic response. Anesthesia may provoke the entire process by itself; when trauma is not surgical, pain and emotional factors may also aggravate the metabolic response.

Weight loss during convalescence may be the result of many associated factors, among them the loss of tissue resulting from the operation itself, which in extensive mutilations may eliminate important amounts, blood and fluid loss as exudates, protein catabolism, atrophy of muscular masses because of inactivity and decreased food ingestion through lack of appetite, which in many patients may be the most important factor.[356]

5. Pathogenesis. The complexity of the metabolic response to trauma, with the three stages described and the various changes in cardiovascular physiology, in balance of body fluids and electrolytes, in composition of blood, in energetic metabolism, in endocrine functions, etc., render any single and simple explanation very unlikely. When studies in this field were in their beginnings the situation was different; the number of known facts was limited and theories proposed served to orient research. But at present there is an enormous accumulation of facts which grows almost every day and the old theories are no longer satisfactory, without vastly complicated additions, deletions and reservations. Such theories may easily become more complex than the phenomena they attempt to explain. It is always possible to find a suggestive pattern in nature and establish certain correlations, but in this respect, "such explanations have the air of being excuses, and one begins to wonder if the pattern itself is real. In any group of randomly disposed phenomena a pattern can always be seen by an effort of the imagination, just as one can see faces and figures in the chance outlines of a tree or a cloud. This is merely a selection of the things which seem to make sense, and rejection of those which seem not to do so."[357] It has been contended that the first phase of the metabolic response to trauma prepares the subject for an emergency situation, that the second is an attempt to preserve circulatory volume at the same time that materials necessary for repair are mobilized, and that the third phase represents another type of mobilization, this time of protein, necessary for building tissues and fluids lost during injury. How much is explained with this type of thinking is not clear, but at any rate reference is made only to the apparent results of homeostatic processes and not to their physiologic mechanisms or integration.

The pathogenesis of the first phase of the metabolic response to trauma was clarified by Cannon,[323] in classic papers which are a model of scientific research. Stimulation of the autonomic nervous system and epinephrine secretion are responsible for the initiation and part of the manifestations of this phase. Furthermore, it was mentioned before that other physiologic changes are caused by stimulation of the hypothalamus and pituitary gland, with secretion of ACTH and increased adrenal-cortical production of corticoids. Some details of this phase are not clearly explained as yet, such as hypoferremia[358] and increased fibrinolysis,[359] but it is doubtful that future research will bring about fundamental changes in the basic mechanism postulated above.

The second phase or shock has many aspects much more difficult to interpret, and for some of them there is no satisfactory explanation as yet. While circulatory changes are the result of homeostatic mechanisms regulating circulation through presso- and osmoreceptors, no adequate mechanism is known for the depression of energetic metabolism. Moon's "circle of death"[360] invoked the presence of toxic factors and increased capillary permeability, but the existence of toxins has not been validated by numerous studies[361] and there are direct demonstrations of normal capillary permeability in shock.[362] In cases of severe blood loss, anoxia may be considered as the cause of decreased energy release through a deviation of carbohydrate metabolism towards anaerobiosis and accumulation of lactic acid. When there is no hemorrhage, however, this explanation is not valid and an "enzymatic lesion" must be postulated,[363] although the nature and actual existence of such a change are purely hypothetical.

Disturbances in water and electrolytes are probably secondary to increased hormonal secretion, sodium retention caused by aldosterone and water retention by antidiuretic hormone, since they fail to appear in hypophysectomized or adrenalectomized subjects.[364] Some data on the regulation of aldosterone secretion and volume receptors are presented in Chapter IX.

The third phase or recovery is surrounded by even more darkness. Administration of ACTH or cortisone will faithfully reproduce most of the metabolic changes in trauma and for this reason almost all hypotheses consider the adrenals as the central organ, from which eventually everything will be explained. Nevertheless, the recovery phase is complex and has resisted all attempts at clarification. Selye's suggestion, that nitrogen loss results from adrenal cortical hyperactivity, was soon shown to be untenable by the demonstration of the same accelerated protein catabolism in adrenalectomized animals supported by a constant dose of cortisone,[365, 366] and by the observation of Robson, et al.[367] who found increased urinary nitrogen loss in a patient with bilateral adrenalectomy. Ingle[368] and others[369] developed the theory of the "permissive" action of corticoids, where these hormones are not directly responsible for the disturbance in protein metabolism, but must be present in concentrations above a certain minimum to provide the conditions in which metabolic processes can occur. A somewhat different idea has been expressed by Dudley et al.[370] who would consider "permissive" as meaning that, although the metabolic response to trauma takes place without measurable change in the secretory rate of the endocrine gland under study, changes in blood concentration of the hormone, arising as a result of extraglandular influences, may provide sufficient stimulus for increased metabolic activity. Selye believes that the permissive effect might be due to the synergistic action of corticoids and other factors acting in the peripheral tissues.[371] Steenburg and Ganong[372] suggest that modifications in circulating adrenocortical steroids result from factors such as hepatic conjugation or renal excretion. Finally, Engel[373] proposed that the function of adrenal glands is to maintain homeostasis in the organism, and considers the metabolic response to trauma as the manifestation of homeostatic mechanisms at play to return the organism to normal conditions. Adrenal corticoids would facilitate these mechanisms, and for this role only minimal amounts would be necessary in the blood. On the other hand, the level of hormones in peripheral blood may be abnormally high and the response may then acquire pathologic features.

It should be clear by now that the metabolic response to injury is a normal process comparable to other adaptations of the organism to stressful situations, as exercise induces tachycardia or excessive heat results in sweating. Only in cases in which it is unduly prolonged after surgery or when its manifestations are severe should the response to injury be considered pathologic. Even then, the metabolic response to trauma is only part of the entire clinical picture of the patient. As long as it remains within normal limits, the metabolic response to trauma should not be treated; a close and careful watch is all that is necessary, in order to be sure that it remains innocuous and is not complicating the general picture of the patient. Although stated in relation to problems of water and electrolytes, the following words by Moore[345] can find wider application: "The most important single factor in care of the patient is a concern for his whole pathological situation and his clinical management: the total problem, not just the chemical aspects, must be solved."

IV. NUTRITION

In order to maintain a normal metabolic exchange and be able to reproduce itself, the organism must take from the surrounding environment a series of substances varying widely in composition, from oxygen and some inorganic elements to the most complex proteins. Although "respiration is nutriment too," the science of nutrition limits itself to the relations between foods and metabolism. In this section reference will be made to the normal food requirements and to the two general disturbances in nutrition, namely malnutrition and obesity.

A. NORMAL FOOD REQUIREMENTS

A normal diet supplies sufficient food for optimal growth, for maintenance of metabolism and for reproduction. Foods belong to three general types, according to the way in which they are used by the organism: (a) those providing energy for metabolism, (b) those contributing to the structure of cells and intercellular substances and (c) those participating directly in neither of the two previous functions, but regulating the reactions whereby energy is released and structure is built. It has been mentioned that energy and intermediary metabolism are closely related and that distinction between them is purely descriptive, since there is a continuous exchange between "structural" substances and those ingested as foods.

The extent to which a given food contributes to energy exchange is known as its "caloric value," while its participation in building the structure of the organism is referred to as its "nutritive value." In general, carbohydrates and fats are the most important energy providers, while proteins are primarily involved in making up the architecture of cells. Nevertheless, the free transformation of proteins into carbohydrates and fats decreases the sharpness of this distinction, although a well balanced diet requires certain minimal amounts of each of these three basic foods. Although carbohydrates and fats are composed of the same elements and are oxidized in the same common metabolic cycle, some tissues can use only the energy derived from carbohydrates, as is the case with the cells of the central nervous system. When carbohydrates are missing from the diet the organism uses its glycogen reserves in liver and muscle, and after these have been exhausted proteins are used for glucose synthesis (glyconeogenesis). Another reason for the requirement of minimal amounts of the three basic foods in any diet is the existence of certain compounds necessary for metabolism, which cannot be synthesized by the organism, at least with the speed necessary to supply the metabolic demands. These "essential" foods are of three types, namely amino acids, fatty acids and vitamins; a varied diet has more probabilities of containing sufficient amounts of each one of these essential foods.[374]

A normal diet is that providing the organism with the necessary amount of energy, the material for synthesis of structural compounds and the agents necessary for the chemical reactions involved in the two preceding processes. Therefore, there are no absolute figures for different foods but rather they vary according to the needs of the organism. A sufficient supply of energy for an adult may be inadequate for a growing child or a pregnant woman, and there are variations according to height, sex, temperature, occupation, etc. When the energy provided is less than adequate for the organism, it will use its own energy reserves in a certain order, first carbohydrate, then fat and last protein. On the other hand, if supply of energy material is more than sufficient, the excess will be stored mainly as fat. Finally, it should be remembered that not all foods ingested are utilized; some are not absorbed in the intestine and are eliminated with the feces, others contribute to maintenance of the normal body temperature, and the process of assimilation requires some expenditure of calories, the so-called "specific dynamic action" of foods. With all these limitations present it is possible to determine certain optimal amounts for different foods, according to age, sex, weight, height and physiologic conditions (pregnancy or lactation). Table 69 contains the daily recommendations of the Food and Nutrition Committee of the National Research Council, revised in 1958; the figures quoted include wide safety margins to cover the usual variation in activity of normal subjects. The caloric and nutritive value of each food will depend on the extent to which it will contribute to supply the optimal quantities quoted in Table 69, but calculation is difficult because many foods are formed by variable combinations of carbohydrates, fats and proteins; the ingested amount is almost never recorded with exactness, and water is present in variable amounts. Therefore, it is necessary to establish, even in an approximate manner, the caloric and nutritive value of different foods as they are ingested in different parts of the world.

Vitamins are chemical compounds existing in plants and animals, and necessary for maintenance of growth, metabolism and reproduction.[375] They differ from hormones in that the organism is unable to synthesize them from simpler compounds, at least in amounts adequate for its requirements. In some cases part of the vitamin requirement may be filled from other compounds, as with niacin derived from tryptophan. In other cases intestinal bacteria supply the most important part, as happens with vitamin K; when bacteria decrease the organism may become adapted to a lower level, but this adaptation has not been measured objectively. The role of vitamins is that of coenzymes[376] necessary for enzymatic action in certain chemical reactions of intermediary metabolism, as with pantothenic acid, which participates in the combination of acetyl-coenzyme A with citric acid, or niacin, which plays a role in the transformation of

Table 69. Recommended Daily Dietary Allowances,[1] Food and Nutrition Board, National Research Council, Revised 1958

DESIGNED FOR THE MAINTENANCE OF GOOD NUTRITION OF HEALTHY PERSONS IN THE U.S.A.

(Allowances are intended for persons normally active in a temperate climate)

	AGE YEARS	WEIGHT KG. (LB.)	HEIGHT CM. (IN.)	CALORIES	PROTEIN GM.	CALCIUM GM.	IRON MG.	VITAMIN A I.U.	THIAM. MG.	RIBO. MG.	NIACIN[2] MG. EQUIV.	ASC. ACID MG.	VITAMIN D I.U.
Men..........	25	70 (154)	175 (69)	3200[3]	70	0.8	10	5000	1.6	1.8	21	75	
	45	70 (154)	175 (69)	3000	70	0.8	10	5000	1.5	1.8	20	75	
	65	70 (154)	175 (69)	2550	70	0.8	10	5000	1.3	1.8	18	75	
Women..........	25	58 (128)	163 (64)	2300	58	0.8	12	5000	1.2	1.5	17	70	
	45	58 (128)	163 (64)	2200	58	0.8	12	5000	1.1	1.5	17	70	
	65	58 (128)	163 (64)	1800	58	0.8	12	5000	1.0	1.5	17	70	
	Pregnant (second half)			+300	+20	1.5	15	6000	1.3	2.0	+3	100	400
	Lactating (850 ml. daily)			+1000	+40	2.0	15	8000	1.7	2.5	+2	150	400
Infants[4].......... 0–1/12[4]	2/12–6/12	6 (13)	60 (24)	kg. × 120	See Footnote 4	0.6	5	1500	0.4	0.5	6	30	400
	7/12–12/12	9 (20)	70 (28)	kg. × 100		0.8	7	1500	0.5	0.8	7	30	400
Children..........	1–3	12 (27)	87 (34)	1300	40	1.0	7	2000	0.7	1.0	8	35	400
	4–6	18 (40)	109 (43)	1700	50	1.0	8	2500	0.9	1.3	11	50	400
	7–9	27 (60)	129 (51)	2100	60	1.0	10	3500	1.1	1.5	14	60	400
	10–12	36 (79)	144 (57)	2500	70	1.2	12	4500	1.3	1.8	17	75	400
Boys..........	13–15	49 (108)	163 (64)	3100	85	1.4	15	5000	1.6	2.1	21	90	400
	16–19	63 (139)	175 (69)	3600	100	1.4	15	5000	1.8	2.5	25	100	400
Girls..........	13–15	49 (108)	160 (63)	2600	80	1.3	15	5000	1.3	2.0	17	80	400
	16–19	54 (120)	162 (64)	2400	75	1.3	15	5000	1.2	1.9	16	80	400

[1] The allowance levels are intended to cover individual variations among most normal persons as they live in the United States under usual environmental stresses. The recommended allowances can be attained with a variety of common foods, providing other nutrients for which human requirements have been less well defined.

[2] Niacin equivalents include dietary sources of the preformed vitamin and the precursor, tryptophan. 60 milligrams tryptophan equals 1 milligram niacin.

[3] Calorie allowances apply to individuals usually engaged in moderate physical activity. For office workers or others in sedentary occupations they are excessive. Adjustments must be made for variations in body size, age, physical activity, and environmental temperature.

[4] The Board recognizes that human milk is the natural food for infants and feels that breast feeding is the best and desired procedure for meeting nutrient requirements in the first months of life. No allowances are stated for the first month of life. Breast feeding is particularly indicated during the first month when infants show handicaps in homeostasis due to different rates of maturation of digestive, excretory and endocrine functions. Recommendations as listed pertain to nutrient intake as afforded by cows' milk formulas and supplementary foods given the infant when breast feeding is terminated. Allowances are not given for protein during infancy.

glucose to pyruvic acid, etc. Nevertheless, in many cases their participation in metabolism is not known, and this is the main reason for the present impossibility of bridging the gap between a vitamin deficiency and its clinical manifestations.[377] For instance, lack of thiamine results in beriberi, characterized by lesions in the central and peripheral nervous system, myocardium, or both. It is known that thiamine is a coenzyme of decarboxylase, the enzyme catalyzing oxidative decarboxylation of pyruvic acid and its transformation into "active acetate," in addition to participating in other decarboxylations, such as that of α-ketoglutaric acid in Krebs' cycle, etc. But between chemical defects and clinical manifestations no satisfactory correlation can be established, and the reasons why the brain or the myocardium suffers are not clear. Furthermore, experimental vitamin deficiencies are pure in type and many times are created under very rigid conditions, whereas clinical avitaminosis is usually multiple and only part of a more generalized picture of malnutrition.

B. DISTURBANCES OF NUTRITION

1. Malnutrition. This is the state in which nutritional supply is inadequate for the needs of the organism. According to this definition malnutrition is a relative concept, depending not only on the amount of food ingested, but also on the actual requirements of the individual; both factors are subject to independent variations.[378] Furthermore, malnutrition is a dynamic process, changing from day to day, which may produce irreversible lesions in advanced stages, although during part of its evolution it is curable by means of adequate diet.

Between the insufficient supply of a given food and the clinical manifestations derived from it, there is a series of sequential steps which must be taken: (a) decrease in adequate supply, which may be the result of an absolute decrease in ingestion, or an increase in the needs of the organism; (b) decrease in the tissue concentration of the substance or substances present in that particular food; (c) deficiency in the biochemical process or processes which require the presence of such elements; (d) establishment of the "biochemical lesion" which,

according to Peters,[379] is a molecular disturbance accompanied by functional changes; (e) development of anatomical changes. Clinically, the diagnosis is apparent only when anatomic changes are manifest, i.e., in the last stage of the sequence.

Malnutrition may be acute or chronic and of very varied severity, although in children it tends to follow a more acute and severe course (*vide infra*), while in adults it is chronic and frequently inapparent. Furthermore, malnutrition may be primary, when the food supply is below normal without any conditioning causes, or else secondary, as a complication of diseases interfering with one or several of the different steps in the normal assimilation of foods. The most frequent causes of malnutrition appear in Table 70 where it can be seen that conditioning factors make up a longer list than the causes of primary malnutrition. Unfortunately, throughout the world the two most frequent causes of malnutrition are ignorance and poverty. They are the main enemies faced by the physician when, in his practice, ". . . he attempts to apply knowledge obtained in laboratories and medical centers, is frequently frustrated by coarse ignorance of practical techniques to deal with traditions, prejudices, attitudes, superstitions, and human convictions surrounding the production, use, and consumption of food. These aspects hinder the work of the physician, whether he is counselling a private patient or influencing the nutritional policy of a country." The areas more closely related to the biologic instincts of self preservation and reproduction, namely food and sex, are the ones more deeply ingrained in individuals and communities, and around them an elaborate mesh of the most unmovable traditions, blind beliefs and elaborate superstitions have been piled up for many generations.

The problem of malnutrition has two different facets. One, of a highly scientific nature, is the relationship existing between the different food principles and the clinical manifestations of their deficiencies. Although there are still many gaps to be bridged, in the last forty years many data have been accumulated which permit the diagnosis and treatment of most disturbances caused by dietary insufficiencies. The

Table 70. **Factors Which Can Produce Undernutrition**

A. By Interference with Food Consumption
  1. Impaired appetite—infectious disease, cardiac disease, surgery and anesthesia, pain and drugs used in its treatment, thiamine deficiency, alcohol
  2. Gastrointestinal disease—peptic ulcer, diarrheas, biliary and liver disease, acute gastroenteritis, obstructive lesions
  3. Traumatic and neurologic disorders interfering with self feeding
  4. Neuropsychiatric disorders—neurosis, psychosis, migraine
  5. Pregnancy—anorexia and vomiting
  6. Food allergy
  7. Therapy—drugs which cause anorexia, diet restricting essential foods
B. By Increasing Destruction
  1. In gastrointestinal tract—achlorhydria, alkali therapy
  2. After absorption—heavy metals, trinitrotoluene, sulfonamides
C. By Interference with Absorption
  1. Absence of normal digestive secretions—achlorhydria, obstructive jaundice, pancreatic achylia, gastric resection
  2. Intestinal hypermotility—ulcerative colitis, bacillary and amebic dysentery, other diarrheal diseases
  3. Reduction of effective absorbing surface—intestinal resections, short-circuiting operations, small bowel disease
  4. Impairment of intrinsic mechanism of absorption—sprue, vitamin deficiencies
  5. Drugs preventing absorption—mineral oil, drastic cathartics, colloidal absorbents
D. By Interference with Utilization or Storage
  1. Impaired liver function—in hepatitis, cirrhosis, uncontrolled diabetes, alcoholism
  2. Hypothyroidism
  3. Neoplasm of gastrointestinal tract
  4. Therapy—sulfonamide, roentgen therapy
E. By Increasing Excretion or Loss
  1. Lactation
  2. Loss in serous exudates, as in severe burns
  3. Glycosuria and albuminuria
  4. Acute or chronic blood loss
F. By Increasing Nutritive Requirements
  1. Increased physical activity—strenous exertion, delirium, certain psychoses
  2. Periods of rapid growth
  3. Pregnancy and lactation
  4. Fever
  5. Hyperthyroidism
  6. Therapy—thyroid medication, fever therapy, high carbohydrate diets, insulin, parenteral dextrose administration

(Keys[378])

other facet of the problem is social and educational in character, and consists in teaching the large masses of undernourished people of the world a small group of principles to modify their stereotyped and rigid habits of eating and favor a more varied ingestion of food in adequate amounts. But even if these principles were known, and the techniques for their introduction were available, the economic problems involved in raising the average income in the undernourished areas of the world would require more decision and intelligence than those employed today for other purposes, such as the rapid destruction of equally large masses of people.

Conditioning factors interfering with food consumption are the following: (a) decrease in appetite accompanies many infectious diseases, surgical and anesthetic stress, pain and drugs used in their treatment, alcoholism, etc. Many diseases of the gastrointestinal tract are causes of malnutrition, such as stomatitis, peptic ulcer, diarrhea, intestinal obstruction, etc.; in some neuroses food ingestion may decrease considerably, the same as in the first months of pregnancy, in which anorexia may be accompanied by vomiting, thus creating a more complicated problem since food requirements are increased. (b) Another mechanism by which gastrointestinal disease may interfere with normal assimilation of food is by defects in absorption, which may result from achlorhydria, pancreatic insufficiency, ulcerative colitis, extensive intestinal resections, sprue, etc. (c) Chronic liver disease, diabetes, cancer, hypothyroidism and many other diseases are also accompanied by defects in intermediary metabolism of foods. (d) Frequently, substances important in metabolism are lost through the influence of some physiologic state, such as lactation, or some pathologic situations, such as glycosuria, albuminuria, acute or chronic hemorrhage, etc. (e) Finally, ingestion of food may be adequate for basal metabolic conditions but with increase in somatic needs it may become insufficient, as in rapid growth, fever, hyperthyroidism, certain psychoses, pregnancy and lactation, etc. Indeed, few conditions will fail to influence nutrition, and whatever their specialty physicians should always be concerned with the principles and mechanisms regulating normal ingestion and utilization of food.

Pathologic changes secondary to malnutrition are very variable. It must be emphasized again that combined deficiencies are the rule, and that even apparently pure pictures are usually established on the basis of a gross deficiency of all other dietary elements. The patient with pellagra who has glossitis and diarrhea is not selectively eliminating from his diet all those foods containing niacin, but simply refuses to eat, and the little that he does eat he loses through diarrhea. Anyhow, it is important to call attention to a group of studies published from the Hospital de Enfermedades de la Nutrición in Mexico, in which certain aspects of primary malnutrition in adults are analyzed.[381] This study was carried out in 80 patients with 50 per cent deficiency in all recommended foods, especially in proteins. The main clinical disturbances were glossitis and diarrhea, accompanied by nonspecific radiologic changes in the intestine and by atrophy and edema of the intestinal mucosa, atrophy of the muscular layer and, occasionally, ulcerations in the mucosa of the small intestine. Furthermore, there were few anatomic changes in the exocrine portion of the pancreas.[382] The skin was dry, thin, brilliant, pigmented and scaly, with generalized atrophy and vascular changes such as telangiectasis, ecchymoses, petechiae, etc.; the hair was dry and scarce.[383] In a larger group of patients there were several

neurologic manifestations such as polyneuritis, Wernicke's syndrome and pellagra encephalopathy.[384] Endocrine changes were characterized by panhypopituitarism with retarded somatic growth, decreased muscular development, decreased sexual activity and lower fertility, as well as by decreased urinary secretion of adrenal corticoids.[385] Anatomically there was atrophy or involution of the pituitary gland, adrenals, testes, ovaries and thyroid, and clinically there was depression of the entire endocrine system;[386] 50 per cent of young women had amenorrhea and atrophy of the breasts, while men had decreased libido and impotency. There were also manifestations of adrenal hypofunction such as absence of axillary hair, increased pigmentation of skin and mucosa, arterial hypotension and asthenia; there were no signs of hypothyroidism.[387] All these data point to a marked insufficiency of the anterior pituitary gland, which is also demonstrable by a series of hormonal determinations and functional endocrine tests: the elimination of urinary estrogens and vaginal smears revealed decreased estrogenic activity, even in cases with cirrhosis of the liver; urinary 17-ketosteroids were also depressed indicating testicular and adrenal hypofunction. The latter was confirmed by positive water tests, flat glucose tolerance curves and hypoglycemia in many patients.

Sepúlveda et al.[388] studied liver biopsies in 80 patients with primary malnutrition and found clinical and laboratory evidence of moderate hepatic insufficiency, fatty deposition, fibrosis and inflammatory infiltration, all of them slight to moderate in intensity.

2. Experimental Hepatic Necrosis. It would be surprising if the liver did not participate in nutritional deficiencies. Fatty deposition caused by dietary and other conditions has been discussed (p. 22); here, reference will be made only to experimental dietary necrosis of the liver.

Several experimental diets may produce necrosis of the liver[389] and this phenomenon may be prevented by means of sulphur amino acids, vitamin E and selenium (the casein factor).[390] The first studies were difficult to interpret because diets would produce fatty deposition, cirrhosis and necrosis of the liver. This was a result of the composition

Table 71. Factors Responsible for Liver Necrosis and Fatty Liver Cirrhosis

	LIVER NECROSIS	FATTY LIVER CIRRHOSIS
Disease process	Degenerative metabolic change of the liver parenchyma leading to sudden, acute attack of massive necrosis	Fatty metamorphosis of liver with slowly developing fibrosis, cirrhosis
	No fatty infiltration	*No* (massive)
	No fibrosis	Necrosis
Residual signs	Postnecrotic scarring	Cirrhosis
Protective factors		
Cystine	Protects	*Enhances*
Vitamin E	Protects	Without effect
Factor 3	Protects	Not known
Choline	*Enhances*	Protects
Betaine	*Enhances*	Protects
Methyl group precursors	*Enhances*	Protects
Vitamin B$_{12}$	*Enhances*	Protects
Folic acid/citrovorum factor	*Enhances*	Protects

(Schwartz[391])

of the diets, which were characterized by having low concentrations of protein and all lipotropic factors, and high concentrations of fat,[391] but at present several factors responsible for either fatty deposition or necrosis have been identified and may be listed as in Table 71. Hepatic necrosis may be due not only to a deficiency, but also to an excess of cystine,[392] which is in favor of an enzymatic effect, since it is well known that many enzymatic systems are inhibited by an excess of substrate. Intoxication with bromobenzene acts to eliminate cystine since it combines with cysteine, is acetylated and finally excreted as mercapturic acid;[393] this phenomenon represents an instance of a "toxic" substance whose effect is interference with an enzymatic action. Bromobenzene eliminates not only cystine but also its precursor methionine, and induces massive liver necrosis by a deficiency of sulphur amino acids. Selenium also inhibits cystine by replacing the sulphur in the molecule and forming an analogue competing with this amino acid in liver metabolism;[394] the result is hepatic necrosis. For some time it was suspected that intestinal bacteria played a role in dietary necrosis of the liver, partly because this phenomenon is more severe and frequent in the left half of the organ. It was believed that sulphur amino acids and vitamin E produced by saprophytes in the intestine would reach mainly the right half of the liver and would protect it, whereas the left half would receive bacterial toxins from

the colon and the result would be necrosis. Furthermore, antibiotics protect against this type of dietetic destruction but their effect is transitory, and this was correlated with the development of resistant strains in the intestinal lumen.[395] Nevertheless, studies with germ-free rats have shown that with identical diets they also show massive necrosis of the left half of the liver, so at present it is believed that intestinal bacteria play a secondary role, perhaps destroying sulphur amino acids.[396]

Vitamin E protects the liver against dietary and other forms of necrosis, including that produced by carbon tetrachloride, pyridine, naphthalene, etc.[397] There are many indirect data suggesting that such poisons act by precipitating oxidation of systems unsaturated with lipids while vitamin E increases the respiratory quotient, the same as the compounds mentioned. Lepkovsky and Borsoon[398] concluded that toxic hydrocarbons may accelerate the utilization of oxygen by cells, stimulating oxidation of unsaturated fatty acids and creating a relative local anoxia which would be higher in the liver than in other tissues, mainly because this organ has a greater concentration of phospholipids. The protective effect of vitamin E would be to preserve oxygen for the cell through antioxidant action and thus prevent massive necrosis. In the same fashion, lack of selenium depresses tissue respiration and decreases the amount of acetyl-coenzyme A and oxidation of pyruvic acid, thus leading to hepatic necrosis; the effect may be prevented with vitamin E or cystine.[399] This is an instance of the participation of dietary elements in enzymatic systems catalyzing oxidoreduction reactions, and gives support to the concept that vitamin E participates in metabolism of sulphur amino acids, which lead to synthesis of acetyl-coenzyme A. In its absence, oxygen is used faster than it can be supplied by the circulation and the resulting anoxia is the cause of experimental necrosis of the liver.

3. Malnutrition in Infancy and Childhood, and "Kwashiorkor." Gómez *et al.*[400, 401] have published a series of papers on infantile malnutrition, analyzing different clinical, biochemical and therapeutic aspects, that should be read to gain a better idea of this problem. The most important feature of malnutrition in infancy is inhibition of the process of growth and development, not only of height, but also of the skeleton and mental capacity. This defect in growth and development appears in 90 per cent of the cases between 6 months and 5 years of age, and is usually caused by the ingestion of diets deficient in protein, fat and vitamins, and rich in carbohydrates.[402] According to the amount of weight loss there are three degrees of malnutrition in children, which are as follows: (1) first degree malnutrition, when body weight is between 85 and 75 per cent of the ideal weight for the age of the child; (2) second degree malnutrition, when the body weight is between 65 to 75 per cent of the ideal body weight; (3) third degree malnutrition, when the body weight is below 60 per cent of the ideal. All tissues show alterations, with the possible exception of teeth and gums; the most conspicuous changes occur in the skin, and here they vary greatly in intensity and aspect. Skin lesions frequently appear as fissures, dryness and changes in pigmentation, which in the beginning is erythematous and disappears with pressure, but later changes to purple and reddish-brown, with darker margins and exfoliation. These lesions appear in areas exposed to sunlight, and may be symmetrical and extensive or macular and coalescent.[403] The hair, which shows changes in texture and color, is yellowish-brown and may even appear red or brownish-red; it falls very easily.

There are mucous lesions such as cheilosis, xerophthalmia and vulvitis. Mental disturbances are very varied and may appear as apathy or irritability; there are episodes of abnormal behavior, "the child with third degree malnutrition does not smile; when he does, it is a sign of recovery." Diarrhea is the rule, and in close to 30 per cent of the cases it is of bacterial origin, while in the rest it has not been found associated with enteric pathogens and it is probably caused by atrophy of the intestinal tract. Infections of the respiratory tract are frequent, especially bronchopneumonia, and it is significant that there is little or no systemic resistance to these infections.

Biochemical changes are many and very varied. There is hypoproteinemia with hypoalbuminemia, decrease in the α and β fractions of globulins and increase in the γ fraction. Liver function tests are usually normal. The extracellular fluid compartment is increased, and there is anemia with eosinopenia. Duodenal enzymes are decreased but return to normal during recovery.[402]

The most frequent anatomic change is fatty deposition in the liver, which may be accompanied by portal fibrosis; nutritional cirrhosis in malnourished infants must be extremely rare if it really exists. Other changes involving the connective tissue in the liver have been described by Hill *et al.*[404] in Jamaica. Skin changes are characterized by diffuse or perifollicular hyperkeratosis, focal parakeratosis, atrophy of the malpighian layers with hyperpigmentation of the basal layer, edema of the dermis and atrophy of the skin adnexae.

Malnutrition in infancy and childhood is also known by the exotic and inadequate term of "kwashiorkor." This name was first used by Williams,[380] who remarks: "This cumbersome word was merely a confession of ignorance. It was the name given to the disease by the Accra people, to whom it was well known. Some say the word means 'red Kwashi.' Kwashi is the name for a boy born on a Sunday, but it is used as a generic name as we would use Johnny or Tommy. . . . In this name, I believe the redness refers to the raw areas where the skin has peeled off in the severe and acute cases and not to the hair. . . . The supreme virtue of the word kwashiorkor is that it does not make any unwarranted assumptions with respect to etiology or pathology . . . it has the merit of neutrality." Gómez, et al.[405] have shown in a rather definitive way that kwashiorkor and infantile malnutrition are the same thing, so it is no longer appropriate to continue the use of the term, as it is no longer necessary, except for sensationalism, to continue calling bubonic plague "the black death" or malaria "fevers."

Infantile malnutrition has accompanied poverty and ignorance for many centuries, and it will continue to do so as long as the wishes of many people, adequately expressed by Williams, are not fulfilled: "All over the world the medical authorities have been dazzled by the ease and by the results of mass methods of prevention and by the heroics of therapeutic miracle. It is urgently necessary for the leaders of medicine to cultivate that rare and most necessary factor, common sense, and to decide . . . that society must measure its well-being in terms of the health of its children."

4. Obesity. Obesity is not the opposite of malnutrition, since an individual may be obese and malnourished.[406] Obesity is defined as an abnormal increase in body weight due to accumulation of fat. Brozek and Keys[407] have pointed out that determination of body weight is not an exact index of obesity, since it is necessary to take into account the chemical composition of tissues responsible for increased body weight. Nevertheless, methods required for these determinations are rather complicated and have little practical application in clinical work.[408, 409] As long as water retention is considered, body weight is still an adequate measure of obesity. A loss of equilibrium between energy supplied by foods and its expenditure in metabolism is at the base of all cases of obesity. If the fundamental defect is a positive energy balance, it may be the result of excessive ingestion of food without a parallel increase in metabolism, of decrease in energy expenditure without a similar cut down in food ingestion, or to a combination of both mechanisms.[410]

Although it is generally admitted that there are no metabolic disturbances in obesity, Pennington[411] has challenged this idea with the suggestion that the basic metabolic defect lies in an exaggerated transformation of foods to fat and its immobilization in the depots, where it cannot be reached by the tissues; thus, peripheral tissues would be in a state of "malnutrition" in obese patients. Pennington believes that the biochemical disturbance is decreased oxidation of pyruvic acid, which accumulates as lactic acid in the organism. The excess of lactic acid would inhibit the transformation of fatty acids into ketone bodies, the oxidation of fatty acids by tissues and the oxidation of acetate, which instead of being used in energy metabolism is then stored as fat.[412] This represents a vicious circle called the "dynamic phase of obesity," where the ingestion of energy-producing material exceeds expenditure until a new level is reached, the "static phase of obesity," represented by an equilibrium between supply and expenditure of energy, and increase in body weight ceases. The final result is a "compensatory hypertrophy of adipose tissue," where a limited fraction of fat is used to provide energy during the postabsorptive phase. This attractive hypothesis has the support of effective therapeutic results and the demonstration of increased lactic acid in the circulation of many obese subjects, but the cause of the metabolic defect is still obscure.

The classification of obesity proposed by Van Itallie[413] is based on possible conditioning mechanisms. The two main groups are: regulatory obesity, where there is a disturbance in the equilibrium between supply and expenditure of energy, with excess of substrate and without primary metabolic abnormalities; and metabolic obesity, in which the disturbance is enzymatic, the substrate is found in normal amounts but is improperly handled, so food ingestion increases. In this group would be Pennington's "compensatory hypertrophy of adipose tissue" (Table 72).

Whatever the mechanism or classification of obesity, it can always be interpreted as a disturbance between the amount of energy ingested and the amount utilized;[414] therefore, it is of interest to examine some of the hypotheses suggested to explain the regulation of the amount of food ingested. Brobeck[415] has reduced most hypotheses to the following three: (a) It has been postulated

Table 72. Tentative Grouping of Forms of Obesity According to Mechanism

I. Regulatory obesity (No primary metabolic abnormality)
  A. Psychologic
    1. Neurotic overeating
    2. Nonneurotic overeating (cultural dietary pattern)
  B. Physiologic
    1. Increased intake—hypothalamic disorder
    2. Decreased output—forced immobilization
II. Metabolic obesity
  A. Enzymatic—? genetic obesity in mice
  B. Hormonal—hyperadrenocorticism
  C. Neurologic—? lipodystrophy (autonomic)

(Van Itallie[413])

that the factor regulating food ingestion is the caloric value of the diet, which is the same as saying that "animals and men eat to maintain a normal caloric level"; however, no receptor of potential energy of foods has been identified.[416] (b) It has been proposed that the regulating factor is the body temperature, i.e., "animals and men eat to keep warm."[417] It has been observed that when diets of variable composition are offered to experimental animals the amount consumed is better correlated with the specific dynamic action of foods than with any other factor; furthermore, there are centers sensitive to temperature changes in the hypothalamus, which would provide a complete homeostatic cycle.[418] On the other hand, it is surprising that the organism should use this particular mechanism to regulate its temperature when it is provided with many others much finer and better adjusted; furthermore, no correlation has been established between the specific dynamic action and the energetic requirements of the organism. (c) Finally, Mayer has suggested the "glucostatic" theory,[419] which postulates that hunger appears when there is a decrease in the glucose blood level, and with the ingestion of food glucose would rise again and the driving sensation responsible for food ingestion would cease. Therefore, carbohydrates would be the regulating factor of the energetic supply to the organism. The "glucostatic" theory is based on the experimental demonstration that hunger appears when there are important differences between arterial and venous blood glucose concentrations, and disappears when these values tend to become equal.[420] Further-

more, cells sensitive to glucose concentration have been demonstrated in the hypothalamus, which in this sense resemble more the cells of the rest of the organism than their congenerous nervous cells, which use carbohydrates for their metabolism independently of the rest of the organism. On the other hand, Bornstein and Grossman[421] failed to suppress food intake in animals or subjective desire for food in humans by means of intravenous infusions of glucose.

Obesity is accompanied by an average shorter life span,[422] because of its complications;[423] it is difficult to decide, however, if obesity and its complications are not the result of another, more basic alteration. The most important complications of obesity are cardiovascular, cardiorespiratory and general.

a. Cardiovascular Complications. Obesity may be the direct cause of some diseases of the cardiovascular system, may predispose to a higher frequency of others and may aggravate still other diseases etiologically unrelated to overweight or nutrition in general.[424] Saphir and Corrigan[425] mentioned some autopsy cases of sudden death in obese people in which no anatomic explanation was found except extensive fatty infiltration of the myocardium, but it is doubtful that this change could be the cause of any functional disturbance. In cases of heart failure from other causes, obesity creates an extra load for the heart because it increases the area that must be irrigated. In these cases it is necessary to reduce body weight as one of the measures in treatment of heart failure.[426] Coronary insufficiency is also made worse by obesity, although perhaps the most important relation between obesity and coronary circulation is the higher frequency of atherosclerosis in overweight subjects. In a study of 80 cases of death due to coronary insufficiency in subjects between 20 and 36 years old, French and Dock[427] found that 91 per cent were obese. Arterial hypertension is frequent in obese patients, and decrease in body weight is usually accompanied by an improvement in the general condition of hypertensives. Furthermore, there are statistical data supporting the idea that obesity predisposes to arterial hypertension.[428] Postoperative vascular complications, such as thrombosis and

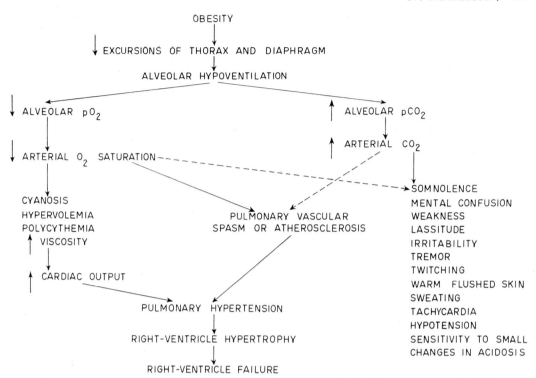

FIG. 10–14. Mechanism of hypoventilation syndrome in extreme obesity (Courtesy of Dr. M. J. Seide and the Editor, New England Journal of Medicine.)

embolism, are more frequent in obese subjects, and the same is true of pulmonary infarcts.[429]

b. Cardiorespiratory Complications. Extreme obesity may result in a syndrome characterized by marked somnolence, pruritus, cyanosis, periodic respiration, polycythemia, right ventricular hypertrophy and heart failure. Laboratory studies reveal arterial unsaturation of oxygen, increased carbon dioxide concentration and decreased respiratory volume and alveolar ventilation.[430, 431] No anatomic changes have been described in either heart or lungs. In an excellent review of the dynamic aspects of obesity, Kerr and Lagen[432] suggested that thoracic kyphosis was the most important factor in the production of this syndrome. The curve of the vertebral column elevates the ribs and produces a funnel chest; the diaphragm is flattened and widened, and its movement hindered by visceral ptosis and by the thick fat pad. Tidal air decreases because of the permanent inspiratory position of the chest, and passive respiration is impeded, forcing the patient to perform superficial and active respirations. This leads to alveolar hypoventilation, decreased partial tension of oxygen and increased partial tension of carbon dioxide in the alveolar air, with resulting hypoxia and hypercapnia. This explains cyanosis, polycythemia and pulmonary hypertension, with the consequent right ventricular hypertrophy and right heart failure. Hypercapnia accounts for symptoms of carbon dioxide intoxication such as somnolence, mental confusion, weakness, irritability, sweating, etc.[433] (Fig. 10–14).

c. General Complications. It has been mentioned that obese individuals have a statistically shorter life span than people with normal body weight, and reference has also been made to the higher frequency of diabetes in obese patients. Toxemia of pregnancy has been observed with more frequency in obese women, as well as menstrual disorders. Mortality caused by diseases of the gallbladder and extrahepatic biliary tract is approximately three times higher in overweight than in normal subjects.[434]

REFERENCES

1. Stetten, D., Jr.: The levels of disorganization, Am. J. Med. 20:817, 1956.
2. Cameron, G. R.: New Pathways in Cellular Pathology, London, Edward Arnold, 1956.
3. Oliver, J.: The structure of the metabolic process in the nephron, J. Mt. Sinai Hosp. 15:175, 1948.
4. Schrödinger, E.: What is Life? The Physical Aspect of the Living Cell, New York, Cambridge University Press, 1951.
5. Stetten, D., Jr.: Thermodynamic, kinetic, and biological stability, Am. J. Med. 13:251, 1952.
6. Stetten, D., Jr.: The nature of the engine, Am. J. Med. 16:307, 1956.
7. Neuman, W. F., and Neuman, M. W.: The nature of the mineral phase of bone. Chem. Rev. 53:1, 1953.
8. Harkness, R. D., Marko, A. M., Muir, H. M., and Neuberger, A.: The metabolism of collagen and other proteins of the skin of the rabbit, Biochem. J. 56:558, 1954.
9. Stetten, D., Jr.: Certain Aspects of Hormonal Regulation of Carbohydrate Metabolism, in Kinsell, L. W. (Ed.): Hormonal Regulation of Energy Metabolism, Springfield, Charles C Thomas, 1957.
10. Schoenheimer, R.: The Dynamic State of Body Constituents, Cambridge, Harvard University Press, 1942.
11. Brobeck, J. R.: Energy Exchange, in Fulton, J. F. (Ed.): Textbook of Physiology, ed. 17, Philadelphia, W. B. Saunders. 1957.
12. Rabinowitch, E. I.: Photosynthesis and Related Processes, New York, Interscience Publishers, 1956.
13. Pardee, A. B.: Free Energy and Metabolism, in Greenberg, D. M. (Ed.): Chemical Pathways of Metabolism, New York, Academic Press, 1954.
14. Lehninger, A. L.: Oxidative phosphorylation, Harvey Lect. 49:176, 1955.
15. Szent-Györgyi, A.: Bioenergetics, Science 124:873, 1956.
16. Best, C. H., and Taylor, N.: The Physiological Basis of Medical Practice, ed. 5, Baltimore, Williams and Wilkins, 1950.
17. Duncan, G. G.: Introductory Considerations, in Duncan, G. G. (Ed.): Diseases of Metabolism, ed. 3, Philadelphia, W. B. Saunders, 1956.
18. Wilhelmj, C. M.: Specific dynamic action of food, Physiol. Rev. 15:202, 1935.
19. Mayer, J., and Bullen, B.: Nutrition and athletic performance, Physiol. Rev. 40:369, 1960.
20. Brobeck, J. R.: Regulation of Energy Exchange, in Fulton, J. F. (Ed.) Textbook of Physiology, ed. 17, Philadelphia, W. B. Saunders Co., 1957.
21. Mayer, J., Marshall, N. B., Vitale, J. J., Christensen, J. H., Mashayekhi, M. B., and Stare, F. J.: Exercise, food intake, and body weight in normal rats and in genetically obese adult mice, Am. J. Physiol. 177:544, 1954.
22. Johnson, M. L., Burke, B. S., and Mayer, J.: Relative importance of inactivity and overeating in the energy balance of obese high school girls, Am. J. Clin. Nutr. 4:37, 1956.
23. Stefanik, P. A., Heald, F. P., Jr., and Mayer, J.: Caloric intake in relationship to energy output of obese and non-obese adolescent boys, Am. J. Clin. Nutr. 7:55, 1959.
24. Hetherington, A. W., and Ranson, S. W.: Spontaneous activity and food intake of rats with hypothalamic lesions, Am. J. Physiol. 136:609, 1942.
25. Ruch, T. C., and Shenkin, H. A.: Relation of area 13 on orbital surface of frontal lobe to hyperactivity and hyperphagia in monkeys, J. Neurophysiol. 6:349, 1943.
26. Masoro, E. J., Chaikoff, I. L., and Dauben, W. G.: Lipogenesis from glucose in the normal and liverless animal as studied with C^{14}-labeled glucose, J. Biol. Chem. 179:1117, 1949.
27. Anand, B. K., and Brobeck, J. R.: Hypothalamic control of food intake in rats and cats, Yale J. Biol. & Med. 24:2, 1951.
28. Grossman, S. P.: Eating or drinking elicited by direct adrenergic or cholinergic stimulation of hypothalamus, Science 132:301, 1960.
29. Villee, C. A.: Intermediary metabolism, New Eng. J. Med. 251:21, 64, 1954.
30. Peters, J. P.: Carbohydrate Metabolism. Lipid Metabolism. Protein Metabolism, in Grollman, E. (Ed.): Clinical Physiology, New York, McGraw-Hill, 1957.
31. Quastel, J. H.: Intestinal absorption of sugars and amino acids, Am. J. Clin. Nutr. 8:137, 1960.
32. Shannon, J. A., and Fisher, S.: The renal tubular reabsorption of glucose in the normal dog, Am. J. Physiol. 122:765, 1938.
33. Wick, A. N., Drury, D. R., and MacKay, E.: Glucose space of the body, Am. J. Physiol. 163:224, 1950.
34. Cori, C. F.: Enzymatic reactions in carbohydrate metabolism, Harvey Lect. 41:253, 1945.
35. Ross, E. J.: Insulin and the permeability of cell membranes to glucose, Nature 171:125, 1953.
36. Goldstein, M. S., Henry, W. L., Huddlestun, B., and Levine, R.: Action of insulin on transfer of sugars across cell barriers: common chemical configuration of substances responsive to action of the hormone, Am. J. Physiol. 173:207, 1953.
37. Wilbrandt, W., Frei, S., and Rosenberg, T.: The kinetics of glucose transport through the human red cell membrane, Exper. Cell Res. 11:59, 1956.
38. Stetten, D., Jr., and Stetten, M. R.: Glycogen metabolism, Physiol. Rev. 40:505, 1960.
39. Recant, L.: Recent developments in the field of glycogen metabolism and the diseases of glycogen storage, Am. J. Med. 19:610, 1955.
40. Wolfe, S. J.: A recently recognized pathway for glucose metabolism—pentose phosphate pathway, Arch. Int. Med. 102:493, 1958.
41. Siperstein, M. D.: Inter-relationship of glucose and lipid metabolism, Am. J. Med. 26:685, 1959.
42. Horecker, B. L., and Mehler, A. H.: Carbohydrate metabolism, Ann. Rev. Biochem. 24:207, 1955.
43. Wood, H. G.: Significance of alternate pathways in the metabolism of glucose, Physiol. Rev. 35:841, 1955.
44. Weinhouse, S.: Carbohydrate metabolism: some aspects of the intermediary metabolism of carbohydrates and lipids, Ann. Rev. Biochem. 23:125, 1954.
45. Long, C. N. H.: The Endocrine Regulation of Carbohydrate Metabolism, in Newer Concepts of the Causes and Treatment of Diabetes, New York, National Vitamin Foundation, 1955.
46. Stadie, W. C.: Current views on the mechanism of insulin action, Am. J. Med. 19:257, 1955.
47. Park, C. R., Reinwein, D., Henderson, M. J., Cadenas, E., and Morgan, H. E.: The action of insulin on the transport of glucose through the cell membrane, Am. J. Med. 26:674, 1959.
48. Winegrad, A. I., and Renold, A.: Studies on rat adipose tissue in vitro. I. Effects of insulin on the metabolism of glucose, pyruvate, and acetate, J. Biol. Chem. 233:267, 1958.
49. Stadie, W. C.: Aspects of carbohydrate and phosphate metabolism in diabetes, Bull. New York Acad. Med. 34:5, 1958.

50. Berthet, J.: Some aspects of the glucagon problem, Am. J. Med. 26:703, 1959.
51. Elrick, H., Staub, A., and Maske, H.: Recent developments in glucagon research, New Eng. J. Med. 256:742, 1957.
52. Long, C. N. H., Katzin, B., and Fry, E. G.: The adrenal cortex and carbohydrate metabolism, Endocrinology 26:309, 1940.
53. Houssay, B. A.: Advancement of knowledge of the role of the hypophysis in carbohydrate metabolism during the last twenty-five years, Endocrinology 30:884, 1948.
54. Ingram, W. R., and Barris, R. W.: Evidence of altered carbohydrate metabolism in cats with hypothalamic lesions, Am. J. Physiol. 114:562, 1936.
55. Alvarez Bullya, R.: Intervención del sistema nervioso en la regulación de la glicemia, Acta physiol. latino-am. 8:56, 1958.
56. Hill, R., Baker, N., and Chaikoff, I. L.: Altered metabolic patterns induced in the normal rat by feeding an adequate diet containing fructose as sole carbohydrate, J. Biol. Chem. 209:705, 1954.
57. Darragh, J. H., Womersley, R. A., and Meroney, W. H.: Fructose in the treatment of diabetic ketosis, J. Clin. Invest. 32:1214, 1953.
58. Moorhouse, J. A., and Kark, R. M.: Fructose and diabetes, Am. J. Med. 23:46, 1957.
59. Lynen, F.: Lipid metabolism, Ann. Rev. Biochem. 24:653, 1955.
60. Bergström, S., and Borgström, B.: Metabolism of lipids, Ann. Rev. Biochem. 25:177, 1956.
61. Borgström, B.: On the mechanism of the intestinal fat absorption. V. The effect of bile diversion on fat absorption in the rat, Acta physiol. scandinav. 28:279, 1953.
62. Zilversmith, D. B.: Current concepts of lipid metabolism, Am. J. Med. 23:120, 1957.
63. Borgström, B.: Randomization of glyceride fatty acids during absorption from the small intestine of the rat; J. Biol. Chem. 214:671, 1955.
64. Fernandes, J., van den Kamer, J. H., and Weigers, H. A.: The absorption of fat studied in a child with chylothorax, J. Clin. Invest. 34:1026, 1955.
65. Friedman, M., Byers, S. O., and St. George, S.: Cholesterol metabolism, Ann. Rev. Biochem. 25:613, 1956.
66. Wertheimer, E., and Shapiro, B.: The physiology of adipose tissue, Physiol. Rev. 28:451, 1948.
67. Anker, H. S.: On the mechanism of fatty acid synthesis in vivo, J. Biol. Chem. 194:177, 1952.
68. Brady, R. O., and Gurin, S.: Biosynthesis of fatty acids by cell-free or water-soluble enzyme systems, J. Biol. Chem. 199:421, 1952.
69. White, A., Handler, P., Smith, E. L., and Stetten, D., Jr.: Principles of Biochemistry, New York, McGraw-Hill, 1954.
70. Favarger, P., and Gerlach, J.: Recherches sur la synthese des graisses a partir d'acétate ou de glucose. II. Les roles respectifs du foie, du tissue adipeux et des certains autres tissus dans la lipogènese chez la souris, Helvet. physiol. et pharmacol. acta 13:96, 1955.
71. Zilversmith, D. B., McCandless, E. L., and Shore, M. L.: Plasma phospholipid synthesis in the eviscerated rabbit, Proc. Soc. Exper. Biol. & Med. 93:542, 1956.
72. Bloch, K., and Rittenberg, D.: On the utilization of acetic acid for cholesterol formation, J. Biol. Chem. 145:625, 1942.
73. Srere, P. A., Chaikoff, I. L., Treitman, S. S., and Burstein, L. S.: The extrahepatic synthesis of cholesterol, J. Biol. Chem. 182:629, 1950.
74. Green, D. E.: Fatty acid oxidation in soluble systems of animal tissues, Biol. Rev. 29:330, 1954.
75. Lehninger, A. L.: Enzymatic Oxidations and Synthesis of Fatty Acids, in Najjar, V. A. (Ed.) Fat Metabolism. A Symposium on the Clinical and Biochemical Aspects of Fat Utilization in Health and Disease, Baltimore, Johns Hopkins University Press, 1954.
76. Lynen, F.: Acetyl coenzyme A and the "fatty acid cycle," Harvey Lect. 48:210, 1954.
77. Weinhouse, S., Millington, R. H., and Friedman, B.: The effect of carbohydrate on the oxidation of fatty acids by liver slices, J. Biol. Chem. 181:489, 1949.
78. Weinhouse, S., Medes, G., and Floyd, N. F.: The mechanism of fatty acid oxidation, J. Biol. Chem. 153:689, 1944.
79. Lossow, W. J., and Chaikoff, I. L.: Carbohydrate sparing of fatty acid oxidation. I. The relation of fatty acid chain length to the degree of sparing. II. The mechanisms by which carbohydrate spares the oxidation of palmitic acid, Arch. Biochem. 57:23, 1955.
80. Dole, V. P.: Fat metabolism in diabetes, Bull. New York Acad. Med. 34:21, 1958.
81. Eder, H. A.: The lipoproteins of human serum, Am. J. Med. 23:269, 1957.
82. Bragdon, J. H., Havel, R. J., and Boyle, E.: Human serum lipoproteins. I. Chemical composition of four fractions, J. Lab. & Clin. Med. 48:36, 1956.
83. Havel, R. J., Eder, H. A., and Bragdon, J. H.: The distribution and chemical compositions of ultracentrifugally separated lipoproteins in human serum, J. Clin. Invest. 34:1345, 1955.
84. Hahn, P. F.: Abolishment of alimentary lipemia following injection of heparin, Science 98:19, 1943.
85. Anderson, N. G., and Fawcett, B.: An antichylomicronemic substance produced by heparin injections, Proc. Soc. Exper. Biol. & Med. 63:768, 1950.
86. Robinson, D. S., and French, J. E.: The heparin clearing reaction and fat transport, Quart. J. Exper. Physiol. 42:151, 1957.
87. Robinson, D. S.: The heparin clearing reaction, Am. J. Clin. Nutr. 8:7, 1960.
88. French, J. E., and Morris, B.: The removal of C^{14}-labelled chylomicron fat from the circulation in rats, J. Physiol. 138:326, 1957.
89. Engelberg, H.: Heparin lipemia clearing reaction and fat transport in man. Summary of available knowledge, Am. J. Clin. Nutr. 8:21, 1960.
90. Korn, E. D.: Clearing factor, a heparin-activated lipoprotein lipase. I. Isolation and characterization of the enzyme from normal rat heart, J. Biol. Chem. 215:1, 1955.
91. Havel, R. J.: Transport and metabolism of chylomicra, Am. J. Clin. Nutr. 6:662, 1958.
92. Overbeek, G. A.: Fat-splitting enzymes in blood, Clin. chim. acta 2:1, 1957.
93. Fredrickson, D. S., and Gordon, R. S., Jr.: Transport of fatty acids, Physiol. Rev. 38:585, 1958.
94. Peters, J. P., and Man, E. B.: The interrelations of serum lipids in normal persons, J. Clin. Invest. 22:707, 1953.
95. Deuel, H. J., Jr.: The Lipids—Their Chemistry and Biochemistry, vol. 2, New York, Interscience Publishers, 1955.
96. Zilversmith, D. B.: Metabolism of complex lipids, Ann. Rev. Biochem. 24:157, 1955.
97. Eckles, N. E., Taylor, C. B., Campbell, D. J., and Gould, R. G.: The origin of plasma cholesterol and the rates of equilibration of liver, plasma,

and erythrocyte cholesterol, J. Lab. Clin. Med. *46:*359, 1955.

98. Friedman, M., Byers, S. O., and St. George, S.: Cholesterol metabolism, Ann. Rev. Biochem. *25:* 613, 1956.

99. Hotta, S., and Chaikoff, I. L.: The role of the liver in the turnover of plasma cholesterol, Arch. Biochem. *56:*28, 1955.

100. Weil, R., and Stetten, D., Jr.: The urinary excretion of a fat-mobilizing agent, J. Biol. Chem. *168:*129, 1947.

101. Best, C. H.: The lipotropic agents in the protection of the liver, kidney, heart, and other organs in experimental animals, Proc. Roy. Soc. London s. B *145:*151, 1956.

102. Artom, C.: Role of choline in the oxidation of fatty acids by the liver, J. Biol. Chem. *205:*101, 1953.

103. Engel, F. L.: The influence of the endocrine glands on fatty acid and ketone body metabolism, Arch. Int. Med. *100:*18, 1957.

104. Wertheimer, E., and Shapiro, B.: The physiology of adipose tissue, Physiol. Rev. *28:*451, 1948.

105. Perry, W. F., and Bowen, H. F.: Fatty acid utilization by adrenalectomized rats, Am. J. Physiol. *186:*190, 1956.

106. Payne, R. W.: Studies on the fat-mobilizing factor of the anterior pituitary gland, Endocrinology *45:*305, 1949.

107. Petersen, V. P., and Lotspeich, W. D.: Further aspects of the endocrine regulation of ketogenesis, Am. J. Physiol. *182:*273, 1955.

108. Weil, R.: Metabolic function of the pituitary growth hormone, Arch. Int. Med. *95:*739, 1955.

109. Ehrensvärd, G.: Metabolism of amino acids and proteins, Ann. Rev. Biochem. *24:*275, 1955.

110. Korelitz, B. I., and Janowitz, H. D.: The physiology of intestinal absorption, J. Mt. Sinai Hosp. *24:* 181, 1957.

111. Meister, A.: Biochemistry of the Amino Acids, New York, Academic Press, 1957.

112. Fruton, J. S., and Simmonds, S.: General Biochemistry, ed. 2, New York, John Wiley and Sons, 1958.

113. Davies, B. M. A., and Yudkin, J.: Role of glutaminase in the production of urinary ammonia, Nature *167:*117, 1951.

114. McDermott, W. V., Jr.: Metabolism and toxicity of ammonia, New Eng. J. Med. *257:*1076, 1957.

115. Phear, E. A., Sherlock, S., and Summerskill, W. H. J.: Blood ammonium levels in liver disease and "hepatic coma," Lancet *1:*836, 1955.

116. Riddell, A. C.: Changes in man and animals with portocaval anastomosis, Proc. Roy. Soc. Med. *48:*481, 1955.

117. Rose, W. C., Eades, L. C., Jr., and Coon, M. J.: The amino acid requirements of man. XII. The leucine and isoleucine requirement, J. Biol. Chem. *216:*225, 1955.

118. Krebs, H. A.: Considerations concerning the pathways of synthesis in living matter, Bull. Johns Hopkins Hosp. *95:*19, 1954.

119. Siekevitz, P., and Zamecnick, C. P.: In vitro incorporation of l-C14 DL-alanine in proteins of rat liver granular fractions, Fed. Proc. *10:*246, 1951.

120. Brachet, J. R.: Ribonucleic acid and the synthesis of cellular proteins, Nature *186:*194, 1960.

121. Kit, S.: Intermediary Metabolism of Building Blocks Involved in Growth, in Nowinski, W. W. (Ed.): Fundamental Aspects of Normal and Malignant Growth, Amsterdam, Elsevier Publishing, 1960.

122. Geiger, E.: Role of time factor in protein synthesis, Science *111:*594, 1950.

123. Axelrod, A. E.: Role of vitamins in antibody formation, Metabolism *2:*1, 1953.

124. Meister, A.: Transamination in amino acid metabolism, Fed. Proc. *14:*683, 1955.

125. Drury, D. R.: The significance of D:N ratio and its bearing on the mechanism of diabetes mellitus, J. Clin. Invest. *21:*153, 1942.

126. Bollman, J. L., Mann, F. C., and Magath, T. B.: Studies on the physiology of the liver. VIII. Effect of total removal of the liver on the formation of urea, Am. J. Physiol. *69:*371, 1924.

127. Russell, J. A.: Hormonal control of amino acid metabolism, Fed. Proc. *14:*696, 1955.

128. Bartlett, P. D., and Gaebler, O. H.: Studies on the mechanism of nitrogen storage. VI. Rate of protein synthesis and size of the nitrogen pool, J. Biol. Chem. *196:*1, 1952.

129. Krebs, H. A.: Intermediary stages in biological oxidations of carbohydrate, Advances Enzymol. *3:*191, 1953.

130. Krebs, H. A.: The tricarboxylic acid cycle, Harvey Lect. *44:*165, 1949.

131. Duncan, G. G.: The modern aspects of the diabetic problem, Bull. New York Acad. Med. *34:*73, 1958.

132. Wilder, R. M.: Reflections on the causation of diabetes mellitus, J.A.M.A. *144:*1234, 1950.

133. O'Brien, J. J., and Thayer, T. R.: Pancreatitis: observations on 131 patients, New Eng. J. Med. *253:*355, 1955.

134. Bell, E. T.: Carcinoma of the pancreas, Am. J. Path. *33:*499, 1957.

135. Kleckner, M. S., Kark, R. M., Baker, L. A., Chapman, A. Z., and Kaplan, E.: Clinical features, pathology, and therapy of hemochromatosis, J.A.M.A. *157:*1471, 1955.

136. Lawrence, R. D.: Three types of human diabetes, Ann. Int. Med. *43:*1199, 1955.

137. Schwartz, R., Schafer, I. A., and Renold, A. E.: Generalized lipoatrophy, hepatic cirrhosis, disturbed carbohydrate metabolism and accelerated growth (lipoatrophic diabetes). Longitudinal observations and metabolic studies, Am. J. Med. *28:*973, 1960.

138. Hartroft, W. S.: Islet pathology in diabetes, Diabetes *5:*98, 1956.

139. Bell, E. T.: Hyalinization of islands of Langerhans in diabetes mellitus, Diabetes *1:*341, 1952.

140. Mirsky, I. A.: Insulinase, insulinase-inhibitors, and diabetes mellitus, Rec. Progr. Hormone Res. *13:* 429, 1957.

141. Mirsky, I. A.: The etiology of diabetes mellitus in man, Rec. Progr. Hormone Res. *7:*437, 1952.

142. Berson, S. A., Yalow, R. S., Bauman, A., Rothschild, M. A., and Newerly, K.: Insulin-I[131] metabolism in human subjects: demonstration of insulin-binding globulin in the circulation of insulin-treated subjects, J. Clin. Invest. *35:*170, 1956.

143. De Bodo, R. C., and Altzuler, N.: Insulin hypersensitivity and physiological insulin antagonists, Physiol. Rev. *38:*389, 1958.

144. Lawrence, R. D.: Lipodystrophy and hepatomegaly with diabetes, lipemia, and other metabolic disturbances, Lancet *1:*724, 1946.

145. Lukens, F. D. W.: Experimental diabetes and its relation to diabetes mellitus, Am. J. Med. *19:* 790, 1955.

146. Houssay, B., and Biasotti, A.: La diabétes pancréatica de los perros hipofisoprivos, Rev. Soc. argent. biol. *6:*251, 1930.

147. Harvey, J. C., and de Klerk, J.: The Houssay phenomenon in man, Am. J. Med. *19:*327, 1955.

148. Ross, E. J.: The influence of insulin on the perme-

ability of the blood aqueous barrier to glucose, J. Physiol. *116:*414, 1952.

149. Levine, R., Goldstein, M. S., Huddlestun, B., and Klein, S. P.: Action of insulin on the "permeability" of cells to free hexoses, as studied by its effect on the distribution of galactose, Am. J. Physiol. *163:*170, 1950.

150. Soskin, S., and Levine, R.: Carbohydrate Metabolism, Chicago, Chicago University Press, 1952.

151. Field, J. B.: On the nature of the metabolic defect(s) in diabetes, Am. J. Med. *26:*662, 1959.

152. Butterfield, J., Kelsey-Fry, I., and Holling, E.: Effects of insulin, tolbutamide, and phenethyldiguanidine on peripheral glucose uptake in man, Diabetes *7:*449, 1958.

153. Feller, D., Chaikoff, I. L., Strisower, E H., and Searle, G. L.: Glucose utilization in the diabetic dog studied with C¹⁴ glucose, J. Biol. Chem. *188:*865, 1951.

154. Shreeve, W. W., Baker, N., Miller, M., Shipley, R. A., Incefy, G. E., and Craig, J. W.: C¹⁴ studies in carbohydrate metabolism. II. The oxidation of glucose in diabetic human subjects, Metabolism *5:*22, 1956.

155. Walaas, A., and Walaas, O.: Effect of insulin on rat diaphragm under aerobic conditions, J. Biol. Chem. *195:*367, 1952.

156. Levine, R., and Goldstein, M.: On the mechanism of action of insulin, Rec. Progr. Hormone Res. *11:*343, 1955.

157. Danowski, T. S., and Elkinton, J. R.: Exchanges of potassium related to organs and systems, Physiol. Rev. *3:*42, 1950.

158. Stadie, W. C., Haugaard, N., and Vaughan, M.: Studies on insulin binding with isotopically labelled insulin, J. Biol. Chem. *199:*729, 1952.

159. Chernick, S. S., and Chaikoff, I. L.: Two blocks in carbohydrate utilization in the liver of the diabetic rat, J. Biol. Chem. *193:*793, 1951.

160. Hoberman, H. D.: Endocrine regulation of amino acid and protein metabolism during fasting, Yale J. Biol. & Med. *22:*341, 1950.

161. Dole, V. P.: Fat metabolism in diabetes, Bull. New York Acad. Med. *34:*21, 1958.

162. Rodríguez, R., and Casarín, R. E.: Acidosis y coma diabético, Rev. invest. clín. *6:*21, 1954.

163. Warren, S., and LeCompte, P. M.: The Pathology of Diabetes Mellitus, ed. 3, Philadelphia, Lea and Febiger, 1952.

164. Ricketts, H. T.: The problem of degenerative vascular disease in diabetes, Am. J. Med. *19:*933, 1955.

165. Bell, E. T.: Atherosclerotic gangrene of the lower extremities in diabetic and non-diabetic persons, Am. J. Clin. Path. *28:*27, 1957.

166. Faber, M., and Lund, F.: Human aorta. IV. Aorta in diabetes mellitus, Arch. Path. *52:*239, 1951.

167. Ricketts, H. T.: Serum lipids and atherosclerosis, Diabetes *2:*316, 1953.

168. Adlersberg, D., Wang, C. I., Rifkin, H., Berkman, J., Ross, G., and Weinstein, C.: Serum lipids and polysaccharides in diabetes mellitus, Diabetes *5:*116, 1956.

169. Gofman, J. W., Jones, H. B., Lyon, T. P., and Strisower, B.: Lipoproteins and atherosclerosis, J. Gerontol. *6:*105, 1951.

170. Baldwin, A. D., and Root, H. F.: Infection of the urinary tract in the diabetic patient, New Eng. J. Med. *223:*244, 1940.

171. Lauler, D. P., Schreiner, G. E., and David, A.: Renal medullary necrosis, Am. J. Med. *29:*132, 1960.

172. Bell, E. T.: Renal vascular disease in diabetes mellitus, Diabetes *2:*376, 1953.

173. Rogers, J., and Robbins, S. L.: Intercapillary glomerulosclerosis: clinical and pathological study. I. Specificity of clinical syndrome, Am. J. Med. *12:*688, 1952.

174. Rogers, J., Robbins, S. L., and Jeghers, H.: Intercapillary glomerulosclerosis: clinical and pathological study. II. Clinical study of 100 anatomically proven cases, Am. J. Med. *12:*692, 1952.

175. Robbins, S. L., Rogers, J., and Wolleman, O. J., Jr.: Intercapillary glomerulosclerosis: clinical and pathological study. III. Pathologic study of 100 cases, Am. J. Med. *12:*700, 1952.

176. Gellman, D. D., Pirani, C. L., Soothill, J. F., Muehrcke, R. C., and Kark, R. M.: Diabetic nephropathy: a clinical and pathologic study based on renal biopsies, Medicine *38:*321, 1959.

177. McManus, J. F. A.: The development of intercapillary glomerulosclerosis, Proc. Am. Diabetes A. *9:*303, 1949.

178. Ashton, N.: Arteriolar involvement in diabetic retinopathy, Brit. J. Ophth. *37:*282, 1953.

179. Ashton, N.: Diabetic retinopathy: relation to glomerulosclerosis, Brit. M. J. *1:*1002, 1957.

180. Wilson, L., Root, H. F., and Marble, A.: Prevention of degenerative vascular lesions in young patients by control of diabetes, Am. J. Med. Sc. *221:*479, 1951.

181. Ellenberg, M.: Diabetic neuropathy presenting as the initial clinical manifestation of diabetes, Ann. Int. Med. *49:*620, 1958.

182. Ellenberg, M.: Diabetic neuropathy: a consideration of factors in onset, Ann. Int. Med. *52:*1067, 1960.

183. Garland, H., and Taverner, D.: Diabetic myelopathy, Brit. M. J. *1:*1405, 1953.

184. Lang, C. A., Becker, B., Gleysteen, D., and Chow, B. F.: Diabetic retinopathy and urinary excretion of vitamin B_{12}, Fed. Proc. *12:*420, 1953.

185. Engel, F. L.: Role of the adrenal cortex in intermediary metabolism, Am. J. Med. *10:*556, 1951.

186. Conn, J., and Seltzer, H. S.: Spontaneous hypoglycemia, Am. J. Med. *19:*460, 1955.

187. Thompson, C. M., and Hilferty, D. J.: Primary carcinoma of the liver (cholangioma) with hypoglycemic convulsions, Gastroenterology *20:*158, 1952.

188. Tucker, H. St. G., Jr., and Porter, W. B.: Hypoglycemia following alcoholic intoxication, Am. J. Med. Sc. *204:*559, 1942.

189. Mellinkoff, S. M., and Tumulty, P. A.: Hepatogenic hypoglycemia: its occurrence in congestive heart failure, New Eng. J. Med. *247:*745, 1952.

190. Rogers, F. A.: Islet cell tumors of the pancreas and hyperinsulinism, Am. J. Surg. *99:*268, 1960.

191. Sieracki, J., Marshall, R. B., and Horn, R. C.: Tumors of the pancreatic islets, Cancer *13:*347, 1960.

192. Lopez-Kruger, R., and Dockerty, M. D.: Tumors of islets of Langerhans, Surg. Gynec. & Obst. *85:*495, 1947.

193. Friesen, S. R., and Miller, D. R.: Fibrogenic mesodermal tumors, an unusual cause of hyperinsulinism, Am. J. Surg. *99:*420, 1960.

194. Schaefer, L. E., Adlersberg, D., and Steinberg, A. G.: Serum phospholipids: genetic and environmental influences, Circulation *18:*341, 1958.

195. Schaefer, L. E., Adlersberg, D., and Steinberg, A. G.: Heredity, environment, and serum cholesterol, Circulation *17:*537, 1958.

196. Frazer, A. C.: Steatorrhea, Brit. M. J. *2:*805, 1955.

197. Paterson, J. C. S.: The sprue syndrome, Am. J. Med. Sc. *231:*92, 1956.

198. Salvesen, H. A., and Böe, J.: Osteomalacia in sprue, Acta med. scandinav. *146:*290, 1953.

199. Girdwood, R. H.: The megaloblastic anaemias: their investigation and classification, Quart. J. Med. *25:*87, 1956.

200. Adlersberg, D. (Ed.): The Malabsorption Syndrome, New York, Grune and Stratton, 1957.

201. Volwiler, W.: Gastrointestinal malabsorptive syndromes, Am. J. Med. *23:*250, 1957.

202. Dixon, K. C.: Fatty deposition, Quart. J. Exper. Physiol. *43:*139, 1958.

203. King, D. W., Socolow, E. L., and Bensch, K. G.: The relation between protein synthesis and lipid accumulation in L strain cells and Ehrlich ascites cells, J. Biophys. Biochem. Cytol. *5:*421, 1959.

204. Popper, H., and Schaffner, F.: Liver: Structure and Function, New York, McGraw-Hill, 1957.

205. Tannhauser, S. J.: Lipidoses. Diseases of the Intracellular Lipid Metabolism, ed. 3, New York, Grune and Stratton, 1958.

206. Katz, L. N., and Staemmler, J.: Experimental Atherosclerosis, Springfield, Charles C Thomas, 1953.

207. Tuna, N., Reckers, L., and Franctz, I., Jr.: The fatty acids of total lipids and cholesterol esters from normal plasma and atheromatous plaques, J. Clin. Invest. *37:*1153, 1958.

208. Gore, I., Robertson, W. B., Hirst, A. E., Hadley, G. G., and Koseki, Y.: Geographic differences in the severity of aortic and coronary atherosclerosis. The United States, Jamaica, W. I. South India, and Japan, Am. J. Path. *36:*559, 1960.

209. Pérez Tamayo, R., Brandt, H., and Ontiveros, E.: Pathology of atherosclerosis in Mexico, Arch. Path. *71:*113, 1961.

210. Briggs, R. D., Rubenberg, M. L., O'Neal, R. M., Thomas, W. A., and Hartroft, W. S.: Myocardial infarction in patients treated with Sippy and other high milk diets. An autopsy study of fifteen hospitals in the U. S. A. and Great Britain, Circulation *21:*538, 1960.

211. Page, I. H.: Atherosclerosis. An Introduction, Circulation *10:*1, 1954.

212. Duff, G. L., and McMillan, G. C.: Pathogenesis of atherosclerosis, Am. J. Med. *11:*92, 1951.

213. Weinhouse, S., and Hirsch, E. F.: Atherosclerosis. II. The lipids of the serum and tissues in experimental atherosclerosis in rabbits, Arch. Path. *30:*856, 1940.

214. Kellner, A.: Lipid metabolism and atherosclerosis, Bull. New York Acad. Med. *28:*11, 1952.

215. Hirsch, E. F.: An analysis of the causal factors of atherosclerosis, Arch. Int. Med. *102:*1024, 1958.

216. Gofman, J., Lindgren, F., Elliot, H., Mantz, W., Hewitt, J., Strisower, B., and Herring, V.: Role of lipids and lipoproteins in atherosclerosis, Science *111:*166, 1950.

217. Barr, D. P.: Some chemical factors in the pathogenesis of atherosclerosis, Circulation *8:*641, 1953.

218. Siperstein, M. D., Chaikoff, I. L., and Chernick, S. S.: Significance of endogenous cholesterol in arteriosclerosis: synthesis in arterial tissue, Science *113:*747, 1951.

219. Ahrens, E. H.: Nutritional factors and serum lipid levels, Am. J. Med. *23:*928, 1957.

220. Klein, P. D.: Dietary fat and plasma cholesterol. A speculative review, Am. J. Clin. Nutr. *8:*104, 1960.

221. Ahrens, E. H., Hirsch, J., Insull, W., Tsaltas, T. T., Blomstrand, R., and Peterson, M.: Dietary control of serum lipids in relation to atherosclerosis, J.A.M.A. *164:*1905, 1957.

222. Kumerow, F. A., Ueno, A., Nishida, T., and Kokatnur, M.: Unsaturated fatty acids and plasma lipids, Am. J. Clin. Nutr. *8:*62, 1960.

223. Kinsell, L. W., Michaels, G. D., and Friskey, R. W.: Essential fatty acids, lipid metabolism, and atherosclerosis, Lancet *1:*334, 1958.

224. Katz, L. N., Stamler, J., and Pick, R.: The Role of the Hormones in Atherosclerosis, in Symposium on Atherosclerosis, Nat. Acad. Sc., U.S.A., 1954.

225. Adlersberg, D.: Hormonal influences on the serum lipids, Am. J. Med. *23:*769, 1957.

226. Furman, R. H., Howard, R. P., Norcia, L. N., and Keaty, E. C.: The influence of androgens, estrogens, and related steroids on serum lipids and lipoproteins, Am. J. Med. *24:*80, 1958.

227. Mammorstoh, J., Magidson, O., Lewis, J. J., Mehl, J., Moore, F. J., and Bernstein, J.: Effect of small doses of estrogen on serum lipids in female patients with myocardial infarction, New Eng. J. Med. *258:*583, 1958.

228. Schroepfer, G. J., Jr.: Lipid factors in atherosclerosis, New Eng. J. Med. *257:*1223, 1275, 1957.

229. Labecki, T. D.: Lipoproteins in atherosclerosis, Am. J. Clin. Nutr. *8:*332, 1960.

230. Albrink, M. J., Man, E. B., and Peters, J. P.: The relation of neutral fat to lactescence of the serum, J. Clin. Invest. *34:*147, 1955.

231. Friedman, M., and Byers, S. O.: Role of hyperphospholipidemia and neutral fat increase in plasma in the pathogenesis of hypercholesterolemia, Am. J. Physiol. *186:*13, 1956.

232. Jones, R. J., Cohen, L., and Corbus, H.: The serum lipid pattern in hyperthyroidism, hypothyroidism, and coronary atherosclerosis, Am. J. Med. *19:*71, 1955.

233. Poole, J. C. F.: The effect of certain fatty acids on the coagulation of plasma *in vitro*, Brit. J. Exper. Path. *36:*248, 1955.

234. Buzina, R., and Keys, A.: Blood coagulation after fat meal, Circulation *14:*854, 1956.

235. Duguid, J. B.: The arterial lining, Lancet *2:*202, 1952.

236. Fullerton, W. H.: The role of diet in the pathogenesis of coronary artery disease, Proc. Roy. Soc. Med. *48:*664, 1955.

237. Swank, R. L.: Effects of fat on blood viscosity in dogs, Circulation Res. *4:*579, 1956.

238. Haust, M. D., More, R. H., and Movat, H. Z.: The mechanism of fibrosis in arteriosclerosis, Am. J. Path. *35:*265, 1959.

239. Steiner, A., and Kendall, F. E.: Atherosclerosis and arteriosclerosis in dogs following ingestion of cholesterol and thiouracil, Arch. Path. *42:*433, 1946.

240. Kaplansky, S. Y.: Disorders of amino acid metabolism in protein-deficiencies and their correction, Clin. Chem. *5:*186, 1959.

241. Gutman, A. B.: The expanding pattern of the inborn errors of metabolism, Bull. New York Acad. Med. *35:*419, 1959.

242. Gutman, A. B.: Primary and secondary gout, Ann. Int. Med. *39:*1062, 1953.

243. Smyth, C. J., Cotterman, C. W., and Freyberg, R. H.: The genetics of gout and hyperuricemia—an analysis of 19 families, J. Clin. Invest. *27:*749, 1948.

244. Tannhauser, S. J.: The pathogenesis of gout, Metabolism *5:*582, 1956.

245. Wyngaarden, J. B.: Overproduction of uric acid as the cause of hyperuricemia in primary gout, J. Clin. Invest. *36:*1508, 1957.

246. Benedict, J. D., Roche, M., Yu, T. F., Bien, E. J.,

Gutman, A. B., and Stetten, D. W., Jr.: Incorporation of glycine nitrogen into uric acid in normal and gouty man, Metabolism *1:*3, 1952.

247. Combined Staff Clinics: Metabolic and clinical aspects of gout, Am. J. Med. *22:*807, 1957.

248. Lichtenstein, L., Scott, H. W., and Levin, M. H.: Pathologic changes in gout. Survey of eleven necropsied cases, Am. J. Path. *32:*871, 1956.

249. Owen, J. A., and Got, C.: The biological significance of the anomalous serum and urinary proteins of myelomatosis lymphomas and other conditions, J. Clin. Path. *13:*58, 1960.

250. Osserman, E. F., and Lawlor, D. P.: Abnormal serum and urine proteins in thirty-five cases of multiple myeloma as studied by filter paper electrophoresis, Am. J. Med. *18:*462, 1955.

251. Teilum, G.: Periodic acid-Schiff positive reticuloendothelial cells producing glycoprotein. Functional significance during formation of amyloid, Am. J. Path. *32:*945, 1956.

252. Gross, P. A. M., Gitlin, D., and Janeway, C. A.: The gamma globulins and their clinical significance, New Eng. J. Med. *260:*21, 72, 121, 170, 1959.

253. Feinstein, A. R., and Petersdorf, R. G.: Clinical significance of hyperglobulinemia. I. Diagnostic implications, Ann. Int. Med. *44:*899, 1956.

254. Young, I. I., Wolfson, W. Q., and Cohn, C.: Studies in serum proteins. Agammaglobulinemia in the adult, Am. J. Med. *19:*222, 1955.

255. Domz, C. A., and Dickson, D. R.: The agammaglobulinemias. Relations and implications, Am. J. Med. *23:*917, 1957.

256. Garrod, A. E.: Inborn Errors of Metabolism, London, Henry Frowde, 1909.

257. Hsia, D. Y. Y.: Inborn Errors of Metabolism, Chicago, Year Book Publishers, 1959.

258. Dent, C. E.: Symposium on Inborn Errors of Metabolism. Introduction, Am. J. Med. *22:*671, 1957.

259. Stetten, D. W., Jr.: A current view of metabolic errors, Am. J. Med. *26:*659, 1959.

260. Harris, H.: Human Biochemical Genetics, Cambridge, Cambridge University Press, 1959.

261. Hsia, D. Y. Y.: Medical Genetics, New Eng. J. Med. *262:*1172, 1222, 1273, 1318, 1960.

262. Landing, B. H.: Hereditary metabolic diseases—general considerations, Metabolism *9:*208, 1960.

263. von Gierke, E.: Hepato-Nephromegalia Glycogenica (Glycogenspeicherkrankheit der Leber und Nieren). Beitr. path. Anat. u. allg. Path. *82:*497, 1929.

264. di Sant'Agnese, P. A.: Diseases of glycogen storage with special reference to cardiac type of generalized glycogenosis, Ann. New York Acad. Sci. *72:*439, 1959.

265. Cori, G. T., and Cori, C. F.: Glucose-6-phosphatase of the liver in glycogen storage disease, J. Biol. Chem. *199:*661, 1952.

266. Illingworth, B., and Cori, G. T.: Structure of glycogens and amylopectins. III. Normal and abnormal human glycogen, J. Biol. Chem. *199:*653, 1952.

267. Schwartz, R., Ashmore, J., and Renold, A. E.: Galactose tolerance in glycogen storage disease, Pediatrics *19:*585, 1957.

268. Hauk, R., Illingworth, B., Brown, D. H., and Cori, C. F.: Enzymes of glycogen synthesis in glycogen-deposition disease, Biochim. et biophys. acta *33:*554, 1959.

269. di Sant'Agnese, P. A., Anderson, D. H., Mason, H. H., and Bauman, W. A.: Glycogen storage disease of the heart. II. Critical review of the literature, Pediatrics *6:*607, 1950.

270. Kirkman, H. N.: Galactosemia, Metabolism *9:*316, 1960.

271. Holzel, A., Komrower, G. M., and Schwartz, V.: Galactosuria, Am. J. Med. *22:*703, 1957.

272. Isselbacher, K. J.: Galactose metabolism and galactosemia, Am. J. Med. *26:*715, 1959.

273. Komrower, G. M., Schwartz, V., Holzel, A., and Goldberg, L.: A clinical and biochemical study of galactosemia, Arch. Dis. Child. *31:*254, 1956.

274. Edmonds, A. M., Hennigan, G. R., and Crooks, R.: Galactosemia, report of a case with autopsy, Pediatrics *10:*40, 1952.

275. Reubi, F. C.: Glucose Titration in Renal Glycosuria, in Ciba Foundation Symposium on The Kidney, Boston, Little, Brown, 1954.

276. Touster, O.: Pentose metabolism and pentosuria, Am. J. Med. *26:*724, 1959.

277. van Creveld, S.: The Lipoidoses, Advances Pediat. *6:*190, 1953.

278. Farber, S., Cohen, J., and Uzman, L. L.: Lipogranulomatosis: new lipo-glycoprotein storage disease, J. Mt. Sinai Hosp. *24:*816, 1957.

279. Lichtenstein, L.: Histiocytosis "X," Arch. Path. *56:*84, 1953.

280. Adlersberg, D., and Schaefer, L. E.: The interplay of heredity and environment in the regulation of circulating lipids and in atherogenesis, Am. J. Med. *26:*1, 1959.

281. Epstein, F. H., Block, W. D., Hand, E. A., and Francis, T., Jr.: Familial hypercholesterolemia, xanthomatosis and coronary heart disease, Am. J. Med. *26:*39, 1959.

282. Knox, W. E., and Hsia, D. Y. Y.: Pathogenetic problems in phenylketonuria, Am. J. Med. *22:*687, 1957.

283. Hsia, D. Y. Y.: Recent developments in the study of hereditary diseases in children, Postgrad. Med. *22:*203, 1957.

284. Mitoma, C., Auld, R. M., and Undefriend, S.: On the nature of enzymatic defect in phenylpyruvic oligophrenia, Proc. Soc. Exper. Biol. & Med. *94:*634, 1957.

285. Jervis, G. A.: Phenylpyruvic oligophrenia, Nerv. & Ment. Dis. *33:*259, 1954.

286. Pauling, L., Intano, H. A., Singer, S. J., and Wells, I. C.: Sickle cell anemia, a molecular disease, Science *110:*543, 1949.

287. Undefriend, S., and Bessman, S. P.: Hydroxylation of phenylalanine and antipyrine in phenylpyruvic oligophrenia, J. Biol. Chem. *203:*961, 1953.

288. Jervis, G. A.: Excretion of phenylalanine and derivatives in phenylpyruvic oligophrenia, Proc. Soc Exper. Biol. & Med. *75:*83, 1950.

289. Paine, R. S.: Evaluation of familial biochemically determined mental retardation in children with special reference to aminoaciduria, New Eng. J. Med. *262:*658, 1960.

290. Weil-Malherbe, H.: The level of adrenaline in human plasma and its relation to mental activity, J. Ment. Sc. *101:*733, 1955.

291. Himwich, H. E., and Fazekas, J. F.: Cerebral arteriovenous oxygen difference. II. Mental deficiency, Arch. Neurol. & Psychiat. *51:*72, 1944.

292. Armstrong, M. D., and Tyler, F. H.: Studies in phenylketonuria. I. Restricted phenylalanine intake in phenylketonuria, J. Clin. Invest. *34:*565, 1955.

293. Harris, H., and Robson, E. B.: Cystinuria, Am. J. Med. *22:*774, 1957.

294. Korn, D.: Demonstration of cystine crystals in peripheral white blood cells in a patient with cystinosis, New Eng. J. Med. *262:*545, 1960.

295. Dent, C. E., and Harris, H.: Genetics of cystinuria, Ann. Eugenics *16*:60, 1951.

296. Dent, C. E., Senior, B., and Walshe, J. M.: Pathogenesis of cystinuria, J. Clin. Invest. *33*:1210, 1954.

297. Stein, W. H., and Moore, S.: The free amino acids of human blood plasma, J. Biol. Chem. *211*:915, 1954.

298. Doolan, P. D., Harper, H. A., Hutchin, M. E., and Alpen, E. L.: Renal clearance of lysine in cystinuria. Pathogenesis and management of this abnormality, Am. J. Med. *23*:416, 1957.

299. Robson, E. B., and Rose, G. A.: The effect of intravenous lysine on the renal clearances of cystine, arginine, and ornithine in normal subjects, in patients with cystinuria and Fanconi syndrome and their relatives, Clin. Sc. *16*:75, 1957.

300. Dent, C. E., and Rose, G. A.: Amino acid metabolism in cystinuria, Quart. J. Med. *20*:205, 1951.

301. Lightwood, R., Payne, W. W., and Black, J. A.: Infantile renal acidosis, Pediatrics *12*:629, 1953.

302. Clay, R. D., Darmady, E. M., and Hawkins, M.: The nature of the renal lesion in the Fanconi syndrome, J. Path. & Bact. *65*:591, 1953.

303. Jackson, W. P. U., and Linder, G. C.: Innate functional defects of renal tubules, with particular reference to Fanconi syndrome, Quart. J. Med., *22*:133, 1953.

304. Stowers, J. M., and Dent, C. E.: Studies on the mechanism of Fanconi syndrome, Quart. J. Med. *16*:275, 1947.

305. Bickel, H., Smallwood, W. C., Smellie, J. M., Baar, H. S., and Hickmans, E. M.: Cystine storage disease with aminoaciduria and dwarfism, Acta paediat. *42*: (Suppl. 90), 1952.

306. Dent, C. E., and Harris, H.: Hereditary forms of rickets and osteomalacia, J. Bone & Joint Surg. *38B*:204, 1956.

307. Fraser, D.: Hypophosphatasia, Am. J. Med. *22*:730, 1957.

308. McCance, R. A., Fairweather, D. V. I., Barret, A. M., and Morrison, A. B.: Genetic, clinical, biochemical, and pathological features of hypophosphatasia, Quart. J. Med. *25*:523, 1956.

309. Fraser, D., Yendt, E. R., and Christie, F. H. E.: Metabolic abnormalities in hypophosphatasia, Lancet *1*:286, 1955.

310. Bearn, A. G.: Wilson's disease. An inborn error of metabolism with multiple manifestations, Am. J. Med. *22*:747, 1957.

311. Bearn, A. G.: Genetic and biochemical aspects of Wilson's disease, Am. J. Med. *15*:442, 1953.

312. Scheinberg, I. H., and Gitlin, D.: Deficiency of ceruloplasmin in patients with hepatolenticular degeneration, Science *116*:484, 1952.

313. Bearn, A. G., and Kunkel, H. G.: Localization of Cu⁶⁴ in serum fractions following oral administration: an alteration in Wilson's disease, Proc. Soc. Exper. Biol. & Med. *85*:242, 1954.

314. Bearn, A. G., Yu, T. F., and Gutman, A. B.: Renal function in Wilson's disease, J. Clin. Invest. *36*:1107, 1957.

315. Anderson, P. J., and Popper, H.: Changes in hepatic structure in Wilson's disease, Am. J. Path. *36*:483, 1960.

316. Lichtenstein, B. W., and Gore, I.: Wilson's disease —chronic form; clinical-pathological observations in brother and sister, Arch. Neurol. & Psychiat. *73*:13, 1955.

317. Adams, R. D., and Foley, J. M.: The neurological disorder associated with liver disease, Res. Publ. A. Nerv. & Ment. Dis. *32*:198, 1953.

318. Uzman, L. L., Iber, F. L., Chalmers, T. C., and Knowlton, M.: The mechanism of copper deposition in the liver in hepatolenticular degeneration (Wilson's disease), Am. J. Med. Sc. *231*:511, 1956.

319. Moore, F. D.: Metabolic Care of the Surgical Patient, Philadelphia, W. B. Saunders, 1960.

320. Hardy, J. D.: Metabolic response to surgery, Ann. New York Acad. Sc. *73*:401, 1958.

321. Hume, D. M.: The neuroendocrine response to injury: present status of the problem, Ann. Surg. *138*:547, 1953.

322. Selye, H.: The general adaptation syndrome and the diseases of adaptation, J. Clin. Endocrinol. *6*:117, 1946.

323. Cannon, W. B.: Bodily Changes in Pain, Hunger, Fear, and Rage, ed. 2, Boston, Charles T. Banford, 1953.

324. Davis, W. M., Davis, A. K., Lee, W., and Alpen, E. L.: The combined effects of thermal burns and whole body X-radiation. III. Study of blood coagulation, Ann. Surg. *142*:66, 1955.

325. Moore, F. D.: Endocrine changes after anesthesia, surgery, and unanesthetized trauma in man, Rec. Progr. Hormone Res. *13*:511, 1957.

326. McCann, S. M.: Effect of hypothalamic lesions on adrenal cortical response to stress in rats, Am. J. Physiol. *175*:13, 1953.

327. Vogt, M.: Plasma adrenalin and release of ACTH in normal and demedullated rats, J. Physiol. *118*:588, 1952.

328. Hardy, J. D.: Metabolic Reaction to Staged Operations in Man, in Hardy, J. D. (Ed.): Surgical Physiology of the Adrenal Cortex, Springfield, Charles C Thomas, 1955.

329. Moore, F. D.: Metabolism in trauma: the meaning of definitive surgery. The wound, the endocrine glands, and metabolism, Harvey Lect. *52*:74, 1958.

330. Richards, D. W., Jr.: Effects of hemorrhage on circulation, Ann. New York Acad. Sc. *49*:534, 1948.

331. Clowes, G. H. A., Jr., and del Guercio, L. R.: Circulatory response to trauma of surgical operations, Metabolism *9*:67, 1960.

332. Johnson, S. R.: The effect of some anesthetic agents on the circulation in man, Acta chir. scandinav. (Suppl.) *158*:1, 1951.

333. Born, G. V. R.: Some Effects of Injury on Metabolism, in Florey, H. W. (Ed.): General Pathology, ed. 2, Philadelphia, W. B. Saunders Co., 1958.

334. Green, H. N., and Stoner, H. B.: Effect of injury on carbohydrate metabolism and energy metabolism, Brit. M. Bull. *10*:38, 1954.

335. LePage, G. A.: Effects of hemorrhage on tissue metabolites, Am. J. Physiol. *147*:446, 1946.

336. Wilhelmi, A. F.: Metabolic aspects of shocks, Ann. Rev. Physiol. *10*:259, 1948.

337. Stoner, H. B., and Threlfall, C. J.: The effect of nucleotide and ischemic shock on the level of energy-rich phosphates in the tissues, Biochem. J. *58*:115, 1954.

338. Stoner, H. B., Threlfall, C. J., and Green, H. N.: Studies on the mechanism of shock. Carbohydrate metabolism in nucleotide and ischaemic shock, Brit. J. Exper. Path. *33*:131, 1952.

339. Engel, F. L.: Mechanism of fainting, J. Mt. Sinai Hosp. *12*:152, 1945.

340. Russell, J. A., Long, C. N. H., and Engel, F. L.: Biochemical studies in shock; role of peripheral tissues in metabolism of protein and carbohydrate during hemorrhagic shock in rat, J. Exper. Med. *79*:1, 1944.

341. Wiggers, C. J.: Physiology of Shock, Cambridge, Harvard University Press, 1950.

342. Threlfall, C. J., Stoner, H. B., and Green, H. N.:

Kidney citrate level in nucleotide shock, Nature *168:*297, 1951.

343. Cuthbertson, D. P.: Interrelationship of metabolic changes consequent to injury, Brit. M. Bull. *10:*33, 1954.

345. Moore, F. D.: Common patterns of water and electrolyte changes consequent to injury, surgery, and disease, New Eng. J. Med. *258:*277, 325, 377, 427, 1958.

346. Cuthbertson, D. P.: The influence of prolonged muscular rest on metabolism, Biochem. J. *23:* 1328, 1929.

347. Moore, F. D.: The significance of weight changes after trauma, Ann. Surg. *141:*141, 1955.

348. Paquin, A. J., Jr.: The rate of body weight loss following surgical stress of uniform intensity, Ann. Surg. *141:*383, 1955.

349. Munro, H. N., and Cuthbertson, D. P.: Response of protein metabolism to injury, Biochem. J. *37:* xii, 1943.

350. Munro, H. N., and Chalmers, M. I.: Fracture metabolism at different levels of protein intake, Brit. J. Exper. Path. *26:*396, 1945.

351. Borsook, H., and Dubnoff, J. W.: The metabolism of proteins and amino acids, Ann. Rev. Biochem. *12:*183, 1943.

352. Cuthbertson, D. P.: Protein metabolism in relation to energy needs, Metabolism *8:*787, 1959.

353. Yuile, C. L., Lucas, F. V., Jones, C. K., Chopin, S. J., and Whipple, G. H.: Inflammation and protein metabolism. Studies of carbon[14]-labeled proteins in dogs with sterile abscesses, J. Exper. Med. *98:*173, 1953.

354. Moore, F. D.: Getting well: the biology of surgical convalescence, Ann. New York Acad. Sc. *73:* 387, 1958.

355. Moore, F. D., and Ball, M. B.: The Metabolic Response to Trauma, ed. 2, Springfield, Charles C Thomas, 1957.

356. Kinney, J. M.: Influence of intermediary metabolism on nitrogen balance and weight loss, some considerations basic to an understanding of surgery, Metabolism *8:*809, 1959.

357. McFarlane, R. G.: The Reactions of Blood to Injury, in Florey, H. W. (Ed.): General Pathology, ed. 2, Philadelphia, W. B. Saunders, 1958.

358. Feldthusen, V., Lassen, V., and Lassen, N. A.: Serum iron and operative stress, Acta med. scandinav. *147:*311, 1954.

359. Cooper, J. F.: The surgical aspects of fibrinolysis, Surg. Gynec. & Obst. (Internat. Abst. Surg.) *108:*417, 1959.

360. Moon, V. H.: Disturbances of Circulation, in Anderson, W. A. D. (Ed.): Pathology, ed. 3, St. Louis, C. V. Mosby, 1957.

361. Frank, H. A.: Present day concepts of shock, New Eng. J. Med. *249:*445, 486, 1953.

362. Fine, J., and Seligman, A. M.: Traumatic shock: experimental study including evidence against capillary leakage hypothesis, Ann. Surg. *118:* 238, 1943.

363. Judah, J. D., and Spector, W. G.: Reactions of enzymes to injuries, Brit. M. Bull. *10:*42, 1954.

364. Hammond, W. G., Vandam, L. D., Davis, J. M., Carter, R. D., Ball, M. R., and Moore, F. D.: Studies in surgical endocrinology, Ann. Surg. *148:*199, 1958.

365. Ingle, D. J., Ward, E. O., and Kuizenga, M. H.: Relationship of the adrenal glands to changes in urinary non-protein nitrogen following multiple fractures in force-fed rat, Am. J. Physiol. *149:* 510, 1947.

366. Ingle, D. J., Meeks, R. C., and Thomas, K. E.: The effect of fractures upon urinary electrolytes in non-adrenalectomized rats and adrenalectomized rats treated with adrenal cortex extract, Endocrinol. *49:*703, 1951.

367. Robson, J. S., Dudley, H. A. F., Horn, D. B., and Stewart, C. P.: Metabolic response to adrenalectomy, Lancet *2:*632, 1955.

368. Ingle, D. J.: The role of the adrenal cortex in homeostasis, Pediatrics *17:*407, 1956.

369. Sayers, G.: The adrenal cortex and homeostasis, Physiol. Rev. *30:*241, 1950.

370. Dudley, H. A. F., Robson, J. S., Smith, M., and Stewart, C. P.: The permissive role of adrenal cortical hormones after injury in man. Metabolism *8:*885, 1959.

371. Selye, H.: Stress, Montreal, Acta, 1950.

372. Steenburg, R. W., and Ganong, W. F.: Observations on the influence of extra-adrenal factors on circulating 17-hydroxycorticosteroids, Surgery *38:* 92, 1955.

373. Engel, F. L.: A consideration of the roles of the adrenal cortex in stress and in the regulation of protein metabolism, Rec. Progr. Hormone Res. *6:*277, 1951.

374. Kampmeier, R. H.: Nutrition in internal medicine, Am. J. Med. *25:*662, 1958.

375. Griffith, W. H.: The physiologic role of vitamins, Am. J. Med. *25:*666, 1958.

376. Rosenberg, H. R.: Vitamins, New York, Interscience Publishers, 1942.

377. Bean, W. B.: The Vitamins, in Grollman, A. (Ed.): Clinical Physiology, New York, McGraw-Hill, 1955.

378. Keys, A.: Undernutrition, in Duncan, G. G. (Ed.): Diseases of Metabolism, ed. 3, Philadelphia, W. B. Saunders Co., 1954.

379. Peters, R. A.: Development of theoretical significance of British anti-lewisite (BAL), Brit. M. Bull. *5:*313, 1948.

380. Williams, C. D.: Kwashiorkor, J.A.M.A. *153:*1280, 1953.

381. Zubirän, S.: Consideraciones generales y antecedentes de la alimentación de enfermos desnutridos, Rev. invest. clín. *9:*11, 1957.

382. Rivera, A., and Esquivel, F.: Alteraciones del tubo digestivo en la desnutrición, Rev. invest. clín. *9:* 17, 1957.

383. Millán, J.: Alteraciones dermatológicas en la desnutrición, Rev. invest. clín. *9:*25, 1957.

384. Hernández Peniche, J.: Manifestaciones neurológicas de la desnutrición, Rev. invest. clín. *9:*29, 1957.

385. Gómez Mont, F., and Zubirán, S.: Alteraciones de la función endócrina en la desnutrición Rev. invest. clín. *9:*33, 1957.

386. Zubirán, S., and Gómez Mont, F.: Endocrine disturbances in chronic human malnutrition, Vitamins & Hormones *11:*97, 1953.

387. Zubirán, S., Gómez Mont, F., and Laguna, J.: Endocrine disturbances and their dietetic background in undernourished in Mexico, Ann. Int. Med. *42:*1259, 1955.

388. Sepúlveda, B., Hernández de la Portilla, R., Rojas, E., and Macías, J. J.: Las alteraciones del hígado en la desnutrición, Rev. invest. clín. *9:* 445, 1957.

389. Goettsch, M.: Dietary methods for induction of necrotic liver degeneration, Ann. New York Acad. Sc. *57:*839, 1954.

390. Schwartz, K.: Factors protecting against dietary necrotic liver degeneration, Ann. New York Acad. Sc. *57:*878, 1954.

391. Schwartz, K.: Liver necrosis versus fatty liver and cirrhosis, Ann. New York Acad. Sc. *57:*617, 1954.

392. Earle, D. P., Jr., and Victor, J.: Effect of various

diets on liver damage caused by excess cystine, J. Exper. Med. *75:*179, 1942.

393. Koch-Wesser, D., de la Huerga, J., Yesinick, C., and Popper, H.: Hepatic necrosis due to bromobenzene and its dependence upon available sulfur amino acids, Proc. Soc. Exper. Biol. & Med. *79:* 196, 1953.

394. Schwartz, K., and Foltz, C. A.: Selenium as an integral part of Factor 3 against dietary necrosis and liver degeneration, J. Am. Chem. Soc. *79:* 3292, 1957.

395. Györgyi, P.: Antibiotics and liver injury, Ann. New York Acad. Sc. *57:*925, 1957.

396. Luckey, T. D., Reyniers, J. P., Györgyi, P., and Forbes, M.: Germ-free animals and liver necrosis, Ann. New York Acad. Sc. *57:*932, 1954.

397. Goettsch, M.: The role of vitamin E in the production of nutritional liver injury on low casein diets, J. Nutrition *44:*443, 1951.

398. Lepkovsky, S., and Borsoon, H. J.: Nutrition and nutritional diseases, Ann. Rev. Med. *6:*93, 1955.

399. Gitler, C.: Studies in vitamin B deficiency in the rat and the chick, Doctoral Thesis, University of Wisconsin, 1958.

400. Gómez, F., Ramos-Galván, R., Cravioto, J., and Frenk, S.: Prevention and treatment of chronic severe malnutrition (kwashiorkor), Ann. New York Acad. Sc. *69:*969, 1958.

401. Gómez, F., Ramos-Galván, R., Cravioto, J., and Frenk, S.: Malnutrition in infancy and childhood with special reference to kwashiorkor, Advances Pediat. *7:*131, 1955.

402. La Desnutrición en el Niño, Bol. Hosp. Infant. México *15:*753, 1958.

403. Moore, R. A., Spies, T. D., and Cooper, Z. K.: Histopathology of skin in pellagra, Arch. Dermat. & Syph. *46:*100, 1942.

404. Hill, K., Rhodes, K., Stafford, J., and Aub, R.: Serous hepatosis A. Pathogenesis of hepatic fibrosis in Jamaican children, Brit. M. J. *2:*117, 1953.

405. Gómez, F., Ramos-Galván, R., Cravioto, J., and Frenk, S.: Desnutrición de tercer grado en México (kwashiorkor en Africa), Bol. Hosp. Infant. México *9:*281, 1952.

406. Murphy, R.: The complexities of the problem of obesity, Med. Clin. North Am. *44:*439, 1960.

407. Brozek, J., and Keys, A.: The evaluation of leanness-fatness in man, norms and interrelationships, Brit. J. Nutrition *5:*194, 1951.

408. Behnke, A. R., Osserman, E. F., and Wellham, W. C.: Lean body mass. Its clinical significance and estimation from excess fat and total body water determinations, Arch. Int. Med. *91:*585, 1953.

409. Edwards, D. A.: Estimation of the proportion of fat in the body by measurements of skin-fold thickness, Am. J. Clin. Nutr. *4:*35, 1956.

410. Newburgh, L. H.: Obesity. I. Energy metabolism, Physiol. Rev. *24:*18, 1944.

411. Pennington, A. W.: A reorientation on obesity, New Eng. J. Med. *248:*959, 1953.

412. Pennington, A. W.: Pyruvic acid metabolism in obesity, Am. J. Digest. Dis. *22:*33, 1955.

413. Combined Staff Clinics: Obesity, Am. J. Med. *19:* 111, 1955.

414. Booyens, J., and McCance, R. A.: Individual variations in expenditure of energy, Lancet *1:*225, 1957.

415. Brobeck, J. R.: Obesity, Nutr. Symp. Series *6:*36, 1953.

416. Edholm, O. G., Fletcher, J. G., Widdowson, E. M., and McCance, R. A.: The energy expenditure and food intake of individual men, Brit. J. Nutrition *9:*286, 1955.

417. Brobeck, J. R.: Food intake as a mechanism of temperature regulation, Yale J. Biol. & Med. *20:* 545, 1948.

418. Brobeck, J. R.: Neural regulation of food intake, Ann. New York Acad. Sc. *63:*44, 1955.

419. Mayer, J.: Regulation of energy intake and the body weight; the glucostatic theory and the lipostatic hypothesis, Ann. New York Acad. Sc. *63:* 15, 1955.

420. Mayer, J.: Glucostatic mechanisms of regulation of food intake, New Eng. J. Med. *249:*13, 1953.

421. Bornstein, L. M., and Grossman, M. I.: An experimental test of the glucostatic theory of regulation of food intake, J. Clin. Invest. *35:*626, 1956.

422. Kurlander, A. B., Abraham, S., and Rion, J. W.: Obesity and disease, Human Biol. *28:*203, 1956.

423. Dublin, L. I.: Relation of obesity to longevity, New Eng. J. Med. *248:*971, 1953.

424. Marks, H. H.: Influence of obesity on morbidity and mortality, Bull. New York Acad. Med. *36.* 296, 1960.

425. Saphir, O., and Corrigan, M.: Fatty infiltration of the myocardium, Arch. Int. Med. *52:*410, 1933.

426. Aceves, S.: Obesidad y enfermedades cardiovasculares, Principia Cardiol. *3:*27, 1956.

427. French, A. J., and Dock, W.: Fatal coronary arteriosclerosis in young soldiers, J.A.M.A. *124:* 1233, 1944.

428. Adlersberg, D., Coler, H. R., and Laval, J.: Effect of weight reduction on course of arterial hypertension, J. Mt. Sinai Hosp. *12:*984, 1946.

429. Hartroft, W. S.: The pathology of obesity, Bull. New York Acad. Med. *36:*313, 1960.

430. Carroll, D.: Peculiar type of cardiopulmonary failure associated with obesity, Am. J. Med. *21:*819, 1956.

431. Burwell, C. S., Robin, E. D., Whaley, R. D., and Bickelman, A. G.: Extreme obesity associated with alveolar hypoventilation: pickwickian syndrome, Am. J. Med. *21:*811, 1956.

432. Kerr, E. J., and Lagen, J. B.: Postural syndrome related to obesity leading to postural emphysema and cardiorespiratory failure, Ann. Int. Med. *10:* 569, 1936.

433. Seide, M. J.: Heart failure due to extreme obesity, New Eng. J. Med. *257:*1227, 1957.

434. Walker, H. C.: Obesity. Its complications and sequelae, Ann. Int. Med. *93:*951, 1954.

THE NATURE OF DISEASE

Throughout the entire period of recorded history, man has attempted to understand himself and his surroundings. Results of these efforts have been the development of magical concepts, of religious convictions, of philosophic systems and of scientific theories. Each one of those avenues of understanding is composed of both emotional and rational elements, the difference lying in their relative proportions: magical ideas are almost entirely emotional, while science might be characterized as a serious attempt to explain Nature on rational grounds. Whatever the content of irrational and objective elements in any conception of life and the universe, it has always been construed within the limitations of the epoch; in a very important sense, such systems mirror the intellectual and emotional climate of their historical period. For the same reason no system, be it fantastic or scientific, is likely to be either complete or permanent, nor is it entirely abandoned when newer concepts become popular. On the contrary, out-of-fashion theories become incorporated in a more or less disguised manner into the new system, sometimes as a basis upon which further elaborations are built, other times as an integrated and indistinguishable part of bolder speculations, faithfully conforming to hegelian synthesis. To the many differences already discovered between man and other animals, philosophers should add the human inclination and ability to collect things and live by tradition; it may not be as generalized as his featherlessness, but it is certainly more distinctive. It might be wise to question whether human explanations of life and Nature serve any purpose other than the gratification of man's craving

for significance. Indeed, most religions and many philosophic systems proclaim the world a magnificent stage for the solemn performance of man's comedy; a brief and almost instantaneous episode preceding eternities of different degrees of bliss and temperature. Should this be the only role of theorizing on these matters, such speculations could be considered as interesting but not very important. But there is another sense in which interpretations of life and "Weltanschauung" contribute to human development. Man needs a theory, for the phenomena that come under his observation are so manifold that in the absence of a theory they would elude his grasp. Generalizations are necessary as frames of reference for experience, as master prints where the "irreducible and stubborn facts" of Nature may be accommodated in an intelligible and harmonic sequence. Theories provide events with meaning within the context in which they occur.

Disease is as old as life, and in his attempts at understanding life and the world man has also suggested different explanations for disease. Such explanations reflect the historical moment in which they were suggested; they go no farther than the forefront of knowledge of the epoch, although as all manifestations of intellectual activity they may also serve to influence the further development of a culture at a given time. This seems to be the case at the present time. Since the aim of this book is to serve as an introduction to the study of disease, it does not appear out of place to review briefly some historical concepts of disease before discussing the present trend. If the reader is inclined to continue his examination of these paragraphs (a bold decision, to say the least) he is advised to keep in mind that they are offered in the main as a suggestion, as a working hypothesis which claims only to be an attempt at providing a general frame of reference for the understanding of disease in terms of a modern concept of life. The heuristic value of this concept is openly acknowledged. Support has been obtained from Rous' words: "But since in Medicine, as in everything else, what one does is determined by what one thinks, it is well to think something."

I. THE BEGINNING OF THE STORY, OR THE MAGICAL CONCEPT OF DISEASE

In his scholarly analysis of the identity of all forms of ancient and primitive medicine, Garrison points out that savage man made use of three different viewpoints of disease. First, he confused life with motion, was "puzzled if not awed by the rustling of leaves in the forest, the crash and flash of thunder and lightning, the flicker and play of sunlight and firelight, and he could see no causal relation between a natural object and its moving shadow, a sound and its echo, flowing water and the reflections on its surface. Winds, clouds, storms, earthquakes, or unusual sights and sounds in nature were to him the outward and visible signs of malevolent gods, demons, spirits, or other supernatural agencies." Therefore, he considered disease as an evil spirit or the work of an evil spirit, and his therapy was aimed at either pleasing or frightening away such demons. Second, savage man believed his enemies to have supernatural powers and to use them to produce disease. Third, the offended spirits of the dead, whether of men, animals or plants, were accepted as causal agents of several ailments. The close association of these concepts with primitive religion explains the appearance of "medicine men" or shamans among the priests, who treated their patients with psychotherapeutic techniques and attempted prophylaxis with amulets to be worn by the ailing subject or his scared relations.

An instance of this magical concept of disease, described by Guthrie, is the custom of "pointing the bone," which to this day prevails in Australia. The native of central Australia is considered the most primitive type of man today, and although there is no obvious reason to believe that he is the same as his ancestors of 5000 years ago, his idea of disease is entirely magical. The "bone" is a long slender stick marked with rings to indicate the number of victims, and when used with malevolent intent it is held in a special position pointing towards the victim. A song may accompany the ritual, which ends with the burial of the bone. The first sign of having been "boned" may be the onset of illness, upon which the friends of the patient look for the bone, and if they find it, recovery is rapid. If the search proves useless the medicine man is summoned and he proceeds to extract the evil influence by suction and other means; after much incantation the medicine man expectorates in his hand and proceeds to show the patient a small stone or crystal rock (conveniently prepared in anticipation) the very cause of the disease. Immediate improvement is the rule, and health is soon restored to the sick man.

Egyptian medicine has always been considered as essentially magic or magico-religious and for good reasons, since it began with the priests and remained stationary for many centuries. Although the absence of religious or magical elements in the Edwin Smith papyrus is not entirely surprising, since it is primarily a surgical treatise (throughout history, surgeons seem to have held closer to the ground than physicians), in problems of internal disease the early physician was faced with baffling mystery and resorted to all sorts of spells and incantations. A cold, for instance, could be exorcised by such magic words as "Depart, cold, son of a cold, thou who breakest the bone, destroyest the skull, makest ill the seven openings of the head! . . . Go out on the floor, stink, stink, stink!" This cure was probably as effective as the more elaborate, present-day treatments for this ancient disease. Nevertheless, the transition from magico-religious concepts to empirical observations and natural causes was probably started by the Egyptians with their concept of wdhw, which has been explored in a scholarly fashion by Steuer and Saunders. Briefly, wdhw was an etiologic principle derived from the intestinal putrefaction of foods which passed from the bowel to the circulatory system. Here it acted upon the blood and was transformed, together with part of the circulating fluid, into pus. Finally, as the last stage of this pathologic process, the blood underwent coagulation, establishing a local lesion or making the blood unfit to support the physiologic mechanisms of the body. From this concept physicians, as well as the common citizens, derived their keen interest in cleansing the gastrointestinal tract with admirable though somewhat exaggerated repetition, causing Herodotus to say, referring to the Egyptians, "They purge themselves every month, three days in succession, seeking to preserve health by emetics and clysters, for they suppose that all diseases to which men are subjected proceed from the food they use."

The Egyptian departure from magical ideas is the beginning of a transition from imaginary to objective concepts of disease. That this is no simple feat for man is testified by the whole history of medicine, which is little more than the tale of repeated attempts to break away from supernatural beliefs and construct a rational system, based on Nature itself. No rash condemnation of magical ideas should result from this passing glimpse of ancient concepts. For magic is really an attempt to obtain specific results on the basis of certain rigidly defined rites, sometimes entirely irrelevant but always firmly adhered to by either medicine man or patient. Magic entails the recognition of the principle of causality, that given the same antecedent conditions, the same results will follow. In a very profound sense, magic is really early science. On the other hand, religion springs from an entirely different source. Here, the whole system is based on the achievement of results against, or in spite of, regular sequence. Religion functions in the region of the miraculous and anti-natural, which requires the violation of causality. Although frequently mixed in primitive thought, these two ways of thinking are thus quite different; civilization, and with it most of the lofty conquests of the human spirit, represents the slow but progressively successful rejection of positions demanding the sacrifice of man's intellect in variously disguised Moloch's shrines.

The purely religious concept of disease is embodied in the Old Testament. There, disease is the expression of the wrath of God, to be removed only by painful moral reform, prayers and sacrifice, and it is God who confers both health and disease according to His divine and unpredictable will: "I will put none of these diseases upon thee, which I have brought upon the Egyptians: for I am the Lord that healeth thee." A clear example of the relation between divinely caused disease and prayer is the case of Hezekiah, who was severely ill and prayed to God for his health. His prayers were overheard by the prophet Isaiah, who begged and obtained divine acquiescence to help him; Isaiah ordered that a lump of figs be applied to Hezekiah's afflicted parts, with the result that the ailing man was restored to health.

Early Greek medicine was also dominated by superstition. The legend of Aesculapius is worth retelling since it shows the prevailing atmosphere preceding the appearance of the great revolution represented by Hippocrates. According to Sigerist, Apollo surprised Coronis (a beautiful virgin of the Lapithae) bathing in Lake Boebeis. The god conceived a passion for such a charming figure and possessed her. Coronis became with child, but her father had chosen her cousin Ischus for her husband, and she was forced to obey him. Upon learning this, Apollo wrathfully slew Ischus, while Coronis suffered the same fate by Apollo's sister Artemis. But as the god contemplated the dead body of his lover he felt sorrow for his unborn son, whereupon he proceeded to liberate the child from the mother's womb and to take him to the cave of Chiron the Centaur in Mount Pelion. Chiron was the son of Saturn, and skilled in music, surgery and ancient lore. For his knowledge, Chiron had been entrusted with the education of Jason, Hercules and Achilles; above all, he was now in charge of guiding the first steps of Apollo's son by Coronis, Aesculapius.

The boy grew into a man so proficient in the healing arts that Pluto accused him of diminishing the number of shades in Hades, so Zeus destroyed him with a thunderbolt. It was inevitable that Aesculapius would become an object of worship, and so it was. A special group of physicians was eventually formed who called themselves the Asclepiads; one of them, mentioned by Plato, was Hippocrates.

II. THE HELLENIC CONTRIBUTION, OR THE BIRTH OF REASON

Thales of Miletus, one of the Seven Wise Men of Greece, is considered to have begun both philosophy and science by saying, "All things are made of water." The significance of this dictum is not embodied in itself, but in the fact that it represents an answer to one question that had been asked since the beginning of history. The question, however, consistently had been answered by taking recourse to entirely different ways of thinking. The question was, "What is the universe made of?" and the answers had been either magical or religious. Thales' answer inaugurates the use of reason as a powerful method of looking at Nature; such a system of thought has had its ups and downs, and although it may seem somewhat incredible, it was totally discredited for over twelve centuries after it was introduced. Reason was not to regain its proper place in human affairs until unreason had had its day, which was not a short one; but for a brief period of a few hundred years, the Greeks held the stage and mankind had a quick vision of wisdom. Thales, however, was only the first man of whom there is any record of attempting to explain the world without recourse to anthropomorphic or moral ideas. Other Milesians, such as Anaximander and Anaximenes, had suggestions of their own concerning the basic stuff of the universe and its organization. Anaximander believed the world to be made of an infinite fund of material extending in all directions, called the Boundless, from which the world arises and into which it will in the end return. Anaximenes held air as the basic substance of the universe, the different forms of matter arising through processes of condensation and rarefaction. The soul is air; fire is rarefied air; when condensed, air becomes first water, then earth and finally stone.

The Milesians are important not for the actual contents of their respective theories, but for the nature of the questions they asked and, above all, for the general trend of their answers. Anaximander presaged the Hippocratic idea of Eukrasia or equilibrium of bodily components in health when he stated that there should be a certain proportion of fire, earth and water in the world, and that each element is perpetually attempting to enlarge its empire; nevertheless, there is a kind of necessity or natural law which perpetually redresses the balance, so that the eternally fixed bounds are not overstepped. Greek drama is full of this concept of equilibrium, represented by Fate. The similarity is more than simply metaphoric; in a very important sense, the laws of Nature which rule also in Olympian realms, are the limitations imposed on man and the world by the way things are made.

A closer relation can be envisaged between Pythagoras and the Hippocratic concept of disease. The Pythagoreans were a religious sect with mystical elements derived from the orphic revival, which among other things held that the soul is subject to a series of transmigrations. Philosophy (understood as adherence to Pythagoreanism) provided an escape from this wheel of birth. Purification was necessary, and a powerful agent was music. Whether the Pythagorean interest in music derived from this mystical aspect of their doctrines or from their intense interest in mathematics is a subject of conjecture. According to the legend, Pythagoras discovered that a tuned string will sound the octave if the length is halved, that if the length is reduced to three quarters the sound is a fourth, and if shortened two thirds the sound is a fifth. The tuned string played a central role in Greek philosophic thought. The notion of harmony, in the sense of balance, the adjustment of opposites like high and low, and the doctrine of the four temperaments, all these in the end go back to Pythagoras' discovery. The number emerged as the essence of all things.

Unity was perfection and represented God; twelve was the whole material universe; four were the primordial elements and at the same time the perfection of eternally flowing nature. Corresponding with the four elements, earth, air, fire and water, were the qualities dry, cold, moist and hot, which were later combined as follows:

hot + dry   = fire
hot + moist = air
cold + dry   = earth
cold + moist = water

These four elements had been introduced by Empedocles as "the four-fold root of all things." Empedocles was a Pythagorean for some time, but was expelled from the group because he revealed some of their esoteric doctrine. He believed in transmigration, and announced that he had been "in bygone times a youth, a maiden, and a flowering shrub; a bird, yes, and a fish that swims in silence through the deep sea." He further believed that the human body was made of the four primordial substances earth, air, fire and water, health resulting from their balance, disease from their imbalance. Alcmeon probably anticipated Empedocles in the doctrine that health is the equilibrium (*isonomia*) and disease the preponderance (*monarchia*) of heat, cold, moisture, dryness, acidity, sweetness, etc. Long before Aristotle it was held that there were four humors in the body, namely blood, phlegm, yellow bile and black bile. The stage was set, then, for the doctrine of the balance of humors, which became prominent in Hippocratic teachings and, adopted and modified by Galen and the "Arabian" physicians, reigned supreme until the Renaissance.

Hippocrates represents the culmination of Hellenic medicine. Time has consecrated him as the perfect physician, embodied with both the most sagacious clinical abilities and the highest ethical standards. Among his eternal contributions are the dissociation of the healing arts from theology and philosophy, the recognition of the value of clinical observation and the teaching of disease as a natural phenomenon. Humility and honesty are not the least of his virtues. Of his 42 cases in *Epidemics,* 25 are reported as fatal, which by modern standards cannot be considered as an enviable statistic. Osler quotes

Hippocrates as saying, "I have written this down deliberately, believing it is valuable to learn of unsuccessful experiments and to know the causes of their failure."

In the Hippocratic writings disease is considered as due to natural causes. The book on *The Sacred Disease* (probably epilepsy) begins with these words: "It is not in my opinion any more divine or more sacred than other disease, but has a natural cause, and its supposed divine origin is due to man's inexperience." A little later he states: "Every disease has its own nature and arises from external causes, from cold, from the sun, or from changing winds." This sentence is as valid today as it was then. As with Alcmeon and Empedocles, health was considered a matter of equilibrium, disease resulting from disturbances in the equilibrium. The forces or qualities contributory to this equilibrium are variously named in the different Hippocratic writings; the juices or "humors" are repeatedly mentioned. Sometimes many humors are admitted, other times there seem to be only two, bile and mucus. Again, in one of the later books, it is stated that there are two pairs of humors with opposed qualities, blood and black bile, mucus and yellow bile. Should one of these humors be present in excess, or corrupted in any way, the organism endeavors, by means of its natural healing forces (*Vis Medicatrix Naturae*) to restore the balance. The peccant humor undergoes a process which may be compared with boiling (coction) and when this process is finished, the peccant material is eliminated in the urine or in the stools, in the vomit or in pus.

The essential contribution of the Greeks to culture was a movement towards enlightment and liberation from supernatural or magico-religious bonds. In philosophy, in art, in science, the trend is the same, to center man's attention on the world as it is, and to attempt to interpret it by means of reason. Although they did not discover the value of experiment, the Greek's insistence on adherence to observation was a magnificent step forward, a radical departure from primitive habits of thought and life. That the Hellenic lead was not followed with the same fervor, and that for over a thousand years man returned to his conformity to dogma and his recourse to supernatural explanations can be understood by the turn of history after Alexander's death, but it is nevertheless appalling. Fortunately, the Greek seed remained dormant and suddenly burst out and grew vigorously from the Renaissance onwards, first in art, then in philosophy, finally in science. Man lived again by Socrates' dictum, that the unexamined life is not worth living, and by Aristotle's idea that what is important is not to live long but to live well. But before this upsurge of classic values, twelve centuries had to elapse. And during all this period disease continued to accompany man faithfully, "like the shadow follows the body." What ideas were held on disease during all these weary and unhappy years?

III. GALENIC INTERLUDE

Galen was born in Pergamum, the son of Nicon, a well-to-do, widely educated engineer. From his father he probably inherited an inclination towards culture in all its manifestations, while from his mother ("so ill-tempered that she sometimes bit her servant maids, was continually screaming, was a scold, berating her husband more savagely than Xanthippe did Socrates") he probably derived his great gusto and ability for controversy, and his boundless self assurance. After a brief period of study in Pergamum, Galen traveled in various lands for nine years, visiting Smyrna, Greece, Corinth and Alexandria. In 157 A.D. he returned to Pergamum, where for three years he was the gladiatorial surgeon, leaving an unsurpassed record since not a single fatality occurred in this period. Nevertheless, in 162 A.D. Galen was already in Rome, and for the next four years he rose in fame and wealth, no simple feat for an unknown stranger in the world's capital. For unknown reasons he returned to Pergamum, and remained there for a brief spell, until a royal summons took him back to Rome, where he stayed for the next and last thirty years of his life.

Although Galen lived in what Gibbon considered the most happy period of humanity (the second century) the seeds of the Dark Ages were planted in his very time. During the first century B.C., Asia Minor, Syria, Egypt and Gaul fell to the Roman legions, and in the first century A.D. Britain followed the same fate. It came to be that the lands of the Roman Empire were bounded in the North by the Rhine and the Danube, in the East by the Euphrates and the Arabian desert, in the South by the Sahara and in the West by the ocean. In this setting, the Roman Empire lived in comparative peace for the first two centuries A.D. It is true that there was some internal trouble, and that warfare continued along the borders, but neither was of such proportions as to disturb the Imperial rule seriously.

But with the passing of the Greek world, the general spirit of freshness and vitality was lost. The Greeks had a cheerful attitude towards life, a sort of bold and adventurous stand. Problems faced them from all directions, but the stimulating challenge awakened such interesting and keen speculation that the world was viewed as a rather nice place to live in. Alexander's expansion brought with it a decay of this attitude, so that the philosophic trend was changed to an over-all pessimism and a sense of insecurity. The cynics, emerging as a response to this feeling, turned away from worldly goods and concentrated on virtue as the only good worth having. They were followed by the skeptics, who influenced the Academy for at least 200 years and in the end demanded a more definite and systematic set of beliefs. Men were looking for peace in an age where the old framework of society had collapsed, so virtue became a way of coping with troubles that could not be eschewed. But the most influential philosophic movement in hellenistic times was Zeno's stoicism, a predeterministic and pessimistic philosophy in which the foremost virtue is to live at one with the world. Virtue was considered the only inalienable possession of the individual, which could not be taken away by tyrants and conquerors.

A new element in these variations on Greek philosophy was introduced by the neoplatonist Plotinus, who lived in Alexandria in the third century A.D. This new element was mysticism, and it was to become one of the predominant ingredients of Medieval philosophy. The mystic experience cannot be wholly communicated, it is considered unique and untransferable, to be bestowed only upon those who have submitted themselves to prolonged and difficult preparations. In this aspect, mysticism is quite the opposite of Greek philosophy, which was entirely public and accessible to both slave and sage. In Plotinus there is a Trinity made up of the One, Nous or Spirit, and Soul, which sets up the pattern of much that was later adopted by Christianity. Still, Plotinus allowed for Nature to be beautiful and enjoyable, whereas later mystics came to curse beauty and pleasure as base and evil.

From Thales to Plotinus some nine centuries elapsed. Political strife was accompanied by a loss of the Greek contribution, a capacity to be struck with amazement and wonder at the ways of Nature. The Greek enterprise resulted in liberation from fear of the unknown through the logos and the pursuit of knowledge for itself. At the threshold of the Dark Ages such enterprise was abandoned for religious mysteries with an aura of ineffability. When mysticism becomes central in man's preoccupations he betrays the possibility of explaining the world through reason and exchanges his faith in a natural order for another faith in a divine and inscrutable will. The stage is set for religious intolerance, for persecution and bigotry, for the rule of authority over speculation. This is the spirit that made Galen the undisputed ruler of medicine for twelve centuries.

Galen's writings are the most voluminous of all ancient history; he composed nine books on anatomy, seventeen on physiology, six on pathology, fourteen on therapeutics, thirty on pharmacy, sixteen on the pulse, etc. He searched with great zeal for a complete system, an integrated body of theory that would account for all and every aspect of medicine. With characteristic cocksureness Galen gives an answer to every problem, has a reason for every phenomenon. Thus, he produced not one, but several all-embracing schemes, which were later on added to and interpreted by a host of translators and commentators, becoming the ulti-

mate court of appeal for all discussions up to the time of Vesalius. Combining the humoral ideas of Hippocrates with the Pythagorean theory of the four elements and his own conception of an all-pervading pneuma, Galen proceeded to explain everything in the light of his personal medical philosophy. He abandoned the careful notation of facts, so dear to Hippocrates, quoting only his miraculous cures. Perhaps he was the first to present distorted and biased statistics to back his pet theories and favorite therapeutics. His main pathologic doctrine is based on an adequate balance of naturals, non-naturals, and contranaturals.

And yet, one cannot but marvel at Galen's industry and breadth of knowledge. He explored every field, upturned every medical stone, leaving his mark of genius before moving to other areas. Anatomy, dissection, pharmacology, experimental neurology, physiology, were all explored by this restless physician and enriched with many original observations and more baseless theorizing, claiming always complete knowledge with disarming sufficiency. According to Garrison, "The effect of this dogmatism and infallibility upon after-time was appalling; for while Galen's monotheism and piety appealed to the Moslems, his assumption of omniscience was specially adapted to appease the mental indolence and flatter the complacency of those who were swayed entirely by reverence for authority. . . . After his death, European medicine remained at a dead level for nearly fourteen centuries."

IV. THE MEDIEVAL PERIOD, OR THE REIGN OF DOGMA AND UNREASON

This period of civilization represents an almost complete relapse to supernatural ideas of disease. The all-pervading power of the Church claimed that nothing should interfere with the influence of the one Great Physician. Disease was a divine punishment, the best remedies prayer and fasting. The early Christian view of disease was a backward step. Thus, St. Basil of Cesarea denied that there were natural causes for any ailment, holding at the same time that many diseases were sent as punishments for sin; St. Ambrose declared that "the precepts of medicine are contrary to celestial science, watching, and prayer." The bitter opposition to secular learning had its climax when a mob of Christian fanatics set fire to the great library at Alexandria in 391 A.D., destroying forever many priceless treasures. In this respect, the Byzantine period was important mainly because many of the classical writings were preserved until western Europe became again capable of understanding and using them. The old idea that disease was caused by God's anger and diabolic influence came back and was widely held. Origen said, "It is demons which produce famine, unfruitfulness, corruptions of the air, pestilences; they hover concealed in clouds in the lower atmosphere, and are attracted by the blood and incense that the heathen offer to them as gods."

Singer says that, early in the Dark Ages, belief in possession by demons was not shared by Teutonic tribes, disease being attributed among them to the action of supernatural beings, elves, smiths and witches. Suffering was brought about by shooting the passer-by with poisoned darts, and for this reason Singer describes it as the doctrine of the elf-shot. This theory on the nature of disease was shared by the English for a long time, at first in unmodified form and later in many different combinations with flying venoms and diabolic possession, until the elves were completely displaced and left to practice their malignant attacks on beings of lesser importance, the cattle, "whom the more self-respecting demons might be expected to regard as providing but a poor field for their accomplishments."

In 1248, the Council of Le Mans forbade surgery to monks. This was a shocking blow to the public at large, since frequent condemnations of the healing arts had relegated their practice to the lowest social strata, and with all due exceptions it was primarily in the hands of quacks and nomadic mountebanks. At the same time, it was the culmination of a campaign against all forms of knowledge, started some time before by St. Bernard when he admonished certain monks

that to seek relief from disease in medicine was in harmony neither with their religion nor with the honor and purity of their order. Nevertheless, many of the classical texts were preserved in monasteries, where for years some ignored benefactors of mankind patiently copied and recopied Greek and Latin books, including some of Galen's. But in 1243 the Dominican order forbade medical treatises to be brought into their monasteries, and the practice dwindled down until it nearly vanished.

Important as they were in the preservation and further elaboration of Hippocratic and Galenic concepts, the Jewish and Arabic scholars added little of significance to medieval ideas of disease. Salerno, Montpelier, Bologna, and all other early universities were even more conservative, as they represented established authority and were strongly influenced by ecclesiastics. Teaching consisted of reading and commentaries on Galen, Avicenna, Aristotle, and perhaps one or two other authors who rose to fame by copying and repeating the classics and each other. An idea of the status of medical teaching in the Middle Ages may be gained from the following curriculum of the University of Tübingen in 1481.

HOUR	FIRST YEAR	SECOND YEAR	THIRD YEAR
8 a.m.	Galen's *Ars Medica*	First book of Avicenna (anatomy and physiology)	*Aphorisms* of Hippocrates
1 p.m.	First and second sections of Avicenna's *Treatise on Fevers*	Ninth book of Rhazes (local pathology)	Galen

The dearth of bedside teaching was such that at Oxford it was possible for a fully qualified doctor to leave school without ever having laid a hand upon a patient. Even Antonio Benivieni, who is usually held to be the "father of pathology" because he performed autopsies in search of the causes of symptoms and death, remarks in his discussion of the treatment of Morbus Gallicus, ". . . you should seek to produce a balance of the humors. . . ." These words were written a few years before 1506, showing Galen's influence in full operation.

V. PARACELSUS

If these lines were devoted to a cold analysis of different theories on the nature of disease, Paracelsus would be worth a brief remark as a medievalist who, unhappy with the prevailing Galenic beliefs of his time, rebelled against them and in their stead created others still more incredibly obscure and dogmatic. In his work, Paracelsus was not even attempting a revival of Hippocratic doctrines, despite his battle cry, "The patients are your textbook, the sickbed is your study." Like the Ionian philosophers, Paracelsus is important not for what he did, but for what he attempted. Standing at the threshold of the Renaissance, he belongs body and soul to the Dark Ages. His claim to immortality is his lone and desperate fight against blind authority, a fight that took him to the confines of the known world of his time, that endeared him neither to secular nor religious authorities, quacks nor physicians, friends nor followers, and was probably the cause of his premature death. In the end, Paracelsus lost his fight but the world gained a glimpse of the future, when freedom from orthodoxy and dogmatism would favor independent research into the ways of Nature. This future was not far, since two years after Paracelsus' death publication of Vesalius' *Fabrica* and Copernicus' *Dialogues* hailed the dawn of the Renaissance.

Phillippus Theophrastus Aureolus Bombastus ab Hohenheim, Eremita, called Paracelsus, Doctor of both Medicines and Professor of Theology, also Adept of the Holy Cabbala and Expert of the Alchemical Art, Friend of the Common Man and Defender of Liberty, was born with a shorter name and no titles in Einsiedeln, Switzerland, in 1493. When he was ten years old his mother died and he moved with his father to Villach, in the neighborhood of a lead mining district and Count Füger's smelting works. Here, Paracelsus developed a keen and lasting interest in chemistry which was to show in many of his writings and was to make him one of the founders of biochemistry; it was also in the mines that many of his theories of disease, to be developed in later years, found their inception. When the time came Paracelsus went to Italy to study medicine, but he did not remain in school for long; indeed, he never finished school nor received a medical degree. When accused that he had no right to practice medicine, since he had not entered this science through the right door, Paracelsus retorted, "But which one is the truly legitimate door —Galen and Avicenna, or Nature? I have entered through the door of Nature. Her light, not the lamp of an apothecary's shop, has illuminated my way." He continued to travel throughout his life, always repeating the same strange sequence of events, like a well rehearsed play. Wherever he went he was preceded by tales of miraculous cures, so he was received with open arms; his knowledge of medicine would bring about some successful treatments and for a short period it would seem that the traveling physician had found a secure and permanent place. But his pugnacious nature decreed otherwise, and with haughty and obscene language he would accuse other practitioners of being quacks, ignoramuses, sworn fools, swindlers, accredited asses, etc. He would associate with peasants and vagabonds, was accused by his secretary Oporinus of drinking and eating too much, and when the town doctors were ready for a fight, Paracelsus would lose the support of the authorities and in the end would have to move to another town, sometimes leaving all his possessions and writings behind. He was associated with the figure of Dr. Faustus, and legend would have him the possessor of the "elixir of life." His life was hard, marked by many failures and few moments of self satisfaction; he died in Salzburg, in 1541. Sudhoff believes he died of cancer; his disciples attributed his death to an overdose of the famous elixir that was supposedly in his possession and which he carried in the pommel of his enormous sword; his enemies spread the rumor that he died from blows received in a tavern brawl.

In his youth, Paracelsus published a small volume called *Paramirum,* which perhaps means "Beyond the Miraculous." Here he sets up his major theory on the nature of disease, an open challenge to the prevailing Galenic humoral pathology. Paracelsus believed that the Galenic guild was only a small part of medicine, that the field was much larger and, therefore, disease has causes other than humoral imbalance. He disinguished five major causes of disease, which were considered as five principles or spheres (*Entia*). They were *Ens Astri,* the influence of the stars, which was envisaged as caused by exhalations of the stars which poison the air and may produce epidemics or wars; furthermore, such a meteorological environment was also capable of producing any other systemic disease. There followed the *Ens Veneni,* the relation between man and his environment, from which he must derive sustenance and which may provoke disturbances of metabolism. The third element is very interesting because it introduces heredity as a pathologic mechanism. It was known as *Ens Naturale* and was supposed to determine the "natural cycle of the body," its "complexion." When a child is born under the luckiest stars and receives the richest gifts, yet he suffers a disease, "Who is to blame? The blood which comes by generation." The fourth cause of disease is *Ens Spirituale,* since man's life has important spiritual elements which may be deranged and cause mental disease. Finally, *Ens Dei* stands for those illnesses sent by God which are, obviously, incurable. There follows a list of doctors supposed to fit the five categories of disease, beginning with Naturales, who treat contrary with contrary in the Galenic tradition, and ending in Christ and the Apostles.

A more elaborate development of these ideas was produced some four years later under the name of *Opus Paramirum.* Of special interest here was Paracelsus' answer to the cause of decay of matter, which led to an entirely different, all embracing theory of disease. He believed that the cause of growth and decay was not the stars nor the humors, but the material which pervades the whole universe. Although Paracelsus did not know the elements of modern chemistry, he advanced medieval alchemy by adding one basic substance to the other two already accepted, sulphur (spirits) and mercury (liquids). Paracelsus insisted that salt (the ashes) was also a basic component of all bodies. Sulphur represented the gaseous and combustible elements, but also the forces of the soul, or the principle of energy; mercury stood for the fluid elements and for the forces of the intellect; while salt was the stuff of solid things and the principle of matter. These three substances were the link of man with the universe and through them he partook of the great metabolism of nature. Disease followed disturbances in the equilibrium of these substances. If the mercury in man "volatilizes" he may lose his mind, if the salt "sublimates" in the body it corrodes the organism and causes pain, etc. Behind all this and more high flown verbiage, some of his own and more spuriously attributed to him, Paracelsus was astonishingly modern. His concept of disease as a disharmony of normal functions, which represents the rejection of most medieval theories and a far-sighted vision of ideas held at present, was the result of his violent opposition to orthodox teachings. Unfortunately, it lies hidden in one of his early works, later to be superseded by several other visionary and baseless pronouncements more in keeping with his times and philosophic inclinations.

And yet, it is intriguing to look, though only in passing, into the philosophic allegiance of Paracelsus and its influence on his work. Early in his career, while studying in Tübingen, Paracelsus had been swept into the fight between "old school" and "modern" professors. The former were followers of John the Scot, who preached Free Will and was closer to Plato, while the latter were influenced by William of Occam, a critical disciple of Aristotle who believed in predistination and held that faith alone could save a man's soul. Paracelsus was sworn into the "old school" followers of John the Scot, and throughout his life he felt attracted to Plato's idealism and speculative assertiveness. He looked for certainty, not about particular facts but about the essence of all things; in his theorizing, Paracelsus was interested in "evidence," the world appearing as reasonable and harmonious. From this philosophy he probably derived the idea that belief in personal judgment of the good and the sublime was the supreme authority, which was obstinately denied by Occamists, who held (and still hold) that man is constantly in error. Paracelsus' whole life was to be an outcry against servitude to destiny and the limitations of individual speculation; "What is nature if not philosophy?" Many similarities can be traced between Paracelsus' utterings and Scotist doctrines, but they need not detain this brief survey. Suffice it to say that to the very end Paracelsus was faithful to his destiny, that in his visionary guesses he was "correct more often than anyone else, but without knowing anything correctly," and that by his valiant and stubborn defense of man's right to freedom of thought he fiercely carved his name in history. After Paracelsus, science was reborn and grew, slowly at first and then with ever increasing speed, bringing with it the promise of a freer and better life. Though hardly the midwife of this happy birth, Paracelsus was the bearer of good news to the world. In order to play this role in civilization he paid a heavy price. It is to be hoped that the show he is enjoying from his high seat is not a sorry one.

VI. FROM THE RENAISSANCE TO CLAUDE BERNARD

So far this survey has been rather biographical, arbitrarily choosing those mythical beings or historical individuals who have marked a change in prevailing concepts of disease. But for the following three centuries a different approach has been adopted, both because the subject becomes rather complex and because significant contributions were short-lived in the progressively ascending flight of human understanding. The introduction of the printing press in the middle of the fifteenth century, which enabled scholars to reproduce classical works and displace the corrupted texts accumulated throughout centuries of medieval stagnation; the discovery of the New World, which expanded the earth and suddenly released western man from the close boundaries of Europe; the dethronement of the earth as the center of the universe by Copernicus, which violated one basic dogma of medieval scholasticism and greatly advanced knowledge of the heavens; the publication of Vesalius' *De Humanis Corpori Fabrica* by Oporinus (a former secretary of Paracelsus), ranked by Singer as "The first

positive achievement of science itself in modern times"; all these bold and brave adventures helped to usher in the Renaissance and, with it, the scientific era. These were not light-hearted and happy times; on the contrary, the Church bitterly fought a lost battle, highlighted by "autos de fé" in Seville and Madrid, the flames of Giordano Bruno, Etienne Dolet, Miguel Servet, Paleario Aonio and many others, the seclusion of Galileo, the massacre of St. Bartholomew, etc. And yet, from this trial by fire there emerged a profound humanism, an immortal art and an enlightened science, as a three-headed Phoenix arising from medieval ashes, which soared without fear in the light and limitless heavens of new discovery. The climate was propitious; the Maecenases were generous, and the people were anxiously waiting for literary and artistic creations. And the world was blessed with an outpouring of genius.

The Renaissance in science came a little later, as the most tender and delicate product of human intellect. Galileo was born on the day of Michelangelo's death, Descartes was his contemporary, and Borelli, one of his students, was a teacher of Malpighi; these were also the times of Harvey, and therefore of the birth of modern medicine. The introduction of experiment as a means of exploring nature, voiced by Francis Bacon but accomplished by Harvey, was probably the most important positive step in the evolution of humanity during the seventeenth century. Although first and foremost a philosopher and mathematician, Descartes also contributed to physiology with his *De homine,* and helped to establish the Iatromathematical or Iatromechanical School, also represented by Sanctorius, Borelli and Baglivi, the last of whom observed that, "The two chief pillars of Physick are Reason and Observation." Moderns might add "Experimentation" and this view is essentially correct. To this school man was a machine made up of many smaller machines, and disease was simply the derangement of some mechanical contraption. Another school developed with van Helmont, that of the Iatrochemists, who considered the human body as a test tube. Van Helmont was a mystic follower of Paracelsus, who "in choosing a profession, he declined to take Holy Orders because his livelihood would be derived from the sins of the people. Law he also rejected, as it was not always based on truth and justice." As his last recourse van Helmont entered medicine. He envisaged the body force, or "Blas," as an all pervasive element which caused both health and disease; it produced fever, cough, etc., but sometimes it overdid itself and had to be pacified by treatment. Others, such as Sylvius and Willis, followed van Helmont in these and many other theories, which together with those of Iatromechanicists were attempts at breaking away from the past. But the lead in this liberation was not to come from too much theorizing. On the contrary, it was necessary to abandon the idea of an all inclusive scheme and to look into disease as it appeared in the sick; a return to the methods of Hippocrates was necessary, and this was championed by Thomas Sydenham.

For this "English Hippocrates," disease was the result of a fight between the nature of the sick person and the noxious influences producing the ailment; symptoms were the expressions of such a struggle. Sydenham issued a classification of manifestations of disease into "symptomata essentialia," resulting from the action of pathogenic influences on the organism, and "symptomata accidentalia," arising from the reaction of the body's efforts to overcome the agent of disease and return the organism to normal. But for Sydenham all theorizing, his as well as that of others, was useless when the doctor came to his business, the healing of the sick. He believed that, the human mind being fallible and limited, ultimate causes of disease were to remain unknown forever. And all that was of only secondary importance, since the role of physicians was not the building of systems but the care of patients. His disregard for books was so great that his well known retort to one of his students has survived to this day. When asked to recommend a textbook of medicine, Sydenham answered, "Read Don Quixote, a very good book; I read it myself still" (an excellent bit of advice).

This healthy attitude of attention to the book of medicine represented by the sick was not without criticism. Another school developed which was to contribute greatly to the confusion of the eighteenth century, namely animism. It was born with Stahl, who believed that the soul or "anima" gave life to inanimate matter, all vital processes being under its dominance. And since disease was just a vital manifestation, it was also controlled by the "anima." Thus, when chills, fever, vomiting, etc., were produced by the soul, the physician should not counteract them; no record exists, however, of the interpretation of phenomena not clearly purposive. This tendency changed in name but not in spirit with Barthez, who called it "vitalism," and survived adopted by distinguished men such as Bichat and Driesch. Related to animism was Hoffman's theory, which was not baptized with any "ism" but held that the universe (and the human body) was pervaded by a vital substance, a true *élan vital,* finer than everything else and not exactly soul, spirit or mind. Such a substance maintained the body in a status of equilibrium or tonus. Disease resulted from a deficiency or excess of tonus; an exaggeration of tonus, or spasm, was the cause of acute disease, while a relaxation of tonus, or atony, brought about chronic disease. Brown's system regarded living tissues as excitable, and life the result of external stimuli upon an organized body. Diseases were then caused by either increased or decreased stimulation, and treatment consisted of counteracting the existing condition; the favorite therapeutic elements were opium and alcohol, respectively. Since doses were rather high, it is contended that Brunonianism destroyed more people than the French Revolution and the Napoleonic wars combined, a record quite difficult to supersede.

But the frenzy of theory continued. Kämpf produced the "theory of infarctus" in which the cause of most human diseases was simply fecal impaction. This was indeed a poor revival of the principle of wdhw, introduced by the Egyptians some fifteen centuries before, with the difference that Kämpf's forerunners were more elaborately physiologic and more imaginatively therapeutic. Garrison sums up the *reductio ad absurdum* of this cult in the following satyric verse:

"And fell all prostrate at Cloaca's shrine."

Another speculation of interest here,

mainly because of its Hegelian influence in the later development of the modern concept of disease, was the ontological theory. Derived through somewhat distorted interpretations of Sydenham, Pinel and Broussais, it held that disease was not only an entity but an actual "thing," a parasite infesting the organism and causing all signs and symptoms. Broussais said: "Surely, if diseases are not within the organs, then what is it that is within them?" Accordingly, the patient supposedly contained within himself another organism, sometimes localized in certain tissues or organs, at other times diffusely pervading the entire economy. The ontologic theory of disease was adopted by natural philosophers in Germany, and became a powerful stimulus for the emergence of its antithesis, namely the physiologic concept of disease.

The recitation of many other systems of medicine, which characterized the eighteenth century, would occupy several more pages and would serve no useful purpose. Those cited so far should convince the reader that after the Renaissance the medical world found itself released from the mental chains imposed for so long a period by Galen and Avicenna, and that as a counteraction theorizing went overboard. Here is a list of the different schools at the middle of the eighteenth century in Europe, quoted from Pagel: Metaphysicians, Idealists, Iatromechanics, Iatrochemists, Experimental Physiologists, Natural Philosophers, Mystics, Magnetizers, Exorcisers, Galenists, Modern Paracelsian Homunculi, Stahlianists, Humoral Pathologists, Gastricists, Infarct-Men, Broussaists, Contrastimulists, Natural Historians, Physiatricists, Ideal-Pathologists, German Christian Theosophists, Schoenleinian Epigones, Pseudo-Schoenleinians, Homeobiotics, Homeopathists, Isopathists, Homeopathic Allopathists, Psorists and Scorists, Hydropathists, Electricity-Men, Physiologists after Hamberger, Heinrothians, Sachsians, Kieserians, Hegelians, Morisonians, Phrenologists, Iatrostatisticians. This list is far from being complete, and even farther from being a thing from the past. Many names can be easily recognized, as either identical to, or under flimsy disguises as some of the "modern" systems introduced or upheld by contemporary philosophers of nature. This was the theoretical environment in medicine in the middle of the eighteenth century; Claude Bernard was born in 1813.

VII. BERNARD, VIRCHOW AND CANNON, OR THE MODERN CONCEPT OF DISEASE

"The organism is only a living machine constructed in such a fashion that, on the one hand, there is full communication between the external environment and the *milieu intérieur,* and on the other, there are protective functions of organic elements holding living materials in reserve and maintaining without interruption humidity, heat, and other conditions indispensable to vital activity. Sickness and death are only dislocations or perturbations of that mechanism." Here, succinctly expressed, is the modern view of disease. This paragraph appears in Bernard's celebrated *"Introduction a l'Etude de la Médicine Expérimentale,"* published in 1865. It is an additional credit to Bernard's genius that, through the maze of philosophico-pseudoscientific theories of his epoch, he saw disease as clearly and as simply as he did. For further refinements and additions to this pregnant statement have only confirmed its validity. Another sentence in his book might be quoted: "It is by the normal activity of organic elements that life manifests itself in the state of health; it is by the abnormal manifestations of the same elements that diseases are characterized." This sounds obvious to the modern reader, but a minute of reflection will show that no such comprehensive theory of disease had been suggested before. It was a great revolution, one of the greatest in medical science. For centuries physicians had been searching, first in superstition, then in magic and religion, now in mysticism, later in philosophy, finally in pseudoscientific concepts, *entia* and entelechiae, for the nature of disease. But this elusive concept had always been there, in the very patients that stimulated such speculations; the signs and symptoms of illness, the turns towards health or death, the favorable response to empirical treatments or the relentless progression towards the grave despite all efforts, everything was embodied in life itself, and not in spirits, divine punishments, stars, humors or ineffable entities. Disease is not, has never been a "thing." It is a process, neither adding nor subtracting anything from the individual; it gains a transient personality by distorting normal anatomic and physiologic features, but when properly analyzed it remains the very same mystery: life.

Bernard suggested that the condition of independent life was the constancy of the *milieu intérieur*. It is impossible to resist the temptation to quote him once more: "The stability of the milieu intérieur is the primary condition for freedom and independence of existence; the mechanism which allows this is that which ensures in the *milieu intérieur* the maintenance of all conditions necessary for the life of the elements." Thus defined, many physiologic mechanisms acquire significance within the context of the organism. In this manner the "how" of many phenomena are answered, and countless observations can be placed neatly in their meaningful pigeon holes as contributing to the preservation of this *sine qua non* condition of life. And obviously, not a single "why" has found an adequate answer, since questions phrased in this manner are not scientific. When framing a hypothesis, when attempting to explain a given scientific phenomenon, when trying to establish the meaning of an observation, finalism becomes a useful instrument. It is as useful as an electric stimulator or a Warburg apparatus; but it is still an instrument, which plays no role in the explanation of phenomena, only in their investigation. This is what Bernard had in mind when he admonished investigators to, "Put off your imagination, as you take off your overcoat, when you enter the laboratory; but put it on again, as you do your overcoat, when you leave the laboratory."

Although the king of physiologists ("Ce n'est pas un gran physiologiste; c'est la physiologie même"), Bernard was also a pathologist, and a very able one, not perhaps as a morbid anatomist, performing autopsies and looking down the microscope to fixed tissues, but in the wider sense as a student of disease. Those who are not limited by technique or chained by the manifold beauties of straight morphology look upon Bernard as a forefather of modern pathology, as one who, joined by another giant prophet of modern medicine, handed down to posterity the basic concepts with which to build a dynamic science of disease. This other scientist, a contemporary of Bernard, was Rudolf Virchow.

In fighting the ontologic concept of disease, Virchow stated in 1849, ". . . disease is only the orderly manifestation of definite phenomena of life (normal in themselves) under abnormal conditions, with deviations which are simply quantitative. . . ." This sentence, indeed, precedes the one quoted from Bernard by sixteen years. At that time, Virchow was only 28 years old; two years before, in his inaugural lecture at the Collège de France, Bernard had said that his task was to develop the physiologic basis of scientific medicine, a statement interpreted by his eulogizers as implying already a grasp of this idea. Priority of concept is of no significance here, especially since Bernard held fast to his idea to the very end while Virchow in 1895 reverted to an ontologic concept of disease by stating that cellular pathology was ". . . expressively ontological. That is its virtue, not its fault. There actually is an *ens morbi,* just as there is an *ens vitae.*" But here Virchow was defending his immortal contribution, that of cellular pathology. He believed, as most of us do now, that the seat of disease was the cell, and at the same time he held that disease was just life under abnormal conditions. A group of diseased cells would be, therefore, ". . . . a parasite in the sense of the natural-historical school . . ."

The modern concept of disease was thus established. It was first expounded as a hypothesis, and to this day it remains a hypothesis. From the middle of the nineteenth century to the present day, facts have been piled upon facts to support and expand this concept. Nevertheless, such sweeping generalizations require permanent critical analysis. It is in the nature of hypotheses that they measure their usefulness by the number of data they help to uncover and by the degree of meaningfulness they impart on facts. If a single observation is found in conflict with a given hypothesis, the entire theoretical construction is held under suspicion, to be replaced by another conceptual building showing no such flaw and offering a satisfactory explanation for all adequately confirmed facts. Simplicity and elegance are additional qualities existing in, and demanded from, reigning scientific concepts. They concur in an admirable way in the theory under discussion, which holds disease to be life under abnormal conditions. But once proposed, this hypothesis was not to remain unexplored. Further elaborations awaited it, this time coming from America. Faithful to its physiologic tradition (proposed by a physiologist, supported by a pathologist who considered pathologic physiology as "destined to replace general pathology"), the hypothesis holding disease to be abnormal life was adorned and expanded by Cannon's concept of physiologic homeostasis.

W. B. Cannon, late Professor of Physiology at Harvard University, is to be the last station in this brief survey of the evolution of the concept of disease. His main contribution in this field was to make possible the analysis of life on objective terms. This he did by defining the general mechanisms governing self preserving and self reproducing organisms as follows: "The coördinated physiological processes which maintain most of the steady states in the organism are so complex and so peculiar to living beings—involving, as they may, the brain and nerves, the heart, lungs, kidneys and spleen, all working coöperatively—that I have suggested a special designation for these states, *homeostasis*. The word does not imply something set and immobile, a stagnation. It means a condition—a condition which may vary, but which is relatively constant." Bernard taught that the constancy of the *milieu intérieur* was the condition of independent life; both Bernard and Virchow established that disease is precisely the disturbance of this constancy, but Cannon showed what the *mechanisms* of such disturbances are. The difference is of emphasis, but at the same time has great significance because it passes from a general hypothesis to terms susceptible of experimental analysis. Cannon's work made possible questions regarding the "how" of disease, since it gives meaning to questions directed to the "how" of life. The influence of the sympathetic nervous system and the adrenals was central in many of Cannon's investigations into reactions to fear, rage and other emotions. He showed that tachycardia, arterial hypertension, hyperglycemia, dilation of pupils, etc., were all caused by "adrenalin" discharge, brought about by sympathetic stimulation, which in turn was caused by perception of external stimuli. It seemed as if the organism was physiologically prepared for the emergency, either for fight or for flight. There is no narrow finalism in this interpretation, which can be expressed easily in the most rigidly deterministic and evolutionary terms. But the concept requires no defense any longer, since its firmness is now beyond shortsighted attacks. What is significant here is that disease may be construed as a disturbance in homeostasis, and with further elaboration as an uncompensated disturbance in homeostasis.

In his major statement on homeostasis, *"The Wisdom of the Body,"* Cannon shows that most physiologic processes can be interpreted as contributing to the welfare of the organism, to the constancy of the *milieu intérieur*. He goes on to say that: ". . . the means employed by the more highly evolved animals for preserving uniform and stable their internal economy (i.e., for preserving homeostasis) may present some general principles for the establishment, regulation, and control of steady states. . . ." This hint at a master plan in life, at a common general pattern of organization in living beings (or even "other kinds of organization, even social and industrial") which operates throughout Nature, is proving to have been correct.

Thus, a homeostatic mechanism requires the presence of adequate stimuli, of sensitive receptors, of an afferent communication to a regulating center, of an efferent pathway from such a center to the effector cell or tissue, and of a response or responses tending to return conditions to their normal state of equilibrium. There are many physiologic processes illustrating that this is precisely the organization found in living beings: the maintenance of temperature, the elimination of water and sodium by the kidney, the regulation of blood calcium levels, the formation of adaptive enzymes, etc. Many of the problems involved in the elucidation of homeostatic mechanisms refer to communication, to the conveyance of information obtained through receptors to integrating centers, and from the latter to effector organs. The nervous system and the endocrine glands are preeminent in this function, but other possibilities of communication between distant areas of the organism are beginning to emerge from concentrated research. This communication is no simple transfer of stimuli; on the contrary, it plays a very important role in the regulation of the whole homeostatic system.

Electronic engineers introduced the idea of negative "feed-back" mechanisms into biology, meaning that performance is self regulated by a process which uses deviations from the normal to correct itself; they are negative because they tend to produce an effect cancelling an original error in performance. The entire field has been baptized as "Cybernetics" by Wiener, one of Cannon's most forceful and biologically minded proponents, and has served not only to produce a better understanding of physiology but also for building complicated machines based on the same principles, such as automatic dial telephone systems or electronic computers.

But where does this "negative feed-back" play a role in pathology? The answer is, "everywhere." Wherever one looks in pathology, at any level of organization, disturbance of self regulation emerges as one unmistakable mechanism of disease. In fever, in edema, in parkinsonism, in cancer, in the metabolic response to injury, in heart failure, even in death, phenomena can be interpreted, and useful hypotheses can be erected, on the basis of disturbed homeostasis, of misfired self regulation. No examples will be cited, as this whole book is an attempt at presenting disease on this basis. Pathogenesis, the mechanism of disease, that "most delicate flower of Medicine," can be usefully approached in this manner.

In papers full of wit and wisdom, Richards has further developed the concept of disease as disturbed homeostasis, adding names to phenomena arising half uncovered by the new insight, half hidden by the novelty of interpretation: *hyperexis,* or the excessive homeostatic response: *ellepsis,* or the deficient response; *akairia,* or the inadequate response; *taraxis,* or the disorderly response. Whether these names will be used or not I will not venture to guess. They are only "indicative of the old familiar role of man as his own most exquisite torturer, implacable enemy, violent and relentless inquisitor." . . . They refresh the old adage *"Homo lupus hominis,"* this time with more disturbing, more concrete evidence. For after all these centuries of recorded history, and many more preceding our short and ridiculous attempt at keeping track of all human frailties and greatness, it has emerged that disease, as all other manifestations of living beings, is life itself, and nothing more.

INDEX

Folios in *italic type* refer to illustrations.